Nanobiomaterials in Soft Tissue Engineering

Applications of Nanobiomaterials

Nanobiomaterials in Soft Tissue Engineering

Applications of Nanobiomaterials

Edited by

Alexandru Mihai Grumezescu

Department of Science and Engineering of Oxide Materials and Nanomaterials, Faculty of Applied Chemistry and Materials Science, University Politehnica of Bucharest, Bucharest, Romania

Department of Biomaterials and Medical Devices, Faculty of Medical Engineering, University Politehnica of Bucharest, Bucharest, Romania

ELSEVIER

AMSTERDAM • BOSTON • HEIDELBERG • LONDON
NEW YORK • OXFORD • PARIS • SAN DIEGO
SAN FRANCISCO • SINGAPORE • SYDNEY • TOKYO
William Andrew is an imprint of Elsevier

William Andrew is an imprint of Elsevier
The Boulevard, Langford Lane, Kidlington, Oxford, OX5 1GB, UK
50 Hampshire Street, 5th Floor, Cambridge, MA 02139, USA

ISBN: 978-0-323-42865-1

British Library Cataloguing-in-Publication Data
A catalogue record for this book is available from the British Library.

Library of Congress Cataloging-in-Publication Data
A catalog record for this book is available from the Library of Congress.

For Information on all William Andrew publications
visit our website at http://store.elsevier.com/

Typeset by MPS Limited, Chennai, India
www.adi-mps.com

Contents

List of contributors

Gustavo A. Abraham
Research Institute for Materials Science and Technology, INTEMA (UNMdP-CONICET), Mar del Plata, Argentina

Madalina Georgiana Albu
National Research & Development Institute for Textiles and Leather (INCDTP) – Leather and Footwear Research Institute, Bucharest, Romania

Ecaterina Andronescu
Department of Science and Engineering of Oxide Materials and Nanomaterials, Faculty of Applied Chemistry and Materials Science, University Politehnica of Bucharest, Bucharest, Romania

Florencia Montini Ballarin
Research Institute for Materials Science and Technology, INTEMA (UNMdP-CONICET), Mar del Plata, Argentina

Vaishali Bambole
Department of Physics, University of Mumbai, Santacruz (E), Mumbai, India

Pierre Basmaji
Innovatec's—Biotechnology Research and Development, São Carlos, SP, Brazil

Cornelia Bejenaru
Department of Vegetal & Animal Biology, Faculty of Pharmacy, University of Medicine and Pharmacy of Craiova, Craiova, Romania

Ludovic Everard Bejenaru
Department of Pharmacognosy & Phytotherapy, Faculty of Pharmacy, University of Medicine and Pharmacy of Craiova, Craiova, Romania

Şerban Vifor Gabriel Beresteanu
Head & Neck Surgery Clinic, Colţea Clinical Hospital, Bucharest, Romania

Pablo C. Caracciolo
Research Institute for Materials Science and Technology, INTEMA (UNMdP-CONICET), Mar del Plata, Argentina

Michele Carrabba
Research Center E. Piaggio, University of Pisa, Pisa, Italy

Mariana Carmen Chifiriuc
Microbiology Immunology Department, Faculty of Biology, University of Bucharest, Bucharest, Romania; Research Institute of the University of Bucharest, Bucharest, Romania

Pablo R. Cortez Tornello
Research Institute for Materials Science and Technology, INTEMA (UNMdP-CONICET), Mar del Plata, Argentina

Ligia Maria Manzine Costa
Department of Chemistry – USP/FFCLRP, Brazil

Giuseppe Criscenti
Research Center E. Piaggio, University of Pisa, Pisa, Italy

Carmen Curutiu
Microbiology Immunology Department, Faculty of Biology, University of Bucharest, Bucharest, Romania; Research Institute of the University of Bucharest, Bucharest, Romania

Yaser Dahman
Department of Chemical Engineering, Ryerson University, Toronto, Canada

Gildásio de Cerqueira Daltro
College Hospital Complex Prof. Edgard Santos (COM-HUPES), UFBA, Salvador, Brazil

Paula Braga Daltro
Department of Physical Chemistry – UNESP/Araraquara-SP, Brazil

Aurora De Acutis
Research Center E. Piaggio, University of Pisa, Pisa, Italy

Carmelo De Maria
Research Center E. Piaggio, University of Pisa, Pisa, Italy; Department of Ingegneria dell'Informazione, University of Pisa, Pisa, Italy

Lia-Mara Ditu
Microbiology Immunology Department, Faculty of Biology, University of Bucharest, Bucharest, Romania; Research Institute of the University of Bucharest, Bucharest, Romania

Filová Eva
Department of Tissue Engineering, Institute of Experimental Medicine of the ASCR, v. v. i., Prague, Czech Republic

Prosecká Eva
Department of Tissue Engineering, Institute of Experimental Medicine of the ASCR, v. v. i., Prague, Czech Republic

Anton Ficai
Department of Science and Engineering of Oxide Materials and Nanomaterials, Faculty of Applied Chemistry and Materials Science, University Politehnica of Bucharest, Bucharest, Romania

Denisa Ficai
Department of Inorganic Chemistry, Faculty of Applied Chemistry and Materials Science, University Politehnica of Bucharest, Bucharest, Romania

Garazi Gainza
NanoBioCel Group, Laboratory of Pharmaceutics, University of the Basque Country (UPV/EHU), School of Pharmacy, Vitoria, Spain; Biomedical Research Networking Center in Bioengineering, Biomaterials and Nanomedicine (CIBER-BBN), Vitoria, Spain

Itxaso Garcia-Orue
NanoBioCel Group, Laboratory of Pharmaceutics, University of the Basque Country (UPV/EHU), School of Pharmacy, Vitoria, Spain; Biomedical Research Networking Center in Bioengineering, Biomaterials and Nanomedicine (CIBER-BBN), Vitoria, Spain

Maryam Ghaffari
Biomaterials Group, Faculty of Biomedical Engineering (Center of Excellence), Amirkabir University of Technology, Tehran, Iran

Mustafa Abu Ghalia
Department of Chemical Engineering, Ryerson University, Toronto, Canada

Mazaher Gholipourmalekabadi
Biotechnology Department, School of Advanced Technologies in Medicine, Shahid Beheshti University of Medical Sciences, Tehran, Iran

Aaron S. Goldstein
Department of Chemical Engineering, Virginia Tech, Blacksburg, VA, USA; School of Biomedical Engineering and Sciences, Virginia Tech, Blacksburg, VA, USA

Raluca Grigore
Head & Neck Surgery Clinic, Colţea Clinical Hospital, Bucharest, Romania

Alexandru Mihai Grumezescu
Department of Science and Engineering of Oxide Materials and Nanomaterials, Faculty of Applied Chemistry and Materials Science, University Politehnica of Bucharest, Bucharest, Romania

Antonio Carlos Guastaldi
Department of Physical Chemistry – UNESP/Araraquara-SP, Brazil

Rosa Maria Hernandez
NanoBioCel Group, Laboratory of Pharmaceutics, University of the Basque Country (UPV/EHU), School of Pharmacy, Vitoria, Spain; Biomedical Research Networking Center in Bioengineering, Biomaterials and Nanomedicine (CIBER-BBN), Vitoria, Spain

Alina Maria Holban
Department of Science and Engineering of Oxide Materials and Nanomaterials, Faculty of Applied Chemistry and Materials Science, University Politehnica of Bucharest, Bucharest, Romania; Microbiology Immunology Department, Faculty of Biology, University of Bucharest, Bucharest, Romania; Research Institute of the University of Bucharest, Bucharest, Romania

Manoli Igartua
NanoBioCel Group, Laboratory of Pharmaceutics, University of the Basque Country (UPV/EHU), School of Pharmacy, Vitoria, Spain; Biomedical Research Networking Center in Bioengineering, Biomaterials and Nanomedicine (CIBER-BBN), Vitoria, Spain

Carmen Iordache
Microbiology Immunology Department, Faculty of Biology, University of Bucharest, Bucharest, Romania; Research Institute of the University of Bucharest, Bucharest, Romania

Vahid Jajarmi
Biotechnology Department, School of Advanced Technologies in Medicine, Shahid Beheshti University of Medical Sciences, Tehran, Iran; Cellular and Molecular Biology Research Center, Shahid Beheshti University of Medical Sciences, Tehran, Iran

Veronica Lazar
Microbiology Immunology Department, Faculty of Biology, University of Bucharest, Bucharest, Romania; Research Institute of the University of Bucharest, Bucharest, Romania

Plencner Martin
Department of Tissue Engineering, Institute of Experimental Medicine of the ASCR, v. v. i., Prague, Czech Republic

Daniela Meliţă
Department of Science and Engineering of Oxide Materials and Nanomaterials, University Politehnica of Bucharest, Bucharest, Romania

Rampichová Michaela
Department of Tissue Engineering, Institute of Experimental Medicine of the ASCR, v. v. i., Prague, Czech Republic

Holeček Miroslav
New Technologies Research Centre, University of West Bohemia, Pilsen, Czech Republic

Laurenţiu Mogoantă
Research Center for Microscopic Morphology and Immunology, University of Medicine and Pharmacy of Craiova, Craiova, Romania

George Dan Mogoşanu
Department of Pharmacognosy & Phytotherapy, Faculty of Pharmacy, University of Medicine and Pharmacy of Craiova, Craiova, Romania

Masoud Mozafari
Bioengineering Research Group, Nanotechnology and Advanced Materials Department, Materials and Energy Research Center (MERC), Tehran, Iran

Gabriel Molina de Olyveira
Department of Physical Chemistry – UNESP/Araraquara-SP, Brazil

Satish Patel
University Institute of Pharmacy, Pt. Ravishankar Shukla University, Raipur, Chhattisgarh, India

Jose Luis Pedraz
NanoBioCel Group, Laboratory of Pharmaceutics, University of the Basque Country (UPV/EHU), School of Pharmacy, Vitoria, Spain; Biomedical Research Networking Center in Bioengineering, Biomaterials and Nanomedicine (CIBER-BBN), Vitoria, Spain

Kochová Petra
European Centre of Excellence NTIS, Faculty of Applied Sciences, University of West Bohemia, Pilsen, Czech Re/public

Marcela Popa
Microbiology Immunology Department, Faculty of Biology, University of Bucharest, Bucharest, Romania; Research Institute of the University of Bucharest, Bucharest, Romania

Gabriela Purcel
Department of Science and Engineering of Oxide Materials and Nanomaterials, University Politehnica of Bucharest, Bucharest, Romania

Zahra Rezvani
Bioengineering Research Group, Nanotechnology and Advanced Materials Department, Materials and Energy Research Center (MERC), Tehran, Iran

Carla dos Santos Riccardi
Department of Physical Chemistry – UNESP/Araraquara-SP, Brazil

Márcio Luiz dos Santos
Department of Physical Chemistry – UNESP/Araraquara-SP, Brazil

Haji Shirinzadeh
Device Fabrication Group, Semiconductors Department, Materials and Energy Research Center (MERC), Tehran, Iran

Deependra Singh
University Institute of Pharmacy, Pt. Ravishankar Shukla University, Raipur, Chhattisgarh, India; NCNPR, School of Pharmacy, University of Mississippi, Oxford, MS, USA

Manju Rawat Singh
University Institute of Pharmacy, Pt. Ravishankar Shukla University, Raipur, Chhattisgarh, India

Maria Sonmez
University Politehnica of Bucharest, Bucharest, Romania; National Research & Development Institute for Textiles and Leather (INCDTP) – Leather and Footwear Research Institute, Bucharest, Romania

Kubíková Tereza
Department of Histology and Embryology, Faculty of Medicine in Pilsen, Charles University, Prague, Czech Republic

Patrick S. Thayer
School of Biomedical Engineering and Sciences, Virginia Tech, Blacksburg, VA, USA

Keshav Deo Verma
Department of Physics, S.V. (P.G.) College, Aligarh, Uttar Pradesh, India

Silvia Villullas
Biopraxis Research AIE, Miñano, Spain

Giovanni Vozzi
Research Center E. Piaggio, University of Pisa, Pisa, Italy; Department of Ingegneria dell'Informazione, University of Pisa, Pisa, Italy

Jatinder Vir Yakhmi
HomiBhabha National Institute (DAE), Mumbai, India

Tonar Zbyněk
Biomedical Centre, Faculty of Medicine in Pilsen, Charles University, Prague, Czech Republic

Preface of the series

The era of nanosized materials is now considered the center of the evolution of future tools and emerging technologies with wide applications in industry, research, health, and beyond. Despite recent scientific progress, biological applications of nanomaterials are far from being depleted and current knowledge is limited by the poor access to significant data, but also by widespread and usually unfounded speculation. Although exhaustive, the current literature is difficult to reach and understand because of the specificity and strict focuses of researchers investigating different applications of nanomaterials.

In this context, the scientific series entitled "Applications of Nanobiomaterials" was motivated by the desire of the Editor, Alexandru Mihai Grumezescu, and others to bring together comprehensive, up-to-date and relevant findings on the field of biological applications of nanostructured materials, to promote the knowledge and expand our vision regarding future perspectives. Even though the approached domain is quite specific and research-oriented, this multivolume set is easily intelligible for a wide audience including: under-graduate and post-graduate students, engineers, researchers, academic staff, pharmaceutical companies, biomedical sector, and industrial biotechnologies. However, some basic knowledge of the field of materials science (nanobiomaterials, pharmaceutical industry, products for medicinal treatments, nanoarchitectonics for delivery of biological active molecules and release, bone implants and stomatology) and engineering is a requisite for understanding technical aspects.

The selected authors of each chapter are outstanding specialists in the field of nanobiomaterials, who have made impressive contributions in a specific area of research or applied area within the scope of this book.

Each of the 11 volumes of the series contains 15 chapters, addressing the most relevant and recent matters on the field of the volume.

The first volume, *Fabrication and Self-Assembly of Nanobiomaterials*, introduces the reader to the amazing field of nanostructured materials and offers interesting information regarding the fabrication and assembly of these nanosized structures. In Volume II, entitled *Engineering of Nanobiomaterials*, readers can easily find the most commonly investigated methods and approaches for obtaining tailored nanomaterials for a particular application, especially those with a great deal of significance in the biomedical field. In the following step, readers will discover the importance and the ways of modifying the surface of nanostructured materials to obtain bioactive materials, by reading Volume III, *Surface Chemistry of Nanobiomaterials*. Starting with Volume IV *Nanobiomaterials in Hard Tissue Engineering* and Volume V *Nanobiomaterials in Soft Tissue Engineering* the biomedical applications of engineered nanomaterials are revealed and discussed, focusing on one of the most impacted fields, tissue engineering. Volume VI, *Nanobiomaterials in Antimicrobial Therapy*, highlights the potential of different nanostructured materials to be utilized in the development of novel efficient antimicrobial approaches to fight the global crisis of antibiotic inefficiency and emerging infectious diseases caused by resistant pathogens. Volume VII moves on to another key biomedical domain—cancer therapy. This volume, *Nanobiomaterials in Cancer Therapy*, describes current issues of cancer therapy and discusses the most relevant findings regarding the impact of nanobiomaterials in cancer management. *Medical Imaging* represents the focus of Volume VIII, while Volume IX deals with applications of *Nanobiomaterials in Drug Delivery*. Volume X, entitled *Nanobiomaterials in Galenic Formulations and Cosmetics*, refers to the perspectives highlighted by the utilization of nanosized functional biomaterials in the development of improved drugs and active principles for different biomedical industries. Finally, Volume XI is dedicated to the impact of *Nanobiomaterials in Dentistry*, which currently represents one of the most investigated and controversial domains related to the biomedical applications of nanostructured materials.

Due to their specific organization, each volume can be treated individually or as a part of this comprehensive series, which aims to bring a significant contribution to the field of research and biomedical applications of nanosized engineered materials.

Ecaterina Andronescu
Department of Science and Engineering
of Oxide Materials and Nanomaterials,
Faculty of Applied Chemistry and Materials Science,
University Politehnica of Bucharest, Bucharest, Romania

Preface

ABOUT THE SERIES (VOLUMES I–XI)

The increased fabrication of nanosized materials with applications on the biomedical field by using biomimetic and bioinspired processes and formulations has recently led to a new concept, nanobiotechnology. This complex research brings together significant knowledge from physical, chemical, biological, and technological sciences in an applicative field.

Medical applications of nanobiomaterials range from the development of adequate scaffolds for tissue engineering to therapeutic nanostructures, such as targeted drug-delivery systems. The purpose of this multivolume set entitled *Applications of NanoBioMaterials* is to offer a broad, updated, and interdisciplinary point of view regarding the applications of these "materials of the future medicine," starting with their fabrication, specific engineering, and characterization and ending with the most investigated applications such as tissue engineering, antimicrobial and cancer therapies, and also the development of different medical and cosmetic products. These books bring together the work of outstanding contributors who have significantly enhanced the basic knowledge and applicative concepts of this research field in their respective disciplines.

The multivolume set *Applications of NanoBioMaterials* contains 165 chapters, organized in 11 volumes which are ready to present a novel and up-to-date approach related to this intriguing domain. Each chapter is carefully composed and illustrated to highlight the relevance of nanobiomaterials on relevant biomedical fields, revealing the most recent applications on each investigated domain. The whole set represents a great material for the academic community, starting with undergraduate and postgraduate students, researchers, engineers, and medical doctors, but also pharmaceutical companies, the industrial sector, and innovative biotechnologies.

These 11 volumes cover almost all aspects related to the *Applications of NanoBioMaterials* as it follows:

Volume I: Fabrication and Self-Assembly of Nanobiomaterials
Volume II: Engineering of Nanobiomaterials
Volume III: Surface Chemistry of Nanobiomaterials
Volume IV: Nanobiomaterials in Hard Tissue Engineering
Volume V: Nanobiomaterials in Soft Tissue Engineering
Volume VI: Nanobiomaterials in Antimicrobial Therapy
Volume VII: Nanobiomaterials in Cancer Therapy
Volume VIII: Nanobiomaterials in Medical Imaging
Volume IX: Nanobiomaterials in Drug Delivery
Volume X: Nanobiomaterials in Galenic Formulations and Cosmetics
Volume XI: Nanobiomaterials in Dentistry

ABOUT VOLUME V

Volume V, *NanoBioMaterials in Soft Tissue Engineering*, is an up-to-date book that presents the recent progress of dedicated nanobiostructures in soft tissue engineering. The book highlights the main conventional and unconventional fabrication methods of typical three-dimensional (3D) scaffolds used in regenerative medicine (such as for muscle, nerve, tendon, ligament disorders, cartilage, neural outgrowth and regeneration, cardiovascular diseases, skin burns, and wounds). Also, in this work is presented an up-to-date overview regarding surface modification, spatial properties, and the newest *in vivo* applications of engineered 3D scaffolds.

Volume V contains 15 chapters, prepared by outstanding international researchers from the United States of America, Argentina, Brazil, Spain, Italy, Czech Republic, Romania, Iran, and India.

In Chapter 1, *Soft Tissue Engineering and Microbial Infections: Challenges and Perspectives*, Carmen Mariana Chifiriuc et al. review the recent progress in tissue engineering applications from the design of multifunctional biomaterials assuring simultaneously the scaffold function, as well as the release of antimicrobial drugs, growth factors, and other bioactive molecules, in order to prevent infections and therefore to accelerate optimal tissue regeneration.

Garcia-Orue Itxaso et al., in Chapter 2, *Nanotechnological Approaches for Skin Wound Regeneration Using Drug-Delivery Systems*, discuss engineered nanomaterials utilized in delivery and controlled release of drugs used in skin wound regeneration, particularly emphasizing with polymeric and also lipid nanoparticles, silver nanoparticles, nanofibrous structures, nanosheets, and nanohybrids.

Chapter 3, *Bacterial Cellulose for Advanced Medical Materials*, prepared by Gabriel Molina de Olyveira et al. describes recent advances regarding the applications of bacterial cellulose in human regenerative medicine and stem cell behavior. The chapter also reveals recent drug-delivery applications and future insights with respect to bacterial cellulose.

In Chapter 4, *Applications of Nanobiopolymers for Soft Tissue Engineering*, George Dan Mogoşanu et al. present details about the main natural and synthetic polymers used for soft tissue engineering: collagen, chitosan, heparin, fibrin, gelatin, alginate, hyaluronic acid, silk; polylactic acid, polyglycolic acid, poly (lactic-*co*-glycolic acid), poly-ε-caprolactone, poly(L-lactic acid-*co*-ε-caprolactone), polyethylene oxide, polyurethane, polyethylene terephthalate, and polymethyl methacrylate, as well as their clinical applications.

Next, C. De Maria et al., in Chapter 5, *Machine Design for Multimaterial Processing*, present the design of a novel parallel manipulator with three translational degrees of freedom for microfabrication of biomaterials. In this work, hydrogel-based composite scaffolds with applications in soft tissue engineering are discussed.

In Chapter 6, *Advanced Nanobiomaterials in Tissue Engineering: Synthesis, Properties, and Applications*, Mustafa Abu Ghalia and Yaser Dahman highlight the variety of organic and inorganic materials used in tissue engineering applications. Fabrication routes and details of the processing techniques used to evaluate interfaces in tissue engineering are also provided.

Gabriela Purcel et al., in Chapter 7, *Collagen-Based Nanobiomaterials: Challenges in Soft Tissue Engineering*, describe the main properties, advantages, and biomedical applications of collagen. The chapter highlights functional nanobiomaterials based on collagen for use in regenerative medicine, not only as a subject for laboratory studies, but also for general clinical use.

In Chapter 8, *Micro/Nanofiber-Based Scaffolds for Soft Tissue Engineering Applications: Potential and Current Challenges*, Pablo R. Cortez Tornello et al. give an overview about recent research advances made in the development of electrospun scaffolds for soft tissue engineering applications focusing on wound dressings, cartilage, muscle, cardiovascular, nerve, and skin tissues.

Chapter 9, *Natural Polymer-Based Hydrogels as Scaffolds for Tissue Engineering*, prepared by Manju Rawat Singh et al., focuses on fabrication and applications of hydrogel scaffolds obtained with natural polymers used in the treatment of wounds and healing, with the ultimate goal of clinical tissue regeneration.

Chapter 10, *Bioactive Nanomaterials for Cartilage and Muscle Regeneration*, prepared by Alina Maria Holban et al., presents the most prevalent cartilage- and muscular tissue-related diseases and highlights the recent scientific progress regarding the development of classical and recent therapeutic approaches, also discussing the impact and advantages of bioactive nanomaterials in designing functional scaffolds for cartilage and muscle repair.

Aaron S. Goldstein and Patrick S. Thayer, in Chapter 11, *Fabrication of Complex Biomaterial Scaffolds for Soft Tissue Engineering by Electrospinning*, present an up-to-date overview about the electrospinning process for the engineering of specific soft tissues, including muscle, nerve, tendon, ligament, skin, and vascular applications. This chapter reviews fabrication methods of microfiber meshes through electrospinning and describe how changing the fiber properties can influence cell behavior through contact guidance and mechanical effects.

Chapter 12, *Oxygen-Generating Nanobiomaterials for the Treatment of Diabetes: A Tissue Engineering Approach*, by M. Gholipourmalekabadi et al., discusses the impact of oxygen-generating nanobiomaterials in the improvement of survival of transplanted cellular products by sustained oxygen delivery within the microenvironment of tissue-engineered sites.

Denisa Ficai et al., in Chapter 13, *Advances in the Field of Soft Tissue Engineering: From Pure Regenerative to Integrative Solutions*, report the recent progress on regenerative systems successfully combined with therapeutic agents in order to design synthetic graft materials used in the treatment of skin infections of skin cancer.

In Chapter 14, *Tissue Engineering: Use of Electrospinning Technique for Recreating Physiological Functions*, Vaishali Bambole and J. V. Yakhmi discuss aspects regarding tissue engineering in the electrospinning process and review the most relevant and recent typical case studies.

In Chapter 15, In Vivo *Microscopic and Mechanical Characteristics of Bioengineered and Biodegradable Tissue Scaffolds and Nanomaterials*, Kubíková Tereza et al. present an up-to-date overview of chemical composition, dimensions, surface modifications, and spatial properties (spacing and porosity) of meshes and fiber scaffolds. The authors discuss the modifications of scaffolds that affect adhesion, migration, proliferation, and differentiation of cells as well as formation of new extracellular matrix.

Alexandru Mihai Grumezescu
Department of Science and Engineering
of Oxide Materials and Nanomaterials,
Faculty of Applied Chemistry and Materials Science,
University Politehnica of Bucharest,
Bucharest, Romania

Department of Biomaterials and Medical Devices,
Faculty of Medical Engineering,
University Politehnica of Bucharest, Romania
http://grumezescu.com/

CHAPTER

1 Soft tissue engineering and microbial infections: challenges and perspectives

Mariana Carmen Chifiriuc[1], Anton Ficai[2], Alexandru Mihai Grumezescu[2], Lia-Mara Ditu[1,4], Marcela Popa[1], Carmen Iordache[1], Alina Maria Holban[1,2,4], Şerban Vifor Gabriel Beresteanu[3], Raluca Grigore[3] and Veronica Lazar[1]

[1]Microbiology Immunology Department, Faculty of Biology, University of Bucharest, Bucharest, Romania [2]Department of Science and Engineering of Oxide Materials and Nanomaterials, Faculty of Applied Chemistry and Materials Science, University Politehnica of Bucharest, Bucharest, Romania [3]Head & Neck Surgery Clinic, Colţea Clinical Hospital, Bucharest, Romania [4]Research Institute of the University of Bucharest, Bucharest, Romania

1.1 INTRODUCTION

Tissue engineering requires an interdisciplinary approach for the achievement of successful strategies dedicated to human tissue reconstruction, regeneration, and restoration of their normal functions in conditions in which their self-repairing capacity is affected by disease or injury (Herbert and Rahul, 2005).

The identified practical solutions require the use of biomaterials as scaffolds and/or delivery systems for cells, growth factors, and other bioactive molecules stimulating the cellular proliferation, differentiation, and integration of new tissue. The term "tissue engineering" refers to bone and cartilage or soft tissue regeneration. This chapter is dedicated to the last of these two categories.

Tissue engineering could represent a solution by the construction of biological substitutes which could be used instead of donated organs (Atala, 2004).

Soft tissue replacement needs can arise for various reasons, such as congenital or chronic diseases (e.g., infections, inflammatory diseases, cystic fibrosis, ciliary dyskinesia, cardiovascular, congenital or acquired diseases), tumor rejection or other traumatic lesions (e.g., corneal scars, severe burns, and deep wounds), and the clinical approach consists more often of autologous tissue grafts, and less frequently in the use of allografts, xenografts, and synthetic materials, in order to avoid undesired complications, such as infection or graft rejection (Stosich et al., 2009).

Some of the limits of conventional approaches are expected to be resolved by tissue engineering technologies, although this will not be an easy task to achieve,

Nanobiomaterials in Soft Tissue Engineering. DOI: http://dx.doi.org/10.1016/B978-0-323-42865-1.00001-5

due to the complexity and diversity of the involved tissues (bone, cartilage, muscle, blood vessels, nerves, connective tissue, dermis, and epidermis), the difficulty of achieving adequate vascularization, and maintaining engineered shape and size (Johnson et al., 2007; Stosich et al., 2007).

To address these drawbacks some strategies have been developed, such as using scaffolds with a microchannel network to facilitate cell seeding and the diffusion of soluble molecules stimulating vascular growth, fabrication of blood vessel analogs which can be connected to the human vascular network during surgery, design of polymeric biomaterials with optimal mechanical properties and degradation kinetics (Garfein et al., 2003; Lu et al., 2009; Hong et al., 2010).

Irrespective of the tissue engineering application, the three main actors involved are the biomaterial, which represents the scaffold of the new tissue, the stem or progenitor cells which proliferate *in vitro* and differentiate in the correct phenotype, being (i) locally applied to the injured tissue or injected or (ii) combined with a scaffold to obtain an engineered tissue, and the bioactive substances stimulating the proliferation and differentiation of the respective cells.

1.2 BIOMATERIALS USED IN SOFT TISSUE ENGINEERING

Biomaterials include “any substance or combination of substances, of natural or synthetic origin, which can be used on a clearly defined time period as a whole or a part of a system that treats, speeds healing or replace tissues, organs or a function of the human body” (Williams, 1990).

Biomaterials of different sizes are currently largely used in different medical fields (orthopedics, cardiology, maxillofacial surgery, plastic surgery, ophthalmology, neurology, tissue engineering) to sustain life, improve or restore a functional structure and improve or restore the contour, without producing side effects in the human body. Therefore, the design of a biomaterial starts with the analysis of the function which it should fulfill, the anatomical location, and the evaluation of the impact exhibited on the human body, the choice of the proper material and manufacturing technology, prototype analysis and examination of its chemical, physical and mechanical properties, biocompatibility assay, cost-effectiveness analysis, clinical studies to clinical tests to prove that their properties are similar with those of tissues/organs that it will replace (Rosiak et al., 2002; Figure 1.1).

In order to be used as a scaffold, a biomaterial should meet a series of requirements, that is, appropriate mechanical and degradation characteristics, low immunogenicity, adequate cellular response to the material, generation of nontoxic degradation products that can be easily resorbed or excreted, flexibility for chemical modification, ease of use in the clinic, and cost-effectiveness (Kim et al., 2000; Puoci et al., 2011; Zhu and Nelson, 2013).

The biocompatibility of biomaterials refers to their property to be accepted by living body tissues without causing immune reactions (Dumitraşcu, 2007) and

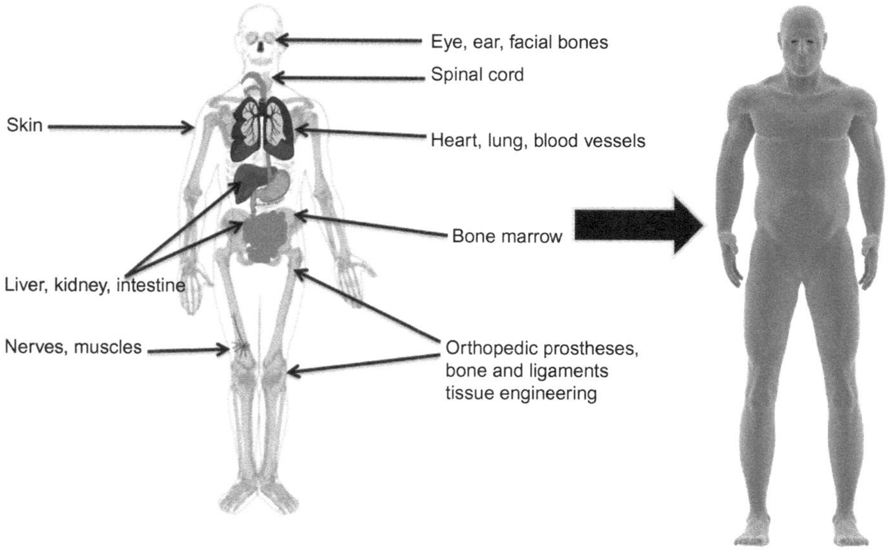

FIGURE 1.1

Graphic representation of biomaterial use for implant and tissue engineering medical applications.

depends on many biological, chemical, physical, and mechanical factors. The human body has an extraordinary ability to recognize foreign bodies and to generate a rejection response mediated by the immune system. Nanoscale objects are recognized by antibodies and rejected, while larger objects produce an inflammatory reaction around them. In order to be biocompatible, a biomaterial must have good corrosion resistance since the composition of the internal environment varies continuously from acid to basic pH and low thermal conductivity to prevent the thermal shock (Brown et al., 1997). Besides the intrinsic properties of the biomaterial, its biocompatibility is also influenced by other factors, such as patient health and age, tissue permeability, and immunological disorders (Wei et al., 2009).

The classification of biomaterials with applications in the medical field can be made according to several criteria. Depending on their nature, they can be polymers, metals, ceramics, or composites (Ratner et al., 2004).

The polymers are organic materials, widely used in the medical materials industry. Since 1960 polymers, such as polyglycolides (PGA) and polylactide (PLA), have been used. Polymers are appropriate for medical applications because they are available in different forms and compositions (solid, fiber, manufactured, gels, and films) and exhibit the advantages of being easy to handle and process, and also cost-effective as compared to metallic and ceramic biomaterials (Dumitraşcu, 2007).

Both natural and synthetic polymer biomaterials offer an excellent versatile design and the possibility to be functionalized with different biomolecules, thus being largely used for tissue engineering (Yuan et al., 2011). In order to increase the biofunctional material–tissue interaction, a biomaterial must undergo surface physicochemical modification for proper modulation of cellular adhesion, proliferation, differentiation, migration, or apoptosis.

The use of biodegradable polymers for biomedical applications has advanced in recent decades, due to their minimal side effects, high biocompatibility, biodegradability (under the enzymatic action of hydrolases, such as proteases, glycosidases, and phosphatases), and flexibility (Kaditi et al., 2012).

The enzymatic degradation is affected by many factors such as the interaction with the polymer chain (diffusion or adsorption of the enzyme), the physicochemical properties of the substrate (molecular weight, surface area), the properties of the enzyme, environmental conditions (pH, temperature), and the presence or absence of catalysts or inhibitors in the local environment (Marin et al., 2013).

Biomaterials which are suitable to be used as scaffolds in soft tissue engineering are represented by natural polymers [derivatives of hyaluronic acid, chitosan, amylose/amylopectin, heparin, dextran, collagen types I and IV, fibrin, fibronectin, silk, elastin, gelatin, adipose-derived extracellular matrix (ECM), matrigel (laminin, collagen-IV, entactin, and perlecan), decellularized human placenta, laminin, keratin, mussel adhesive proteins bearing the amino acid 3,4-dihydroxyphenyl-L-alanine residues which are mediating the underwater chemisorption to different substrata] (Waite, 1992; Flynn et al., 2007; Mano et al., 2007; Vashi et al., 2008; Heim et al., 2010; Connelly et al., 2011; Sapir et al., 2011; Wang et al., 2011a,b; Zhu and Marchant, 2011; Khem et al., 2012), synthetic polymers [PLA, polycaprolactone, elastic biodegradable poly(L-lactide-co-caprolactone), polyethylene glycol (PEG), polyglutamic acid (PGA), poly(L-lactide-co-glycolide) (PLGA), PLLA, poly(propylene) fumarate, β-tricalcium phosphate, poly(propylene fumarate-*co*-ethylene glycol), oligo(poly(ethylene glycol) fumarate), polyethylene terephthalate, polytetrafluoroethylene, polyethylene glycol diacrylate, polyethylene oxide] (Peter et al., 1997; Lu et al., 1998; Suggs et al., 1998; Jo et al., 2001; Hemmrich and von Heimburg, 2006; Kretlow et al., 2007; Speer et al., 2011; Zhu et al., 2007; Zhu and Ong, 2009; Choi et al., 2010; Kim et al., 2011; Sala et al., 2011; Bitar and Zakhem, 2013). For mass organ replacement silicone, nitinol, saline implants, and derivatives of polyurethanes, etc., are used (Fujimoto et al., 2007a).

The combination of synthetic and natural polymer characteristics to obtain hybrid hydrogels proved to be a promising approach for the fabrication of bioactive hydrogel scaffolds for different tissue engineering applications. Examples of such mixed polymers used for hydrogel scaffolds are PEG-, PNIPAm-, synthetic peptide-, pluronic-modified natural polymers (proteins or polysaccharides) (Wang et al., 1999, 2001; Shu et al., 2004; Hiemstra et al., 2007; Jia and Kiick, 2009; Shachar et al., 2011).

Cyclic Arg-Gly-Asp peptides have been used to modify hydrogels in order to enhance the cellular adhesion, due to their affinity to surface integrins (Liu et al., 2001). Genetic engineering opens new perspectives for the development of optimized biomaterial systems, offering the possibility to obtain new protein sequences with tunable properties, to combine specific functional regions into a fusion protein, obtaining multifunctional biomaterials, promoting the cellular adhesion and migration, exhibiting the optimal mechanical properties, and releasing antimicrobial and other bioactive molecules. This approach circumvents the use of chemical methods for covalent binding of bioactive motifs or crosslinking, which can result in undesired protein denaturation or toxicity side effects (Gomes et al., 2012).

If natural polymers exhibit the advantage of being part of the native extracellular matrix, and are therefore more biocompatible (Lavik and Langer, 2004), the synthetic ones are more easily obtained, and have tailored physical, chemical, and mechanical properties (Bertesteanu et al., 2014). However, the synthetic polymers are generally hydrophobic and need additional bulk or surface modifications to increase their biocompatibility (Mark et al., 2010).

In tissue engineering, biomaterials are used not only as scaffolds, but also concomitantly or independently, as delivery systems (micro- and nanoparticles) for bioactive agents and cells. The regenerative pharmacology faces a lot of challenges because it uses mixtures of growth factors with high molecular weights which must be delivered in the active form (protected from enzymatic degradation and hydrolysis), in the appropriate amount, for the desired period of time in a target tissue (Christ et al., 2013). Functionalized and smart biomaterials as well as new delivery systems have been developed (microparticles, nanoparticles, liposomes, polymerosomes, micelles, cation–anion polyplexes) (Atala, 2004).

Some of the mentioned polymeric biomaterials, such as those containing glycolic or lactic acids and caprolactone, are FDA-approved (Kohn et al., 2007).

There are also some commercially available products used in skin repairing in patients with severe wounds, such as Epicel™ (autologous keratinocyte skin graft; Bie, 2007), Apligraf (bovine collagen I matrix seeded with keratinocytes; Zaulyanov and Kirsner, 2007), Atrigel® (biodegradable polymers for drug delivery; Degim and Çelebi, 2007).

However, much research is needed in order to identify the biomaterial scaffolds which perfectly simulate the structural and biological properties of the natural extracellular matrix (composed of collagen type IV, laminin, nidogen, heparan sulfate-rich perlecan glycoprotein), in order to provide the appropriate environment for cellular growth and tissue regeneration, followed by reproducing as closely as possible the complex interactions of different cell types that are necessary to obtain a functional tissue (Mooney and Vandenburgh, 2008; Neal et al., 2009; Vrana et al., 2013).

The emergence of nanotechnology has radically improved this area, because the biological systems have been shown to respond well to nanosized structures. The cellular response occurs at different levels (microscopic, nanometer, or molecular) in the extracellular matrix, where nanosized structures are responsible for the control of many cellular processes. Therefore the use of a nanosized biomaterial will promote better cell growth and proliferation. Through nanotechnology nanosized transport and target delivery systems to produce a specific response can be obtained, to influence the functional expression and cell survival, in order to promote adherence, growth, expansion, and functional expression of cells (Burugapalli et al., 2014). Performant extracellular matrices for tissue engineering constructs can be obtained from polymeric nanofibers. These nanofibers closely resemble, in their size and structure, the natural collagen found in natural cellular matrices. These properties, combined with the physical surface properties and high porosity and biocompatibility, make them ideal for the production of such matrices (Roszek et al., 2005).

1.3 BIOMATERIAL MICROBIAL COLONIZATION AND BIOFILM-ASSOCIATED INFECTIONS

Unfortunately, the increased use of biomaterials in the medical field has resulted in an increased rate of biomaterial-associated microbial infections, which are persistent and very difficult to treat (Augustin et al., 2010; Auler et al., 2010; Gallo et al., 2014).

Shortly after the insertion of a biomaterial into tissue, the biomaterial surface is pelliculized by a conditioning film mainly composed of proteins belonging to the extracellular matrix, the most representative being fibronectin, fibrinogen, and fibrin. These proteins act as anchors for the adherence of free state bacteria (e.g., Gram-positive cocci, Gram-negative rods, and *Candida albicans*) (Samaranayake and Samaranayake, 1994; Samaranayake et al., 1994; Hawser & Islam, 2006; Lazar and Chifiriuc, 2010b).

The source of biomaterials contaminating microorganisms is either exogenous contamination of the respective biomaterial (due to the intrinsic microbial charge or iatrogenic maneuvers) or endogenous (by systemic dissemination or from neighboring infected tissues). The adherence of the microbial cell to the biomaterial surface is mediated by van der Waals forces and hydrophobic interactions. The molecular and atomic interactions involved in the microbial adhesion have been studied for *Staphylococcus aureus* and *Staphylococcus epidermidis* strains, which are the most common microorganisms causing biomaterial-related infections (Arciola et al., 2012).

After adherence to the substrate, both pathogenic and commensal bacteria proliferate rapidly, recruiting other cells and producing an extracellular matrix, forming dense sessile communities, with three-dimensional organization, which are called biofilms (Costerton et al., 1999).

Approximately 80–95% of microbial infections associated with biomaterial implantation involve the formation of biofilms (von Eiff et al., 2005;

Nandakumar et al., 2013). Biomaterial-associated infections are therefore a major public health problem, being an important cause of morbidity and mortality.

The pathogenesis of biofilm-associated infections is multifactorial and is due to the enhanced biofilm-embedded cells' resistance to host defense mechanisms (i.e., clearance mechanisms, lysozyme, phagocytes, complement, antibodies) and to antibiotics and other antimicrobials; tissue injuries due to the occurrence of a pro-inflammatory reaction triggered by Gram-negative bacteria lipopolysaccharides; the increased exponential proliferation of microbial cells inside the rich nutrient microenvironment; detachment and dissemination of biofilm with the occurrence of secondary infection loci or systemic infections (Lazar et al., 2003, 2005a,b; Lazar and Chifiriuc, 2010a; Chifiriuc et al., 2012).

Biofilm-associated infections belong to a very large spectrum, from the Gram-positive (*S. epidermidis* and *S. aureus*) to the Gram-negative pathogens (*Pseudomonas aeruginosa, Escherichia coli*) and to different members of the *Candida* genus (particularly *C. albicans, C. parapsilosis*). Once a biofilm has developed, the chemotherapy must rely on antibiotic doses required to kill bacteria protected by the biofilm matrix, which are significantly higher than those established on planktonic cells, by the standard CLSI (Clinical Laboratory Standards Institute)-approved, antibiotic susceptibility testing methods. The pharmaceutical industry is concerned at present with the development of antimicrobial agents with good biofilm penetration, by studying the microbial biofilms in close relationship with the host. The use of experimental models in which the microbial biofilm or microcolonies are flooded by a liquid with a very similar composition to the natural one is strongly recommended (Ceri et al., 1999). For these reasons, the development of experimental models for detecting the antimicrobial susceptibility of microbial cells included in biofilms is of great importance in order to ensure the *in vivo* efficiency of the tested antimicrobial substances (Lazar, 2011). Therefore, a new parameter, equivalent to the minimal inhibitory concentration, determined by standard assays for free state bacteria, called the minimal biofilm eradication concentration, has been proposed for testing the biofilm-associated bacteria susceptibility to antibiotics (Thomas et al., 2006).

The gene expression of biofilm-associated cells is drastically modified (40–60%) by comparison with the planktonic ones, being coordinated by cell-to-cell signaling mechanisms and having as a consequence the occurrence of significantly more resistant phenotypes to limiting conditions (Davey and O'Toole, 2000; Lazar and Chifiriuc, 2010a). For the same infected organ, the minimal dose required for infection is thousand times lower for biofilm cells as compared with free bacteria which are most susceptible to host defense mechanisms (Blot et al., 1999; Costerton et al., 1999; Lazar, 2003; Rodriguez-Martinez and Pascuala, 2008; Lazar and Chifiriuc, 2010a).

The increased resistance of biofilm cells to antibiotics and biocides is behavioral and, thus, called tolerance, defining the capacity of bacterial cells to survive in the presence of bactericidal substances, due to phenotypic, reversible adaptations, and not necessarily to the expression of a certain resistance gene (Lazar and Chifiriuc, 2010a).

The microbial tolerance is a multifactorial and incompletely elucidated process involving: (i) low penetration rate of antibiotics, antibodies, phagocytes through the extracellular matrix; (ii) higher proliferation rate due to the nutrient reserve assured by the biofilm; (iii) antibiotic degradation by bacterial enzymes accumulated in the biofilm microenvironment; (iv) decreased porin expression/increased efflux pumps activity; and (v) the selection of viable, but nongrowing persister cells which could represent ~1% of the bacterial population in *P. aeruginosa, E. coli*, or *S. aureus* biofilms (Passador and Iglewsi, 1995; Donlan and Costerton, 2002; Keren et al., 2004; Mandsberg et al., 2007) with high adaptation through high genetic mutation rates (*hypermutators*) (Ciofu, 2007; Costerton, 2007) and horizontal gene transfer facilitated by the high bacterial density inside biofilms.

An experimental model for the assessment of phenotypic resistance/tolerance of adherent bacteria forming biofilms on inert substratum specimens immersed in liquid medium has been proposed. Briefly, different biomaterial specimens are introduced in liquid culture medium containing different antimicrobial substance concentrations distributed in plastic wells, inoculated with different bacterial suspensions. The antibiotic could be added from the beginning (assessment of its influence on the first adhesion step) or after an incubation period (assessment of its influence on the adherent cells). After incubation, the biomaterial specimens are gently washed in sterile saline for the removal of nonadherent bacteria, moved in fresh nutrient medium, left for incubation, and then submitted to bacterial cultures density measurement (optical density at A_{600} nm), the obtained values being directly proportional to the adherence process intensity and biofilm development (Lazar et al., 2005a,b).

The contiguous or bloodstream dissemination of microbial cells detached from a mature biofilm could lead to the occurrence of systemic, severe infections. This process is influenced by the growth phase, biofilm development degree, nutrient gradient, and other local factors, such as hemodynamic or mechanical shear forces. The biofilm cells could detach either as single cells or in small aggregates (erosion) or by sloughing, leading to a rapid and massive loss of biofilm. Moreover, if bacterial aggregates are detaching from the implanted biomaterial they could block the small capillary vessels from lung and brain, producing pneumonia or strokes.

More than half of the cases of nosocomial infection that occur annually in the United States are associated with implants. Although they are less frequent than systemic infections associated with catheters, implant-associated infections are more difficult to treat because the involved strains are highly virulent ones, such as methicillin-resistant *Staphylococcus aureus*, requiring complex treatment schemes and repeated surgical procedures (Ma et al., 2012).

Clinical biofilms are generally complex, multispecies consortia integrated through synergistic and antagonistic interactions. The complex interspecific interactions established among the biofilm component species are still insufficiently known (Joint et al., 2002; Hogan, 2006).

The mixed biofilm composed of *C. albicans* and *S. aureus* (the second and, respectively, the third most isolated bloodstream pathogens in hospitalized patients) revealed a particular architecture and an increased protein expression profile, including that of virulence factors (Peters et al., 2010). In polymicrobial biofilm consortia, the "indirect pathogenicity" interaction can also occur, which can lead to treatment failure, although the standard therapeutic scheme consists of a combined therapy, because a resistant, but avirulent microorganism could protect a pathogenic strain from the activity of the antibiotic, as already shown in the case of *S. aureus* vancomycin resistance induced by *C. albicans* co-infections (Jenkinson and Lamont, 2005; Harriott and Noverr, 2009). Alternatively, limited space and nutrients in biofilms can lead to competition between microorganisms resulting in antagonistic interactions, such as the one described between *Pseudomonas* sp. and *Agrobacterium* sp. (An et al., 2006) or between *P. aeruginosa* and *C. albicans*, in which *P. aeruginosa* inhibits the development of *C. albicans* hyphae (McAlester et al., 2008).

The success of any pathogen in the colonization of a sensitive host and the development of an infectious process depend on its ability to sense its environment and to modulate the expression of the genes encoding factors required for the establishment in and adaptation to the new habitate. Inside biofilms, which illustrate the prokaryotic differentiation capacity (Costerton et al., 1999; Hall-Stoodley et al., 2004), the social behavior of bacterial cells is coordinated by a density-dependent, intercellular communication, and signaling mechanisms called *quorum-sensing and response* (QS; Israil and Chifiriuc, 2009), which is ubiquitous in bacterial world. The chemical QS mediators are represented by small molecules (e.g., *N*-acyl-homoserine lactones and derivatives in Gram-negatives, and octapeptides and amino acids in Gram-positive bacteria) (Chifiriuc et al., 2014).

The understanding of the mechanism of crosstalk between the bacterial cells, and bacterial pheromones and host cells may contribute to the elaboration of an efficient strategy for controlling the severity of biofilm-associated infections, called "antipathogenic," because it is not based on interference with bacterial growth (Lazar and Chifiriuc, 2011).

Although the bacterial cell attachment to the implanted biomaterial surface and the existence and development of biofilms was demonstrated, the pathogenesis mechanisms of biofilm-associated infections are not fully elucidated, however they are required for the development of effective strategies that could counteract recurrent infections associated with implanted biomaterials.

Some researchers estimate that the modification of a biomaterial surface can prevent bacterial biofilm formation. In this sense, hydrophilic surfaces, very hydrated and nonpolar, could be an efficient choice. It has been shown *in vitro* that such surfaces could prevent the accession of several bacterial species on the surface of biomaterials, by limiting the contact between bacteria and the material (Rojo et al., 2008). It is estimated that the surface roughness and the pores are prone to bacterial adhesion compared to smooth surfaces. Therefore, bacterial colonization could be prevented by smoothening the biomaterial surfaces (Gallo et al., 2014).

Another option could be to coat biomaterial surfaces with organic molecules (antibiotics, natural substances, quorum-sensing inhibitory compounds, enzymes) to prevent protein adsorption which may also inhibit biofilm formation (Timsit et al., 2011).

The efficiency of essential oils, polyphenolic extracts obtained from plants, and their synergistic effects have been demonstrated against highly resistant bacteria, such as: methicillin-resistant *S. aureus*, extended-spectrum β-lactamase-producing *E. coli*, and multiresistant *P. aeruginosa*. Antimicrobial activity of terpenoids from *Ocimum basilicum* and *Mentha piperita*, such as extracts obtained from Portulaca *oleracea*, was demonstrated against a large range of clinical strains: *S. aureus, Enterococcus faecalis, E. coli, Acinetobacter baumanii, Klebsiella pneumoniae, Salmonella enterica* subsp. enterica serotype Typhimurium, *C. albicans,* and *Trichophyton* (Lachowicz et al., 1998; Smith-Palmer et al., 1998; Hammer et al., 1999; Oh et al., 2000).

Our previous results have shown that the usnic acid renders the exposed bacterial cells sensitive to the usual doses of antimicrobials, probably acting as a QS inhibitor, which interferes with the coordinate expression of the virulence factors, including the synthesis of adhesins and biofilm development (Lazar and Chifiriuc, 2010a).

The formation and stabilization of biofilms are mediated by diffusible QS autoinducers. Taking into account the importance of the formation of microbial biofilms, there is growing interest in the exploitation of QS for developing novel antimicrobial strategies (Wilson, 1995). Metabolites interfering with this process have been identified in plants, animals, and microbes, and synthetic analogs are known.

The inhibition of the QS signaling could take place at different levels: (i) inhibition of QS molecule generation through the utilization of SAM (S-adenosyl-homocysteine, S-adenosyl cysteine, sinefungin, erythromycin) (Hentzer and Givskov, 2003); (ii) inhibition of the homoserine-lactone (HL) signal dissemination by decreasing the extracellular HL concentration through the use of some bacterial enzymes called lactonases or quorum-quenching enzymes, produced by different *Bacillus* species (Yang et al., 2005) or by nonenzymatic, alkaline hydrolysis; and (iii) the inhibition of the signal reception by using competitive molecules (with a homologous structure to that of bacterial pheromones) or uncompetitive (with a different chemical structure) capable of interfering with the HL binding and signal transmission, produced by bacteria, algae, lichens, plants (germinated seeds), and other organisms (Kiewit and Iglewski, 2000; Oggioni et al., 2004; Jayaraman and Wood, 2008; Nash and Thomas, 2008).

It has been shown that soluble compounds produced by probiotics could interfere with the pathogenic bacteria by inducing changes in the expression of surface molecules and, in consequence, affecting their adherence capacity, and by modulating the expression of quorum-sensing genes in two of the most feared opportunistic pathogens, that is, *S. aureus* and *P. aeruginosa* (Cotar et al., 2013a,b).

Another strategy used for fighting biofilms inspired by the capacity of biofilm-embedded cells to escape from biofilms is represented by the use of biofilm-matrix-destroying enzymes (acting on the polysaccharide component or cleaving the extracellular DNA) (Estrela et al., 2010).

However, it must be taken into account that the antipathogenic strategies are targeting a bacterial phenptype, but are not microbicidal. Therefore, an efficient therapeutic scheme in the case of biofilm-associated infections should contain a combination of antibiofilm compounds and antibiotics.

1.4 ANTIMICROBIAL POLYMERS USED IN SOFT TISSUE ENGINEERING

The nanostructures made of biocompatible and biodegradable polymers represent an important source for the manufacture of biomaterials with antimicrobial activity, used for controlled drug release applications in various formulations, such as microspheres, nanospheres, and hydrogels, and for tissue engineering.

Nanofibrillar chitin and chitosan have a wide range of biomedical applications in wound healing, epithelial, bone, and dental tissue regeneration, cell culture, antimicrobial agents, and dermal protection. Their beneficial effects are increased by protection against infections with bacteria, fungi, and viruses (Muzzarelli et al., 2014).

Chitin–nanosilver composite scaffolds proved to be bactericidal against *S. aureus* and *E. coli*, were not cytotoxic, and exhibited good blood clotting, being potentially used in wound-healing applications (Madhumathi et al., 2009).

A hydrosoluble chitosan derivative, quaternized carboxymethyl chitosan conjugated with collagen peptides by a carbodiimide reaction, exhibited an improved hydrogen-peroxide-scavenging activity and cellular viability, which together with the intrinsic antibacterial activity of chitosan is beneficial for the wound-healing process (Zhu et al., 2014).

The incorporation of antibiotics in chitosan could provide a viable alternative for the treatment musculoskeletal infections (Noel et al., 2008).

A 3D collagen–glycosaminogycan–chitosan scaffold containing tetracycline influenced the ultrastructural organization of the newly synthesized collagen I fibrils in a cornea reconstruction model (Builles et al., 2007).

Bilayered crosslinked collagen–hyaluronic acid matrices containing ciprofloxacin or tobramycin antibiotics exhibited an antibacterial effect lasting from 48 to 96 h and the tobramycin-incorporated polymers also enhanced wound healing, being potentially useful in defective skin tissue replacement and infection prevention (Park et al., 2004).

The *N*-(2-hydroxy) propyl-3-trimethylammonium chitosan chloride proved antibacterial efficiency on *E. coli* and *S. aureus* as well as biocompatibility (proving thus that clay could be used for the design of electrospun nanofibers and of other polymeric implants for tissue-engineering applications (Aliabadi et al., 2013).

Cellulose-based hydrogels have wide applications in tissue engineering and controlled delivery systems. Cloramphenicol-loaded 2,3-dialdehyde cellulose hydrogel membranes exhibited a 3-day antibacterial effect, and promoted fibroblast adhesion and proliferation, these effects being favorable for the wound-healing process (Laçin, 2014).

The alternate deposition of negatively charged phosvitin and positively charged chitosan on cellulose mats through a layer-by-layer self-assembly technique resulted in excellent antibacterial activity against *E. coli* and *S. aureus*, recommending them for tissue-engineering applications (Zhou et al., 2014a,b).

A multilayer film consisting of gold nanoparticles and lysozyme-deposited cellulose mats through a layer-by-layer self-assembly technique proved to have excellent antibacterial activity against *S. aureus* and *E. coli*, being promising tools for tissue engineering and wound treatment (Zhou et al., 2014a,b).

An antibacterial silk fibroin scaffold containing gelatin microspheres doped with gentamycin sulfate that was designed as a dermal regeneration template in deep burns has been shown to protect against *P. aeruginosa* infections over a period of 21 days, and also speeded up dermal regeneration and epithelialization rates proving to be a promising candidate for wound treatment and healing in severely burned patients (Lan et al., 2014).

Tetracycline (1% and 5%)-loaded silk fibroin membranes exhibited a significantly higher positive impact on the viability, proliferation, and differentiation of the human mesenchymal stem cells representing suitable variants for stem cell tissue engineering (Jin et al., 2014).

The human antimicrobial peptides neutrophil defensins 2 and 4, and hepcidin were fused to spider silk through bioengineering and showed microbicidal activity against *E. coli* and *S. aureus* as well as biocompatibility with mammalian cells and, therefore, potential for tissue-engineering applications (Gomes et al., 2011).

The phenolic-endowed atelocollagen films might be suitable for tissue-engineering applications, on account of the combined antimicrobial and cell proliferation stimulatory activity of polyphenols extracted from *Allium schoenoprasum, Salvia pratensis, Sambucus nigra* and *Taraxacum officinale* and collagen (López-García et al., 2013).

The surface of a polyurethane subcutaneously implanted energy transmitter was coated with a type I atelocollagen and rifampicine composite, which prevented the infection occurrence at the interfacial space between the tissue and the device in the first 7 weeks and stimulated dermal tissue regeneration and the obstruction of the interfacial space concomitantly with polymer degradation (Suh et al., 1994).

An antibacterial collagen film containing tobramycin crosslinked by 1-ethyl-3-(3-dimethyl aminopropyl) carbodiimide and *N*-hydroxysuccinimide was designed for corneal repair. The film showed excellent antibacterial effect and could be sutured in rabbit eyes and completely epithelialized in 10–20 days, without the occurrence of a corneal rejection reaction, neovascularization, or keratoconus in the following 3 months (Liu et al., 2014).

An infection-preventing membrane composed of a dense and porous collagen network has been developed. A bilayered membrane composed of hyaluronan microparticles loaded with silver-sulfadiazine was fabricated by gelling and was then incorporated into collagen layers. The collagen membrane assured a sustained release of the antimicrobial agent in active form, as revealed by its inhibitory activity against *P. aeruginosa* sustained for 4 days, while *in vivo*, the use of such membrane was associated with increased tissue regeneration (Lee et al., 2002).

A dual-functional composite with anticoagulant and antibacterial properties based on heparinized silk fibroin and chitosan was synthesized showing antimicrobial activity against *S. aureus*, proving its potential to be used as a composite biomaterial for blood contact devices (Wang et al., 2011a,b).

Lactoferrin is a bioactive globular protein with antimicrobial activity but also with potent antiapoptotic and osteogenic activity mediated by the Wnt5a/PKA pathway and the stabilization of β-catenin by rhLF dependent on the PKA/LRP6 signaling pathway. Recombinant human lactoferrin gels have been shown to support MC3T3 osteoblast cell viability, proliferation, and differentiation, as well as phosphorylation of signaling proteins (Amini and Nair, 2014).

Poly(ε-caprolactone) and gelatin blended with metronidazole designed for guided tissue regeneration revealed a good release of the antibiotic, which successfully prevented colonization with anaerobic bacteria (Xue et al., 2014).

Fibrous structures and synthetic polymer blends are promising candidates for variate tissue-engineering applications (scaffolds for stem cells, engineered grafts, vascular stents, drug delivery systems, transdermal patches, wounds, and burn care).

The polyvinyl alcohol combination with chitosan also exhibited a large spectrum of antibacterial activities, thus protecting against infection (Bhullar et al., 2015).

A bionanofilm consisting of homogeneous silver nanoparticles coated on single-walled carbon nanotubes, which were later hybridized with DNA and stabilized in poly(vinyl alcohol), proved to be biocompatible and displayed antimicrobial activity (Subbiah et al., 2011).

Bioactive adhesive materials containing dimethylaminododecyl methacrylate exhibited a marked antibiofilm activity against *Streptococcus mutans, Streptococcus gordonii*, and *Streptococcus sanguinis* biofilms (Zhang et al., 2015).

The pH-sensitive, negatively charged layer-by-layer hydrogel films, consisting of poly(2-alkylacrylic acids) crosslinked with varying polymethacrylic acid, poly(2-ethylacrylic acid), poly(2-*n*-propylacrylic acid), and poly(2-*n*-butylacrylic acid), have been proved to turn from hydrophilic to hydrophobic, becoming dehydrated and thus bactericidal in response to acidic conditions induced by bacterial multiplication. The films were also highly biocompatible, proving to be promising candidates for the development of biomaterials with low infection risk (Lu et al., 2015).

Biocompatible propolis-loaded polyurethane nanofibers exhibited significant antibacterial activity, revealing a great potential for wound dressing and skin tissue engineering (Kim et al., 2014).

Citrate-based polymers have unique properties recommending them for biomedical applications: citric acid is a natural biocompatible product with antimicrobial activity and also provides multiple functional groups for crosslinking and for conjugation of biomolecule antimicrobial properties. Citric acid polymers significantly reduced *S. aureus* and *E. coli* proliferation, this activity representing a great advantage of this type of polymer for use in tissue engineering (Su et al., 2014).

It has been shown that doxycycline antibiotic treatment for 1 month after hernia repair reduced the matrix metalloproteases and increased the collagen I:collagen III ratios, and the tensile strength of repaired interface fascia (Tharappel et al., 2014).

An antiadhesive polymer–peptide conjugate composed of block copolymer Pluronic F-127 and functionalized with antimicrobial peptides exhibited a contact bactericidal effect against *S. aureus, S. epidermidis*, and *P. aeruginosa*, while the arginine–glycine–aspartate peptides promoted the adhesion and spreading of human fibroblast cells (Muszanska et al., 2014).

In situ forming hydrogels containing poloxamer grafted on the hyaluronic acid were designed for tissue-engineering applications (i.e., ophthalmic delivery system) and proved to assure a sustained release of ciprofloxacin (Cho et al., 2003).

Silver-nanoparticle-loaded nanofibrous PLGA scaffolds were obtained by electrospinning and showed good biocompatibility and antimicrobial and antibacterial activity against *S. aureus* and *K. pneumoniae* at silver nanoparticle concentrations >0.5 wt%, proving their potential for tissue-engineering applications (Xing et al., 2011).

Usnic acid-loaded PLGA-PVA-loaded microspheres proved to inhibit both the initial *S. aureus* adherence phase as well as the development of mature biofilm rendering them as competitive candidates for the development of scaffolds for stem cell cultivation and tissue engineering (Grumezescu et al., 2014).

A nanostructured PLGA membrane designed to be used as a next-generation antibacterial skin graft material proved to exhibit an intrinsic anti-*S. aureus* activity and, at the same time, promoted keratinocyte proliferation, without increasing the density of dermal fibroblasts implicated in scar tissue formation, proving its effectiveness in limiting scar tissue formation and bacterial invasion, while promoting wound-healing (Karahaliloğlu et al., 2014).

Poly(D,L-lactide-co-glycolide) porous microspheres containing silver-releasing degradable phosphate glass or metronidazole proved to exhibit antimicrobial properties against *S. aureus, E. coli*, and *Bacteroides fragilis*, which normally colonize the perianal fistulae. Moreover, microspheres became rapidly integrated within the host tissue after subcutaneous implantation into a rodent wound model, demonstrating their utility as scaffolds for guided tissue regeneration (Blaker et al., 2008).

Polylactic acid nanofibers loaded with highly porous Ag microparticles exhibited good antimicrobial activity and low cytotoxicity, showing great promise for using as skin substitutes or wound dressings (Mohiti-Asli et al., 2014a,b), while poly(D,L-lactide) sponges loaded with chloramphenicol assured the release of the incorporated drug in both degradation and diffusion-controlled routes (Kozluca et al., 1995).

Nanofibers, due to their morphological similarity to the skin extracellular matrix components, have great potential for skin tissue engineering. A silver ion nanocoating of biocompatible, biodegradable poly(L-lactic acid) nanofibrous scaffolds led to the achievement of excellent antimicrobial efficacy activity against *S. aureus* and *E. coli*, maintaining human skin cell viability and proliferation at silver ion concentrations lower than 62.5 μg/ml (Mohiti-Asli et al., 2014a,b).

Biopolymeric 3D open-channeled scaffolds of poly(lactic acid) with microporous structure exhibited significantly enhanced ampicillin-loading capacity as compared to the nonmicroporous scaffolds, as well as biphasic release, with an initial fast one (*ca.* 85% for 1 week), followed by a slow one lasting 1 month, rendering them potentially useful for tissue engineering and regenerative pharmacology (Dorj et al., 2014).

Dissolvable polymeric nanofilms containing silver nanoparticles exhibited excellent antimicrobial activity, allowing normal and complete wound closure by re-epithelialization (Herron et al., 2014).

Electrospun nanofibrous scaffolds of polyurethane, cellulose acetate, and zein were proved to exhibit good hydrophilicity, promoted cell attachment and proliferation and also prevented Gram-positive bacterial colonization through the release of streptomycin sulfate (Unnithan et al., 2014).

Blended synthetic and natural polymer nanofiber scaffolds composed of polyurethane and gelatin, mixed with silver-sulfadiazine were incorporated into nanofibers after electrospinning, proving the capacity to be used as a substrate for skin regeneration, to prevent the microbial growth and, consequently, to accelerate wound healing (Heo et al., 2013).

Biodegradable biomaterials composed of mixtures of polycaprolactone and polyvinyl pyrrolidone-iodine were shown to be more resistant in terms of biofilm formation by *E. coli*.

The hydrogels formed by crosslinking polylysine and PEG showed significant antibacterial activity against *E. coli* and *S. aureus*, and superior cell adhesion and increased cell proliferation activity, recommending them as "matrices" in the healing process of skin wounds (Bertesteanu et al., 2014).

Poly(ethylene) combined with TRITON (1:1 mM:mM) was found to provide strong antibacterial properties to the collagen scaffolds prepared for tissue regeneration applications (Mandal et al., 2012).

Hyperbranched epoxy nanocomposites prepared with *Homalomena aromatica* rhizome oil-modified bentonite and with organically modified montmorillonite clay have shown excellent antimicrobial activity against *S. aureus, E. coli, Mycobacterium smegmatis*, and *C. albicans* as well as *in vivo* proven bicompatibility and stimulatory activity on dermatocyte proliferation, recommending these nanocomposites as nontoxic biomaterials for tissue regeneration (Barua et al., 2014).

Halloysite nanotubes/poly(lactic-co-glycolic acid) composite nanofibers doped with tetracycline obtained through electrospinning proved to be biocompatible and able to release tetracycline in a sustained manner and display antimicrobial activity for 42 days, showing promise as scaffolds for tissue-engineering and drug-delivery applications (Qi et al., 2013).

Encapsulating amoxicillin in laponite-doped poly(lactic-co-glycolic acid) nanofibers enabled a sustained and slower release of the drug, also correlated with a good cytocompatibility, showing their potential applications in tissue engineering (Wang et al., 2012).

Nanohydroxyapatite particles loaded with amoxicillin were dispersed into poly (lactic-co-glycolic acid) solution to form electrospun hybrid nanofibers, which proved to be cytocompatible and displayed a sustained-release profile of the antibiotic against *S. aureus*, proving their potential applications in tissue engineering (Zheng et al., 2012).

Silver nanoparticles have been incorporation in electrospun degradable 50:50 poly(L-lactide-co-epsilon-caprolactone) scaffolds designed for skin tissue engineering applications. The scaffolds containing between 0.5 and 1.0 mg Ag proved good biocompatibility towards human epidermal keratinocytes and wide-spectrum antibacterial activity against Gram-positive and negative strains (Samberg et al., 2014).

Nanofiber poly(caprolactone) tissue scaffolds fabricated by electrospinning and loaded with the rifampicin antibiotic inhibited the development of *P. aeruginosa* and *S. epidermidis* in suspension, as well as biofilm development in the first 6 h (Ruckh et al., 2012).

Bonded fibrous matrices have great potential for tissue-engineering applications due to their unique 3D and porous structure. The antibacterial polymer polyhexamethylene biguanide was applied on the fiber surface of a bonded poly (ε-caprolactone) fibrous matrix using a layer-by-layer assembly technique. The obtained composite was proved to have antimicrobial activities and a good biocompatiblity, showing promise for using as an anti-infective scaffold (Tang et al., 2012).

Self-assembling peptides composed of two antibacterial peptides and a central tetrapeptide linker undergoing structural transition from a random coil to a stable unimolecular β-hairpin conformation, subsequently forming an elastic hydrogel when stimulated by pH, ionic strength and heat proved intrinsic antibacterial activity against *E. coli*, being adequate for drug delivery, tissue engineering, and regenerative medicine (Liu et al., 2013). Genetically engineered elastin-like polymers used to prepare a hydrogel scaffold by ultrasonication proved to successfully release antibiotics and other proteins, which are critical for a successful tissue-engineering application (Amruthwar and Janorkar, 2012).

Fibrous materials containing poly(3-hydroxybutyrate), nanosized TiO_2 and chitosan were prepared by electrospinning, electrospraying, and impregnation techniques, and exhibited a significant inhibitory activity against *E. coli*, being at the same time compatible with human mesenchymal stem cells, proving to be a favorable scaffold for their development (Korina et al., 2013).

Hyperbranched poly(NIPAM) polymers functionalized with vancomycin and polymyxin B exhibited antimicrobial activity against *P. aeruginosa* and *S. aureus* in the infected skin model, proving potential for use as scaffolds and wound dressings (Shepherd et al., 2011).

Silver nanoparticle thin films (*ca.* 0.4 $\mu g/cm^2$) immobilized on poly(allylamine hydrochloride) and poly(acrylic acid) polymeric surfaces were not toxic and allowed attachment and proliferation of mammalian cells, while exhibiting a bactericidal effect against *S. epidermidis*, allowing proper management of microbial infections in wound beds without affecting the wound-healing process (Agarwal et al., 2010).

Low nitric oxide (NO)-releasing carbon-based coatings of monofilament polypropylene meshes have shown bactericidal activity against *S. aureus, E. coli, P. aeruginosa*, and cogulase-negative staphylococci biofilms, proving to be efficient in preventing the infection of surgical meshes used in abdominal wall reconstructions (Engelsman et al., 2009).

Drug-eluting medical implants (e.g., drug-eluting vascular stents and wound dressings and protein-eluting scaffolds for tissue regeneration, bone cements, fillers, and coatings for orthopedic applications, periodontal devices) are bioactive implants which have both healing effects achieved by the controlled release of pharmacologically active substances and support functions. Composite core/shell fibers and structured films can be used to fabricate antibiotic-eluting devices, which could prevent biomaterial-associated infections and therefore favor tissue regeneration (Zilberman and Elsner, 2008; Zilberman et al., 2010).

Drug-eluting porous structures were fabricated by freeze-drying of inverted emulsions, a process enabling the incorporation of antibiotics and the obtaining of an active implant that releases them to the surrounding tissue in a controlled desired manner, preventing infection and favoring wound healing or other tissue regeneration processes (Elsner et al., 2012).

Some microbial strains survive after the pulsed electric field decontamination of labile matrices used in tissue-engineering applications. The use of the bacteriocin nisin proved to generate a synergistic effect on the inactivation of *S. epidermidis* in collagen gels, decreasing the risk of exogenous infections during clinical applications (Griffiths et al., 2011).

1.5 CONCLUSIONS

Despite the huge progresses made in the design of competitive biomaterials for soft tissue engineering however, their use in clinical applications is conditioned and sometimes limited by the increased risk of biomaterial-associated infections with an important impact on present and future clinical applications. Recent progress in the field of biomaterials suggests that biomaterials could exhibit excellent and long-lasting intrinsic antimicrobial properties, which, in some cases, are coupled with an excellent biocompatibility. Moreover, biomaterials dedicated for soft tissue engineering could be functionalized or doped with antimicrobial substances, either inorganic (metallic nanoparticles) or organic (natural and synthetic compounds) using adequate scaffold-processing methods. However, a clear elucidation of the interaction between the antimicrobial substances and the other host components implicated in tissue formation would certainly contribute to the identification of the optimal solutions. Tissue-engineering applications could therefore benefit from the design of multifunctional biomaterials assuring simultaneously the scaffold function, as well as the release of antibiotics, growth factors, and other bioactive molecules, in order to prevent infections and therefore to accelerate optimal tissue regeneration.

ACKNOWLEDGMENT

This work was supported by a grant of the Romanian National Authority for Scientific Research and Innovation, CNCS–UEFISCDI, project number PN-II-RU-TE-2014-4-2269.

REFERENCES

Agarwal, A., Weis, T.L., Schurr, M.J., Faith, N.G., Czuprynski, C.J., McAnulty, J.F., et al., 2010. Surfaces modified with nanometer-thick silver-impregnated polymeric films that kill bacteria but support growth of mammalian cells. Biomaterials 31 (4), 680–690.

Aliabadi, M., Dastjerdi, R., Kabiri, K., 2013. HTCC-modified nanoclay for tissue engineering applications: a synergistic cell growth and antibacterial efficiency. Biomed. Res. Int. 2013, 749240.

Amini, A.A., Nair, L.S., 2014. Recombinant human lactoferrin as a biomaterial for bone tissue engineering: mechanism of antiapoptotic and osteogenic activity. Adv. Health Mater. 3 (6), 897–905.

Amruthwar, S.S., Janorkar, A.V., 2012. Preparation and characterization of elastin-like polypeptide scaffolds for local delivery of antibiotics and proteins. J. Mater. Sci. Mater. Med. 23 (12), 2903–2912.

An, D., Danhorn, T., Fuqua, C., Parsek, M.R., 2006. Quorum sensing and motility mediate interactions between *Pseudomonas aeruginosa* and *Agrobacterium tumefaciens* in biofilm cocultures. Proc. Natl Acad. Sci. U.S.A. 103 (10), 3828–3833.

Arciola, C., Campoccia, D., Speziale, P., Montanaro, L., Costerton, J., 2012. Biofilm formation in *Staphylococcus* Implant Infections. A review of molecular mechanisms and implications for biofilm-resistant materials. Biomaterials. Available from: http://dx.doi.org/10.1016/j.biomaterials.2012.05.031.

Atala, A., 2004. Tissue engineering and regenerative medicine: concepts for clinical application. Rejuv. Res. Spring 7 (1), 15–31.

Augustin, M., Balotescu-Chifiriuc, C., Lazar, V., Stănescu, R., Burlibaşa, M., Ispas, D.C., 2010. Microbial biofilms in dental medicine related to prosthetic rehabilitation. Revista Chirirurgia Oro-Maxilo-Faciala 1 (1), 9–13.

Auler, M.E., Morreira, D., Rodrigues, F.F., Abr Ao, M.S., Margarido, P.F., Matsumoto, F.E., et al., 2010. Biofilm formation on intrauterine devices in patients with recurrent vulvovaginal candidiasis. Med. Mycol. 48 (1), 211–216.

Barua, S., Dutta, N., Karmakar, S., Chattopadhyay, P., Aidew, L., Buragohain, A.K., et al., 2014. Biocompatible high performance hyperbranched epoxy/clay nanocomposite as an implantable material. Biomed. Mater. 9 (2), 025006.

Bertesteanu, S., Chifiriuc, M.C., Grumezescu, A.M., Printza, A.G., Marie-Paule, T., Grumezescu, V., et al., 2014. Biomedical applications of synthetic, biodegradable polymers for the development of efficient anti-infective strategies. Curr. Med. Chem. 21 (29), 3383–3390.

Bhullar, S.K., Özsel, B.K., Yadav, R., Kaur, G., Chintamaneni, M., Buttar, H.S., 2015. Antibacterial activity of combination of synthetic and biopolymer non-woven structures. J. Complement Integr. Med. Available from: http://dx.doi.org/10.1515/jcim-2015-0027.

Bie, C.D., 2007. Genzyme: 15 years of cell and gene therapy research. Regen. Med. 2, 95–97.

Bitar, K.N., Zakhem, E., 2013. Tissue engineering and regenerative medicine as applied to the gastrointestinal tract. Curr. Opin. Biotechnol. 24 (5), 909–915.

Blaker, J.J., Pratten, J., Ready, D., Knowles, J.C., Forbes, A., Day, R.M., 2008. Assessment of antimicrobial microspheres as a prospective novel treatment targeted towards the repair of perianal fistulae. Aliment. Pharmacol. Ther. 28 (5), 614–622.

Bleotu, C., Lazar, V., Chifiriuc, C.M., Mogosanu, G.D., 2014. Usnic acid-loaded biocompatible magnetic PLGA-PVA microsphere thin films fabricated by MAPLE with increased resistance to staphylococcal colonization. Biofabrication 6 (3), 035002.

Blot, F., Nitenberg, G., Chachaty, E., Raynard, B., Germann, N., Antoun, S., et al., 1999. Diagnosis of catheter-related bacteraemia: a prospective comparison of the time to positivity of hub-blood versus peripheral-blood cultures. Lancet 354, 1071–1077.

Brown, T.L., LeMay, H.E., Bursten, B.E., 1997. Chemistry, the Central Science, seventh ed. Prentice Hall, Upper Saddle River, NJ.

Builles, N., Justin, V., André, V., Burillon, C., Damour, O., 2007. Reconstructed corneas: effect of three-dimensional culture, epithelium, and tetracycline hydrochloride on newly synthesized extracellular matrix. Cornea 26 (10), 1239–1248.

Burugapalli, K., Burugapalli, K., Chan, J.C.Y., Kelly, J.L., Pandit, A.S., 2014. Efficacy of crosslinking on tailoring *in vivo* biodegradability of fibro-porous decellularized extracellular matrix and restoration of native tissue structure: a quantitative study using stereology methods. Macromol. Biosci. 14 (2), 244–256.

Ceri, H., Olson, M.E., Stremick, C., Read, R.R., Morck, D., Buret, A., 1999. The calgary biofilm device: new technology for rapid determination of antibiotic susceptibilities of bacterial biofilms. J. Clin. Microbiol. 37, 1771–1776.

Chifiriuc, C., Grumezescu, V., Grumezescu, A.M., Saviuc, C., Lazar, V., Andronescu, E., 2012. Hybrid magnetite nanoparticles/*Rosmarinus officinalis* essential oil nanobiosystem with antibiofilm activity. Nanoscale Res. Lett. 7 (1), 209.

Chifiriuc, C.M., Grumezescu, A.M., Lazar, V., 2014. Quorum sensing inhibitors from the sea: lessons from marine symbiotic relationships. Curr. Org. Chem. 18 (7), 823–839.

Cho, K.Y., Chung, T.W., Kim, B.C., Kim, M.K., Lee, J.H., Wee, W.R., et al., 2003. Release of ciprofloxacin from poloxamer-graft-hyaluronic acid hydrogels *in vitro*. Int. J. Pharm. 260 (1), 83–91.

Choi, J.H., Gimble, J.M., Lee, K., Marra, K.G., Rubin, J.P., Yoo, J.J., et al., 2010. Adipose tissue engineering for soft tissue regeneration. Tissue Eng. Part B Rev. 16 (4), 413–426.

Christ, G.J., Saul, J.M., Furth, M.E., Andersson, K.-E., 2013. The pharmacology of regenerative medicine. Pharmacol. Rev. 65 (3), 1091–1133.

Ciofu, O., 2007. *Pseudomonas aeruginosa* hypermutability and oxidative stress in biofilms. Abstracts book of The International Symposium and the 43rd ESCMID Post-Graduate Course—Bacterial Adaptation Mechanisms.

Connelly, J.T., Petrie, T.A., García, A.J., Levenston, M.E., 2011. Fibronectin- and collagen-mimetic ligands regulate bone marrow stromal cell chondrogenesis in three-dimensional hydrogels. Eur. Cell. Mater. 22, 168–176.

Costerton, J.W., 2007. Biofilms: the bacterial way to persist. Abstracts book of The International symposium and the 43rd ESCMID post-graduate course- Bacterial Adaptation Mechanisms: Biofilms, Hypermutability and Antibiotic Resistance, Palma de Mallorca, Spain, p. 9.

Costerton, J.W., Stewart, P.S., Greenberg, E.P., 1999. Bacterial biofilms: a common cause of persistent infections. Science 284, 1318–1322. Available from: http://dx.doi.org/10.1126/science.284.5418.1318.

Cotar, A., Saviuc, C., Nita, A., Bezirtzoglou, E., Lazar, V., Chifiriuc, M.C., 2013a. Anti-pathogenic strategies for fighting *Pseudomonas aeruginosa* infections- probiotic soluble compounds as inhibitors of quorum sensing genes expression. Curr. Organ. Chem. 17 (2), 155–161.

Cotar, A., Ionescu, B., Pelinescu, D., Voidarou, C., Lazar, V., Bezirtzoglou, E., et al., 2013b. Current solutions for the interception of quorum sensing in *Staphylococcus aureus*. Curr. Organ. Chem. 17 (2), 97–104.

Davey, M.E., O'Toole, G.A., 2000. Microbial biofilms: from ecology to molecular genetics. Microbiol. Mol. Biol. Rev. 64, 847–867.

Degim, I.T., Çelebi, N., 2007. Controlled delivery of peptides and proteins. Curr. Pharm. Des. 13, 99–117.

Donlan, R.M., Costerton, J.W., 2002. Biofilms: survival mechanisms of clinically relevant microorganisms. Clin. Microbiol. Rev. 15, 167–193.

Dorj, B., Won, J.E., Purevdorj, O., Patel, K.D., Kim, J.H., Lee, E.J., et al., 2014. A novel therapeutic design of microporous-structured biopolymer scaffolds for drug loading and delivery. Acta Biomater. 10 (3), 1238–1250.

Dumitraşcu, N., 2007. Biomaterials and Biocompatibility. Alexandru Ioan Cuza University Press, Iasi, ISBN 978-973-703-235-5.

Elsner, J.J., Kraitzer, A., Grinberg, O., Zilberman, M., 2012. Highly porous drug-eluting structures: from wound dressings to stents and scaffolds for tissue regeneration. Biomatter 2 (4), 239–270.

Engelsman, A.F., Krom, B.P., Busscher, H.J., van Dam, G.M., Ploeg, R.J., van der Mei, H.C., 2009. Antimicrobial effects of an NO-releasing poly(ethylene vinylacetate) coating on soft-tissue implants *in vitro* and in a murine model. Acta Biomater 5 (6), 1905–1910.

Estrela, A.B., Abraham, W., Berte, F., 2010. Combining biofilm-controlling compounds and antibiotics as a promising new way to control biofilm infections. Pharmaceuticals 3 (5), 1374–1393.

Flynn, L., Prestwich, G.D., Semple, J.L., Woodhouse, K.A., 2007. Adipose tissue engineering with naturally derived scaffolds and adipose-derived stem cells. Biomaterials 28, 3834–3842.

Fujimoto, K.L., Guan, J., Oshima, H., Sakai, T., Wagner, W.R., 2007a. *In vivo* evaluation of a porous, elastic, biodegradable patch for reconstructive cardiac procedures. Ann. Thorac. Surg. 83, 648–654.

Gallo, J., Martin, H., Călin, S.M., 2014. Antibacterial surface treatment for orthopaedic implants. Int. J. Mol. Sci. 15 (8), 13849–13880.

Garfein, E.S., Orgill, D.P., Pribaz, J.J., 2003. Clinical applications of tissue engineered constructs. Clin. Plast. Surg. 30 (4), 485–498.

Gomes, S.C., Leonor, I.B., Mano, J.F., Reis, R.L., Kaplan, D.L., 2011. Antimicrobial functionalized genetically engineered spider silk. Biomaterials 32 (18), 4255–4266.

Gomes, S.C., Leonor, I.B., Mano, J.F., Reis, R.L., Kaplan, D.L., 2012. Natural and genetically engineered proteins for tissue engineering. Prog. Polym. Sci. 37 (1), 1–17.

Griffiths, S., Maclean, M., Macgregor, S.J., Anderson, J.G., Helen Grant, M., 2011. Decontamination of collagen biomatrices with combined pulsed electric field and nisin treatment. J. Biomed. Mater. Res. B Appl. Biomater. 96 (2), 287–293.

Grumezescu, V., Holban, A.M., Grumezescu, A.M., Socol, G., Ficai, A., Vasile, B.S., et al., 2014. Usnic acid loaded biocompatible magnetic PLGA-PVA microspheres thin films fabricated by MAPLE with increased resistance to staphylococcal colonization. Biofabrication. 6, 035002.

Hall-Stoodley, L., Costerton, J.W., Stoodley, P., 2004. Bacterial biofilms: from the natural environment to infectious diseases. Nat. Rev. Microbiol. 2, 95–108.

Hammer, K.A., Carson, C.F., Riley, T.V., 1999. Antimicrobial activity of essential oils and other plant extracts. J. Appl. Microbiol. 86, 985–990.

Harriott, M.M., Noverr, M.C., 2009. *Candida albicans* and *Staphylococcus aureus* form polymicrobial biofilms: effects on antimicrobial resistance. Antimicrob. Agents Chemother. 53 (9), 3914–3922.

Hawser, S., Islam, K., 2006. Candida. In: Pace, J.L., Rupp, M., Finch, R.G. (Eds.), Biofilms, Infection and Antimicrobial Therapy. Taylor & Francis Group, Boca Raton, FL, pp. 171–184.

Heim, M., Römer, L., Scheibel, T., 2010. Hierarchical structures made of proteins. The complex architecture of spider webs and their constituent silk proteins. Chem. Soc. Rev. 39, 156–164.

Hemmrich, K., von Heimburg, D., 2006. Biomaterials for adipose tissue engineering. Exp. Rev. Med. Devices 3 (5), 635–645.

Hentzer, M., Givskov, M., 2003. Pharmacological inhibition of quorum sensing for the treatment of chronical infections. J. Clin. Invest., 1300–1307.

Heo, D.N., Yang, D.H., Lee, J.B., Bae, M.S., Kim, J.H., Moon, S.H., et al., 2013. Burn-wound healing effect of gelatin/polyurethane nanofiber scaffold containing silver-sulfadiazine. J. Biomed. Nanotechnol. 9 (3), 511–515.

Herbert, E., Rahul, S., 2005. Impact of Nanotechnology on Biomedical Sciences: Review of Current Concepts on Convergencs of Nanotechnology with Biology. Available from: http://dx.doi.org/10.5772/8510.

Herron, M., Agarwal, A., Kierski, P.R., Calderon, D.F., Teixeira, L.B., Schurr, M.J., et al., 2014. Reduction in wound bioburden using a silver-loaded dissolvable microfilm construct. Adv. Health Mater. 3 (6), 916–928.

Hiemstra, C., van der Aa, L.J., Zhong, Z., Kijkstra, P.J., Feijen, J., 2007. Rapidly *in situ*-forming degradable hydrogels form dextran thiols through Michael addition. Biomacromolecules 8 (5), 1548–1556.

Hogan, D.A., 2006. Talking to themselves: autoregulation and quorumsensing in fungi. Eukaryot Cell 5 (4), 613–619.

Hong, Y., Guan, J., Fujimoto, K.L., Hashizume, R., Pelinescu, A.L., Wagner, W.R., 2010. Tailoring the degradation kinetics of poly(ester-carbonate urethane)urea thermoplastic elastomers for tissue engineering scaffolds. Biomaterials 31 (15), 4249–4258.

Israil, A.M., Chifiriuc, M.C., 2009. Inter-bacteria communication phenomena: new concepts in anti-infective therapy. Asclepius (Ed.), 110 p. ISBN 978-973-88785-7-0579.6.

Jayaraman, A., Wood, T.H., 2008. Bacterial quorum sensing: signals, circuits, and implications for biofilms and disease. Ann. Rev. Biomed. Eng. 10, 145–167.

Jenkinson, H.F., Lamont, R.J., 2005. Oral microbial communities in sickness and in health. Trends Microbiol. 13 (12), 589–595.

Jia, X., Kiick, K.L., 2009. Hybrid multicomponent hydrogels for tissue engineering. Macromol. Biosci. 9 (2), 140–156.

Jin, S.H., Kweon, H., Park, J.B., Kim, C.H., 2014. The effects of tetracycline-loaded silk fibroin membrane on proliferation and osteogenic potential of mesenchymal stem cells. J. Surg. Res. 192 (2), e1–e9.

Jo, S., Shin, H., Shung, A.K., Fisher, J.P., Mikos, A.G., 2001. Synthesis and characterization of oligo(poly(ethylene glycol) fumarate) macromer. Macromolecules 34 (9), 2839–2844.

Johnson, P.C., Mikos, A.G., Fisher, J.P., Jansen, J.A., 2007. Strategic directions in tissue engineering. Tissue Eng. 13 (12), 2827–2837.

Joint, I., Tait, K., Callow, M.E., Callow, J.A., Milton, D., Williams, P., et al., 2002. Cell-to-cell communication across the prokaryote-eukaryote boundary. Science 298 (5596), 1207.

Kaditi, E., Mountrichas, G., Pispas, S., Demetzos, C., 2012. Block copolymers for drug delivery nano systems [DDnSs]. Curr. Med. Chem. 19, 5088–5100.

Karahaliloğlu, Z., Ercan, B., Chung, S., Taylor, E., Denkbaş, E.B., Webster, T.J., 2014. Nanostructured anti-bacterial poly-lactic-co-glycolic acid films for skin tissue engineering applications. J. Biomed. Mater. Res. A 102 (12), 4598–4608.

Keren, I., Shah, D., Spoering, A., Kaldalu, N., Lewis, K., 2004. Specialized persister cells and the mechanism of multidrug tolerance in *Escherichia coli*. J. Bacteriol. 186, 8172–8180.

Khem, E., Raghavan, S., Gilmont, R.R., Bitar, K.N., 2012. Chitosan-based scaffolds for the support of smooth muscle constructs in intestinal tissue engineering. Biomaterials 33, 4810–4817.

Kiewit, T.R., Iglewski, B.H., 2000. Bacterial quorum-sensing in pathogenic relationship. Infect. Immun. 68, 4839–4859.

Kim, B.S., Baez, C.E., Atala, A., 2000. Biomaterials for tissue engineering. World J. Urol. 18, 2–9.

Kim, H.I., Ishihara, K., Lee, S., Seo, J.H., Kim, H.Y., Suh, D., et al., 2011. Tissue response to poly(L-lactic acid)-based blend with phospholipid polymer for biodegradable cardiovascular stents. Biomaterials 32 (9), 2241–2247.

Kim, J.I., Pant, H.R., Sim, H.J., Lee, K.M., Kim, C.S., 2014. Electrospun propolis/polyurethane composite nanofibers for biomedical applications. Mater. Sci. Eng. C Mater. Biol. Appl. 44, 52–57.

Kohn, J., Welsh, W.J., Knight, D., 2007. A new approach to the rationale discovery of polymeric biomaterials. Biomaterials 28, 4171–4177.

Korina, E., Stoilova, O., Manolova, N., Rashkov, I., 2013. Multifunctional hybrid materials from poly(3-hydroxybutyrate), TiO2 nanoparticles, and chitosan oligomers by combining electrospinning/electrospraying and impregnation. Macromol. Biosci. 13 (6), 707–716.

Kozluca, A., Denkbaş, E.B., Pişkin, E., 1995. A potential soft tissue filling material: chloramphenicol loadedpoly(D,L-lactide) sponges. Artif. Organs. 19 (9), 902–908.

Kretlow, J.D., Klouda, L., Mikos, A.G., 2007. Injectable matrices and scaffolds for drug delivery in tissue engineering. Adv. Drug Deliv. Rev. 59 (4–5), 263–273.

Lachowicz, K.J., Johns, G.P., Briggs, D.R., Bienvenu, F.E., Wan, J., Wilcock, A., et al., 1998. The synergistic preservative effects of essential oils of Sweet Basil (*Ocimum basilicum* L.) against acid-tolerant food microflora. Lett. Appl. Microbiol. 206, 209–214.

Laçin, N.T., 2014. Development of biodegradable antibacterial cellulose based hydrogel membranes for wound healing. Int. J. Biol. Macromol. 67, 22–27.

Lan, Y., Li, W., Jiao, Y., Guo, R., Zhang, Y., Xue, W., et al., 2014. Therapeutic efficacy of antibiotic-loaded gelatin microsphere/silk fibroin scaffolds in infected full-thickness burns. Acta Biomater. 10 (7), 3167–3176.

Lavik, E., Langer, R., 2004. Tissue engineering: current state and perspectives. Appl. Microbiol. Biotechnol. 65, 1–8.

Lazar, V., 2003. Aderenta microbiana. Editura Academiei Romane, Bucuresti.

Lazar, V., 2011. Quorum sensing in biofilms-how to destroy the bacterial citadels or their cohesion/power? Anaerobe 17, 280–285.

Lazar, V., Chifiriuc, C., 2010a. Medical significance and new therapeutical strategies for biofilm associated infections. Rom. Arch. Microb. Immunol. 69 (3), 125–138 (ISSN 1222-3891; Indexed in MEDLINE).

Lazar, V., Chifiriuc, M.C., 2010b. Architecture and physiology of microbial biofilms. Roum. Arch. Microbiol. Immunol. 69 (3), 92–98.

Lazar, V., Chifiriuc, M.C., 2011. Mechanisms and experimental models for the assessment of microbial biofilms phenotypical resistance/tolerance. In: Méndez-Vilas, A. (Ed.), Science against microbial pathogens: communicating current research and technological advances. Formatex Research Center, pp. 906–911.

Lazar, V., Balotescu, C., Cernat, R., Bulai, D., Niþu, G., Ilina, L., 2003. Phenotypic antibioticresistance of some enterobacterial strains adhered to an inert substratum. *In vitro* models for biofilm formation in liquid and solid media. Clin. Microbiol. Infect. 9 (Suppl. 1), 227.

Lazar, V., Balotescu, C., Bucur, M., Banu, O., Cernat, R., Bulai, D., 2005a. Comparative study of antibiotic susceptibility levels of some clinical strains of *P. aeruginosa* as planktonic and adherent growing in biofilms cells. Clin. Microbiol. Inf. 11 (Suppl. 3), 540.

Lazar, V., Balotescu, C., Cernat, R., Bulai, D., 2005b. Patent no. A/1089 Experimental model for determining the susceptibility to antibiotics for biofilms immersed in liquid medium.

Lee, J.E., Park, J.C., Lee, K.H., Oh, S.H., Kim, J.G., Suh, H., 2002. An infection-preventing bilayered collagen membrane containing antibiotic-loaded hyaluronan microparticles: physical and biological properties. Artif. Organs 26 (7), 636–646.

Liu, G., Eskin, S.G., Mikos, A.G., 2001. Integrin alpha(v)beta(3) is involved in stimulated migration of vascular adventitial fibroblasts by basic fibroblast growth factor but not platelet-derived growth factor. J. Cell Biochem. 83 (1), 129–135.

Liu, Y., Yang, Y., Wang, C., Zhao, X., 2013. Stimuli-responsive self-assembling peptides made from antibacterial peptides. Nanoscale 5 (14), 6413–6421.

Liu, Y., Ren, L., Long, K., Wang, L., Wang, Y., 2014. Preparation and characterization of a novel tobramycin-containing antibacterial collagen film for corneal tissue engineering. Acta Biomater. 10 (1), 289–299.

López-García, J., Kuceková, Z., Humpolíček, P., Mlček, J., Sáha, P., 2013. Polyphenolic extracts of edible flowers incorporated onto atelocollagen matrices and their effect on cell viability. Molecules 18 (11), 13435–13445.

Lu, L., Garcia, C.A., Mikos, A.G., 1998. Retinal pigment epithelium cell culture on thin biodegradable poly(DL-lactic-co-glycolic acid) films. J. Biomater. Sci. Polym. Ed. 9 (11), 1187–1205.

Lu, G., Sheng, B., Wang, G., Wei, Y., Gong, Y., Zhang, X., et al., 2009. Controlling the degradation of covalently cross-linked carboxymethyl chitosan utilizing bimodal molecular weight distribution. J. Biomater. Appl. 23 (5), 435–451.

Lu, Y., Wu, Y., Liang, J., Libera, M.R., Sukhishvili, S.A., 2015. Self-defensive antibacterial layer-by-layer hydrogel coatings with pH-triggered hydrophobicity. Biomaterials 45, 64–71.

Ma, Y., Chen, M., Jones, J.E., Ritts, A.C., Yu, Q., Sun, H., 2012. Inhibition of *Staphylococcus epidermidis* biofilm by Trimethylsilane plasma coating. Antimicrob. Agents Chemother. 56, 5923–5937.

Machado, I., Simões, M., Vieira, M.J., Pereira, M.O., 2007. Persisters, in the news yesterday, on our labs today: the world together for a safer tomorrow in Biofilms, Hypermutability and Antibiotic Resistance. Palma de Mallorca, Spain, p. 24.

Madhumathi, K., Sudheesh Kumar, P.T., Abhilash, S., Sreeja, V., Tamura, H., Manzoor, K., et al., 2009. Development of novel chitin/nanosilver composite scaffolds for wound dressing applications. J. Mater. Sci. Mater. Med. 21 (2), 807–813.

Mandal, A., Meda, V., Zhang, W.J., Farhan, K.M., Gnanamani, A., 2012. Synthesis, characterization and comparison of antimicrobial activity of PEG/TritonX-100 capped silver nanoparticles on collagen scaffold. Colloids Surf. B Biointerfaces 90, 191–196.

Mandsberg, L.F., Ciofu, O., Kirkby, N., Philipsen, K.R., Høibi, N., 2007. Development of antibiotic resistance in weak *Pseudomonas aeruginosa* mutators with impaired DNA oxidative repair system. Abstracts book of The International Symposium and the 43rd ESCMID Post-Graduate Course—Bacterial Adaptation Mechanisms: Biofilms, Hypermutability and Antibiotic Resistance, p. 52.

Mano, J.F., Silva, G.A., Azevedo, H.S., Malafaya, P.B., Sousa, R.A., Silva, S.S., et al., 2007. Natural origin biodegradable systems in tissue engineering and regenerative medicine: present status and some moving trends. J. R. Soc. Interface 4, 999–1030.

Marin, E., Briceño, M.I., Caballero-George, C., 2013. Critical evaluation of biodegradable polymers used in nanodrugs. Int. J. Nanomed. 8, 3071–3091.

Mark, K., Park, J., Bauer, S., Schmuki, P., 2010. Nanoscale engineering of biomimetic surfaces: cues from the extracellular matrix. Cell Tissue Res. 339, 131–153.

McAlester, G., O'Gara, F., Morrissey, J.P., 2008. Signal-mediated interactions between *Pseudomonas aeruginosa* and *Candida albicans*. J. Med. Microbiol. 57, 563–569.

Mohiti-Asli, M., Pourdeyhimi, B., Loboa, E.G., 2014a. Novel, silver-ion-releasing nanofibrous scaffolds exhibit excellent antibacterial efficacy without the use of silver nanoparticles. Acta Biomater. 10 (5), 2096–2104.

Mohiti-Asli, M., Pourdeyhimi, B., Loboa, E.G., 2014b. Skin tissue engineering for the infected wound site: biodegradable PLA nanofibers and a novel approach for silver ion release evaluated in a 3D coculture system of keratinocytes and *Staphylococcus aureus*. Tissue Eng. Part C Methods 20 (10), 790–797.

Mooney, D.J., Vandenburgh, H., 2008. Cell delivery mechanisms for tissue repair. Cell Stem Cell 2, 205.

Muszanska, A.K., Rochford, E.T., Gruszka, A., Bastian, A.A., Busscher, H.J., Norde, W., et al., 2014. Antiadhesive polymer brush coating functionalized with antimicrobial and RGD peptides to reduce biofilm formation and enhance tissue integration. Biomacromolecules 15 (6), 2019–2026.

Muzzarelli, R.A., El Mehtedi, M., Mattioli-Belmonte, M., 2014. Emerging biomedical applications of nano-chitins and nano-chitosans obtained via advanced eco-friendly technologies from marine resources. Mar. Drugs 12 (11), 5468–5502.

Nandakumar, V., Chittaranjan, S., Kurian, V.M., Doble, M., 2013. Characteristics of bacterial biofilm associated with implant material in clinical practice. Polymer. J. 45, 137–152. Available from: http://dx.doi.org/10.1038/pj.2012.130.

Nash, I.I.I., Thomas, H. (Eds.), 2008. Lichen Biology. second ed. Cambridge University Press, Cambridge.

Neal, R.A., McClugage, S.G., Link, M.C., Sefcik, L.S., Ogle, R.C., Botchwey, E.A., 2009. Laminin nanofiber meshes that mimic morphological properties and bioactivity of basement membranes. Tissue Eng. Part C Methods 15, 11.

Noel, S.P., Courtney, H., Bumgardner, J.D., Haggard, W.O., 2008. Chitosan films: a potential local drug delivery system for antibiotics. Clin. Orthop. Relat. Res. 466 (6), 1377–1382.

Oggioni, M.R., Iannelli, F., Ricci, S., Chiavolini, D., Parigi, R., Trappetti, C., et al., 2004. Antibacterial activity of a competence-stimulating peptide in experimental sepsis caused by *Streptococcus pneumonia*. Antimicrob. Agents Chemother 48 (12), 4725–4732.

Oh, K.B., Chang, I.M., Hwang, K.J., Mar, W., 2000. Detection of antifungal activity in *Portulaca oleracea* by a single-cell bioassay system. Phytother. Res. 14 (5), 329–332.

Park, S.N., Kim, J.K., Suh, H., 2004. Evaluation of antibiotic-loaded collagen-hyaluronic acid matrix as a skin substitute. Biomaterials 25 (17), 3689–3698.

Passador, L., Iglewsi, B., 1995. Quorum sensing and virulence gene regulation in *Pseudomonas aeruginosa*. In: Roth, J.A., Bolin, C.A., Brogden, K.A., Minion, F.C., Wannemuehler, M.J. (Eds.), Virulence Mechanisms of Bacterial Pathogens.

Peter, S.J., Yaszemski, M.J., Suggs, L.J., Payne, R.G., Langer, R., Hayes, W.C., et al., 1997. Characterization of partially saturated poly(propylene fumarate) for orthopaedic application. J. Biomater. Sci. Polym. Ed. 8 (11), 893–904.

Peters, B.M., Jabra-Rizk, M.A., Scheper, M.A., Leid, J.G., Costerton, J.W., Shirtliff, M.E., 2010. Microbial interactions and differential protein expression in *Staphylococcus aureus* and *Candida albicans* dual-species biofilms. FEMS Imm. Med. Microbiol. 59, 493–503.

Prigent-Combaret, C., Lejeune, P., 1999. Genetics of the biofilms development and fomation. În: «les biofilms (2)». Bull. Soc. Fr. Microbiol. 14, 121–126.

Puoci, F., Cirillo, G., Curcio, M., Parisi, O.I., Iemma, F., Picci, N., 2011. Molecularly imprinted polymers in drug delivery: state of art and future perspectives. Exp. Opin. Drug Deliv. 8 (10), 1379–1393.

Qi, R., Guo, R., Zheng, F., Liu, H., Yu, J., Shi, X., 2013. Controlled release and antibacterial activity of antibiotic-loaded electrospun halloysite/poly(lactic-co-glycolic acid) composite nanofibers. Colloids Surf. B Biointerfaces 110, 148–155.

Ratner, B.D., Hoffman, A.S., Schoen, F.J., Lemons, J.E., 2004. second ed. Biomaterials Science. An Introduction to Materials in Medicine, 1-32. Elsevier Academic Press, San Diego, CA, pp. 137–151.

Rodriguez-Martinez, J.M., Pascuala, A., 2008. Antimicrobial activity in bacterial biofilms. Ediciones Doyma SA 26, 107–114.

Rojo, L., Barcenilla, J.M., Vazquez, B., Gonzalez, R., San Roman, J., 2008. Intrinsically antibacterial materials based on polymeric derivatives of eugenol for biomedical applications. Biomacromolecules 9, 2530–2535.

Rosiak, J.M., Janik, I., Kadlubowski, S., Kozicki, M., Kujawa, P., Ulanski, P., 2002. Radiation formation of hydrogels for biomedical applications.. Inst. Appl. Radiat. Chem. Tech. Univ. Lodz Wroblewskiego 15, 93–590.

Roszek, B., De Jong, W.H., Geertsma, R.E., 2005. Nanotechnology în medical applications: state-of-the-art in materials and devices, RIVM report 265001001.

Ruckh, T.T., Oldinski, R.A., Carroll, D.A., Mikhova, K., Bryers, J.D., Popat, K.C., 2012. Antimicrobial effects of nanofiber poly(caprolactone) tissue scaffolds releasing rifampicin. J. Mater. Sci. Mater. Med. 23 (6), 1411–1420.

Sala, F.G., Matthews, J.A., Speer, A.L., Torashima, Y., Barthel, E.R., Grikscheit, T.C., 2011. A multicellular approach forms a significant amount of tissue-engineered small intestine in the mouse. Tissue Eng. Part A 17 (13–14), 1841–1850.

Samaranayake, Y.H., Samaranayake, L.P., 1994. Candida Krusei: biology, epidemiology, pathogenicity and clinical manifestations of an emerging pathogen. J. Med. Microbiol. 41, 295–310.

Samaranayake, Y.H., Wu, P.C., Samaranayake, L.P., So, M., Yuen, K.J., 1994. Adhesion and colonization of *Candida krusei* on host surfaces. J. Med. Microbiol. 41, 251–258.

Samberg, M.E., Mente, P., He, T., King, M.W., Monteiro-Riviere, N.A., 2014. *In vitro* biocompatibility and antibacterial efficacy of a degradable poly(L-lactide-co-epsilon-caprolactone) copolymer incorporated with silver nanoparticles. Ann. Biomed. Eng. 42 (7), 1482–1493.

Sapir, Y., Kryukov, O., Cohen, S., 2011. Integration of multiple cell-matrix interactions into alginate scaffolds for promoting cardiac tissue regeneration. Biomaterials 32, 1838–1847.

Shachar, M., Tsur-Gang, O., Dvir, T., Leor, J., Cohen, S., 2011. The effect of immobilized RGD peptide in alginate scaffolds on cardiac tissue engineering. Acta Biomater 7 (1), 152–16.

Shepherd, J., Sarker, P., Rimmer, S., Swanson, L., MacNeil, S., Douglas, I., 2011. Hyperbranched poly(NIPAM) polymers modified with antibiotics for the reduction of bacterial burden in infected human tissue engineered skin. Biomaterials 32 (1), 258–267.

Shirtliff, M.E., Peters, B.M., Jabra-Rizk, M.A., 2009. Cross-kingdom interactions: *Candida albicans* and bacteria. FEMS Microbiol. Lett. 299 (1), 1–8.

Shu, X.Z., Ghosh, K., Liu, Y., Palumbo, F.S., Clark, R.A., Prestwich, G.D., 2004. Attachment and spreading of fibroblasts on an RGD peptide-modified hyaluronan hydrogel. J. Biomed. Mater. Res. A 68 (2), 365–375.

Smith-Palmer, A., Stewart, J., Fyfe, L., 1998. Antimicrobial properties of plant essential oils and essences against five important food-born pathogens. Lett. Appl. Microbiol. 26, 118–122.

Speer, A.L., Sala, F.G., Matthews, J.A., Grikscheit, T.C., 2011. Murine tissue-engineered stomach demonstrates epithelial differentiation. J. Surg. Res. 171 (1), 6–14.

Stosich, M.S., Bastian, B., Marion, N.W., Clark, P.A., Reilly, G., Mao, J.J.D.D.S., 2007. Vascularized adipose tissue grafts from human mesenchymal stem cells with bioactive cues and microchannel conduits. Tissue Eng. 13 (12), 2881–2890.

Stosich, M.S., Moioli, E.K., Wu, J.K., Lee, C.H., Rohde, C., Yoursef, A.M., et al., 2009. Bioengineering strategies to generate vascularized soft tissue grafts with sustained shape. Methods 47 (2), 116–121.

Su, L.C., Xie, Z., Zhang, Y., Nguyen, K.T., Yang, J., 2014. Study on the antimicrobial properties of citrate-based biodegradable polymers. Front Bioeng. Biotechnol. 2, 23.

Subbiah, R.P., Lee, H., Veerapandian, M., Sadhasivam, S., Seo, S.W., Yun, K., 2011. Structural and biological evaluation of a multifunctional SWCNT-AgNPs-DNA/PVA bio-nanofilm. Anal. Bioanal. Chem. 400 (2), 547–560.

Suggs, L.J., Krishnan, R.S., Garcia, C.A., Peter, S.J., Anderson, J.M., Mikos, A.G., 1998. *In vitro* and *in vivo* degradation of poly(propylene fumarate-co-ethylene glycol) hydrogels. J. Biomed. Mater. Res. 42 (2), 312–320.

Suh, H., Suh, S., Min, B., 1994. Anti-infection treatment of a transcutaneous device by a collagen-rifampicine composite. ASAIO J. 40 (3), M406–M411.

Tang, Y., Zhao, Y., Wang, H., Gao, Y., Liu, X., Wang, X., et al., 2012. Layer-by-layer assembly of antibacterial coating on interbonded 3D fibrous scaffolds and its cytocompatibility assessment. J. Biomed. Mater. Res. A 100 (8), 2071–2078.

Tharappel, J.C., Bower, C.E., Whittington Harris, J., Ramineni, S.K., Puleo, D.A., Roth, J.S., 2014. Doxycycline administration improves fascial interface in hernia repair. J. Surg. Res. 190 (2), 692–698.

Thomas, J.G., Litton, I., Rinde, H., 2006. Economic impact of biofilms on treatment costs. In: Pace, J.L., Rupp, M., Finch, R.G. (Eds.), Biofilms, Infection and Antimicrobial Therapy. Taylor & Francis Group, Boca Raton, FL, pp. 21–38.

Timsit, J., Dubois, Y., Minet, C., Bonadona, A., Lugosi, M., Ara-Somohano, C., et al., 2011. New materials and devices for preventing biofilm associated infections. Ann. Intensive Care 1, 34.

Unnithan, A.R., Gnanasekaran, G., Sathishkumar, Y., Lee, Y.S., Kim, C.S., 2014. Electrospun antibacterial polyurethane-cellulose acetate-zein composite mats for wound dressing. Carbohydr. Polym. 102, 884–892.

Vashi, A.V., Keramidaris, E., Abberton, K.M., Morrison, W.A., Wilson, J.L., O'Connor, A.J., et al., 2008. Adipose differentiation of bone marrow-derived mesenchymal stem cells using Pluronic F-127 hydrogel *in vitro*. Biomaterials 29, 573–579.

von Eiff, C., Jansen, B., Kohnen, W., Becker, K., 2005. Infections associated with medical devices: pathogenesis, management and prophylaxis. Drugs. Available from: http://dx.doi.org/10.2165/00003495-200565020-00003.

Vrana, N.E., Lavalle, P., Dokmeci, M.R., Dehghani, F., Ghaemmaghami, A.M.M.D., Khademhosseini, A., 2013. Engineering functional epithelium for regenerative medicine and *in vitro* organ models: a review. Tissue Eng. Part B Rev. 19 (6), 529–543.

Waite, J.H., 1992. The DOPA ephemera: a recurrent motif in invertebrates. Biol. Bull. 183, 178–184.

Wang, C., Stewart, R.J., Kopecek, J., 1999. Hybrid hydrogels assembled from synthetic polymers and coiled-coil protein domains. Nature 397 (6718), 417–420.

Wang, C., Kopecek, J., Stewart, R.J., 2001. Hybrid hydrogels cross-linked by genetically engineered coiled-coil block proteins. Biomacromolecules 2 (3), 912–920.

Wang, C.C., Yang, K.C., Lin, K.H., Liu, H.C., Lin, F.H., 2011a. A highly organized three-dimensional alginate scaffold for cartilage tissue engineering prepared by microfluidic technology. Biomaterials 32 (29), 7118–7126.

Wang, J., Hu, W., Liu, Q., Zhang, S., 2011b. Dual-functional composite with anticoagulant and antibacterial properties based on heparinized silk fibroin and chitosan. Colloids Surf. B Biointerfaces 85 (2), 241–247.

Wang, S., Zheng, F., Huang, Y., Fang, Y., Shen, M., Zhu, M., et al., 2012. Encapsulation of amoxicillin within laponite-doped poly(lactic-co-glycolic acid) nanofibers: preparation, characterization, and antibacterial activity. ACS Appl. Mater. Interfaces 4 (11), 6393–6401.

Wei, X., Gong, C., Gou, M., Fu, S., Guo, Q., Shi, S., et al., 2009. Biodegradable poly[epsilon-caprolactone]-poly[ethylene glycol] copolymers as drug delivery system. Int. J. Pharm. 381, 1–18.

Williams, D.F., 1990. An Introduction to Medical and Dental Materials, Concise Encyclopedia of Medical & Dental Materials. Pergamon Press and the MIT Press, Oxford.

Wilson, K.H., 1995. Ecological concepts in the control of pathogens. In: Roth, J.A., Bolin, C.A., Brogden, K.A., Minion, F.C., Wannemuehler, M.J. (Eds.), Virulence Mechanisms of Bacterial Pathogens. Cap. V. Strategies to Overcome Bacterial Virulence Mechanisms, second ed. ASM Press, Washington, DC, pp. 245–256.

Xing, Z.C., Chae, W.P., Huh, M.W., Park, L.S., Park, S.Y., Kwak, G., et al., 2011. *In vitro* anti-bacterial and cytotoxic properties of silver-containing poly(L-lactide-co-glycolide) nanofibrous scaffolds. J. Nanosci. Nanotechnol. 11 (1), 61–65.

Xue, J., He, M., Liu, H., Niu, Y., Crawford, A., Coates, P.D., et al., 2014. Drug loaded homogeneous electrospun PCL/gelatin hybrid nanofiber structures for anti-infective tissue regeneration membranes. Biomaterials 35 (34), 9395–9405.

Yang, F., Wang, L.-H., Wang, J., Dong, Y.-H., Hu, J.Y., Zhang, L.-H., 2005. Quorum quenching enzyme activity is widely conserved in the sera of mammalian species. FEBS Lett. 579, 3713–3717.

Yuan, Z., Nie, H., Wang, S., Hun Lee, C., Li, A., Susan, Y., et al., 2011. Biomaterial selection for tooth regeneration. Tissue Eng. Part B Rev. 17, 373–388.

Zaulyanov, L., Kirsner, R.S., 2007. A review of a bi-layered living cell treatment (Apligraf) in the treatment of venous leg ulcers and diabetic foot ulcers. Clin. Interv. Aging. 2, 93–98.

Zhang, K., Wang, S., Zhou, X., Xu, H.H., Weir, M.D., Ge, Y., et al., 2015. Effect of antibacterial dental adhesive on multispecies biofilms formation. J. Dent. Res. 94 (4), 622–629.

Zheng, F., Wang, S., Wen, S., Shen, M., Zhu, M., Shi, X., 2012. Characterization and antibacterial activity of amoxicillin-loaded electrospun nano-hydroxyapatite/poly(lactic-co-glycolic acid) composite nanofibers. Biomaterials 34 (4), 1402–1412.

Zhou, B., Hu, Y., Li, J., Li, B., 2014a. Chitosan/phosvitin antibacterial films fabricated via layer-by-layer deposition. Int. J. Biol. Macromol. 64, 402–408.

Zhou, B., Li, Y., Deng, H., Hu, Y., Li, B., 2014b. Antibacterial multilayer films fabricated by layer-by-layer immobilizing lysozyme and gold nanoparticles on nanofibers. Colloids Surf. B Biointerfaces 116, 432–438.

Zhu, J., Marchant, R.E., 2011. Design properties of hydrogel tissue-engineering scaffolds. Exp. Rev. Med. Devices 8 (5), 607–626.

Zhu, W., Nelson, C.M., 2013. Adipose and mammary epithelial tissue engineering. Biomatter 3 (3), e24630.

Zhu, Y., Ong, W.F., 2009. Epithelium regeneration on collagen (IV) grafted polycaprolactone for esophageal tissue engineering. Mater. Sci. Eng. C 29, 1046–1050.

Zhu, Y., Leong, M.F., Ong, W.F., Chan-Park, M.B., Chian, K.S., 2007. Esophageal epithelium regeneration on fibronectin grafted poly(L-lactide-co-caprolactone) (PLLC) nanofiber scaffold. Biomaterials 28 (5), 861–868.

Zhu, X., Zhou, X., Yi, J., Tong, J., Wu, H., Fan, L., 2014. Preparation and biological activity of quaternized carboxymethyl chitosan conjugated with collagen peptide. Int. J. Biol. Macromol. 70, 300–305.

Zilberman, M., Elsner, J.J., 2008. Antibiotic-eluting medical devices for various applications. J. Control Release 130 (3), 202–215.

Zilberman, M., Kraitzer, A., Grinberg, O., Elsner, J.J., 2010. Poly (ε-caprolactone) scaffolds containing silver nanoparticles 0.1% (w/w) revealed antimicrobial activity against Gram-positive and Gram-negative strains, while being non cytotoxic on endothelial cells. Handb. Exp. Pharmacol. 197, 299–341.

CHAPTER

Nanotechnology approaches for skin wound regeneration using drug-delivery systems

2

Itxaso Garcia-Orue[1,2], Garazi Gainza[1,2], Silvia Villullas[3], Jose Luis Pedraz[1,2], Rosa Maria Hernandez[1,2] and Manoli Igartua[1,2]

[1]NanoBioCel Group, Laboratory of Pharmaceutics, University of the Basque Country (UPV/EHU), School of Pharmacy, Vitoria, Spain [2]Biomedical Research Networking Center in Bioengineering, Biomaterials and Nanomedicine (CIBER-BBN), Vitoria, Spain [3]Biopraxis Research AIE, Miñano, Spain

2.1 INTRODUCTION

Nonhealing wounds have dramatically increased and have become a great problem for healthcare professionals and patients, as pain, diminished quality of life, frequent hospitalization, and increased morbidity and mortality are associated with chronic ulceration. In developed countries, up to 2% of the population may be affected by a chronic wound at least once in their lifetime, which results in a major healthcare and economic burden, representing around 2% of the healthcare expenditure (Menke et al., 2007). In fact, chronic wounds are a current and future challenge for healthcare systems as the demographic change is leading to a much older population. Many factors other than age, associated with a delay in wound healing, can increase the risk of developing chronic wounds, such as obesity, smoking, and chronic diseases, including diabetes mellitus and vascular disorders (Menke et al., 2007). In addition, infection is a common complication that also needs to be addressed when dealing with chronic wounds as it can delay or impair the wound-healing process.

Current therapies involve costly and long-lasting treatments that are often insufficient and are associated with high ulcer recurrence (estimated at up to 70%). Thus, more effective novel treatments are required to solve this unmet need so that the related tremendous healthcare costs and resources can be optimized. For that purpose, the scientific community has focused many of its efforts on developing new therapies to promote wound healing and on improving already-available treatments to, ultimately, accelerate and achieve wound closure.

Nanobiomaterials in Soft Tissue Engineering. DOI: http://dx.doi.org/10.1016/B978-0-323-42865-1.00002-7

To this aim, the use of nanotechnology has provided a great tool to develop new drug-delivery systems (DDSs) for the sustained release of therapeutic agents in order to achieve more cost-effective therapies.

This chapter will provide a general overview of useful therapeutic agents, such as growth factors (GFs) and antimicrobials, employed in wound-healing therapy, and the nanotechnology approaches developed so far to improve treatment effectiveness. A detailed insight into the current advances on DDS development for wound-healing therapy will be given, mainly focusing on polymeric and lipid nanoparticles (NPs), silver nanoparticles (AgNPs), nanofibrous structures, nanosheets, and nanohybrids.

2.2 CUTANEOUS WOUND HEALING AND SKIN LESIONS

The skin, the outer tissue protecting against the environment, is exposed to chemical, physical, and biological harms as well as being the subject of genetic, inflammatory, or metabolic diseases. Aging is associated with a loss or decrease of some of the protective properties of the skin as it becomes drier, less elastic, thinner, and thus more likely to suffer damage and infection. Senescent cells accumulated in aging tissues lead to a decline in several functions of the human skin, such as barrier efficacy, sensory perception, wound healing, immune response, and DNA repair. Furthermore, changes in collagen formation, flattening of the basement membrane, a reduction in blood supply to the skin, and a slower inflammatory response reduce the ability to achieve skin repair (Farage et al., 2009).

Cutaneous wound healing is a well-coordinated biological process that involves the integrated interaction of different GFs, cytokines, enzymes, and cell types, such as inflammatory cells, keratinocytes, fibroblasts, and endothelial cells. Tissue repair is accomplished by tightly regulated processes that overlap in space and time, including an initial inflammatory response, a proliferative phase, and a final remodeling phase (Martin, 1997; Singer and Clark, 1999). Chronic wounds fail to proceed through those sequential phases, subsequently resulting in delayed or incomplete healing.

Multiple factors contribute to poor wound healing. Among them, a major role has been attributed to an abnormal and persistent inflammatory response, a hallmark of nonhealing skin wounds, that leads to an excessive proteolytic activity due to protease inhibitor degradation, and ultimately to inflammation-mediated tissue damage (Trengove et al., 1999). A decreased vascular supply is also a common cause of ulcer formation. In addition, a reduction in the amount of available and biologically active GFs in the wound environment particularly affects wound repair.

One of the most common complications of chronic wounds is infection. In open wounds, there is a disruption of the intact skin that is the first mechanical line of defense against infection. Elevated levels of bacterial load are typically present on open wounds and can stimulate a proinflammatory environment. Hence, the wound-healing process can be impaired partially due to an elongation of the inflammatory phase that suppresses the regenerative phase (Hernandez, 2006; Lipsky and Hoey, 2009). Bacteria not only compete for the limited oxygen and nutrients present in the wound, they also release toxins and induce an increased production of enzymes that can further lead to cellular failure.

Chronic wounds include pressure, vascular (venous or arterial), and diabetic foot ulcers (DFUs). A pressure ulcer is defined as an area of localized damage on the skin and/or underlying tissue, usually over a bony prominence, occurring as a consequence of pressure or shear and/or a combination of these (Black et al., 2007). Vascular ulcers, usually localized on the lower limbs, are caused by a circulation disorder that leads to a reduction in the arterial blood flow or an impaired venous blood return. Vascular ulcers constitute a group of lesions of particular relevance due to their high prevalence. In addition, these ulcers are a leading cause of morbidity among patients suffering from peripheral vascular disease (Markova and Mostow, 2012). Lastly, DFU is a major complication of diabetes because of the high level of consequences produced on the patients' quality of life. DFUs are caused by a number of contributing factors, such as mechanical changes in conformation of the bony architecture of the foot, peripheral neuropathy (damaged nerves), and peripheral vascular disease (blocked arteries), all of which occur with higher frequency and intensity in the diabetic population (Eldor et al., 2004). In addition, DFUs are highly associated with nontraumatic lower-extremity amputations in the industrialized world.

On the other hand, major burns produced by heat, chemicals, electricity, or radiation can also became chronic wounds. A burn injury affects the skin integrity, leading to fluid loss and being a portal for bacterial infection. The severity of a burn depends on the depth, location, and body surface area injured.

2.3 THERAPEUTIC AGENTS FOR WOUND-HEALING THERAPY

2.3.1 GROWTH FACTORS

GFs are biologically active polypeptides which regulate cell growth, differentiation, proliferation, and migration, as well as, protein expression and enzyme production. In addition, GFs have a potential ability to heal wounds by stimulating angiogenesis, modulating the inflammatory response, and intervening in the production and degradation of the extracellular matrix and the granulation tissue (Barrientos et al., 2008; Bodnar, 2013). The main GFs involved in the healing process and skin regeneration are platelet-derived growth factor (PDGF), epidermal growth factor (EGF), basic fibroblast growth factor (bFGF), insulin-like growth factor (IGF), and vascular endothelial growth factor (VEGF) families. Their functions are summarized in Table 2.1.

Table 2.1 Summary of the Main Functions of Different GFs Involved in Wound Healing and Skin Regeneration

Growth Factor	Main Functions	References
PDGF	Chemotactic for neutrophils, monocytes and fibroblasts Promotes extracellular matrix production	Werner and Grose (2003), Li et al. (2008)
EGF	Induces re-epithelialization by the promotion of keratinocyte proliferation and migration Promotes angiogenesis Stimulates wound remodelation and protein production such as fibronectin	Barrientos et al. (2008), Tiaka et al. (2012), Hong et al. (2008)
bFGF	Activates local macrophages up to the remodeling phase. Promotes angiogenesis Stimulates the extracellular matrix metabolism and growth	Robson (1997), McGee et al. (1988), Akita et al. (2008)
IGF	Stimulates wound re-epithelialization and fibroblast proliferation Dampens the local inflammatory response	Provenzano et al. (2007), Emmerson et al. (2012)
VEGF	Promotes angiogenesis, granulation tissue formation, and epithelialization	Losi et al. (2013), Bao et al. (2009)

The external administration of GFs has become one of the most interesting strategies to promote wound healing and skin regeneration, as a decrease in the GF levels has been reported in chronic wounds (Barrientos et al., 2008, 2014). Nevertheless, the proteases present in the lesion, able to degrade the GFs, along with the low *in vivo* stability of these molecules have limited their clinical applications (Mast and Schultz, 1996; Baldwin and Mark Saltzman, 1998; Ulubayram et al., 2001). In this regard, in recent years the nanotechnology approaches for the release of GFs have been expansively investigated in order to improve the stability of GFs at the wound site, allowing their sustained release, and, ultimately, optimizing treatment effectiveness.

2.3.2 ANTIMICROBIAL AGENTS

One of the most common complications in the treatment of chronic wounds is bacterial infections. In fact, 75% of the mortality associated with burn injuries are due to infections, mostly caused by Gram-negative (such as *Pseudomonas aeruginosa*) or Gram-positive bacteria (such as methicillin-resistant *Staphylococcus aureus*) (Saito et al., 2012). Therefore, a suitable strategy for the treatment of chronic wounds involves the administration of antimicrobial agents, such as antibiotics or silver. This section will focus on the latest advances on DDSs devoted to properly formulate antimicrobials for wound infection treatment.

2.3.2.1 Antibiotics

In clinical practice, the choice of antibiotic will depend on the microorganisms present within the wound, the bacterial susceptibility to antimicrobials, and patient characteristics. The main broad-spectrum antibiotics effective against the majority of bacteria commonly found in infected wounds are gentamicin, an aminoglycoside that is effective against many Gram-negative bacteria, especially *Pseudomonas* spp. and certain Gram-positives (such as *S. aureus*) (Chen et al., 2012b); mupirocin, commonly used in wound care prophylaxis against *S. aureus* cutaneous infection and against some Gram-negative flora (Thakur et al., 2008); tetracycline, a broad-spectrum antibiotic that, besides being active against a wide range of Gram-positive and Gram-negative bacteria, is effective against *Chlamydia*, *Mycoplasma*, *Rickettsia*, and protozoan parasites (Chopra and Roberts, 2001); and ciprofloxacin, the most potent fluoroquinolone active against a wide range of bacteria, being the most susceptible aerobic Gram-negative bacilli (Sharma et al., 2010).

Narrow-range antibiotics, such as penicillin G, vancomycin, and lysostaphin, are employed for wound-healing treatment. On the one hand, penicillin G is active against non-β-lactamase-producing Gram-positive bacteria, anaerobes, and Gram-negative cocci from the *Neisseria* spp. (Doi and Chambers, 2015). On the other hand, vancomycin is a glycopeptide active against Gram-positive bacteria and is mainly used in recalcitrant staphylococcal infections that are resistant to penicillin or cephalosporin (Chen et al., 2012b). Finally, lysostaphin is a cell-lytic enzyme secreted by *Staphylococcus simulans* that is highly effective and specific against *S. aureus* (Miao et al., 2011).

Another encouraging strategy to overcome wound bacterial infection is the administration of antimicrobial peptides (AMPs). AMPs are part of the innate immunity, providing a first line of defense against a wide range of pathogenic organisms (Vandamme et al., 2012). Currently, there are more than 600 AMPs classified into two families: defensins and cathelicidins (Hancock, 2001). The LL37 peptide, also known as hCAP-18, is the only human cathelicidin identified to date. This peptide exerts antimicrobial activity towards various microorganisms, such as Gram-positive and Gram-negative bacteria, fungi, parasites, and enveloped viruses. Furthermore, LL37 is chemotactic (Vandamme et al., 2012), stimulates the production of proinflammatory cytokines, neutralizes the immune response through the interaction with the LPS endotoxin (Kai-Larsen and Agerberth, 2008), promotes new vessel formation (Koczulla et al., 2003), and stimulates the proliferation and migration of epithelial cells (Anderson et al., 2008). Therefore, LL37 is emerging as a potential therapeutic tool for promoting wound healing and inhibiting bacterial growth. However, peptides have shown limited stability *in vivo* due to the proteases present in the wound. Thus, optimization of LL37 administration using advanced DDSs can enhance its biological function and thus improve treatment effectiveness (Hancock, 2001).

Finally, it should be noted that most of the antimicrobials employed in the treatment of infected wounds are administered through the systemic route.

However, this approach can lead to the appearance of undesirable side effects or to an insufficient dosage on the lesion as the antibiotics can barely penetrate into ischemic tissues (Xu et al., 2010). In addition, the extensive use and misuse of antibiotics can contribute to the development of antibiotic-resistant bacteria. In order to overcome these disadvantages, antibiotics formulated in advanced DDSs can be locally administered to obtain higher concentrations at the wound site due to a high initial drug release followed by a sustained release that can achieve a long-lasting antimicrobial effect (De Cicco et al., 2014).

2.3.2.2 Silver

The use of silver is a widely employed strategy to overcome bacterial infection and prevent wound sepsis. Silver has shown several interesting properties, such as wide spectrum against several microorganisms; multiple mechanisms of action to inhibit bacterial colonization, which reduces the risk of developing resistance; great effectiveness against multidrug-resistant organisms; and low systemic toxicity (Gunasekaran et al., 2011).

Only the soluble form of silver is biologically active, that is, Ag+ or Ag0 clusters. Ag+ ions are present in silver nitrate, silver sulfadiazine (SSD), and other ionic silver compounds. On the other hand, metallic silver (Ag^0) is found in two different crystalline forms, that is, the nanocrystalline (<20 nm) or the subcrystalline (less than eight atoms of silver) forms (Dunn and Edwards-Jones, 2004).

The mechanism of action of soluble silver is still unknown; however, the most widely accepted mode of action is closely related to the interaction of silver with the bacterial cell wall and cell membrane that inhibits the bacterial respiration process (Klasen, 2000). Furthermore, silver is involved in bacterial DNA condensation, which leads to loss of the replication ability and, therefore, to cell death (Feng et al., 2000). As a result of the multiple bactericidal mechanisms of soluble silver, this noble metal does not produce bacterial resistance; thus, becoming an interesting strategy for the treatment of infected wounds.

2.4 NANOTECHNOLOGY APPROACHES FOR THE RELEASE OF THERAPEUTIC AGENTS FOR WOUND HEALING

Currently, several research groups have developed different nanotechnology approaches for the release of therapeutic agents as a novel strategy in wound-healing therapy. Due to the distinct characteristics of wounds and healing stages, different wound dressings and therapeutic agents can be employed to meet most of the needs in a particular wound stage. Therefore, in this section, the current nanotechnology-based strategies used for the controlled release of drugs involved in skin wound regeneration are summarized (Figure 2.1).

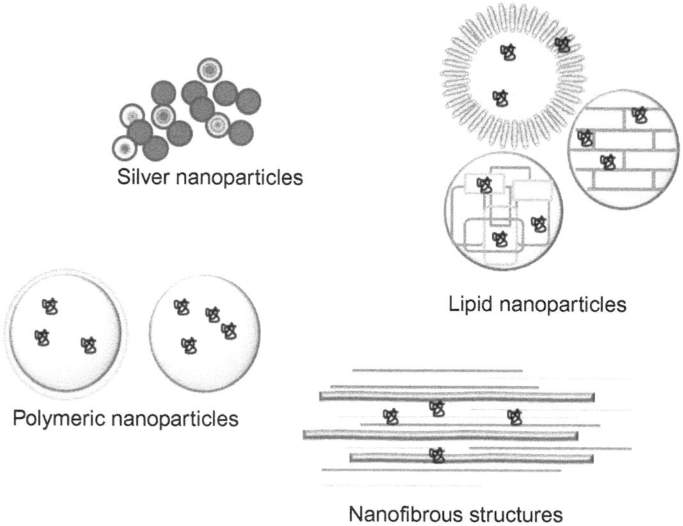

FIGURE 2.1

Schematic illustration of different DDSs used for the treatment of chronic wounds.

2.4.1 NANOTECHNOLOGY APPROACHES FOR GF DELIVERY

As previously mentioned, nanotechnology provides the opportunity to enhance the *in vivo* effectiveness of GFs, preventing proteolytic degradation and prolonging release at the lesion (Kubinová and Syková, 2010). A wide variety of nanoscale delivery systems have been designed to promote wound healing, mainly polymeric NPs, lipid NPs, and nanofibrous structures.

2.4.1.1 Polymeric NPs

Biocompatible polymeric devices have currently become a promising alternative for the controlled release of active compounds, including GFs. These nanometric colloidal systems can be employed in multiple diseases, administration routes, and dosage ranges. Therefore, polymeric carriers have been developed for chronic wound therapy because, apart from allowing controlled drug release over time, they may also reduce drug degradation by the proteases present in the wound environment (Ulubayram et al., 2001; Gainza et al., 2013), and thus, the administration frequency and dose can be decreased. Nanospheres can be prepared using natural or synthetic biomaterials, as well as other polymer combinations (Değim, 2008; Ye et al., 2010; Makadia and Siegel, 2011).

One of the most widely used polymers to prepare nanospheres as DDSs is the synthetic poly-lactic-co-glycolic acid (PLGA), because this polymer allows drug sustained release, and is biocompatible and biodegradable (Makadia and Siegel, 2011). In this regard, Chu and coworkers developed rhEGF-loaded (recombinant human Epidermal Growth Factor) PLGA NPs using a modified double-emulsion method and assessed their effectiveness during 21 days after topical administration in full-thickness wounds created on diabetic rats. The rhEGF-NPs (size around 193.5 nm) showed an encapsulation efficiency (EE) of 85.6% and an rhEGF release for 24 h; therefore, treatments were locally administered once daily. After 7, 14, and 21 days, wounds treated with rhEGF-NPs achieved the greatest wound area reduction of all the experimental groups. In addition, the histopathological examination of lesions showed that the rhEGF-NPs promoted the highest level of fibroblast proliferation and PCNA expression. These results support that the controlled release of rhEGF allows continuous contact of the GF with the wound surface to maintain an effective concentration able to promote healing; and suggest a more appropriate administration for rhEGF (Chu et al., 2010).

The latest advances in drug delivery involved the combination of different technological approaches that may improve dressing integration. In this regard, Losi et al. have developed poly(ether)urethane-polydimethylsiloxane/fibrin-based scaffolds containing VEGF- and bFGF-loaded PLGA NPs that have been demonstrated to be effective in enhancing wound closure by day 15 in *db/db* mice compared with scaffolds not containing GFs. In addition, as observed in the histological evaluation, complete re-epithelialization, improved collagen deposition, and more mature granulation tissue were observed in scaffolds containing GF-loaded NPs, even though no difference between scaffolds containing free GFs and GF-loaded NPs were found. Overall, these results suggest that fibrin-based scaffolds containing GF-loaded NPs are an interesting strategy for the sustained release of VEGF and bFGF because they acted as a double DDS for GF delivery; and therefore, the initial burst release of the GFs and the leak out of the particles from the wound site after topical administration might be reduced, providing a more sustained release of the GFs (Losi et al., 2013).

2.4.1.2 Lipid NPs

Lipid NPs have been intensively studied for dermal application, pharmaceutical, and cosmetic uses (Pardeike et al., 2010). These lipid carriers look promising due to their biocompatibility, ease of preparation, and superior efficacy compared with nonencapsulated drugs (Fan and Zhang, 2013).

The first developed lipid nanocarriers were liposomes, comprising an aqueous core encapsulated by natural or synthetic phospholipids. This structure allows entrapment of hydrophilic drugs in the core, while hydrophobic drugs are entrapped within the lipid bilayers (Fan and Zhang, 2013). Since the first liposomal pharmaceutical product, Doxil® [doxorubicin-polyethylenglycol (PEG)ylated liposome] approved in 1995 for Kaposi's sarcoma, ovarian, and breast cancer, to date, there are a number of commercially available products (Allen and Cullis, 2013).

A few publications have described the use of liposomes as GF carriers for wound healing. First, Brown and collaborators reported the benefits of locally administered EGF-loaded multilamellar liposomes on the tensile strength of experimental incisions on rats. As observed in the measurement of the rate of rhEGF loss from incisions *in vivo*, significantly higher levels of the GF were retained by the multilamellar liposomes (62% after 1 day, 48% after 2 days, and 11% after 5 days). In addition, a single dose of EGF in liposomes significantly prolonged the exposure of EGF, producing a 200% increase in wound tensile strength from days 7 to 14, and increasing collagen formation and fibroblast proliferation. These studies clearly proved that the incororation of EGF in an appropriate vehicle induced more efficient wound healing than local administration of the free GF, since EGF-loaded liposomes improved early tensile strength and therefore promoted wound remodeling and healing (Brown et al., 1988). In a different study published by Pierre and colleagues, very low doses of IGF-I encapsulated in liposomes (0.9 μg/kg/week) administered subcutaneously were as effective at improving re-epithelialization as higher doses of IGF-I (5.0 μg/kg/week) administered together with the growth hormone (GH) and more effective than 5.0 μg/kg/week IGF-I without GH administration (Pierre et al., 1997). These data suggest that nanoencapsulation may improve treatment effectiveness compared with the free GF administration because this technological approach may protect the GFs from the wound environment and degradation (Almeida and Souto, 2007).

However, despite liposomes being well established and extensively investigated, the total number of products in the market is still limited. One of the reasons may be related to the low *in vivo* stability that may induce a rapid uncontrolled release of the drug. Therefore, at the beginning of the 1990s solid lipid nanoparticles (SLNs) and later, nanostructured lipid carriers (NLCs) were developed as alternative carrier systems to liposomes (Müller et al., 2000). SLN preparation requires solid lipids as matrix material while NLCs are prepared using a blend of solid lipids and oils. In addition, both nanoparticulated formulations are ideal for dermal administration because they are able to remain on the skin, improve skin hydration, and release drugs in a sustained manner. However, since SLNs have shown drug expulsion during storage, NLCs may be a more suitable alternative for hydrophilic drug encapsulation due to their enhanced stability (Almeida and Souto, 2007; Pardeike et al., 2010).

Based on this nanotechnology, our research group has demonstrated that rhEGF-loaded SLN and NLC topically administered were more effective at improving healing than a greater dose of free rhEGF intralesionally administered. First, we assessed the effectiveness of both formulations in healing-impaired *db/db* mice. The healing process was improved in terms of wound closure, re-epithelialization and restoration of the inflammatory process in those wounds treated with two weekly doses of topical rhEGF-SLN and rhEGF-NLC over controls, including a significantly higher dose of intralesional free rhEGF (20 μg vs 75 μg) (Gainza et al., 2014). Secondly, we assessed the effectiveness of the rhEGF-developed nanoformulations in a more relevant preclinical model, such as Large White pigs. Because rhEGF-NLC showed an improved EE compared with rhEGF-SLN, the lack of organic solvent needed for their preparation and the same *in vitro*/*in vivo* effectiveness as rhEGF-SLN; the effectiveness of two weekly topical administrations of 20 μg rhEGF-NLC was assessed in a

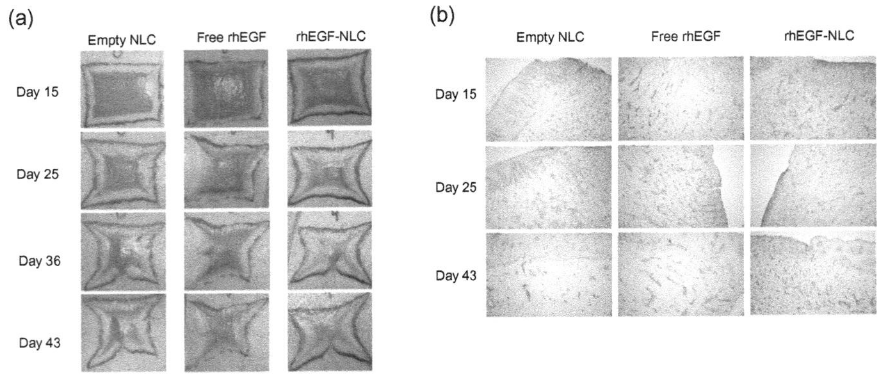

FIGURE 2.2

rhEGF-loaded nanostructured lipid carriers. (a) Wound images obtained from each experimental group on days 15, 25, 36, and 43. (b) Representative pictures of endothelial cells marked with anti-CD 31 antibody on days 15, 25, and 43 (×10 magnification).

Reproduced and adapted with permission from Gainza et al. (2015) (©2014).

full-thickness swine excisional wound model compared with empty NLC and two weekly intralesional administrations of 75 μg free rhEGF. Data obtained from the swine model supported the results previously obtained in rodents, since by day 25, lower doses of rhEGF-NLC increased the wound closure and percentage of healed wounds as much as that exerted by free rhEGF, but more than empty NLC (Figure 2.2a). In addition, the histopathological examination confirmed that rhEGF-NLC promoted fibroblast migration and proliferation, collagen deposition, resolution of the inflammatory response and, as observed in Figure 2.2b, neoangiogenesis (Gainza et al., 2015). Overall, these findings demonstrated that lower doses of topically administered rhEGF-NLC may stimulate healing of full-thickness wounds in rodents and pigs, thereby confirming their potential clinical application for wound management.

2.4.1.3 Nanofibrous structures

Nanofibrous materials are gaining interest for tissue engineering applications, including skin regeneration. Nanofibrous structures mimic the native extracellular matrix and promote the adhesion of various cells and soluble factors that may promote cell function and tissue regeneration. Nanofibers (NFs) for skin tissue regeneration are mainly developed using the electrospinning technique because it allows the production of micro- and nanometric continuous fibers that have shown uniform adhesion to the lesion without fluid accumulation (Chaudhury et al., 2014).

In the last few years, several studies have been performed to assess the effect of NFs in the controlled release of GFs for wound repair. Different materials, natural or synthetic, can be used for the fabrication of electrospun NFs. On the one hand, silk fibroin from *Bombyx mori* silkworm, a natural polymer, has demonstrated adequate mechanical strength and excellent biocompatibility for skin regeneration applications. Silk mats containing EGF have been shown to maintain their structure during the healing process and to enhance healing by inducing the keratinocyte tongue proliferation and thus, promoting re-epithelialization. Therefore, the silk mats offered not only physical protection of the lesion, but also sustained release of EGF to the wound (Schneider et al., 2009). In addition, the effectiveness of silk-protein biomaterials with EGF and SSD has been studied in lesions created on mice. Wound biopsies revealed that those dressings, as well as the other lamellar porous films evaluated in that study, provided the most rapid wound closure, also showing higher healing rate, re-epithelialization, dermis proliferation, and collagen synthesis compared with the air-permeable Tegaderm® (Gil et al., 2013).

Synthetic biomaterials are also widely employed for the preparation of NFs for wound repair. For example, bFGF-loaded electrospun NFs developed using the synthetic poly(ethylene glycol)-poly(DL-lactide) polymer for the treatment of diabetic skin ulcers, compared with NFs infiltrated with free bFGF, significantly improved the healing rate by promoting re-epithelialization and regeneration of skin appendages and the Extracellular matrix (ECM) remodeling. In addition, the obtained sustained release of bFGF enhanced collagen deposition and improved the density and maturity of capillaries for 2 weeks (Yang et al., 2011).

Due to the practicality, easy fabrication, and successful results that NFs have demonstrated, several research groups are currently working on the development of advanced nanofibrous structures combining two or more polymers. In addition, due to the increased recognition of phototherapy in promoting wound healing, photosensitive polymers are also used for NF preparation. In this regard, poly(3-hexylthiophene), a photosensitive polymer, and EGF encapsulated in the core-shell-structured gelatin/poly(L-lactic acid)-co-poly-(ε-caprolactone) (PLLCL) NFs (EGF-Gel/PLLCL/P3GF (cs) prepared by coaxial spinning have been evaluated as skin grafts. EGF-Gel/PLLCL/P3GF(cs) significantly improved human dermal fibroblast proliferation and wound closure under light stimulation in an *in vitro* wound model compared with fibroblasts treated with those NFs but under dark conditions. Moreover, EGF-Gel/PLLCL/P3GF(cs) treatment in adipose stem cells under light stimulation induced keratinocyte differentiation (Jin et al., 2014).

Combinations of poly(ε-caprolactone) and PEG polymers for NF preparation have also been studied. For example, the healing effectiveness of rhEGF surface-immobilized NFs assessed in diabetic burns created on the back of C57BL/6 female mice showed an increased healing rate on days 7 and 14 compared with empty NFs and the untreated control (Choi et al., 2008). Remarkably, wound closure in those wounds treated with rhEGF-NFs was significantly greater than in those treated with a mixture of rhEGF and NFs. These data suggest that the entrapment of rhEGF within NFs may prevent GF degradation from wound proteases. Moreover, the histological examination also confirmed that lesions treated with rhEGF-conjugated NFs showed increased keratinocyte-specific genes and EGF receptor expression; thus, promoting wound healing (Choi et al., 2008). Moreover, two different growth factors, EGF and bFGF, were also incorporated in the coaxial NFs to obtain a biphasic release of the GFs (Choi et al., 2011). EGF was surface immobilized and minimal release, related to the NFs mesh degradation, was shown during 7 days while bFGF, immobilized on the core, showed an initial burst and an approximately 30% release of the encapsulated bFGF in the first 12 h. In addition, studies undertaken in diabetic burns created on the back of C57BL/6 female mice clearly demonstrated that controlled release of EGF and bFGF from NFs further accelerated proliferation of epidermal cells and wound closure than the control groups, EGF-NFs and bFGF-NFs. Moreover, animals treated with EGF/bFGF-NFs improved collagen and keratin accumulation; confirming the nanofibrous matrix as a promising wound dressing to improve wound healing (Choi et al., 2011).

Combinations of different DDSs have also been used as multifunctional wound dressings for wound-healing applications. As an example, a biomimetic nanofibrous scaffold containing PDGF-BB-loaded PLGA NPs and VEGF-loaded chitosan, poly(ethylene oxide) (PEO) NFs were developed to achieve dual release of the two GFs (fast and sustained release) (Xie et al., 2013). This system allowed the quick release of VEGF to promote new vessel formation and provided PDGF-BB sustained release throughout the whole healing process (Figure 2.3a). Studies performed on a rat full-thickness wound model, depicted in Figure 2.3b, revealed an accelerated wound closure of those wounds treated with the biomimetic nanofibrous scaffold compared with the untreated group, empty NFs and the commercial dressing Hydrofera Blue®. In addition, as observed in the histological examination, VEGF

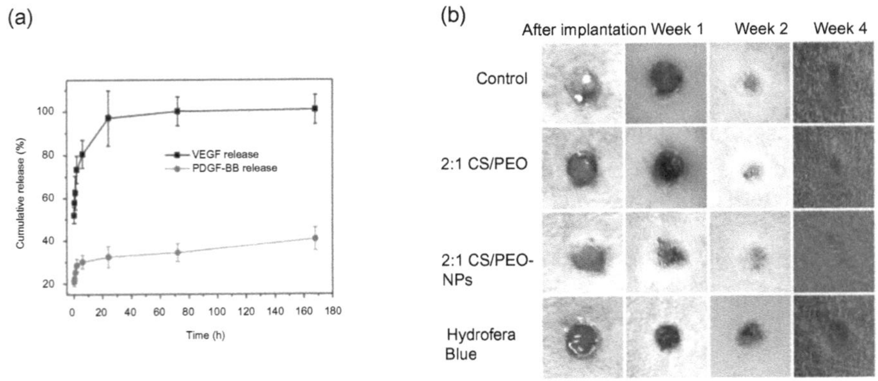

FIGURE 2.3

Biomimetic nanofibrous scaffold containing PDGF-BB-loaded PLGA NPs and VEGF-loaded CS-PEO NFs. (a) Release kinetics of VEGF from NFs and PDGF-nanoparticles within fibers. (b) Representative macroscopic appearance of wound closure on weeks 0, 1, 2, and 4 after wound treatment with two controls (open wound and Hydrofera Blue®) and NF meshes (2:1 CS/PEO) without GFs and NF meshes with nanoparticles and GFs (2:1 CS/PEO-NPs).

Reproduced and adapted with permission from Xie et al. (2013) (©2013).

may be responsible for the increased angiogenesis observed in the early stage of the healing process, while PDFG-BB may improve re-epithelialization, collagen deposition, and tissue remodeling (Xie et al., 2013).

Finally, more complex NP in-fiber structures have also been developed using collagen and hyaluronic acid for programmable multiangiogenic GF release (Lai et al., 2014). In this occasion, bFGF and EGF were directly embedded in the nanofibrous skin equivalent and PDGF-BB and VEGF were encapsulated into gelatine NPs and embedded in the NF meshes. Results obtained from lesions created on sreptozotocin (STZ)-diabetized rats treated with this complex structure revealed that the initial delivery of bFGF and EGF may mimic the early stage of healing by accelerating epithelialization and angiogenesis, while the sustained release of PDGF and VEGF may promote tissue remodeling, blood vessel maturation, and collagen deposition. Overall, these findings demonstrated that this advanced DDS could be a promising bioengineered construct for wound therapy (Lai et al., 2014).

2.4.2 NANOTECHNOLOGY APPROACHES FOR ANTIMICROBIAL AGENTS DELIVERY

2.4.2.1 Antibiotics

Among the current nanotechnology approaches for chronic wound treatment, NPs, NFs, and nanosheets to release antibiotics can be highlighted.

2.4.2.1.1 Polymeric nanoparticles

Polymeric NPs are one of the most promising DDSs for antibiotics (Cortivo et al., 2010). As previously mentioned, it is widely assumed that drug nanoencapsulation can improve drug stability within the wounded area. In this regard, penicillin-G-loaded polyacrylate NPs have been proven to protect penicillin against β-lactamase, since they present an equipotent *in vitro* antibacterial activity against methicillin-susceptible and methicillin-resistant strains of *S. aureus* (Turos et al., 2007). Furthermore, the application of the NP emulsion directly onto skin abrasions in mice accelerated wound healing compared with saline administration and showed no discernible toxicity, that is, no redness, irritation, or inflammation. In addition, the polymeric film formed by the NP emulsion applied over the wound protected the lesion from microorganisms; so that these wound dressings appeared to be an integral part of the forming skin layers, maintaining the skin's mechanical properties, preserving the moisture, and allowing oxygenation of the lesion (Greenhalgh and Turos, 2009).

A different wound dressing based on an *in situ* gelling nanoparticulated dry powder composed of alginate-pectin loaded with gentamicin sulfate has been developed. Remarkably, due to the rapid gelation of the nanoparticulated powder, this nanoformulation was able to absorb large quantities of wound fluid and therefore microorganism colonization could be reduced. Moreover, since the formed hydrogel exhibited proper adhesiveness, easy dressing removal from the wound was allowed. The antimicrobial activity of the gentamicin-sulfate-loaded NPs incorporated into the hydrogel was tested against *S. aureus* and *P. aeruginosa*, the most common bacteria present in infected wounds, revealing a higher antibacterial activity compared with the free drug (De Cicco et al., 2014).

Finally, regarding the controlled delivery of AMPs, Chereddy and collaborators incorporated LL37 in PLGA nanospheres in order to improve the *in vivo* stability of the peptide. As observed in the *in vitro* studies, both PLGA-LL37 and free LL37 were shown not to be cytotoxic and to improve wound healing in the HaCaT cell line; and presented anti-inflammatory activity by downregulating TNF-α in macrophages. However, no significant increase in proliferation was observed in HaCaT and in the fibroblast cell line BJ. In addition, PLGA-LL37 nanospheres improved the wound-healing rate compared with free LL37 in a full-thickness wound model in mice, and presented similar wound closure to wounds treated with the plasmid encoding hCAP-18. Moreover, PLGA-LL37 promoted angiogenesis and diminished inflammatory infiltration, since IL-6 and VEGF were upregulated and the myeloperoxidase activity decreased (Chereddy et al., 2014).

2.4.2.1.2 Nanofibrous structures

Wound dressings based on antibiotic-loaded nanofibrous scaffolds are another encouraging approach for wound treatment.

In a study published by Miao and collaborators, NFs were prepared by electrospinning cellulose, cellulose–chitosan, or cellulose–poly(methylmethacrylate). NFs were then functionalized by conjugation with lysostaphin. In addition, the method of conjugation, which depends on the polymer used, may have a great impact on the antibacterial activity of the antibiotic-loaded NFs. In this regard, the conjugation of lysostaphin and cellulose-NFs by covalent bonds produced the most biostable formulation and the best anti-infective properties, as this formulation showed complete neutralization of *S. aureus*. Furthermore, minimal cytotoxicity in the keratinocyte cell line HaCaT was shown in biocompatibility assays and antimicrobial activity was revealed in a skin-like model consisting of a monolayer of cultured keratinocytes infected with *S. aureus* (Miao et al., 2011).

Additionally, NFs prepared with sodium alginate have also been shown to be suitable for wound treatment due to the biocompatible and biodegradable properties of alginate. Sodium alginate NFs have been prepared by the electrospinning technique, incorporating poly(vinyl acetate) (PVA) into the polymer solution in order to avoid the early gelation of sodium alginate. In this occasion, ciprofloxacin, loaded during the electrospinning process, was employed as the active compound of the wound dressing. Studies carried out in a full-thickness model in rabbits demonstrated that ciprofloxacin-loaded PVA-sodium alginate NFs enhanced wound epithelialization compared with PVA-NFs and a commercial ciprofloxacin formulation (Kataria et al., 2014).

As previously mentioned, NFs can also be prepared using synthetic polymers. For that purpose, a PEG-PLLA nanofibrous membrane loaded with tetracycline had been successfully developed, showing no loss of the tetracycline bioactivity, since the membranes were effective at inhibiting *S. aureus* for 5 days (Xu et al., 2010).

Electrospun scaffolds can also be loaded with several drugs. As an example, a PLLA scaffold containing an antibiotic, mupirocin, and an anesthetic, lidocaine hydrochloride, had been developed. In order to achieve release of both drugs, a dual-spinneret-electrospinning apparatus was used to prepare a single scaffold composed of two types of NFs, that is, mupirocin-loaded NFs and lidocaine-hydrochloride-loaded NFs. The resulting wound dressing presented an initial burst release of lidocaine, for immediate pain relief, and a sustained release of mupirocin, for continuous antibacterial activity. Furthermore, as observed in the *in vitro* activity assays, the antibiotic remained active in the scaffold for at least 3 days (Thakur et al., 2008).

NFs, besides being used as DDSs, can also act as a scaffold for cellular growth and proliferation. In this regard, a sandwich-structured membrane was developed comprising a core layer of PLGA for the release of vancomycin, gentamicin, and lidocaine; and an outer layer of PLGA and collagen, devoted to act as a scaffold for cellular growth and differentiation. As observed in the *in vitro* antibacterial studies performed in *S. aureus* and *Escherichia coli*, gentamicin and vancomycin NFs had above 30% and 37%, respectively, of the maximum activity of each free antibiotic after 3 weeks. Moreover, as observed in the MTT assay, the viability of human fibroblasts was not affected in 21 days (Chen et al., 2012b). The sandwich-structured nanofibrous membranes were effective for the treatment of *S. aureus* and *E. coli* infected wounds in a full-thickness wound model in rats, especially in the early stages of healing. As described by the authors, 2 and 3 weeks after grafting, wounds treated with the developed sandwich-structured membrane presented a newly synthesized fibrous tissue with little infiltration of inflammatory cells, covered by a re-epithelialized epidermis, in contrast with the incomplete re-epithelialization and prominent inflammatory cell infiltration shown in those wounds treated with drug-free scaffolds (Chen et al., 2012a).

Similar sandwich-structured membranes had also been developed for antibiotic release, such as NFs prepared using a needleless electrospinning technology (Nanospider™). Those NFs were composed of a core layer of PVA loaded with gentamicin and cover layers of polyurethane. The *in vitro* antibacterial assay conducted to prove the bioactivity of the gentamicin-loaded NFs did not show any loss of the gentamicin activity after its incorporation in the nanofibrous structure (Sirc et al., 2012).

2.4.2.1.3 Nanosheets

Nanotechnology has also allowed the development of nanosheets. Remarkably, these polymeric ultrathin two-dimensional films have been demonstrated to be useful as wound dressings. In this regard, Saito and collaborators developed a nanosheet consisting of three functional layers; a layer-by-layer nanosheet composed of chitosan and sodium alginate, a tetracycline layer, and a PVAc layer, that acted as a hydrophobic protecting layer. The nanosheets improved the survival rate of *P. aeruginosa*-infected burn injured mice by up to 100%. Moreover, as was observed by the viable bacterial count in the wound site and in liver biopsies, the *P. aeruginosa* infection was suppressed 3 days after wound induction. Finally, the histopathological examinations revealed the resolution of the inflammatory response as the infiltration of inflammatory cells significantly decreased by day 3 in the tetracycline-loaded nanosheet-treated group (Saito et al., 2012).

2.4.2.2 Silver NP

Initially, silver was employed in the ionic form and was directly administered on burns. However, one of the major limitations of ionic silver is that it may be neutralized by anions in body fluids, limitating its effectiveness, and may show several side effects, such as cosmetic abnormalities and impaired healing after prolonged topical use (Gunasekaran et al., 2011).

In order to improve the effectiveness of ionic silver, AgNPs composed of nanocrystalline metallic silver were developed. The improved effectiveness of AgNPs can be attributed to the decreased size of the NP that provides a larger surface area to volume ratio and, thus, improves the antibacterial activity (Rai et al., 2009; Gunasekaran et al., 2011). Moreover, in order to facilitate their administration and reduce the site effects associated with excessive exposure to silver, AgNPs are usually formulated in both traditional dressings and novel DDSs.

AgNPs can be prepared in different manners, such as wet chemical, physical and biological methods, all of them based on a redox reaction, where silver ions ($Ag+$) are reduced to metallic silver (Ag^0). The resulting silver NPs are effective against a wide range of microorganisms, such as Gram-positive and Gram-negative bacteria including methicillin-resistant *S. aureus* and vancomycin-resistant enterococci, yeast, and mold (Atiyeh et al., 2007).

In order to avoid high concentrations of silver in the lesion, and thus reduce associated side effects, Hebeish and colleagues developed silver NPs loaded in cotton fabrics through the pad-dry-cure technique. The 250-ppm AgNP cotton dressing showed antimicrobial activity against *S. aureus, E. coli*, and to a lesser extent against *Candida albicans*. Furthermore, studies in rats revealed that the dressing presented a similar wound-healing rate to that induced by the marketed 1% micronized SSD cream (Dermazin®) in a burn injury model. Furthermore, the dressing possessed similar anti-inflammatory activity to indomethacin, since the inhibition of carrageenan-induced edema was similar in animals that received a single oral dose of either formulation (Hebeish et al., 2014).

AgNPs-loaded NF membranes can also be prepared *in situ* using bacterial cellulose, a natural biopolymer, with high water content, high wet strength, and chemical purity. These membranes were biocompatible with epidermal cells, since cell growth was observed microscopically, and were able to inhibit bacterial growth *of*

S. aureus, E. coli, and *P. aeruginosa* in a similar extent to the commercially available silver-containing dressing Coloplast® (Wu et al., 2014b). The subsequent *in vivo* studies, performed in a second-degree skin burn wound model in Wistar rats, showed that the membranes reduced bacterial proliferation in the wound, reaching preoperative levels on day 21, as observed in the culture of swab samples collected from the wound bed. Furthermore, the membrane demonstrated excellent healing effects as complete healing was reached by day 28 (Wu et al., 2014a).

Guar gum alkylamine (GGAA), a novel cationic biopolymer, can also be employed to develop an antimicrobial wound dressing embedding AgNPs. This polymer presents a great water-absorbing capacity that may facilitate wound exudate absorption. The resulting nanobiocomposite presented an enhanced wound-healing rate in a full-thickness wound rat model, compared with a silver alginate cream, as both achieved complete healing on days 10 and 12, respectively. Moreover, the biochemical markers, such as increased total DNA and protein content, indicated an increase in cellular proliferation, and thus, enhanced healing. Remarkably, the AgNPs-GGAA formulation achieved an improved healing quality since the tensile strength and the hydroxyproline content, both directly related to the collagen content of the wound, were higher than that induced by the silver alginate cream. Additionally, a primary skin irritation study conducted in rabbits showed no irritation after 4 h of dermal exposure to AgNPs-GGAA (Ghosh Auddy et al., 2013).

Chitosan is a suitable polymer widely used due to its remarkable properties for wound healing, such as a pain reliever, bacterial growth inhibitor, and hemostasis and epidermal cell growth inducer. In this regard, Lu and coworkers developed a novel wound dressing composed of AgNPs and chitosan (Silver nanocrystalline chitosan, SNC), by self-assembly technology. SNC-dressing-treated wounds, in a deep-partial thickness wound model in Sprague–Dawley rats, were almost recovered 10 days after the injury, whereas wounds treated with SSD presented a pseudo-scar, and wounds treated with a chitosan film presented some postoperative infection. Furthermore, the SNC group presented an increased wound-healing rate since the average healing time was 3.94 days shorter than in the SSD group. Additionally, the rats treated with SNC presented a lower silver systemic content than those rats treated with SSD at any time, reaching normal levels on day 13, as observed by blood sample determination (Lu et al., 2008).

Other chitosan-based wound dressings have been developed, such as a nanobiocomposite consisting of chitosan and sargo starch impregnated with AgNPs, with and without gentamicin. In addition, alginate and sago starch dressing impregnated with AgNPs and a regenerated cellulose–chitosan biocomposite impregnated with AgNP, both with and without gentamicin, have been developed. The wound dressings were evaluated in an open excision wound in Wistar rats obtaining similar results in the three studies, with faster healing of wounds treated with the tested biocomposites in comparison to the control wounds, as observed in Figure 2.4 for chitosan and sago starch biocomposites. No significant differences were observed in the gross healing pattern among the dressings containing or lacking gentamicin,

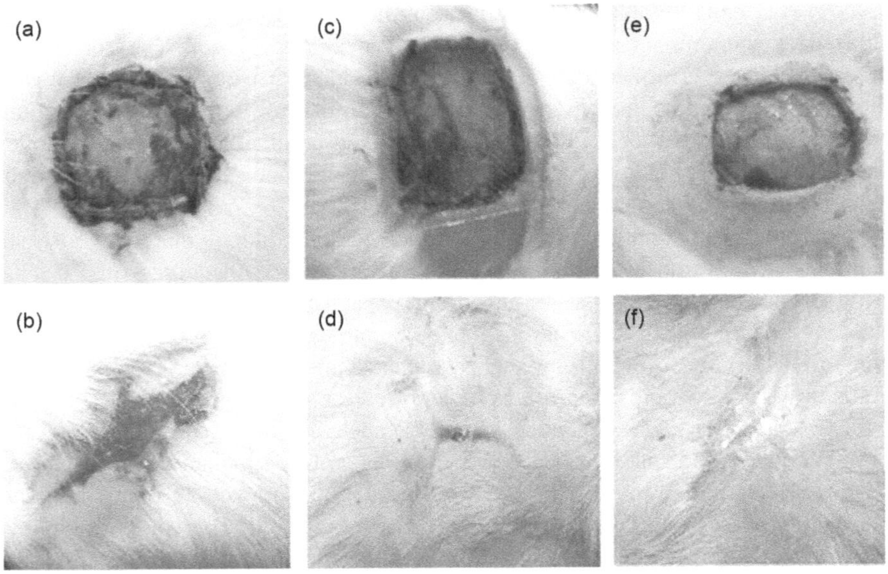

FIGURE 2.4

Photographic representation of wound contraction rate on different days of healing: (a, c, e) are control, chitosan-sago starch-AgNP, and chitosan-sago starch-AgNP-gentamicin-treated groups on 0th day, respectively. (b, d, f) are control, chitosan-sago starch-AgNP, and chitosan-sago starch-AgNP-gentamicin-treated groups on the 16th day, respectively.

Reproduced and adapted with permission from Arockianathan et al. (2012a) (©2012).

and the presence of the antibiotic only reduced the number of inflammatory cells. However, as confirmed by the histological studies, the formulations containing gentamicin achieved complete healing before the control groups (rats treated with a gauze dipped with gentamicin). The biochemical parameters, such as the increase in collagen, DNA, total protein account, hexosamine, and uronic acid, demonstrated that the experimental groups presented faster wound healing than the controls (Arockianathan et al., 2012a, 2012b; Ahamed et al., 2015).

AgNPs can be formulated by ecofriendly procedures. Bhuvaneswari and collaborators prepared AgNPs using plant extracts, as the aqueous extract of *Naringi crenulata*, due to the great affinity of silver to sulfur- or phosphorus-containing biomolecules of plant cells. The resulting AgNPs possessed various phytochemical constituents and were included in an ointment base for topical application in excisional wounds created on Wistar rats. The ointment presented astringent and antimicrobial properties, which enhanced wound contraction and the epithelialization rate, leading to complete wound healing in 15 days (faster than the standard formulation of betadine) (Bhuvaneswari et al., 2014).

AgNPs using either chondroitin sulfate or acharan sulfate had also been produced with a green synthetic route. Both composites showed bactericidal activity *in vitro* against some of the bacteria that usually infect wounds (*S. aureus, Streptococcus pyogenes, P. aeruginosa, E. coli, Salmonella typhimurium, Klebsiella oxytoca, Klebsiella aerogenes*, and *Enterobacter cloacae*). Moreover, in an incisional wound model in mice, these AgNPs showed comparable results with Silmazin® (1% SSD cream) in terms of the wound-healing rate and histological findings, achieving normal skin morphology by day 21 in all cases (Im et al., 2013).

NFs are another encouraging wound dressing for AgNP incorporation. In that regard, Jin and colleagues developed an electrospun composite of PLLCL containing AgNPs. The scaffolds loaded with 0.25 wt% of AgNPs were not cytotoxic for human skin fibroblasts, and remarkably, maintained the bactericidal activity against *S. aureus* and *Salmonella enterica* after incorporation in the wound dressing (Jin et al., 2012).

Li et al. published the development of two different wound dressings, the first one consisted of AgNP-loaded PVA and chitosan-oligosaccharides electrospun NFs (PVA/COS-AgNPs), whereas the second consisted of $AgNO_3$ loaded in the same type of NFs irradiated with ultraviolet light to form the AgNPs (PVA/COS/$AgNO_3$). Both NFs were demonstrated to be effective in a full-thickness wound model in Sprague–Dawley rats; however, the histological examination showed slightly superior wound healing in the early stages for the PVA/COS-AgNP formulation. Moreover, that scaffold had slightly superior antibacterial activity against *S. aureus* and *E. coli*, and *in vitro* biocompatibility in human skin fibroblasts (Li et al., 2013).

Wound dressings can also be prepared using modified clay minerals. Nanohybrids composed of AgNPs and a nanoscale silicate platelet produced from montmorillonite clay presented lower cytotoxicity than commercial SSD in a primary human foreskin fibroblast cell line (Hs68), and no genotoxicity in Chinese hamster ovary cells at concentrations lower than 70 ppm. The effectiveness of those nanohybrids was tested in *S. aureus*-infected acute burn wounds and full-thickness wounds created on Balb/C mice. By day 7, the nanohybrid treated groups (both burns and excision wounds) showed similar healing rates and VEGF and TGF-β1 concentrations, as lesions treated with commercially available products (Aquacel®, a silver-containing wound dressing, and an SSD commercial product). Furthermore, it should be noted that those burns treated with nanohybrids showed a cleaner surface, an improved appearance, and less scar formation (Chu et al., 2012).

2.5 CONCLUSIONS

Chronic wounds represent a major health problem from an epidemiologic, economic, and social point of view. Current therapies devoted to promote wound healing are often insufficient, showing the great and increasing demand for the improvement of chronic wound management. External administration of therapeutic agents, such as GFs and antimicrobials, to stimulate wound healing and tackle wound infection has been shown to be successful in enhancing skin regeneration. Nevertheless, stability problems of these agents associated with the presence of proteases in the wound bed need to be addressed. For that purpose, development of novel DDSs that allow drug protection, controlled release to prolong the drug effect on the wound site, reduction or eradication of the wound bacterial load, and improvement of re-epithelialization is a very encouraging strategy to ultimately achieve wound closure.

Different approaches involving the use of polymeric, lipid or silver NPs, nanofibrous structures, nanosheets, and nanohybrids have been developed and are promising tools to obtain more cost-effective therapies to improve the wound-healing therapy, with the final aim of improving patient quality of life. However, more efforts should be taken as only a few of them have reached use in humans.

REFERENCES

Ahamed, M.I.N., Sankar, S., Kashif, P.M., Basha, S.K.H., Sastry, T.P., 2015. Evaluation of biomaterial containing regenerated cellulose and chitosan incorporated with silver nanoparticles. Int. J. Biol. Macromol. 72, 680–686.

Akita, S., Akino, K., Imaizumi, T., Hirano, A., 2008. Basic fibroblast growth factor accelerates and improves second-degree burn wound healing. Wound Repair Regen. 16 (5), 635–641.

Allen, T.M., Cullis, P.R., 2013. Liposomal drug delivery systems: from concept to clinical applications. Adv. Drug Deliv. Rev. 65 (1), 36–48.

Almeida, A.J., Souto, E., 2007. Solid lipid nanoparticles as a drug delivery system for peptides and proteins. Adv. Drug Deliv. Rev. 59 (6), 478–490.

Anderson, R.C., Rehders, M., Yu, P.L., 2008. Antimicrobial fragments of the pro-region of cathelicidins and other immune peptides. Biotechnol. Lett. 30 (5), 813–818.

Arockianathan, P.M., Sekar, S., Kumaran, B., Sastry, T.P., 2012a. Preparation, characterization and evaluation of biocomposite films containing chitosan and sago starch impregnated with silver nanoparticles. Int. J. Biol. Macromol. 50 (4), 939–946.

Arockianathan, P.M., Sekar, S., Sankar, S., Kumaran, B., Sastry, T.P., 2012b. Evaluation of biocomposite films containing alginate and sago starch impregnated with silver nano particles. Carbohydr. Polym. 90 (1), 717–724.

Atiyeh, B.S., Costagliola, M., Hayek, S.N., Dibo, S.A., 2007. Effect of silver on burn wound infection control and healing: review of the literature. Burns 33 (2), 139–148.

Baldwin, S.P., Mark Saltzman, W., 1998. Materials for protein delivery in tissue engineering. Adv. Drug Deliv. Rev. 33 (1–2), 71–86.

Bao, P., Kodra, A., Tomic-Canic, M., Golinko, M.S., Ehrlich, H.P., Brem, H., 2009. The role of vascular endothelial growth factor in wound healing. J. Surg. Res. 153 (2), 347–358.

Barrientos, S., Stojadinovic, O., Golinko, M.S., Brem, H., Tomic Canic, M., 2008. Growth factors and cytokines in wound healing. Wound Repair Regen. 16 (5), 585–601.

Barrientos, S., Brem, H., Stojadinovic, O., Tomic-Canic, M., 2014. Clinical application of growth factors and cytokines in wound healing. Wound Repair Regen. 22 (5), 569–578.

Bhuvaneswari, T., Thiyagarajan, M., Geetha, N., Venkatachalam, P., 2014. Bioactive compound loaded stable silver nanoparticle synthesis from microwave irradiated aqueous extracellular leaf extracts of *Naringi crenulata* and its wound healing activity in experimental rat model. Acta Trop. 135, 55–61.

Black, J., Baharestani, M., Cuddigan, J., Dorner, B., Edsberg, L., Langemo, D., et al., 2007. National Pressure Ulcer Advisory Panel's updated pressure ulcer staging system. Dermatol. Nurs. 19 (4), 343–350.

Bodnar, R.J., 2013. Epidermal growth factor and epidermal growth factor receptor: the Yin and Yang in the treatment of cutaneous wounds and cancer. Adv. Wound Care (New Rochelle) 2 (1), 24–29.

Brown, G.L., Curtsinger, L.J., White, M., Mitchell, R.O., Pietsch, J., Nordquist, R., et al., 1988. Acceleartion of tensile strenght of incisions treated with EGF and TGF-beta. Ann. Surg. 208 (6), 788–794.

Chaudhury, K., Kumar, V., Kandasamy, J., RoyChoudhury, S., 2014. Regenerative nanomedicine: current perspectives and future directions. Int. J. Nanomed. 9, 4153–4167.

Chen, D.W., Liao, J.Y., Liu, S.J., Chan, E.C., 2012a. Novel biodegradable sandwich-structured naofibrous drug-eluting membranes for repair of infected wounds: an *in vitro* and *in vivo* study. Int. J. Nanomed. 7, 763–771.

Chen, D.W., Hsu, Y., Liao, J., Liu, S., Chen, J., Ueng, S.W., 2012b. Sustainable release of vancomycin, gentamicin and lidocaine from novel electrospun sandwich-structured PLGA/collagen nanofibrous membranes. Int. J. Pharm. 430 (1–2), 335–341.

Chereddy, K.K., Her, C., Comune, M., Moia, C., Lopes, A., Porporato, P.E., et al., 2014. PLGA nanoparticles loaded with host defense peptide LL37 promote wound healing. J. Control. Release 194, 138–147.

Choi, J.S., Leong, K.W., Yoo, H.S., 2008. *In vivo* wound healing of diabetic ulcers using electrospun nanofibers immobilized with human epidermal growth factor (EGF). Biomaterials 29 (5), 587–596.

Choi, J.S., Choi, S.H., Yoo, H.S., 2011. Coaxial electrospun nanofibers for treatment of diabetic ulcers with binary release of multiple growth factors. J. Mater. Chem. 21, 5258–5267.

Chopra, I., Roberts, M., 2001. Tetracycline antibiotics: mode of action, applications, molecular biology, and epidemiology of bacterial resistance. Microbiol. Mol. Biol. Rev. 65 (2), 232–260.

Chu, Y., Yu, D., Wang, P., Xu, J., Li, D., Ding, M., 2010. Nanotechnology promotes the full-thickness diabetic wound healing effect of recombinant human epidermal growth factor in diabetic rats. Wound Repair Regen. 18 (5), 499–505.

Chu, C.Y., Peng, F.C., Chiu, Y.F., Lee, H.C., Chen, C.W., Wei, J.C., et al., 2012. Nanohybrids of silver particles immobilized on silicate platelet for infected wound healing. PLoS One 7 (6), e38360.

Cortivo, R., Vindigni, V., Iacobellis, L., Abatangelo, G., Pinton, P., Zavan, B., 2010. Nanoscale particle therapies for wounds and ulcers. Nanomedicine 5 (4), 641–656.

De Cicco, F., Porta, A., Sansone, F., Aquino, R.P., Del Gaudio, P., 2014. Nanospray technology for an *in situ* gelling nanoparticulate powder as a wound dressing. Int. J. Pharm. 473 (1–2), 30–37.

Değim, Z., 2008. Use of microparticulate systems to accelerate skin wound healing. J. Drug Target. 16 (6), 437–448.

Doi, Y., Chambers, H.F., 2015. Penicillins and β-lactamase inhibitors. In: Bennett, J.E., Dolin, R., Blaser, M.J. (Eds.), Mandell, Douglas, and Bennett's Principles and Practice of Infectious Diseases, eighth ed. Elsevier Saunders, Canada, pp. 263–277.

Dunn, K., Edwards-Jones, V., 2004. The role of acticoat™ with nanocrystalline silver in the management of burns. Burns 30 (Suppl. 1), S1–S9.

Eldor, R., Raz, I., Ben Yehuda, A., Boulton, A.J., 2004. New and experimental approaches to treatment of diabetic foot ulcers: a comprehensive review of emerging treatment strategies. Diabet. Med. 21, 1161–1173.

Emmerson, E., Campbell, L., Davies, F.C., Ross, N.L., Ashcroft, G.S., Krust, A., et al., 2012. Insulin-like growth factor-1 promotes wound healing in estrogen-deprived mice: new insights into cutaneous IGF-1R/ERalpha cross talk. J. Invest. Dermatol. 132 (12), 2838–2848.

Fan, Y., Zhang, Q., 2013. Development of liposomal formulations: from concept to clinical investigations. Asian J. Pharm. Sci. 8 (2), 81–87.

Farage, M.A., Miller, K.W., Berardesca, E., Maibach, H.I., 2009. Clinical implications of aging skin: cutaneous disorders in the elderly. Am. J. Clin. Dermatol. 10 (2), 73–86.

Feng, Q.L., Wu, J., Chen, G.Q., Cui, F.Z., Kim, T.N., Kim, J.O., 2000. A mechanistic study of the antibacterial effect of silver ions on *Escherichia coli* and *Staphylococcus aureus*. J. Biomed. Mater. Res. 52 (4), 662–668.

Gainza, G., Aguirre, J.J., Pedraz, J.L., Hernández, R.M., Igartua, M., 2013. rhEGF-loaded PLGA-alginate microspheres enhance the healing of full-thickness excisional wounds in diabetised wistar rats. Eur. J. Pharm. Sci. 50 (3–4), 243–252.

Gainza, G., Pastor, M., Aguirre, J.J., Villullas, S., Pedraz, J.L., Hernandez, R.M., et al., 2014. A novel strategy for the treatment of chronic wounds based on the topical administration of rhEGF-loaded lipid nanoparticles: *in vitro* bioactivity and *in vivo* effectiveness in healing-impaired Db/Db mice. J. Control. Release 185, 51–61.

Gainza, G., Bonafonte, D.C., Moreno, B., Aguirre, J.J., Gutierrez, F.B., Villullas, S., et al., 2015. The topical administration of rhEGF-loaded nanostructured lipid carriers (rhEGF-NLC) improves healing in a porcine full-thickness excisional wound model. J. Control. Release 197, 41–47.

Ghosh Auddy, R., Abdullah, M.F., Das, S., Roy, P., Datta, S., Mukherjee, A., 2013. New guar biopolymer silver nanocomposites for wound healing applications. Biomed. Res. Int. 2013, 912458.

Gil, E.S., Panilaitis, B., Bellas, E., Kaplan, D.L., 2013. Functionalized silk biomaterials for wound healing. Adv. Healthc. Mater. 2 (1), 206–217.

Greenhalgh, K., Turos, E., 2009. *In vivo* studies of polyacrylate nanoparticle emulsions for topical and systemic applications. Nanomedicine 5 (1), 46–54.

Gunasekaran, T., Nigusse, T., Dhanaraju, M., 2011. Silver nanoparticles as real topical bullets for wound healing. J. Am. Coll. Clin. Wound Spec. 3 (4), 82–96.

Hancock, R.E., 2001. Cationic peptides: effectors in innate immunity and novel antimicrobials. Lancet Infect. Dis. 1 (3), 156–164.

Hebeish, A., El-Rafie, M.H., EL-Sheikh, M.A., Seleem, A.A., El-Naggar, M.E., 2014. Antimicrobial wound dressing and anti-inflammatory efficacy of silver nanoparticles. Int. J. Biol. Macromol. 65, 509–515.

Hernandez, R., 2006. The use of systemic antibiotics in the treatment of chronic wounds. Dermatol. Ther. 19, 326–337.

Hong, J.P., Kim, Y.W., Lee, S.K., Kim, S.H., Min, K.H., 2008. The effect of continuous release of recombinant human epidermal growth factor (Rh-EGF) in chitosan film on full thickness excisional porcine wounds. Ann. Plast. Surg. 61 (4), 457–462.

Im, A.R., Kim, J.Y., Kim, H.S., Cho, S., Park, Y., Kim, Y.S., 2013. Wound healing and antibacterial activities of chondroitin sulfate- and acharan sulfate-reduced silver nanoparticles. Nanotechnology 24 (39), 395102.

Jin, G., Prabhakaran, M.P., Nadappuram, B.P., Singh, G., Kai, D., Ramakrishna, S., 2012. Electrospun poly(L-lactic acid)-co-poly(varepsilon-caprolactone) nanofibres containing silver nanoparticles for skin-tissue engineering. J. Biomater. Sci. Polym. Ed. 23, 2337–2352.

Jin, G., Prabhakaran, M.P., Ramakrishna, S., 2014. Photosensitive and biomimetic core-shell nanofibrous scaffolds as wound dressing. Photochem. Photobiol. 90 (3), 673–681.

Kai-Larsen, Y., Agerberth, B., 2008. The role of the multifunctional peptide LL-37 in host defense. Front. Biosci. 13, 3760–3767.

Kataria, K., Gupta, A., Rath, G., Mathur, R.B., Dhakate, S.R., 2014. *In vivo* wound healing performance of drug loaded electrospun composite nanofibers transdermal patch. Int. J. Pharm. 469 (1), 102–110.

Klasen, H.J., 2000. A historical review of the use of silver in the treatment of burns. II. Renewed interest for silver. Burns 26 (2), 131–138.

Koczulla, R., von Degenfeld, G., Kupatt, C., Krötz, F., Zahler, S., Gloe, T., et al., 2003. An angiogenic role for the human peptide antibiotic LL-37/hCAP-18. J. Clin. Invest. 111 (11), 1665–1672.

Kubinová, S., Syková, E., 2010. Nanotechnologies in regenerative medicine. Minim. Invasive Ther. Allied Technol. 19 (3), 144–156.

Lai, H., Kuan, C., Wu, H., Tsai, J., Chen, T., Hsieh, D., et al., 2014. Tailored design of electrospun composite nanofibers with staged release of multiple angiogenic growth factors for chronic wound healing. Acta Biomater. 10 (10), 4156–4166.

Li, H., Fu, X., Zhang, L., Huang, Q., Wu, Z., Sun, T., 2008. Research of PDGF-BB Gel on the wound healing of diabetic rats and its pharmacodynamics. J. Surg. Res. 145 (1), 41–48.

Li, C., Fu, R., Yu, C., Li, Z., Guan, H., Hu, D., et al., 2013. Silver nanoparticle/chitosan oligosaccharide/poly(vinyl alcohol) nanofibers as wound dressings: a preclinical study. Int. J. Nanomed. 8, 4131–4145.

Lipsky, B.A., Hoey, C., 2009. Topical antimicrobial therapy for treating chronic wounds. Clin. Infect. Dis. 49, 1541–1549.

Losi, P., Briganti, E., Errico, C., Lisella, A., Sanguinetti, E., Chiellini, F., et al., 2013. Fibrin-based scaffold incorporating VEGF- and bFGF-loaded nanoparticles stimulates wound healing in diabetic mice. Acta Biomater. 9 (8), 7814–7821.

Lu, S., Gao, W., Gu, H.Y., 2008. Construction, application and biosafety of silver nanocrystalline chitosan wound dressing. Burns 34 (5), 623–628.

Makadia, H.K., Siegel, S.J., 2011. Poly lactic-co-glycolic acid (PLGA) as biodegradable controlled drug delivery carrier. Polymers (Basel) 3 (3), 1377–1397.

Markova, A., Mostow, E.N., 2012. US skin disease assessment: ulcer and wound care. Dermatol. Clin. 30, 107–111.

Martin, P., 1997. Wound healing—aiming for perfect skin regeneration. Science 276 (5309), 75–81.

Mast, B.A., Schultz, G.S., 1996. Interactions of cytokines, growth factors, and proteases in acute and chronic wounds. Wound Repair Regen. 4 (4), 411–420.

McGee, G.S., Davidson, J.M., Buckley, A., Sommer, A., Woodward, S.C., Aquino, A.M., et al., 1988. Recombinant basic fibroblast growth factor accelerates wound healing. J. Surg. Res. 45 (1), 145–153.

Menke, N.B., Ward, K.R., Witten, T.M., Bonchev, D.G., Diegelmann, R.F., 2007. Impaired wound healing. Clin. Dermatol. 25 (1), 19–25.

Miao, J., Pangule, R.C., Paskaleva, E.E., Hwang, E.E., Kane, R.S., Linhardt, R.J., et al., 2011. Lysostaphin-functionalized cellulose fibers with antistaphylococcal activity for wound healing applications. Biomaterials 32 (36), 9557–9567.

Müller, R.H., Mäder, K., Gohla, S., 2000. Solid lipid nanoparticles (SLN) for controlled drug delivery—a review of the state of the art. Eur. J. Pharm. Biopharm. 50 (1), 161–177.

Pardeike, J., Schwabe, K., Müller, R.H., 2010. Influence of nanostructured lipid carriers (NLC) on the physical properties of the Cutanova Nanorepair Q10 cream and the *in vivo* skin hydration effect. Int. J. Pharm. 396 (1–2), 166–173.

Pierre, E.J., Perez-polo, J.R., Mitchell, A.T., Matin, S., Foyt, H.L., Hernfon, D.N., 1997. Insuline-like growth factor-I liposomal gene transfer and systemic growth hormone stimulate wound healing. J. Burn Care Rehabil. 18 (4), 287–291.

Provenzano, P.P., Alejandro-Osorio, A.L., Grorud, K.W., Martinez, D.A., Vailas, A.C., Grindeland, R.E., et al., 2007. Systemic administration of IGF-I enhances healing in collagenous extracellular matrices: evaluation of loaded and unloaded ligaments. BMC Physiol. 7, 2.

Rai, M., Yadav, A., Gade, A., 2009. Silver nanoparticles as a new generation of antimicrobials. Biotechnol. Adv. 27 (1), 76–83.

Robson, M.C., 1997. The role of growth factors in the healing of chronic wounds. Wound Repair Regen. 5 (1), 12–17.

Saito, A., Miyazaki, H., Fujie, T., Ohtsubo, S., Kinoshita, M., Saitoh, D., et al., 2012. Therapeutic efficacy of an antibiotic-loaded nanosheet in a murine burn-wound infection model. Acta Biomater. 8 (8), 2932–2940.

Schneider, A., Wang, X.Y., Kaplan, D.L., Garlick, J.A., Egles, C., 2009. Biofunctionalized electrospun silk mats as a topical bioactive dressing for accelerated wound healing. Acta Biomater. 5 (7), 2570–2578.

Sharma, P.C., Jain, A., Jain, S., Pahwa, R., Yar, M.S., 2010. Ciprofloxacin: review on developments in synthetic, analytical, and medicinal aspects. J. Enzyme Inhib. Med. Chem. 25 (4), 577–589.

Singer, A.J., Clark, R.A., 1999. Cutaneous wound healing. N. Engl. J. Med. 341 (10), 738–746.

Sirc, J., Kubinova, S., Hobzova, R., Stranska, D., Kozlik, P., Bosakova, Z., et al., 2012. Controlled gentamicin release from multi-layered electrospun nanofibrous structures of various thicknesses. Int. J. Nanomed. 7, 5315–5325.

Thakur, R.A., Florek, C.A., Kohn, J., Michniak, B.B., 2008. Electrospun nanofibrous polymeric scaffold with targeted drug release profiles for potential application as wound dressing. Int. J. Pharm. 364 (1), 87–93.

Tiaka, E.K., Papanas, N., Manolakis, A.C., Georgiadis, G.S., 2012. Epidermal growth factor in the treatment of diabetic foot ulcers: an update. Perspect. Vasc. Surg. Endovasc. Ther. 24, 37–44.

Trengove, N.J., Stacey, M.C., Macauley, S., Bennett, N., Gibson, J., Burslem, F., et al., 1999. Analysis of the acute and chronic wound environments: the role of proteases and their inhibitors. Wound Repair Regen. 7 (6), 442–452.

Turos, E., Reddy, G.S.K., Greenhalgh, K., Ramaraju, P., Abeylath, S.C., Jang, S., et al., 2007. Penicillin-bound polyacrylate nanoparticles: restoring the activity of B-Lactam antibiotics against MRSA. Bioorg. Med. Chem. Lett. 17 (12), 3468–3472.

Ulubayram, K., Cakar, A.N., Korkusuz, P., Ertan, C., Hasirci, N., 2001. EGF containing gelatin-based wound dressings. Biomaterials 22 (11), 1345–1356.

Vandamme, D., Landuyt, B., Luyten, W., Schoofs, L., 2012. A comprehensive summary of LL-37, the factotum human cathelicidin peptide. Cell. Immunol. 280 (1), 22–35.

Werner, S., Grose, R., 2003. Regulation of wound healing by growth factors and cytokines. Physiol. Rev. 83 (3), 835–870.

Wu, J., Zheng, Y., Wen, X., Lin, Q., Chen, X., Wu, Z., 2014a. Silver nanoparticle/bacterial cellulose gel membranes for antibacterial wound dressing: investigation *in vitro* and *in vivo*. Biomed. Mater. 9 (3), 035005.

Wu, J., Zheng, Y., Song, W., Luan, J., Wen, X., Wu, Z., et al., 2014b. *In situ* synthesis of silver-nanoparticles/bacterial cellulose composites for slow-released antimicrobial wound dressing. Carbohydr. Polym. 102, 762–771.

Xie, Z., Paras, C.B., Weng, H., Punnakitikashem, P., Su, L., Vu, K., et al., 2013. Dual growth factor releasing multi-functional nanofibers for wound healing. Acta Biomater. 9 (12), 9351–9359.

Xu, X., Zhong, W., Zhou, S., Trajtman, A., Alfa, M., 2010. Electrospun PEG–PLA nanofibrous membrane for sustained release of hydrophilic antibiotics. J. Appl. Polym. Sci. 118, 588–595.

Yang, Y., Xia, T., Zhi, W., Wei, L., Weng, J., Zhang, C., et al., 2011. Promotion of skin regeneration in diabetic rats by electrospun core-sheath fibers loaded with basic fibroblast growth factor. Biomaterials 32 (18), 4243–4254.

Ye, M., Kim, S., Park, K., 2010. Issues in long-term protein delivery using biodegradable microparticles. J. Control. Release 146 (2), 241–260.

CHAPTER

Bacterial cellulose for advanced medical materials

3

Gabriel Molina de Olyveira[1], Ligia Maria Manzine Costa[2], Carla dos Santos Riccardi[1], Márcio Luiz dos Santos[1], Paula Braga Daltro[1], Pierre Basmaji[3], Gildásio de Cerqueira Daltro[4] and Antonio Carlos Guastaldi[1]

[1]*Department of Physical Chemistry – UNESP/Araraquara-SP, Brazil*
[2]*Department of Chemistry – USP/FFCLRP, Brazil*
[3]*Innovatec's—Biotechnology Research and Development, São Carlos, SP, Brazil*
[4]*College Hospital Complex Prof. Edgard Santos (COM-HUPES), UFBA, Salvador, Brazil*

LIST OF ABBREVIATIONS

Nanoskin®	bacterial cellulose produced by the company of Innovatec's—Biotechnology Research and Development—Brazil
BC	bacterial cellulose
CLS	corn steep liquor
ECM	extracellular matrix
OTL	otoliths supplied by Innovatec's—Biotechnology Research and Development—Brazil
GBR	guided bone regeneration
GTR	guided tissue regeneration

3.1 INTRODUCTION

Bacterial cellulose (BC) can be used in a wide area of applied science, especially for tissue regeneration and regenerative medicine; lately, bacterial cellulose mats have been used in the treatment of skin conditions such as burns and ulcers, because of the morphology of fibrous biopolymers serving as a support for cell proliferation, its pores allow gas exchange between the organism and the environment. Moreover, the nanostructure and morphological similarities with collagen make BC attractive for cell immobilization, cell support, and natural extracellular matrix (ECM) scaffolds. In this scope, natural ECM is the ideal biological scaffold since it contains all the components of the tissue. The development of mimicking biomaterials and hybrid biomaterial can further advance directed cellular differentiation without specific induction. The

Nanobiomaterials in Soft Tissue Engineering. DOI: http://dx.doi.org/10.1016/B978-0-323-42865-1.00003-9

extracellular matrix (ECM) contains several signals that are received by cell surface receptors and contribute to cell adhesion and cell fate which control cellular activities such as proliferation, migration, and differentiation. As such, regenerative medicine studies often rely on mimicking natural ECM to promote the formation of new tissue by host cells, and characterization of natural ECM components is vital for the development of new biomimetic approaches. Our research group works mainly with fermentation process changes and chemical, physical, and cellular modifications in BC mats for several medicinal areas and applications.

Bacterial cellulose (BC) has become established as a new biomaterial and can be used in several applied scientific areas, especially for medical devices. In addition, biomedical materials have claimed attention because of the increased interest in tissue engineering materials for wound care and regenerative medicine. The BC bioprocess production can be changed by controlling the fermentation process. It has unique properties that make it an exciting candidate as a medical material: strength, good integration within the host tissue, and flexibility of production in various shapes and sizes. This chapter describes a morphological investigation in human regenerative medicine, stem cell behavior on bacterial cellulose, and recent drug delivery applications for medical applications. It also discusses futures insights and research with bacterial cellulose.

3.2 BACTERIAL CELLULOSE

3.2.1 SYNTHESIS

Cellulose is found in several microorganisms including fungi and bacteria. In green algae, cellulose and others may serve as structural polysaccharides (Gatenholm and Klemm, 2010; Czaja et al., 2007). It was also be present in some fungi, including in the inner cell wall layer (Shoda and Sugano, 2005; Richmond, 1991).

Microbial cellulose is produced by several species of bacteria which belong to the genera *Gluconacetobacter* (formerly *Acetobacter*), *Agrobacterium*, *Aerobacter*, *Achromobacter*, *Azotobacter*, *Rhizobium*, *Sarcina*, and *Salmonella* (Bielecki et al., 2005).

In this scope, a Gram-negative bacterium produces extracellular biopolymer material, but only some have been able to produce cellulose. *Acetobacter xylinum*, the most famous bacterial cellulose strain, is a Gram-negative and aerobic bacterium (Ross et al., 1991). It is a more often studied bacterial cellulose strain because of its capacity to generate higher polysaccharide using only carbon and nitrogen (Bielecki et al., 2005).

Bacteria use fruit carbohydrate as food. BC is produced on the air–liquid medium when specific HS liquid medium (consisting of D-glucose, peptone, yeast extract, disodium phosphate, citric acid, and distilled water) is inoculated with bacterial cellulose – *Acetobacter xylinum*. Glucose is used as a carbon source, peptone as a nitrogen source, yeast extract as a vitamin, and citric acid and disodium phosphate as a phosphate buffer for the medium (Forng et al., 1989).

The bacteria population is multiplied using glucose and oxygen in the liquid medium. When there is a lower of oxygen, only surface bacteria continue their bacterial cellulose production. The sub-bacterial cellulose production can be activated with former liquid uses in the culture medium (Forng et al., 1989).

Cellulose synthesis with *Acetobacter xylinum*** is a bioprocess with polymerization of D-glucose into linear β-1,4-glucan chains. The first step in this process is extracellular production of linear chains with crystallization of the glucan chains into ribbons.

Acetobacter xylinum is able to produce two kinds of cellulose: (1) cellulose I, the ribbon-like polymer and (2) cellulose II, a more stable amorphous polymer (Iguchi et al., 2000). Intracellular polysaccharides are inside the cell and cell wall polysaccharides act as the structural cell wall; extracellular polysaccharides are outside the cell wall.

Extracellular polysaccharides are of two types: the first is non-adherent to the cell and imparts bacterial growth with solid medium and the second, microcapsules, which are cell wall-linked. Nanofibrillar bacterial cellulose has properties such as high tensile strength, higher degree of polymerization, and crystallinity index (Iguchi et al., 2000).

3.2.1.1 Biosynthesis mechanism

Cellulose is a polysaccharide which consists of glucose (D-glucose) linked by glycosidic β(1-4). In this connection, the hydroxyl at C-1 (anomeric carbon) of one molecule of glucose reacts with the hydroxyl at C-4 of the second molecule (Fengel and Wegener, 1989).

The size of the cellulose molecule is expressed in terms of its degree of polymerization (DP), that is, the number of glucose units present in a chain (Fengel and Wegener, 1989). The conformation of the repeating unit of cellulose can be explained if we consider the biosynthesis of glucose (Chawla et al., 2009).

The active site of the enzyme cellulose synthase, responsible for the synthesis of cellulose, has two sites of uridine-diphosphoglucose precursor (UDP-glucose) and a site of β-glucan (Koyama et al., 1997). The hydroxyl at C-5 of glucose is linked to these sites using UDP-glucose dephosphorylation and producing new links β(1-4). The resulting β-glucan does not react with UDP-glucose and two new units of UDP-glucose are added, initiating synthesis (Zugenmaier, 2001).

Hydroxyls present in cellulose are equatorially positioned, allowing new linear links (Zugenmaier, 2001) with adjacent chains, which produces one structure with hydrogen bonds (Zugenmaier, 2001). These links result in a rigid crystalline structure with a hydrophilic surface, but a hydrophobic core, which produces insoluble cellulose. Growth thermodynamics of these structures generate crystalline regions with amorphous regions randomly distributed (Koyama et al., 1997). Then, the cellulose production process includes UDP-glucose and glucose polymerization in the β(1-4) glucan chain being expelled outside the cell into fibrils.

The synthesis mechanisms of UDP-glucose are well known, however the molecular knowledge of glucose polymerization still needs more research.

3.3 FERMENTATIVE CHANGES: NEW BIOCOMPOSITES

In regenerative medicine, structural features, compatibility, and properties of microbial cellulose can be changed by modifying the surface using physical (Gupta et al., 2002; Hamerli et al., 2003) and chemical methods (D'Souza et al., 1991; Gabriel et al., 2006), thereby obtaining a biomaterial with less rejection and more cellular and blood interaction. The shaping of bacterial cellulose materials in the culture medium can be controlled by the type of cultivation that changes chain sizes; the origin of the strains which produce different proportions of the crystalline phase of bacterial cellulose, and the kind of bioreactor. The bacterial cellulose is obtained in a hydrogel or dry state form by the freeze-drying method (Iguchi et al., 2000; Matsuoka et al., 1996). There are several factors which affect cellulose production, such as growth medium, environmental conditions, and byproducts. In general, a medium containing a high quantity of carbon, among other elements, such as nitrogen, is favorable for polysaccharide production (Ramana et al., 2000; Masaoka et al., 1993). Sani et al. have improved the production of bacterial cellulose nanofibers by using corn steep liquor (CSL) and molasses as a nitrogen and carbon source, respectively. Molasses is found to be a better carbon source than glucose. Molasses is about 50% sugar in dry weight, predominantly sucrose, but it also contains significant amounts of glucose and fructose. The molasses used in this study was supplied by the Oriental Yeast Co., Ltd. (Tokyo, Japan). The original molasses was diluted fivefold (w/v) with distilled water and centrifuged at 6000 rpm for 20 min to separate solid materials. Moreover, higher yields of BC are obtained using glycerol, acetic acid, hydrolyzate of konjac powder, plant infusions, such as tea (*Camellia sinesis*), and the combined use of fructose, glucose, and acetic acid (Sani and Dahman, 2010).

BC biogenesis control can be a useful approach for producing BC composites with new characteristics. A few researchers have studied this approach, including Cienchanska, who modified a fermentative medium of BC with chitosan for wound dressing application (Cienchanska, 2004).

Bodin et al. obtained BC tubes with several shapes and sizes which has made BC interesting for biomedical applications, including bone tissue and soft tissue regeneration, specifically of cartilage and blood vessels (Bodin et al., 2007).

Backdahl et al. obtained a method to modify microporosity in BC tubes for scaffolds in tissue-engineered applications, using paraffin wax and starch particles in a growth culture of *A. xylinum*; bacterial cellulose materials with different morphologies were prepared. Paraffin particles were incorporated in whole scaffold, while starch particles were positioned only in the outer area of the scaffold (Bäckdahl et al., 2008).

Grande et al. developed nanocomposites of cellulose with different sources of starch. Potato and corn starch were added into the culture medium in order to allow the cellulose nanofibers to grow with starch. Samples were characterized with X-ray diffraction (XRD) and Fourier transform infrared spectroscopy (ATR-FTIR), the crystallinity of the BC was kept with starch, however mechanical properties of the nanocomposites showed little changes (Grande et al., 2009).

However, the success of the scaffolds depends to a great deal on cellular adhesion and growth on the surface, thus, the chemical surface of the biopolymer can change cellular response in cellular adhesion, proliferation, and migration (Helenius et al., 2006). Several cellular activities, such as adhesion, proliferation, migration, and differentiation, are influenced by the environment, which directly depends of extracellular matrix (ECM) secreted by the cells. In spite of different cell types and nanoscale features, some general rules are shared by these cell–substrate interactions (Cherian et al., 2012). Cells identify the exposed surface topography and nanofiber features, just as porous matrices and alignment which influence adhesion, proliferation, and gene expression of various cell kinds seeded on substrate. Several scaffolds can exhibit fibers with different nano- or macrometric dimensions, interconnected pores, and elevated superficial area (Cherian et al., 2013; Nogi and Yano, 2008).

Among various applications studied, there are some related to the electronics industry, specifically acoustic diaphragms, sensor applications, and organic light emitting diodes (Kalia et al., 2011; Szymańska-Chargot et al., 2011; Okahisa et al., 2009). In this chapter, the structural features of microbial cellulose and its properties are discussed. Compatibility of the biomaterial and its green nanocomposites for regenerative medicine are proposed in relation to current and future applications in human regenerative medicine, cell behavior, and drug delivery applications. Future insights and research into bacterial cellulose are also discussed.

3.4 MEDICAL APPLICATIONS OF BACTERIAL CELLULOSE

After the fermentation and freeze-drying processes, microbial cellulose possesses high crystallinity, high tensile strength, extreme insolubility in most solvents, and a high degree of polymerization (Schrecker and Gostomski, 2005; Orts et al., 2005). The thickness of the cellulose fibrils is generally 0.1–10 mm, different to that obtained from plants (Borges et al., 2001). In this section, examples of bacterial cellulose for future medical applications are discussed.

3.4.1 HUMAN MEDICINE

When a material comes into contact with blood, its ability to resist thrombus formation is very important. This is particularly relevant for long-term implantable cardiovascular devices, including vascular grafts and artificial heart valves. Blood–material contact is also constantly present in dialysis, blood transfusion, or for analysis or *in vitro* experiments. The material's surface may activate coagulation, leading to thrombus formation. This adverse effect is prevented by antiplatelet and/or anticoagulation therapy.

Bacterial cellulose mats are important in wound healing, reducing pain, and extracellular production, all of which are important for ideal biological dressings. These membranes can be produced with several surfaces and porosity, which is useful for the treatment of soft and hard tissue engineering. Because of this, bacterial cellulose and bacterial cellulose nanocomposite surfaces have been studied recently. Many strategies have been studied to decrease thrombogenicity, such as modification with albumin (Marchant et al., 1989; Hoffman et al., 1972), antiplatelet agents (Ebert et al., 1982), endothelialization (Andersson et al., 2003), and heparinization (Riesenfeld et al., 1995). Besides, surface physical chemistry properties and morphology are important in biological responses to biomaterials. It is well known that cell orientation and cell proliferation are affected by the surface morphology.

The ability to control cell orientation and bonding is especially important for tissue engineering applications (Basmaji et al., 2011a). The advent of lithographic methods, as used in microelectronics for making structures on the same scale as biological cells, has opened up the possibility of surface engineering of biomaterials. Basmaji et al. obtained bacterial cellulose nanocomposites for green composites with natural properties, different thermal and morphological properties, resulting in the pure 3D structure and with higher molecular weight (Basmaji et al., 2011b). Costa et al. published one recent review with *in vivo* analysis of bacterial cellulose to treat diabetic ulcer and other diseases using biological dressings (Figure 3.1; Costa et al., 2012a).

3.4.2 DENTAL APPLICATIONS

The development of new materials for bone tissue and soft tissue regeneration has been changed by research in the field of biomaterials, contributing significantly to quality of life and longevity of the population (Branemark, 1983). Currently, there are several metallic, ceramic, polymer, and composite biomaterials for use in diverse areas of dentistry and medicine. Experience using biomaterials in implants needs studies of bioactivity and biocompatibility in the human body (Ratner, 1996).

Rapid technological development has brought advances in the dental implants area, which represents an important role in functional materials for patients. Thus, advancements in implant dentistry research in biomaterials for this purpose as well as tissue–implant interfaces are of great value (Willians, 1991).

Pure titanium and its alloys are the main biomaterials for dental implants, due to its biocompatibility, high mechanical strength, and corrosion resistance. The main problem with titanium and titanium alloys (Ti) is the expense of the raw material and processing (Willians, 1981).

Several techniques of surface modification in dental implants have been developed to increase bone tissue growth and therefore decrease implant rejection. The coatings on implants including the characteristics of the surface coating and the

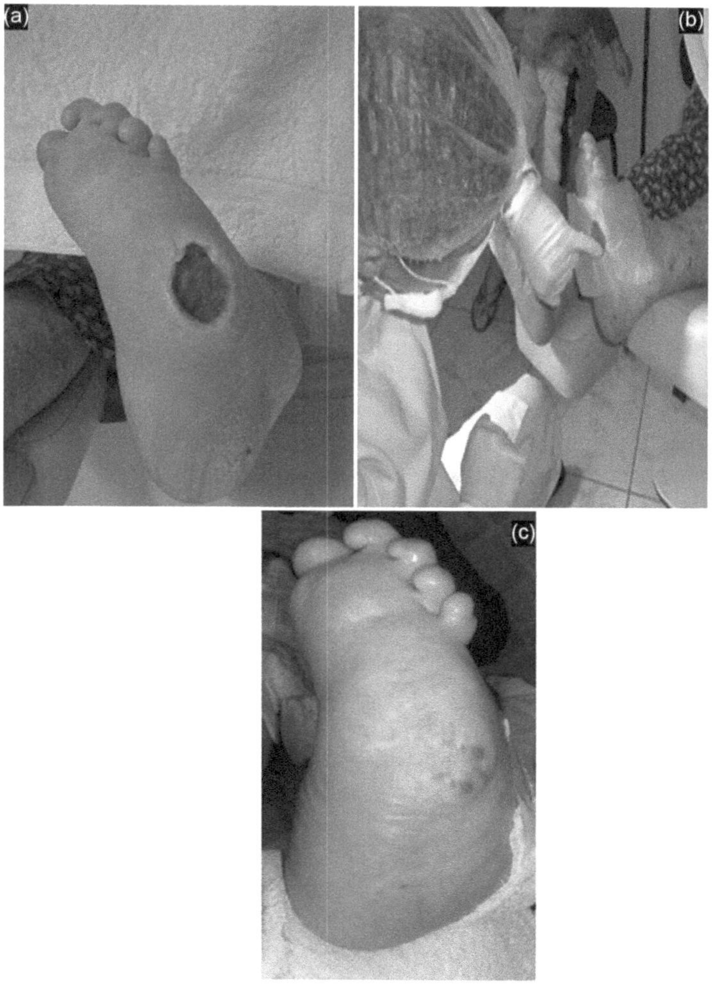

FIGURE 3.1

In vivo behavior of bacterial cellulose mats (Nanoskin) (Costa et al., 2012a).

structural properties of the substrate are extremely important. To increase biocompatibility and decrease rejection of titanium, a coating of hydroxyapatite (HA) has been very well accepted, enabling higher bone tissue growth and increasing timely surgical implants (Ducheyne, 1988; Abe et al., 1990).

HA has the lowest rate of biodegradation or absorption of all the calcium phosphates by animal organisms. As the main mineral constituent of bone (60%), HA has been extensively studied and used as material for permanent inclusion in defective or abnormal bone structure in surgical bone repair, relying on its performance as a biomaterial (biocompatible, bioactive, and osteoconductive) (Le Geros, 2002; Aoki, 1999; Orr et al., 1992).

3.4.2.1 BC/calcium phosphate

The great interest in the search for new biopolymers with the specific intention of use as scaffolds with tissue engineering properties, has increased in recent years, as can be verified by the numerous studies aimed at the development of new biomaterials. It is known that bone tissue is the result of natural minerals, especially apatite nanocrystals and collagen, but there are many reports of problems involving the use of collagen, such as its high cost, difficulty in controlling infection and the number of definitions of commercial sources of this product. On the other hand, bacterial cellulose, when compared to collagen, eliminates the occurrence of infections and has higher mechanical properties such as strength and modulation capacity (Olyveira et al., 2014a).

The benefits of cellulose, the most abundant biopolymer and polysaccharide, were reported in applications for bone repair due to its mechanical properties being similar to the properties of hard tissue. Thus, the modification of cellulose appears to be a prerequisite in the mineralization process, which can be achieved through chemical modification of the hydroxyl groups of cellulose chains of monomeric groups for biomimetic calcium phosphate deposition, resulting in bioactivity of this material (Olyveira et al., 2014b).

A research topic was based on new biocomposites using bacterial cellulose with chondroitin sulfate, hyaluronic acid, and calcium phosphate for guided tissue regeneration (GTR). Chondroitin sulfate and hyaluronic acid influences in bacterial cellulose were analyzed using Fourier transmission infrared (FTIR) spectroscopy, XRD, and scanning electron microscopy (SEM). FTIR analysis showed interaction between bacterial cellulose nanobiocomposites and calcium phosphate and XRD demonstrated amorphous calcium phosphate and sodium chloride on bacterial cellulose nanobiocomposites. SEM images confirmed incorporation of calcium phosphate in the bacterial cellulose nanobiocomposite surface with different calcium phosphate particle morphologies (Olyveira et al. 2014c).

Another recent research studied novel natural nanocomposites with bacterial cellulose for functional dental materials. In order to produce scaffolds with drug delivery ability, porous structure and better cell adhesion, fermentation changes in bacterial cellulose with chondroitin sulfate and gamma irradiation changes were performed. FTIR proved that amorphous calcium phosphate and carbonated apatite are formed and XRD showed that amorphous calcium phosphate with sodium chloride crystals are deposited on nonirradiated sample surfaces. TGA concluded that the effect of radiation on the thermal properties of bionanocomposites presented divergent results with other tested membranes and is therefore not a differential factor with respect to calcium phosphate deposition, possibly the placement of surface groups (hyaluronic acid) was decisive in the deposits of apatite in bionanocomposites (Olyveira et al., 2015a,b). One recent alternative to produce calcium phosphate is the synthesis method. Hyaluronic acid/bacterial cellulose mats were biomimetically modified with calcium phosphate and irradiation; the results showed several apatite crystals on the bacterial cellulose bionanocomposite surfaces (Figure 3.2). In addition, irradiated samples showed higher apatite crystal surface deposition

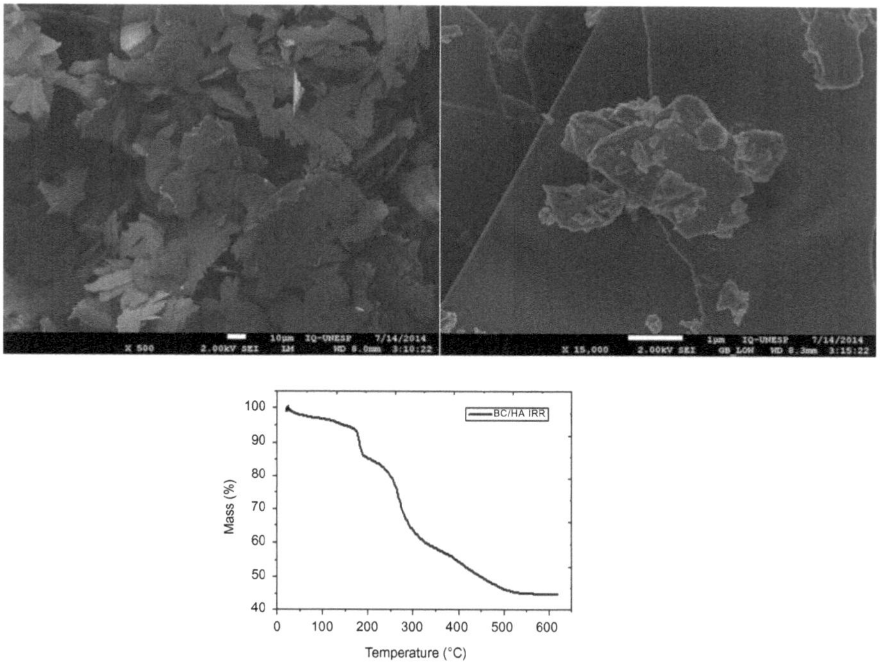

FIGURE 3.2

SEM images of irradiated and biomimetically modified bacterial cellulose/hyaluronic acid mats (Olyveira et al., 2014d).

(45%) than nonirradiated samples, as proved by TGA and SEM (Olyveira et al., 2014d).

3.4.2.2 Cell behavior with nanomaterials—stem cells

Several cellular activities, such as adhesion, proliferation, migration, differentiation, and cell shape, are influenced by the ECM in which they reside. In spite of different cell types and nanoscale features, some general rules are shared by these cell–substrate interactions. Cells identify the exposed surface topography and nanofiber features, like porous matrices, and the alignment influences the adhesion, spreading, proliferation, and gene expression of various cell types which are seeded onto them. Different cell behaviors were found in several surface topographies obtained from lithography (Teixeira et al., 2004; Rajnicek and McCraig, 1997), phase separation (Chen et al., 2006), electrospinning (Kim et al., 2005; Filho et al., 2013), nanoimprinting (Yim et al., 2005), and self-assembly (Harrington et al., 2006).

Nanotopographic features containing varying widths of grooves and ridges, ranging from nano- to microdimensions, provided stimulus for human corneal epithelial cells. Cells were found to align along the grooves and the ridges of the nanodimensions with elongated structures, while rounded cells were observed on smooth surfaces (Teixeira et al., 2003). Cross-linked gelatin nanofibers, with improved mechanical properties and thermal stability, support human dermal fibroblast proliferation and a linear increase in the cell number was observed over time (Zhang et al., 2006).

Mesenchymal stem cells can be obtained in several ways and, specifically, dental tissue is an alternative and interesting source of stem cells. It can be used as a solution for reconstruction of diseased dental tissues, such as dental pulp and periodontal ligament, furthermore it can be used for regeneration of complete or partial tooth structure (Smith et al., 1995).

Isolation and characterization of dental pulp stem cells from the tooth has generated research and the possibility of finding new mesenchymal stem cells. Also, researches showed that dental pulp stem cells were able to differentiate into bone tissue and osteoblasts (Smith and Lesot, 2001).

Dental stem cells have similar properties to mesenchymal stem cells from bone marrow and others, and have potential to be used in various stem cell-based treatments, such as bone and tissue engineering (Grontos et al., 2000).

As a source for new stem cells, the tooth and the dental tissue represent an ideal source of important stem cells for use in medicine and dentistry. Stem cells from exfoliated deciduous teeth are simple and convenient to obtain. Miura et al. identified the cells as highly proliferative, clonogenic cells capable of differentiating into a variety of cell types including neural cells, adipocytes, and odontoblasts (Miura et al., 2003). After *in vivo* transplantation, these cells were able to induce bone formation resulting in dentin (Shi et al., 2005; Sakai et al., 2010). When compared with dental pulp stem cells, these cells exhibited a high proliferation rate, population growth, osteoinductive capacity *in vivo*, and the ability to form spherical clusters. Results of *in vivo* transplantation suggest that stem cells from exfoliated deciduous teeth have a greater capacity for mineralization than dental pulp stem cells.

Cordeiro et al. suggest stem cells from exfoliated deciduous teeth can be a valuable cell source for tissue engineering of dental pulp. They incorporated cells in biodegradable scaffolds prepared from human teeth and transplanted them into immunodeficient mice. The results presented an architecture and cellularity of tissue which resembled that of a physiological dental pulp. Ultrastructural analysis of transmission electron microscopy and immunohistochemistry suggests that the cells are differentiated into *in vivo* odontoblasts (Cordeiro et al., 2008).

Stem cells from exfoliated deciduous teeth have greater proliferation than dental pulp stem cells. *In vivo* studies, where the two types of stem cells have been implanted subcutaneously in rats with HA, revealed that dental pulp stem cells form dentin–pulp complex while stem cells exfoliated from deciduous teeth formed dentin and bone (Seo et al., 2008). Injection of mesenchymal stem cells has also been shown to correct bone defects. Notably, allogeneic bone marrow transplantation or injection of isolated mesenchymal stem cells in children with imperfecta osteogenesis has improved bone formation (Ribitsch et al., 2010).

In this context, Nanoskin® has been studied with dental pulp stem cells. Olyveira et al. tested bacterial cellulose mats with nanotoliths as an inorganic source for bone regeneration, using human dental stem cells. This research shows that the fibers prepared for the study had little initial adhesion and maintenance of viability in the initial stage, besides bacterial cellulose mats with inorganic source have been able to produce an increase in the long term (21 days). After 21 days of culture, the test groups had similar behavior to the control group. Therefore, natural scaffolds with bacterial cellulose and inorganic sources for bone tissue regeneration had little cell adhesion at first; however, during the test its response was ideal, being an effective natural material for bone tissue regeneration (Olyveira et al., 2013a).

Recently, the group's work has studied adhesion and viability behavior with dental pulp stem cells and modified bacterial cellulose mats (hyaluronic acid and gelatin) for tissue engineering. Viability cell data have shown a cell adhesion increase in bacterial cellulose composite scaffolds tested over time, with results different because of the fiber formation process in both scaffolds. Confocal microscopy shows cell adhesion, proliferation, and alignment in the fiber direction in tested scaffolds (Olyveira et al., 2014e).

3.5 GTR MEMBRANES

GTR therapy has been introduced with the aim of achieving a redirection of periodontal ligament fibroblasts and promoting regeneration of periodontal tissues in cases of chronic periodontitis (Nyman et al., 1982). Currently, techniques for GTR have been extensively used both in periodontal surgery, such as in craniotomies in reconstruction of cleft patients, orthopedic surgery, or plastic surgery (Buchardt, 1983).

When GTR relates to the repair of bone structures it is known as guided bone regeneration (GBR), which controls the stimulation of bone formation in bone defects by osteogenesis, osteoconduction, and osteoinduction, restoring the structural and functional characteristics of bone tissue (Oh et al., 2003).

The concept of GTR in periodontology was proposed by Melcher, who described the biological behavior of different tissues (gingival epithelium, connective tissue, periodontal ligament, alveolar bone) during healing.

According to this concept, cells that have the capacity to build bone, cementum, and periodontal ligament defects occupy an appropriate time and sequence that results in tissue regeneration, as opposed to simply repairing the defect. Because progenitor cells reside in the periodontal ligament and alveolar bone, the placement of a physical barrier between the gingival flap and the defect before repositioning of the flap and the suture was proposed to prevent growth of the gingival epithelium and connective tissue (Melcher, 1976).

At the beginning of the use of this therapy, the preferable treatment was GBR, with nonresorbable membranes using expanded polytetrafluoroethylene (e-PTFE), because of its inert characteristics and because of its effective and predictable results as a mechanical barrier. In GTR, for the membrane to be effective it must meet criteria such as biocompatibility, integration with adjacent tissues, mechanical stability, and easy handling. And, with the advent of new substitutes for bone and soft tissue, natural and/or synthetic processed biotechnologically, these have become potential biomaterials for clinical applications in various areas of health (Bosch et al., 1995).

The use of resorbable membrane has been increasing with the development of new biomaterials because the results show no significant difference between the nonresorbable and resorbable GTR, moreover, the resorbable membrane can be used in peri-implant defects. Among the materials used as resorbable membranes are: collagen (types I and III), lactic polyacid, polyacid glycolic acid, and copolymer of polylactic acid/glycolic polyacid (PLGA). These membranes may be associated with bioceramics or growth factors, presenting osteoinductive properties (Jung et al., 2003).

3.5.1 NONRESORBABLE MEMBRANES

3.5.1.1 Expanded polytetrafluoroethylene (e-PTFE)

The e-PTFE membranes are recognized as the principal tested membranes for GTR, especially Gore-Tex®. Reinforced Gore-Tex® membrane is e-PTFE reinforced with titanium. These e-PTFE membranes are available in various forms, thus they can properly maintain the space to be regenerated, and in case of exposure they are easily removed. Applying the principles of GBR using membranes composed of e-PTFE for treatment and/or reconstruction of critical defects or noncritical long bone or craniofacial defects is well established due to their results, over the years, and their high success rate and predictability in the short and long term, especially when these membranes are associated with bone-filling materials, such as grafts, bone substitutes (Macedo et al., 2003), or growth factors (Wikesjo et al., 2004).

Clinical studies support this type of therapy, as GBR can reduce the need for additional surgical interventions, for example, bone graft in patients with inadequate bone volume for implant placement (Jones et al., 2006). Despite the e-PTFE membranes present predictability in its results, has been linked numerous disadvantages along clinical studies with non-resorbable membranes, currently these results lead this type of membrane to the clinical failure ,because bioengineer with new techniques in the development and improvement of mechanical, physical and chemical characteristics of resorbable biomaterials process, mainly polymers of natural origin has more applications in therapies GBR with similar properties than non-resorbable materials (Simion et al., 1994).

With the use of resorbable membranes there is no need for a second surgical procedure for their removal, they also have a lower rate of exposure of the membrane, thereby reducing postoperative infection. In many cases there is no need for fixing screws, furthermore, some of them have osteoinductive properties, improved adhesion, and cell affinity.

Another complication related to the e-PTFE membrane was premature exposure of this type of membrane when exposed to the oral cavity, making the risk of infection and contamination high and thus interfering in tissue regeneration. However, an experimental study by Strietzel et al. (2006), which compared seven types of membranes for GBR, four nonresorbable and three resorbable, observed absence of fistula (Strietzel et al., 2006).

3.5.1.2 Dense polytetrafluoroethylene (d-PTFE)

The use of dense membranes composed of polytetrafluoroethylene in GBR is limited because it prevents adequate blood supply to the site to be regenerated. Therefore, a non-porous barrier is needed during the surgical procedure to place a thin layer of connective tissue beneath the membrane to be able to obtain effective bone healing.

The results obtained with PTFE-d were clinically without exposure and fistula, and histologic without infiltration of the connective tissue within the bone defect because of density of the material and thin layer of connective tissue over and under the membranes; called trabecular bone density (Bartee and Carr, 1995).

3.5.2 RESORBABLE MEMBRANES

3.5.2.1 Natural resorbable membranes

Natural biopolymers have a biological advantage in recognition that can positively support cell adhesion and function. The disadvantages found in the use of such polymers are: (i) induce immunology and transmit pathogens, when the materials are from animal sources or from cadavers, (ii) have less control over the degradation of the polymer and consistency; and (iii) they have low mechanical resistance. The resorption of these polymers occurs by cellular mechanisms or via enzymatic reactions or hydrolysis.

3.5.2.1.1 Collagen

Collagen is the most abundant protein in vertebrates. This class of protein promotes structural support to tissues and is of fundamental importance in the formation of the ECM of connective tissue. In humans, collagen represents more than 30% of total protein, and 80–90% of body collagen constitutes types I, II, and III (Mizuno et al., 1997).

Type I collagen is the most abundant animal protein, and forms the matrix of bone, skin, and other tissues. It is present in tendons, the fibrous cartilage, loose connective tissue, and dense connective tissue. Type I collagen matrix provides a favorable environment for induction of differentiation of *in vitro* osteoblasts and *in vivo* osteogenesis (Mizuno et al., 1997).

Type III collagen is the reticular fibers of tissues, and is also widely used in the manufacture of membranes for GTR, as well as being present in tissues such as skin, aorta, and lungs.

Collagen membranes, when not mineralized, are usually fragile and difficult to handle. The advantage is excellent cell affinity, stimulating fibroblasts, and acting as a support for migration of these cells (osteoconduction). When embedded in the bone matrix they are gradually metabolized by bone remodeling, or may be partially incorporated into the bone matrix (Hurzeler et al., 1998).

The resorption of collagen occurs in parallel with new bone formation, as well as by the formation of new periodontal tissue, such as cementum and periodontal ligament, when GBR is applied to periodontal surgery, over a period of 6–8 weeks (Hurzeler et al., 1998).

The membrane Bio-Gide® was the most widely used membrane for guided bone regeneration, is composed of type I and III collagen of porcine origin, has a bilayer structure with one side compact and another porous.

Collagen membrane in GBR have satisfactory results *in vivo*, for example, the rate of bone regeneration has a similar effect to e-PTFE, this is due to the advent of collagen membranes with good mechanical strength. In the past, it was hard to obtain results due to the difficulty of producing collagen membranes with these characteristics (Pinheiro et al., 2003).

GenDerm® membrane was another widely studied membrane, this membrane is composed of natural bone collagen and laminating bovine cortical bone. It is tolerated by tissues and is reabsorbed completely by mononuclear cells and multinucleated giant cells 30–60 days postoperatively (Oliveira et al., 2006).

Another material that has shown excellent results in the GBR is the Bio-OssCollagen®. This consists of a bone-filling material with approximately 90% of deproteinated bovine bone particles, embedded in a porcine resorbable collagen matrix. Histological studies in humans have shown regeneration of cementum, periodontal ligament, and filling of intraosseous periodontal defects with reduction in probing depth and gain in level of expressive gingival attachment using only Bio-Oss Collagen® or in combination with collagen membranes (GBR). The degradation of this material occurs in the first 6 months, without affecting clinical parameters (Nevis et al., 2003).

3.5.2.1.2 Chitosan

Chitosan is present in significant amounts in marine and terrestrial invertebrates. Currently, deacetylated chitosan exhibits a low degradation rate in an aqueous medium and may take several months to degrade, and is thus a potential material for developing inexpensive and versatile systems for drug carriers (Kuo et al., 2006).

Yeo et al. (2005) synthesized a chitosan membrane and compared it with PLGA membrane (Biomesh®) in GBR, and found that the chitosan membranes provided an increase in bone and cementum tissue, suggesting that this material may hereafter be used to induce periodontal tissue regeneration (Yeo et al., 2005).

Other experimental studies also observed that chitosan enhances bone density and maintains the barrier function for 4 weeks, thus being effective in GBR (Kuo et al., 2006).

3.5.2.2 Natural non-resorbable membranes

3.5.2.2.1 Bacterial cellulose

Currently, it is believed that bacterial cellulose could become one of the most important biotechnology products both in health and for the industrial sector, as it can be obtained on a large scale with a low manufacture cost (Basmaji et al., 2011c). It is obtained by biosynthesis routes through the following genus of bacteria as *Glucanoacetobacter*, *Rhizobium*, *Sarcina*, *Agrobacterium*, and *Alcaligenes*.

In Brazil, in the 1980s, Innovatec's Biotechnological Products Ltd. began producing Nanoskin®, a biosynthetic microfibrillar cellulose film, produced by bacteria of the genus *Acetobacter*, that can be used in the reconstruction and temporary replacement of the skin, burns, and other conditions, such as ulcers and grafts, because their physiological structure is similar to human skin (Olyveira et al., 2011a).

Nanoskin® therefore presents an important biocompatibility and is also nontoxic, inert, and selectively permeable, allowing gaseous exchange. It also acts as a barrier against microorganisms, and in bone tissue it acts as a barrier, preventing fibroblast cells and fibrous tissue from invading the bone defect, thereby promoting effective bone regeneration besides being a low-cost treatment (Olyveira et al., 2011a).

In this context, the company, Innovatec, which researches natural nanomaterials, discovered a new material for bone regeneration tissue called otolith (OTL). This material has the same characteristics as HA but with the advantage that it is a natural material.

Nano-otoliths are osteoinductors or, in other words, they stimulate bone regeneration, enabling more migration of cells for formation of bone tissue. OTLs of *Cynoscion acoupa*, are small particles composed of protein matrix and calcium carbonate, present in the bone of the internal ear of fish and are part of a system which acts as a sensor of depth and balance and also as a detector of sound vibrations. The *C. acoupa* is commercialized throughout the entire coast of Brazil. *C. acoupa* has been shown to be an important source of collagen too; the membranes of collagens can be acquired by acid extraction and posterior saline precipitation (Basmaji et al., 2011c; Olyveira et al., 2011a).

Recently, through research, the ability to regenerate bone nanocomposites with OTLs has been demonstrated. The analysis shows the *in vitro* growth of the bone tissue surface and regularly increased osteoblast activity. In all cases, intense infiltration of polymorphonuclear neutrophils and the formation of microabscesses can be observed in the results (Olyveira et al., 2011b).

The group recently performed *in vivo* analysis of OTL nanocomposites. OTLs presented biocompatibility with the pulp tissue *in vivo* and tissue response to OTL pulp was similar to the group of calcium carbonate. It was concluded that direct dental capping with prepared OTL, similar to calcium hydroxide, preserves the vitality, stimulates the formation of mineralized tissue barrier, and induces the repair pulp response, therefore representing a promising biomaterial to be used in dentistry (Costa et al., 2012b). Membranes stimulated mineralized tissue barrier and induced a reparative response of the dental pulp, making it a potential material for regeneration of dental pulp and GBR.

3.5.3 SYNTHETIC RESORBABLE MEMBRANES

3.5.3.1 *Polylactic acid, polyglycolic acid and poly(lactic-co-glycolic acid)*

Synthetic absorbable polymers based primarily on α-hydroxy acids are used clinically in the form of a suture, derivatives of rigid internal fixation (plates and screws) systems, and matrices for bone regeneration and repair (membranes and scaffolds).

The degradation of these materials occurs for nonenzymatic hydrolysis due to the ester linkages being hydrolytically weak, the products released in this step are metabolic, natural, and nontoxic, and they are converted to water and carbon dioxide (Viljanen and Lindholm, 1998).

During the process of degradation of the bioresorbable polymers, ester bonds are hydrolyzed, resulting in smaller chains (oligomers to monomers) with acid ends. The degradation of these materials is dependent on the chemical composition of each, as well as the crystallinity, molecular weight, and molecular weight distribution (Viljanen and Lindholm, 1998).

PLGA copolymers have an advantage over other bioresorbable polymers such as poly(L-lactic acid) due to the fact that the PLGA copolymers require less time to complete its degradation, with a lower probability of adverse reactions, which often arise from crystalline fragments released for polymers with long degradation time (Motta and Duek, 2006).

The results obtained by several authors demonstrated the clinical effectiveness of these types of membranes in GBR in the long term, with a significant reduction in intrabony defects. When compared with non-resorbable membranes, the membrane Resolut® showed similar regeneration to Gore-Tex®, leading to successful treatment (Stavropoulos et al., 2004).

Gore Resolut® XT consists of a three-layer structure with two arrays of fibers (inner face) and one (outer side) with an occlusive film to the cells. It is composed of synthetic polymers such as polylactic acid, polyglycolic acid, and trimethylene carbonate. Within 8–10 weeks it remains in its intact structure while maintaining its barrier function, with complete absorption within 6–7 months, Gore Resolut Adapt®LT maintains its barrier function between 16 and 24 weeks, gradually being absorbed (Stavropoulos et al., 2004).

3.5.3.1.1 Polyethylene glycol

Polyethylene glycol (PEG) comprises a group of biodegradable synthetic polymers in the form of hydrogels which can be injected into cavities in a minimally invasive way. Hydrogels may be defined as materials that exhibit the ability to absorb water and retain a significant fraction of water within its structure, this capacity of water absorption is due to the presence of hydrophilic groups such as OH, CONH, $CONH_2$, –COOH, and SO_3H (Jung et al., 2006).

The disadvantage of the use of hydrogel in bone tissue engineering is due to its low mechanical strength and the difficulty of handling it *in situ* in the preparation of membranes for GBR.

There are two ways to prepare and apply the biomaterial, first, the application of the hydrogel with certain viscosity on the bone defect to yield a thin layer of PEG, second, preparing a preshaped membrane, capable of sterilizing prior to the surgical procedure. The degradation of the PEG occurs by hydrolysis of ester groups between chains of material in a short period of a few days or weeks *in vivo*, which makes this an impractical material for GBR, because it is necessary for more control over the duration of the membrane acting as a barrier for several months for the procedure to be effective (Hammerle and Jung, 2003).

3.6 ANOTHER APPLICATION: DRUG DELIVERY

Beyond the knowledge of the structure and properties, surface modification, compatibility, and cell interaction of this natural material for regenerative medicine, there is still a need for targeting pharmaceutical drugs to achieve local or systemic drug delivery for controlling diseases and injuries.

BC has chemical groups (OH) in its structure, which enable the stabilization of H bond networks and film-forming properties. However, others features are required for biomedical and pharmaceutical applications, such as superficial charges. Depending on the source and method of obtaining it, polysaccharide has a different chemical structure, molecular weight, and superficial charge. For example, alginate has a superficial negative charge and cellulose has a neutral charge; because of this, bacterial cellulose has limitations for drug delivery applications (Meyers et al., 2008; Chandra and Rustgi, 1998).

Metal nanoparticles have appeared as a new possibility for controlled release of drugs, due to their ability to keep control of necessary therapeutic concentrations and for directing the action of the drug toward certain specific targets, by means of a controlled delivery system. Metal nanoparticles can be produced by chemical and physical methods. Among the chemical methods, the most widely used are those based on reactions in solution, leading to the formation of colloid nanoparticles in a solvent. The biological properties of metal nanoparticles of gold, copper, and platinum have been discovered recently and are already being widely used in various biomedical applications (You et al., 2007). The effects of these nanoparticles have been studied in the treatment of some types of cancer, including ovarian cancer, multiple myeloma, and chronic leukemia, with positive results (Onizawa et al., 2009). Nanoparticles of gold have also been studied to help in the treatment of rheumatoid arthritis (Hong et al., 2009). The platinum nanoparticles have unique properties acting as antioxidants to inhibit various types of inflammation, including pulmonary inflammation caused by cigarette smoking. Another type of nanoparticle with interesting medicinal properties is copper nanoparticles, which can be used in the area of antimicrobes (Bhattacharya and Mukherjee, 2008; Ren et al., 2009).

The release rate can be controlled, depending on the size of the particles and their hydration; the particles can reach nanometric scales. Conjugated polymer drugs have been under study for the last three decades with the aim of solving the aforementioned problems related to chemotherapy. Conventional means, being oral and parenteral administration of drugs, have several disadvantages due to the change of pharmacokinetic parameters and wide distribution throughout the body.

This can be overcome with a nanostructure mediating the delivery of the drug at the desired location of action, offering the opportunity to accumulate in the desired location, thus reducing the treatment toxicity (Sandhiya et al., 2009; Chang et al., 2009). However, researchers in nanoparticle toxicology do not have any conclusive answers yet, so this application area is in development. Costa and colleagues obtained a new platform for catalysis, drug and cell delivery with electrospun bacterial cellulose. In this work, bacterial cellulose mats were acetylated and were then processed by electrospinning to produce artificial symmetrical nanopores (Costa et al., 2012c).

Recently, the group's work has highlighted the potential of gamma irradiation treatment for the modification of BC surface properties, enhancing their potential for biomedical applications. The samples did not show significant variation in thermal properties; however, a higher pore density was produced in the irradiated samples than in the nonirradiated ones, which produced slower diffusion than the nonirradiated membrane (Olyveira et al., 2013b).

3.7 FUTURE MATERIALS—GENETIC MODIFICATIONS

BC for medical applications has been discussed in this chapter; however, for industrial applications it is necessary to improve the cellulose production. The microorganisms from kombucha and their ability for cellulose biosynthesis have been isolated and identified. rDNA genes (16S–28S) of bacteria isolated from kombucha have also been isolated (Gois et al., 2012).

Analysis of the 16S rDNA sequencing gene indicated that three bacteria strains belong to the *Acetobacteraceae* family. One isolated strain (B4) was identified as a *Gluconacetobacter intermedius*, two isolated strains (B2 and B3) were identified as *Acetobacter oeni* and B1, B5, B6, and B7 were identified as belonging to other genus. All fungal isolated strains belong to the *Saccharomycetaceae* family, eight isolated strains (L1–L5 and L7–L9) were identified as *Issatchenkia occidentalis* and one isolated strain (L6) is a *Pichia membranifaciens.*

The 16 isolated strains were tested for cellulose production. Only four isolated strains (B1, B2, B3, and B4) formed pellicle (in stationary culture) or globules (in agitated culture). Real cellulose was confirmed when the pellicle or globules did not dissolve after boiling in NaOH 0.5 M. Among these isolated strains only two (B3 and B4) are cellulose producers. The cellulose yield of these strains was compared under static and agitated culture conditions. The *G. intermedius* gave higher cellulose yield under static culture (8.28 g/l) than under agitated culture (1.05 g/l), whereas the cellulose yield of *A. oeni* in the agitated culture (3 g/l) was not significantly higher than that in the static culture (2.46 g/l) under the conditions of this study.

It were found that the *G. intermedius* microorganisms produced more cellulose with higher levels (14.63 g/l) using static culture conditions. These results shows that the *G. intermedius* strain from kombucha has higher potential for cellulose production.

3.8 CONCLUSIONS

BC properties, such as natural material, biological wound dressing, mechanical properties, and nanostructural morphology, are in the area of tissue engineering. It is the intention of this chapter to disseminate knowledge on this area and to increase the application of bacterial cellulose in regenerative medicine with new natural materials and bionanocomposites obtained with surface modification (chemical and physical). In addition, obtaining a biomaterial with less cellular rejection makes it fit for biomedical applications. However, new studies using genetically modified bacterial cellulose are needed to obtain improved results and higher bacterial cellulose production in biosynthesis.

REFERENCES

Abe, Y., Kobubo, T., Yamamuro, T., 1990. Apatite coatings on ceramics, metals and polymers utilising a biological process. J. Mater. Sci. Mater. Med. 1 (4), 233–238.

Andersson, J., Sanchez, J., Ekdahi, K.N., Elgue, G., Nilsson, B., Larsson, R., 2003. Optimal heparin surface concentration and antithrombin binding capacity as evaluated with human non-anticoagulated blood *in vitro*. J. Biomed. Mater. Res. A 67, 458–466.

Aoki, H., 1999. Science and Medical Applications of Hydroxyapatite. Takayama Press System Center, Tokyo.

Bäckdahl, H., Esquerra, M., Delbro, D., Risberg, B., Gatenholm, P., 2008. Engineering microporosity in bacterial cellulose Scaffolds. J. Tissue Eng. Regen. Med. 2, 320–330.

Bartee, B.K., Carr, J.A., 1995. Evaluation of a high-density polytetrafluoroethylene (*n*-PTFE) membrane as a barrier material to facilitate guided bone regeneration in the rat mandible. J. Oral. Implantol. 21 (2), 88–95.

Basmaji, P., Olyveira, G.M., Costa, L.M.M., Filho, L.X., 2011a. Bacterial Nanocellulose for medicine regenerative. J. Nanotechnol. Eng. Med. 2, 34001–34009.

Basmaji, P., Olyveira, G.M., Costa, L.M.M., Filho, L.X., 2011b. Bacterial cellulose towards functional green composites materials. J. Bionanosci. 5, 167–172.

Basmaji, P., Olyveira, G.M., Costa, L.M.M., 2011c. Nanoskin for medical application. In: Proceeding of Nanotechnology: Bio Sensors, Instruments, Medical, Environment and Energy, June 13–15, Boston, MA, USA.

Bhattacharya, R., Mukherjee, P., 2008. Biological properties of "naked" metal nanoparticles. Adv. Drug Deliv. Rev. 60, 1289–1306.

Bielecki, S., Krystynowicz, A., Turkiewicz, M., Kalinowska, H., 2005. Bacterial cellulose. In: Steinbuchel, A., Rhee, S.K. (Eds.), Polysaccharides and Polyamides in the Food Industry. Wiley VCH Verlag, Germany.

Bodin, A., Bäckdahl, H., Fink, H., Gustafsson, L., Risberg, B., Gatenholm, P., 2007. Influence of cultivation conditions on mechanical and morphological properties of bacterial cellulose tubes. Biotechnol. Bioeng. 97, 425–434.

Borges, J.P., Godinho, M.H., Martins, A.F., Trindade, A.C., Belgacem, M.N., 2001. Cellulose based-composite films. Mech. Compos. Mater. Struct. 37, 257–264.

Bosch, C., Melsen, B., Vargervik, K., 1995. Guided bone regeneration in calvarial bone defects using polytetrafluoroethylene membranes. Cleft Palate Craniofac. 32, 311–317.

Branemark, P.I., 1983. Osseointegration and its experimental background. J. Prosthet. Dent. 50, 399–410.

Burchardt, H., 1983. The biology of bone graft repair. Clin. Orthop. Relat. Res. 174, 28–42.

Chandra, R., Rustgi, R., 1998. Biodegradable polymers. Prog. Polym. Sci. 23, 1273–1335.

Chang, D.K., Chiu, C.Y., Kuo, S.Y., Lin, W.C., Lo, A., Wang, Y.P., et al., 2009. Antiangiogenic targeting liposomes increase therapeutic efficaty for solid tumors. J. Biol. Chem. 284, 12905–12916.

Chawla, P.R., Bajaj, I.B., Shrikant, A.S., Singhal, R.S., 2009. Fermentative production of microbial cellulose. Food Technol. Biotechnol. 47, 107–124.

Chen, V.J., Smith, L.A., Ma, P.X., 2006. Bone regeneration on computer-designed nanofibrous scaffolds. Biomaterials 27, 3973–3979.

Cherian, B.M., Olyveira, G.M., Costa, L.M.M., Leão, A.L., Souza, S.F., 2012. Protein based polymer nanocomposites for regenerative medicine. In: Maya, J.J., Thomas, S. (Eds.), Natural polymers, volume 2: Nanocomposites. Royal Society of Chemistry (RSC Green Chemistry), UK, pp. 255–293.

Cherian, B.M., Leão, A.L., Souza, S.F., Olyveira, G.M., Costa, L.M.M., Brandão, C.V.S., et al., 2013. Bacterial nanocellulose for medical implants. In: Thomas, S., Visakh, P.M., Mathew, A.P. (Eds.), Advances in Natural Polymers, Advanced Structured Materials. Springer, Berlin Heidelberg, pp. 337–359.

Cienchanska, D., 2004. Multifunctional bacterial cellulose/chitosan composite materials for medical applications. Fibres Text. East. Eur. 12, 69–72.

Cordeiro, M.M., Dong, Z., Kaneko, T., Zhang, Z., Miyazawa, M., Shi, S., et al., 2008. Dental pulp tissue engineering with stem cells from exfoliated deciduous teeth. J. Endod. 34, 962–969.

Costa, L.M.M., Olyveira, G.M., Basmaji, P., Filho, L.X., 2012a. Bacterial cellulose towards functional medical materials. J. Biomater. Tissue Eng. 2, 185–196.

Costa, L.M.M., Olyveira, G.M., Basmaji, P., Valido, D.P., Gois, P.B.P., Junior, R.L.A.C., et al., 2012b. Novel otoliths/bacterial cellulose nanocomposites as a potential natural product for direct dental pulp capping. J. Biomater. Tissue Eng. 2, 48–53.

Costa, L.M.M., Olyveira, G.M., Basmaji, P., Filho, L.X., 2012c. Nanopores structure in electrospun bacterial cellulose. J. Biomater. Nanobiotechnol. 3, 92–96.

Czaja, W.K., Young, D.J., Kawecki, M., 2007. The future prospects of microbial cellulose in biomedical applications. Biomacromolecules 8, 1–12.

D'Souza, S.E., Ginsberg, M.H., Plow, E.F., 1991. Arginyl-glycyl-aspartic acid (RGD): a cell adhesion motif. Trends Biochem. Sci. 16, 246–250.

Ducheyne, P., 1988. Titanium and calcium phosphate ceramic dental implants, surfaces, coatings and interfaces. J. Oral Implantol. 14 (3), 325–340.

Ebert, C.D., Lee, E.S., Kim, S.W., 1982. The antiplatelet activity of immobilized prostacyclin. J. Biomed. Mater. Res. 16, 629–638.

Fengel, D., Wegener, G., 1989. Wood: Chemistry, Ultrastructure, Reactions. In: Gruyter, W. (Ed.), Berlin, New York.

Filho, L.X., Olyveira, G.M., Basmaji, P., Costa, L.M.M., 2013. Novel electrospun nanotholits/PHB scaffolds for bone tissue regeneration. J. Nanosci. Nanotechnol. 13, 1–5.

Forng, E.R., Anderson, S.M., Cannon, R.E., 1989. Synthetic medium for *Acetobacter xylinum* that can be used for isolation of auxotrophic mutants ahd study of cellulose biosynthesis. Appl. Environ. Microbiol. 55, 1317–1319.

Gabriel, M., Van Nieuw Amerongen, G.P., Van Hinsbergh, V.W., Amerongen, A.V., Zentner, A., 2006. Direct grafting of RGD-motif-containing peptide on the surface of polycaprolactone films. J. Biomater. Sci. Polym. Ed. 17, 567–577.

Gatenholm, P., Klemm, D., 2010. Bacterial nanocellulose as a renewable material for biomedical applications. MRS Bull. 35, 208–213.

Gois, P.B.P., Olyveira, G.M., Costa, L.M.M., Chianca, C.F., Fraga, I.I.S., Basmaji, P., et al., 2012. Influence of symbioses culture between microorganisms/yeast strain on cellulose synthesis. Int. Rev. Biophys. Chem. 3, 48–54.

Grande, J.C., Torres, F.G., Gomez, C.M., Troncoso, O.P., Canet-Ferrer, J., Martínez-Pastor, J., 2009. Development of self-assembled bacterial cellulose–starch nanocomposites. Mater. Sci. Eng. C 29, 1098–1104.

Gronthos, S., Mankani, M., Brahim, J., Robey, P.G., Shi, S., 2000. Postnatal human dental pulp stem cells(DPSCs) *in vitro* and *in vivo*. Proc. Natl. Acad. Sci. U.S.A. 97, 13625–13630.

Gupta, B., Plummer, C., Bisson, I., Frey, P., Hilborn, J., 2002. Plasma-induced graft polymerization of acrylic acid onto poly(ethylene terephthalate) films: characterization and human smooth muscle cell growth on grafted films. Biomaterials 23, 863–871.

Hamerli, P., Weigel, T., Groth, T., Paul, D., 2003. Surface properties of and cell adhesion onto allylamineplasma-coated polyethylenterephtalat membranes. Biomaterials 24, 3989–3999.

Hammerle, C.H., Jung, R.E., 2003. Bone augmentation by means of barrier membranes. Periodontology 2000 33, 36–53.

Han, G., Ghosh, P., Rotello, V.M., 2007. Functionalized gold nanoparticles for drug delivery. Nanomedicine 2, 113–123.

Harrington, D.A., Cheng, E.Y., Guler, M.O., Lee, L.K., Donovan, J.L., Claussen, R.C., et al., 2006. Branched peptide-amphiphiles as self-assembling coatings for tissue engineering scaffolds. J. Biomed. Mater. Res. 78, 157–167.

Helenius, G., Backdahl, H., Bodin, A., Nannmark, U., Gatenholm, P., Risberg, B., 2006. *In vivo* biocompatibility of bacterial cellulose. J. Biomed. Mater. Res. Part A 76, 431–438.

Hoffman, A.S., Schmer, G., Harris, C., Kraft, W.G., 1972. Covalent binding of biomolecules to radiation grafted hydrogels on inert polymer surfaces. Trans. Am. Soc. Artif. Intern. Organs 18, 10–18.

Hong, M., Wu, L., Tian, L., Zhu, J., 2009. Controlled assembly of Au, Ag, and Pt nanoparticles with chitosan. J. Chem. Eur. J. 15, 5935–5941.

Hurzeler, M.B., Kohal, R.J., Naghshbandi, J., Mota, L.F., Conradt, J., Hutmacher, D., et al., 1998. Evaluation of a new bioresorbable barrier to facilitate guided bone regeneration around exposed implant threads. Int. J. Oral Maxillofac. Surg. 27, 315–320.

Iguchi, M., Yamanaka, S., Budhiono, A., 2000. Bacterial cellulose—a masterpiece of nature's arts. J. Mater. Sci. 35, 261–270.

Jones, A.A., Buser, D., Schenk, R., Wozney, J., Cochran, D.L., 2006. The effect of rhBMP-2 around endosseous implants with and without membranes in the canine model. J. Periodontol. 77 (7), 1184–1193.

Jung, R.E., Glauser, R., Scharer, P., Hammerle, C.H., Sailer, H.F., Weber, F.E., 2003. Effect of rhBMP-2 on guided bone regeneration in humans: a randomized, controlled clinical and histomorphometric study. Clin. Oral Implants Res. 14, 556–568.

Jung, R.E., Zwahlen, R., Weber, F.E., Molenberg, A., Van Lenthe, G.H., Hammerle, C.H.F., 2006. Evaluation of an *in situ* formed synthetic hydrogel as a biodegradable membrane for guided bone regeneration. Clin. Oral Implants Res. 17, 426–433.

Kalia, S., Dufresne, A., Cherian, B.M., Kaith, B.S., Avérous, L., Njuguna, J., et al., 2011. Cellulose based bio and nanocomposites—a review. Int. J. Polym. Sci. 1, 1–35.

Kim, K.H., Jeong, L., Park, H.N., Shin, S.Y., Park, W.H., Lee, S.C., et al., 2005. Biological efficacy of silk fibroin nanofiber membranes for guided bone regeneration. J. Biotechnol. 120, 327–339.

Koyama, M., Helbert, W., Imai, T., Sugiyama, J., Henrissat, B., 1997. Parallel upstructure evidences the molecular directionality during biosynthesis of bacterial cellulose. Proc. Natl. Acad. Sci. U.S.A. 94, 9091–9095.

Kuo, S.M., Chang, S.J., Chen, T.W., Kuan, T.C., 2006. Guided tissue regeneration for using a chitosan membrane: an experimental study in rats. J. Biomed. Mater. Res. 76A, 408–415.

Le Geros, R.Z., 2002. Properties of osteoconductive biomaterials: calcium phosphates. Clin. Orthop. Relat. Res. 395, 81–98.

Macedo, N.L., Macedo, L.G.S., Matuda, F.S., Ouchi, S.M., Monteiro, A.S.F., Carvalho, Y.R., 2003. Guided bone regeneration with subperiosteal implants of PTFE and hydroxyapatite physical barriers in rats. Braz. Dent. J. 14 (2), 119–124.

Marchant, K.K., Anderson, J.M., Umemura, Y., Marchant, R.E., 1989. Effect of albumin coating on the *in vitro* blood compatibility of Dacron arterial prostheses. Biomaterials 10, 147–155.

Masaoka, S., Ohe, T., Sakota, N., 1993. Production of cellulose from glucose by *Acetobacter xylinum*. J. Ferment. Bioeng. 75, 18–22.

Matsuoka, M., Tsuchida, T., Matsushita, K., Adachio, K., Yoshinga, F., 1996. A synthetic medium for bacterial cellulose productionby *Acetobacter xylinum* subsp. sucrofermentans. Biosci. Biotechnol. Biochem. 60, 575–579.

Melcher, A.H., 1976. On the repair potential of periodontal tissues. J. Periodontol. 47, 256–260.

Meyers, M.A., Chen, P.Y., Lin, A.Y.M., Seki, Y., 2008. Biological materials: structure and mechanical properties. Prog. Mater. Sci. 53, 1–206.

Miura, M., Grontos, S., Zhao, M., Lu, B., Fisher, L.W., Robey, P.G., et al., 2003. SHED: stem cells from human exfoliated deciduous teeth. Proc. Natl. Acad. Sci. U.S.A. 100, 5807–5812.

Mizuno, M., Shindo, M., Kobayashi, D., Tsuruga, E., Amemiya, A., Kuboki, Y., 1997. Osteogenesis by bone marrow stromal cells maintained on type I collagen matrix gels *in vivo*. Bone 20, 101–107.

Motta, A.C., Duek, E.A.C., 2006. Síntese, caracterização e degradação *in vitro* do poli (L-ácido láctico-co-ácido glicólico). Matéria 11 (3), 340–350.

Nevins, M.L., Camelo, M., Lynch, S.E., Schenk, R.K., Nevins, M., 2003. Evaluation of periodontal regeneration following grafting intrabony defects with Bio-Oss collagen: a human histologic report. Int. J. Periodontics Restorative Dent. 23, 9–17.

Nogi, M., Yano, H., 2008. Transparent nanocomposites based on cellulose produced by bacteria offer potential innovation in the electronics device industry. Adv. Mater. 20, 1849–1852.

Nyman, S., Lindhe, J., Karring, T., Rylander, D., 1982. New attachment following surgical treatment of human periodontal disease. J. Clin. Periodontol. 22, 290–296.

Oh, T.J., Meraw, S.J., Lee, E.J., Giannobile, W.V., Wang, H.L., 2003. Comparative analysis of collagen membranes for the treatment of implant dehiscence defects. Clin. Oral Implants Res. 14, 80–90.

Okahisa, Y., Yoshida, A., Miyaguch, I.S., Yano, H., 2009. Optically transparent wood–cellulose nanocompositeas a base substrate for flexible organic light-emitting diode displays. Compos. Sci. Technol. 69, 1958–1961.

Oliveira, R.C., Carneiro, E., Cestari, T.M., Taga, R., Granjeiro, J.M., 2006. Dynamics of subcutaneous tissue response to the implantation of tetracycline-treated or untreated membrane of demineralized bovine cortical bone in rats. J. Biomater. Appl. 21 (2), 167–178.

Olyveira, G.M., Costa, L.M.M., Góis, P.B.P., Basmaji, P., Filho, L.X., 2011a. Novel natural transdermal patch for osteoporosis treatment. J. Nanotechnol. Eng. Med. 2, 031011–031015.

Olyveira, G.M., Valido, D.P., Costa, L.M.M., Gois, P.B.P., Filho, L.X., Basmaji, P., 2011b. First otoliths/collagen/bacterial cellulose nanocomposites as a potential scaffold for bone tissue regeneration. J. Biomater. Nanobiotechnol. 2, 239–243.

Olyveira, G.M., Acasigua, G.A.X., Costa, L.M.M., Scher, C.R., Xavier Filho, L., Pranke, P. H., et al., 2013a. Human dental pulp stem cell behavior using natural nanotolith/bacterial cellulose scaffolds for regenerative medicine. J. Biomed. Nanotechnol. 9, 1–8.

Olyveira, G.M., Costa, L.M.M., Basmaji, P., 2013b. Physically modified bacterial cellulose as alternative routes for transdermal drug delivery. J. Biomater. Tissue Eng. 2, 1–6.

Olyveira, G.M., Santos, M.L., Daltro, P.B., Basmaiji, P., Daltro, G.C., Guastaldi, A.C., 2014a. Bacterial cellulose/chondroitin sulfate for dental materials scaffold. J. Biomater. Tissue Eng. 4, 1–5.

Olyveira, G.M., Santos, M.L., Costa, L.M.M., Daltro, P.B., Basmaji, P., Daltro, G.C., et al., 2014b. Bacterial cellulose biocomposites for guided tissue regeneration. Sci. Adv. Mater. 6, 1–6.

Olyveira, G.M., Santos, M.L., Costa, L.M.M., Daltro, P.B., Basmaji, P., Daltro, G.C., et al., 2014c. Bacterial cellulose nanobiocomposites for dental materials scaffolds. J. Biomater. Tissue Eng. 4, 1–7.

Olyveira, G.M., Santos, M.L., Costa, L.M.M., Riccardi, C.S., Basmaji, P., Daltro, G.C., et al., 2014d. Bacterial cellulose nanobiocomposites for periodontolal disease. J. Bionanosci. 8, 1–6.

Olyveira, G.M., Acasigua, G.A.X., Costa, L.M.M., Braghirolli, D.I., Fossati, A.C.M., Guastaldi, A.C., et al., 2014e. Novel chemically modified bacterial cellulose nanocomposite as potential biomaterial for stem cell delivery applications. Curr. Stem Cell Res. Ther. 9, 117–123.

Olyveira, G.M., Santos, M.L., Costa, L.M.M., Riccardi, C.S., Daltro, P.B., Basmaji, P., et al., 2015a. Physically modified bacterial cellulose biocomposites for guided tissue regeneration. Sci. Adv. Mater. 7, 1–8.

Olyveira, G.M., Santos, M.L., Costa, L.M.M., Riccardi, C.S., Daltro, P.B., Basmaji, P., et al., 2015b. Physically modified bacterial cellulose biocomposites for dental materials scaffolds. Mater. Focus 4, 1–7.

Onizawa, S., Aoshiba, K., Kajita, M., Miyamoto, Y., Nagai, A., 2009. Platinum nanoparticle antioxidants inhibit pulmonary inflammation in mice exposed to cigarette smoke. Pulm. Pharmacol. Ther. 22, 340–349.

Orr, R.D., Debruijn, J.D., Davies, J.E., 1992. Scanning electron microscopy of the bone interface with titanium, titanium alloy and hydroxyapatite. Cells Mater. 2, 241–251.

Orts, W.J., Shey, J., Imam, S.H., Glenn, G.M., Guttman, M.E., Revol, J.F., 2005. Application of cellulose microfibrils in polymer nanocomposites. J. Polym. Environ. 13, 301–306.

Pinheiro, A.L.B., Gerbi, M.E.M.M., Júnior, F.A.L., Ramalho, L.M.P., Marzola, C., Ponzi, E.A. C., et al., 2003. Assessment of bone repair associated with the use of organic bovine bone Gen-oxR Organic and membrane irradiated with 830 nm. Int. Congr. Ser. 1248, 441–443.

Rajnicek, A.M., Mc Craig, C.D., 1997. Guidance of CNS growth cones by substratum grooves and ridges: effects of inhibitors of the cytoskeleton, calcium channels and signal transduction pathways. J. Cell. Sci. 110, 2915–2924.

Ramana, K.V., Tomar, A., Singh, L., 2000. Effect of various carbon and nitrogen sources on cellulose synthesis by *Acetobacter xylinum*. World J. Microbiol. Biotechnol. 16, 245–248.

Ratner, D., 1996. In: Ratner, B.D., Hoffman, A.S., Schoen, F.J., Lemons, J.E. (Eds.), Biomaterials Science: An Introduction to Materials in Medicine. Academic Press, San Diego, pp. 1337–1339.

Ren, G., Hu, D., Cheng, E.W., Vargas-Reus, M.A., Reip, P., Allaker, R.P., 2009. Characterisation of copper oxide nanoparticles for antimicrobial applications. Int. J. Antimicrob. Agents 33, 587–590.

Ribitsch, I., Burk, J., Delling, U., Geibler, C., Gittel, C., Julke, H., et al., 2010. Basic science and clinical application of stem cells in veterinary medicine. Adv. Biochem. Eng. Biotechnol. 123, 219–263.

Richmond, P.A., 1991. Occurrence and functions of native cellulose. In: Haigler, C.H., Weimer, P.J. (Eds), Biosynthesis and Biodegradation of Cellulose, New York.

Riesenfeld, J., Olsson, P., Sanchez, J., Mollnes, T.E., 1995. Surface modification with functionally active heparin. Med. Device Technol. 6, 24–31.

Ross, P., Mayer, R., Benziman, M., 1991. Cellulose biosynthesis and function in bacteria. Microbiol. Rev. 55, 35–58.

Sakai, V.T., Zhang, Z., Dong, Z., Neiva, K.G., Machado, M.A.A.M., Shi, S., et al., 2010. SHED differentiate into functional odontoblasts and endothelium. J. Dent. Res. 89, 791–796.

Sandhiya, S., Dkhar, S.A., Surendiran, A., 2009. Emerging trends of nanomedicine—an overview. Fundam. Clin. Pharmacol. 23, 263–269.

Sani, A., Dahman, Y., 2010. Improvements in the production of bacterial synthesized biocellulose nanofibres using different culture methods. J. Chem. Technol. Biotechnol. 85, 151–164.

Schrecker, S., Gostomski, P., 2005. Determining the water holding capacity of microbial cellulose. Biotechnol. Lett. 27, 1435–1438.

Seo, B.M., Sonoyama, W., Yamaza, T., Coppe, C., Kikuiri, T., Akiyama, K., et al., 2008. SHED repair critical size calvarial defects in mice. Oral. Dis. 14, 428–434.

Shi, S., Bartold, P.M., Miura, M., Seo, B.M., Robey, P.G., Gronthos, S., 2005. The efficacy of mesenchymal stem cells to regenerate and repair dental structures. Orthod. Craniofac. Res. 8, 191–199.

Shoda, M., Sugano, Y., 2005. Recent advances in bacterial cellulose production. Biotechnol. Bioprocess Eng. 10, 1–8.

Simion, M., Trisi, P., Maglione, M., Piattelli, A., 1994. A preliminary report on a method for studying the permeability of expanded polytetrafluoroethylene membrane to bacteria *in vitro*: a scanning electron microscopic and histological study. J. Periodontol. 65 (8), 755–761.

Smith, A.J., Lesot, H., 2001. Induction and regulation of crown dentinogenesis: embryonic events as a template for dental tissue repair? Crit. Rev. Oral Biol. Med. 12, 425–437.

Smith, A.J., Cassidy, N., Perry, H., Beguekirn, C., Ruch, J.V., Lesot, H., 1995. Reactionary dentinogenesis. Int. J. Dev. Biol. 39, 273–280.

Stavropoulos, F., Dahlin, C., Ruskin, J.D., Johansson, C., 2004. A comparative study of barrier membranes as graft protectors in the treatment of localized bone defects. An experimental study in canine model. Clin. Oral Implants Res. 15, 435–442.

Strietzel, F.P., Khongkhunthian, P., Khattiya, R., Patchanee, P., Reichart, P.A., 2006. Healing pattern of bone defects covered by different membrane types–a histologic study in the porcine mandible. J. Biomed. Mater. Res. B Appl. Biomater. 78 (1), 35–46.

Szymańska-Chargot, M., Cybulska, J., Zdunek, A., 2011. Sensing the structural differences in cellulose from Apple and bacterial cell wall materials by Raman and FT-IR spectroscopy. Sensors 11, 5543–5560.

Teixeira, A.I., Abrams, G.A., Bertics, P.J., Murphy, C.J., Nealey, P.F., 2003. Epithelial contact guidance on well-defined micro and nanostructured substrates. J. Cell Sci. 116, 1881–1892.

Teixeira, A.I., Nealey, P.F., Murphy, C.J., 2004. Responses of human keratocytes to micro- and nanostructured substrates. J. Biomed. Mater. Res. 71, 369–376.

Viljanen, V.V., Lindholm, T.S., 1998. Background of the early development of absorbable fixation devices. Tech. Orthop. 13, 117–122.

Wikesjo, U.M.E., Qahash, M., Thomson, R.C., Cook, A.D., Rohrer, M.D., Wozney, J.M., et al., 2004. rhBMP-2 significantly enhances guided bone regeneration. Clin. Oral Implants Res. 15, 194–204.

Willians, D.F., 1981. Biocompatibility of Clinical Implant Materials. CRC Press, Boca Raton, FL.

Willians, D.F., 1991. Concise Encyclopedia of Medical and Dental Materials. Pergamon Press, Oxford.

Yeo, Y.-J., Jeon, D.-W., Kim, C.-S., Choi, S.-H., Cho, K.-S., Lee, Y.-K., et al., 2005. Effects of chitosan nonwoven membrane on periodontal healing of surgically created one-wall intrabony defects in beagle dogs. J. Biomed. Mater. Res. B Appl. Biomater. 72, 86–93.

Yim, E.K., Reano, R.M., Pang, S.W., Yee, A.F., Chen, C.S., Leong, K.W., 2005. Nanopattern-induced changes in morphology and motility of smooth muscle cells. Biomaterials 26, 5405–5413.

You, C.C., Miranda, O.R., Gider, B., Ghosh, P.S., Kim, I.B., Erdogan, B., et al., 2007. Detection and identification of proteins using nanoparticle? Fluorescent polymer 'chemical nose' sensors. Nat. Nanotechnol. 2, 318–323.

Zhang, Y.Z., Venugopal, J., Huang, Z.M., Lim, C.T., Ramakrishna, S., 2006. Crosslinking of the electrospun gelatin nanofibers. Polymer 47, 2911–2917.

Zugenmaier, P., 2001. Conformation and packing of various crystalline cellulose fibers. Prog. Polym. Sci. 26, 1341–1417.

CHAPTER

Applications of nanobiopolymers for soft tissue engineering

4

George Dan Mogoşanu[1], Alexandru Mihai Grumezescu[2], Laurenţiu Mogoantă[3], Ludovic Everard Bejenaru[1] and Cornelia Bejenaru[4]

[1]Department of Pharmacognosy & Phytotherapy, Faculty of Pharmacy, University of Medicine and Pharmacy of Craiova, Craiova, Romania [2]Department of Science and Engineering of Oxidic Materials and Nanomaterials, Faculty of Applied Chemistry and Materials Science, University Politehnica of Bucharest, Bucharest, Romania [3]Research Center for Microscopic Morphology and Immunology, University of Medicine and Pharmacy of Craiova, Craiova, Romania [4]Department of Vegetal & Animal Biology, Faculty of Pharmacy, University of Medicine and Pharmacy of Craiova, Craiova, Romania

4.1 INTRODUCTION

Tissue engineering (TE) is an interdisciplinary area aiming to reproduce the native tissue properties, organization, and function at nanoscale dimensions (Langer and Vacanti, 1993). TE combines biology, regenerative medicine (RM), chemistry, engineering, and materials science in order to achieve replacement of damaged tissues or to maintain or enhance tissue functions (Venugopal et al., 2008b). One of the main TE challenges is biomimicking architecture of extracellular matrix (ECM), in order to repair, rehabilitate, and regenerate cells/tissues/organs damaged by injury, disease, or other conditions (Fernandes et al., 2009; Fisher and Mauck, 2013; Harrison et al., 2014).

ECM supports and maintains the cellular microenvironment, providing specific and highly organized "nanofibers," such as proteins (collagen, elastin, fibronectin (FN), laminin (LN)), soluble factors, and cytokines. ECM also supports cell adhesion, migration, and differentiation. Cell adhesion receptors are transmembrane glycoproteins that include integrins, cadherins, selectins, immunoglobulins, and proteoglycan (syndecan). On the other hand, the cellular microenvironment is regulated by cell–cell, cell–ECM, and cell–soluble factors interactions (Khademhosseini and Langer, 2006; Goldberg et al., 2007; Hubmacher and Apte, 2013).

Nanobiomaterials in Soft Tissue Engineering. DOI: http://dx.doi.org/10.1016/B978-0-323-42865-1.00004-0

Soft TE includes different therapeutic/clinical applications, such as neuronal injuries, cardiovascular diseases, cartilage and ligament disorders, skin burns, and wounds (Pradhan and Farach-Carson, 2010; Berthiaume et al., 2011; Bonnans et al., 2014).

Biomimetic nanomaterials, especially biocompatible and biodegradable polymeric nanofibers (scaffolds) produced by electrospinning, molecular self-assembly, or phase separation, are up-to-date acquisitions for TE. In other words, because they tend to replicate the properties of living cells, nanobiomaterials must be safe, nontoxic, nonimmunogenic, biocompatible, and biodegradable, with adequate mechanical properties, high surface area, and a macroporous structure (Hasirci et al., 2006; Venugopal et al., 2008a; Wang et al., 2013; Wang and Wang, 2014).

Electrospinning is the most common technique for the production of nanofibers from 50 nm to 5 μm diameter. Nanofiber morphology and diameter depend on different factors: high voltage (2–40 kV), inner diameter of the needle, temperature, loading rate, humidity, air speed, surface tensioactivity of the solution, molecular weight, and concentration of the polymer, etc. (Cui et al., 2010; Briggs and Arinzeh, 2011, 2014; Rim et al., 2013; Liu et al., 2013).

The main biocompatible and biodegradable nanobiomaterials used for soft TE applications include natural and synthetic polymers, such as collagen, chitosan, heparin, fibrin, gelatin, alginate, hyaluronic acid, silk; polylactic acid (PLA), poly(L-lactic acid) (PLLA), polyglycolic acid (PGA), poly(lactic-*co*-poly(glycolic acid) (PLGA), poly-ε-caprolactone (PCL), poly(l-lactic acid)-*co*-poly(ε-caprolactone) (PLLA–PCL), polyethylene oxide (PEO), polyurethane (PU), polyethylene terephthalate (PET), and polymethyl methacrylate (PMMA).

4.2 NANOBIOPOLYMERS FOR NEURAL TISSUE ENGINEERING

Neural tissue engineering (NTE) is required mainly for the treatment of peripheral nerve (PN) traumatic injuries, by providing connecting bridges between the missing portions, similar to autologous grafts (Schmidt and Leach, 2003; Venugopal and Ramakrishna, 2005b; Wang et al., 2012). In this respect, a wide range of biocompatible and biodegradable nanofibers obtained by electrospinning was investigated as tissue-engineered scaffolds for nerve repair/regeneration. Natural (collagen, chitosan) and synthetic polymers, especially polyesters (PGA, PLLA, PLGA, PCL), are also used as nerve biodegradable matrix filled with the Schwann cells (SCs) or vehicles for neurotrophic growth factor delivery: nerve growth factor (NGF), neurotrophin-5 (NT-5), glial cell line-derived neurotrophic growth factor (GDNF), ciliary neurotrophic factor (CNTF), brain-derived neurotrophic factor (BDNF), FN, and collagen-derived peptides containing arginine–glycine–aspartic acid for cell growth acceleration (Willerth and Sakiyama-Elbert, 2007; Zhang and Uludağ, 2009; Saracino et al., 2013; Ai et al., 2014).

Nanofibrous scaffolds for NTE (PN regeneration) include natural polymers from biological sources, closely related to the ECM and endoneural tube architecture: collagen, chitosan, heparin, gelatin, silk, fibrinogen, fibrin, FN, LN, elastin, hyaluronic acid, and agarose (Biazar et al., 2010; Cunha et al., 2011; Khaing and Schmidt, 2012).

Collagen is used for different NTE applications, such as acetic acid-electrospun photochemical cross-linked collagen nanofibers, with good structural stability (without denaturation) (Liu et al., 2010); random and aligned electrospun-nanofibrous collagen–glycosaminoglycan (GAG) scaffold mimicking ECM, cross-linked with genipin for an improved biocompatibility (Timnak et al., 2011); sustained release of neurotrophin-3 (NT-3) and chondroitinase ABC (ChABC) from electrospun collagen nanofiber scaffolds through microbial transglutaminase mediated cross-linking, for the treatment of spinal cord injuries (SCIs) (Liu et al., 2012); collagen matrices/implants used for the release of neurotrophic factors (NT-3, NT-5, GDNF) in SCIs (Houweling et al., 1998); matrigels with growth factor (GDNF) and SCs, promoting propriospinal axonal regeneration, enhancing myelin formation, and improving graft–host interfaces after SCIs (Iannotti et al., 2003); collagen and LN gel matrices for platelet-derived growth factor BB (PDGF-BB) and insulin-like growth factor I (IGF-I) delivery in nerve gap injuries repaired with silicone tubes (Wells et al., 1997); rapid repair of rat sciatic nerve injury using a nanosilver-embedded collagen scaffold coated with LN or LN plus FN (Ding et al., 2011).

Chitosan membranes, sponges, and fibers are also used for NTE: sponge-like asymmetric chitosan membrane obtained by immersion-precipitation phase-inversion method and tested for a novel wound dressing (Mi et al., 2001); electrospun chitosan nonwoven nano/microfiber mesh tubes as a scaffold for sciatic nerve regeneration in rats (Wang et al., 2008); enhancement of regeneration into sciatic nerve defects in Wistar rats along a chitosan nanofiber mesh tube on which electrically polarized β-tricalcium phosphate (β-TCP) particles are immobilized (Wang et al., 2010); the promotion of neural progenitor cells (NPCs) proliferation by aligned and randomly oriented collagen nanofibers through β1 integrin/MAPK (mitogen-activated protein kinase) signaling pathway (Wang et al., 2011a); a novel nanoparticle growth factor delivery system based on chitosan–heparin for *in vivo* targeting of the sciatic nerve injuries (Gonçalves et al., 2012); microstructured 20-μm-thick polymer filaments used as nerve implants loaded with chitosan–small interfering RNA nanoparticles biofunctionalize nerve implants and enable neurite outgrowth (Mittnacht et al., 2010).

Other researches highlighted the importance of heparin, fibrin, gelatin, silk, and self-assembling peptides for NTE: heparin inhibits ChABC degradation (Liu et al., 2012); heparin-immobilized fibrin-based hydrogels facilitate growth factor controlled release for spinal cord lesions (NT-3) (Taylor et al., 2004) and sciatic nerve regeneration (NGF) (Lee et al., 2003); prolonged protective effect of intravitreally injected basic fibroblast growth factor-impregnated gelatin nanoparticles (bFGF-GNPs) against photoreceptor degeneration in rats (Sakai et al., 2007); electrospun (silkworm) silk fibroin (SF) scaffolds as alternative materials for neural regeneration, due to their biocompatibility and mechanical properties (Altman et al., 2003); regenerated electrospun SF nanofibers promoting SC adhesion, growth, and proliferation (Hu et al., 2012); reknitting the injured dorsal column of rats' spinal cord by transplanted embryonic NPCs and SCs, cultured within self-assembling peptide nanofiber scaffold (SAPNS) (Guo et al., 2007; Chang et al., 2008; Holmes et al., 2000); regeneration of the cavernous nerve by Sonic hedgehog (SHH) proteins using novel aligned peptide amphiphile (PA) nanofibers (Angeloni et al., 2011); cooperative effect of heparan sulfate and LN mimetic peptide nanofibers, even effective in the presence of chondroitin sulfate proteoglycans, on the promotion of neurite outgrowth by PC-12 cells (Mammadov et al., 2012).

Different combinations of natural and synthetic materials are also applied for NTE (PN regeneration), such as electrospinning of ultrathin gelatin (Gt) fibers and Gt–PCL composite nanofibrous scaffolds (Zhang et al., 2005b); random and aligned electrospun (70:30) poly(ε-caprolactone)/gelatin biocomposite nanofibrous scaffolds obtained by polymer blending, enhancing *in vitro* differentiation and proliferation of nerve stem cell (C17.2) culture, and supporting neurite outgrowth (Ghasemi-Mobarakeh et al., 2008); thin films of aligned poly-acrylonitrile methylacrylate (PAN-MA) fibers or solvent casted smooth PAN-MA films, promoting enhanced adsorption of FN and bridging long PN gaps by modulation of SC migration and neurite outgrowth from dorsal root ganglion (DRG) cultures (Mukhatyar et al., 2011); electrospun nerve conduits (NCs) from PLGA-SF bridging 10-mm sciatic nerve gaps of Sprague–Dawley rats, effects similar to those of autologous nerve grafts (Li et al., 2012); random and aligned electrospun poly(L-lactic acid)-*co*-poly (ε-caprolactone) (PLLA-CL))/collagen I/collagen III biocomposite/biocompatible nanofibrous scaffolds prepared by blending, with average diameter of 253 ± 102 nm and a tensile strength of 11.59 ± 1.68 MPa (Kijeńska et al., 2012); (PLLA-PCL)–SF aligned polyblend nanofibrous scaffolds fabricated by electrospinning, which promote PN regeneration and functional recovery of 10-mm sciatic nerve defects in rats, using nerve guidance conduits (Wang et al., 2011c); controlling the survival and maturation of brain neurons through a hybrid nanofibrous scaffold, which combines the structural properties of type I collagen with the epitope-presenting ability of PA nanofibers (Sur et al., 2012). In addition, the axonal regeneration of tubular NCs was significantly stimulated by 2% methylcellulose hydrogel used as vehicle for PDGF-BB and IGF-I growth factors (Wells et al., 1997).

A broad category of synthetic polymers (PLA, PGA, PLGA, PCL, PLCL) are commonly used for NTE, as stated in recent decades' researches: PN regeneration with sustained release of poly(phosphoester) polypropylene fumarate microencapsulated NGF inside silicone tubing within nerve guide conduits (rat sciatic nerve) (Xu et al., 2003); entrapment of migrating hippocampal neural cells (potential neuroprogenitors), from postnatal hippocampal organotypic cultures, in three-dimensional (3D) peptide nanofiber scaffold (Semino et al., 2004; Silva et al., 2004; Gelain et al., 2006); electrospun PLGA and PLGA/PCL biodegradable polymer nanofiber tubes for PN regeneration (Bini et al., 2004; Panseri et al., 2008); electrospinning of nano/microscale PLLA aligned fiber scaffolds with potential applications as cell carriers in NTE (Yang et al., 2005); stimulation of neurite outgrowth by neurotrophins (CNTF) delivered from biodegradable photo-cross-linkable PEG microsphere/hydrogel composites (Burdick et al., 2006); neuronal differentiation of PC-12 cells cultured on nanoscaled 3D scaffolds consisting of growth electrospun aligned poly (ε-caprolactone-*co*-ethyl-ethylene phosphate) (PCLEEP) nanofibrous conduit incorporating growth factors (NGF, GDNF) for sciatic nerve gap regeneration (Chew et al., 2007); anti-Parkinsonian effect (in C57B1/6 mice) of NGFs adsorbed on polybutylcyanoacrylate nanoparticles coated with polysorbate-80 (Kurakhmaeva et al., 2008; Xie et al., 2005); highly aligned electrospun PLLA nanofiber scaffolds compatible with serum-free (axonal) growth of primary motor and sensory neurons at low plating densities, evaluated *in vitro* using embryonic stage nine (E9) chick dorsal root ganglia (DRGs) and rat SCs (Corey et al., 2008; Wang et al., 2009); factor-loaded heparin/poly(L-lysine) nanoparticles coated on PLGA microspheres (Park et al., 2009b); polypyrrole (PPy)-coated electrospun PLGA nanofibers supporting the growth and differentiation of rat pheochromocytoma 12 (PC12) cells and hippocampal neurons (Lee et al., 2009); incorporation of PLGA/PLLA double-walled microspheres into polymer nerve guides, inside the inner surface of single-lumen PCL conduit, for the sustained release of GDNF, promoting migration and proliferation of SCs (Kokai et al., 2010); rat-derived neural stem cells (NSCs) grown on polyhydroxyalkanoate (PHA) nanofiber scaffolds, such as poly(3-hydroxybutyrate) (PHB), copolymer of 3-hydroxybutyrate and 4-hydroxybutyrate (P3HB4HB), and copolymer of 3-hydroxybutyrate and 3-hydroxyhexanoate (PHBHHx), developed for treating central nervous system injuries (Xu et al., 2010); culture of primary motor and sensory neurons in defined media on electrospun PLLA nanofiber scaffolds (Leach et al., 2011); surface modification of PLLA nanofiber with oligo (D-lactic acid) (ODLA) bioactive-peptide conjugates (AG73) for PN regeneration (Kakinoki et al., 2011); electrospun conducting polymer blended nanofibers (85:15), PLLA–polyaniline (PANi) scaffolds, and electrical stimulation of nerve stem cells (Prabhakaran et al., 2011); uniaxially aligned 3D electrospun PLGA nanofibers/scaffolds for neural regeneration (Subramanian et al., 2011); neurite outgrowth of DRGs neurons enhanced on aligned electrospun PLCL nanofibrous biopolymer scaffold with multiwalled carbon nanotube (MWCNT) coating (Jin et al., 2011); aligned electrospun poly(propylene carbonate) nanofibrous scaffolds biocompatible with PN tissues and cells *in vitro* (DRG from Sprague–Dawley rats) (Wang et al., 2011b).

4.3 NANOBIOPOLYMERS FOR CARDIOVASCULAR TISSUE ENGINEERING

4.3.1 CARDIAC TISSUE ENGINEERING

The replacing and regeneration of injured/missing myocardial tissues with natural/synthetic contractile heart tissues represents the main objective of cardiac tissue engineering (CTE) (Vunjak-Novakovic et al., 2010, 2014; Chiu and Radisic, 2013; Hirt et al., 2014). Biocompatible and biodegradable nanobiomaterials, mimicking the structure and chemical properties of cardiac ECM, are used as 3D polymeric scaffolds for cardiomyocytes (CMs) and vascular cells, which are then subjected to the action of some biological and physical (mechanical, electrical, magnetic) stimuli, for the enhancement of tissue maturation and function (Chen et al., 2008; Radisic and Christman, 2013; Georgiadis et al., 2014; Boffito et al., 2014; Huyer et al., 2015).

Natural polymers (alginate, chitosan, heparin, RGD peptide) are usually applied for CTE, as follows: nanowired 3D cardiac patches manufactured from alginate scaffolds incorporating gold nanowires, improving electrical communication between adjacent cardiac cells (Dvir et al., 2011); integration of multiple cell–matrix interactions of two matrix-attached peptides, the adhesion peptide G(4)RGDY and heparin-binding peptide G(4)SPPRRARVTY (HBP), into macroporous alginate scaffolds for promoting cardiac tissue regeneration (Sapir et al., 2011); new magnetically responsive (magnetite-impregnated) alginate scaffold promoting *in vitro* vessel-like organization of aortic endothelial cells (ECs) (Sapir et al., 2012); electrically conductive chitosan/carbon scaffolds prepared by precipitation and seeded with neonatal rat heart cells (Martins et al., 2014); peptide–alginate composites based on intact ECM proteins, such as Arg-Gly-Asp (RGD) sequence from FN and LN, promoting cardiac tissue regeneration through the mediation of cell adhesion and signaling through interactions with integrin receptors on the cell surface (Shin et al., 2003; Rosso et al., 2004; Tsur-Gang et al., 2009; Shachar et al., 2011).

Also, modern researches highlighted the importance of biocompatible and biodegradable synthetic polymers for CTE: electrospun poly(methylglutarimide) nanofibers, with structure similar to ECM, promoting cardiac cell alignment and proliferation into contractile tissue filaments, open-worked tissue meshes and continuous anisotropic cell sheets (Orlova et al., 2011; Zhang et al., 2011); electrically conductive hybrid hydrogel based on thiol-2-hydroxyethyl methacrylate (thiol-HEMA)/HEMA impregnated with homogeneously dispersed gold nanoparticles, with an increased connexin 43 expression at the level of neonatal rat CMs with or without electrical stimulation (You et al., 2011); poly(2-hydroxyethyl-methacrylate-*co*-methacrylic acid) hydrogel as functional template for proangiogenic scaffolds enhancing vascularization and integration of human embryonic stem cell (hESC)-derived CMs (Madden et al., 2010).

4.3.2 VASCULAR TISSUE ENGINEERING

The main target of vascular tissue engineering (VTE) is represented by the development of blood vessel nonimmunogenic artificial substitutes, with suitable biological and mechanical properties, without predisposition to thrombosis (Naito et al., 2011; Cleary et al., 2012; Gui and Niklason, 2014; Li et al., 2014). In recent decades, different nanobiomaterials have been investigated for VTE applications, such as: vascular cell seeding of synthetic polymer scaffolds and the design of bioactive polymers for *in situ* arterial regeneration (Ravi and

Chaikof, 2010); tissue engineered vascular grafts (TEVGs) obtained by seeding autologous bone-marrow-derived mononuclear cells onto biodegradable tubular scaffolds (Naito et al., 2011); immunologically compatible, nonthrombogenic autologous TEVGs, which can grow and can be remodeled, starting from native vessels (preferred vascular conduits) collected during coronary artery bypass or peripheral bypass surgery (Cleary et al., 2012; Seifu et al., 2013); biocompatible and biodegradable scaffold platforms for the regulation and promotion of angiogenesis and vascular network formation, through the control of polymeric network development (chemical composition, dimensional and mechanical properties) (Serbo and Gerecht, 2013); modern TEVGs produced starting from biodegradable synthetic, gel-based or decellularized scaffolds, and self-assembled cell-sheet-based techniques (Tan et al., 2015); surface modification of vascular grafts (hydrophilic PEG, zwitterionic polymers, heparin, other bioactive molecules), and endothelialization of biomaterials as potential nonthrombogenic scaffolds with enhanced hemocompatibility (Ren et al., 2015).

Alginate and collagen are the most used natural polymers for VTE, as follows: spatiotemporal control of vascular endothelial growth factor (VEGF) delivery from injectable alginate hydrogel in ischemic murine (ApoE(−/−)) hindlimbs enhances angiogenesis and returning tissue perfusion to normal levels (Silva and Mooney, 2007); geometrically controlled endothelial tubulogenesis in micropatterned collagen gels, which generate branches during tube formation and more complex capillary architectures (Raghavan et al., 2010); living microvascular networks engineered in 3D tissue type I collagen hydrogel scaffolds with *in vitro* biofunctionality for the study of cardiovascular physiopathology, including complex vascular phenomena, angiogenesis, and thrombosis (Zheng et al., 2012).

Semisynthetic polymers important for VTE include alginate−PCL, PCL−type I collagen, and methacrylated gelatin (GelMA): rat endothelial progenitor cells differentiated from adipose-derived stem cells seeded on the surface of scaffold fabricated by electrospinning PCL through alginate hydrogel conglutinate cells and natural sedimentation seeding cells, developing a novel cell-seeding technique on artificial vascular scaffolds (Sun et al., 2015); *in vivo* biomechanical stability of electrospun PCL−type I collagen scaffolds in vascular reconstruction, in a rabbit aortal−iliac bypass experimental model (Tillman et al., 2009); bilayered nanoscaled electrospun PCL−type I collagen scaffolds for the improvement of engineering cellularized blood vessels (human aortic ECs) (Ju et al., 2010); cell-laden microengineered GelMA hydrogels for complex, cell-responsive microtissues (endothelialized microvasculature), to control the alignment and elongation of fibroblasts, myoblasts, ECs, and cardiac stem cells (Nichol et al., 2010; Aubin et al., 2010).

Biocompatible and biodegradable synthetic polymers with various chemical structures and compositions were searched for up-to-date applications in VTE: proliferation of outgrowth ECs, isolated from rabbit or human peripheral blood, on aligned PLLA nanofibrous scaffolds (Lu et al., 2009); a unique biodegradable nanofibrous structure, aligned poly(l-lactic acid)-*co*-poly(ε-caprolactone) (PLLA-PCL) (75:25) copolymer nanofibrous scaffold, produced by electrospinning

(Xu et al., 2004; Santos et al., 2008, 2009); electrospinning of PLLA-PCL (75:25) copolymer nanofiber tubular scaffold with circumferential alignment and mechanical properties similar to human coronary artery, supporting smooth muscle cell (SMC) adhesion and proliferation (Mo et al., 2004); surface engineering (gelatin-grafted) of electrospun nonwoven PET nanofibers toward development of a new material for blood vessel engineering, improving the spreading and proliferation of ECs (Ma et al., 2005); nanopattern-induced changes in morphology and motility of bovine pulmonary artery SMC on PMMA and poly(dimethylsiloxane) surfaces (Yim et al., 2005); PET and expanded polytetrafluoroethylene synthetic prostheses as tissue-engineered vascular grafts made of decellularized matrices for small-diameter blood vessel regeneration/replacement (Catto et al., 2014; Abruzzo et al., 2014); poly-(D,L-lactide-*co*-glycolide) microsphere formulations containing recombinant human vascular endothelial growth factor, promoting local angiogenesis on ocular disease model (Cleland et al., 2001); poly(*N*-isopropylacrylamide-*co*-propylacrylic acid-*co*-butyl acrylate) (p[NIPAAm-*co*-PAA-*co*-BA]) hydrogel containing basic fibroblast growth factor (bFGF) improved angiogenesis in ischemic hindlimbs (Zhou et al., 2012; Chan et al., 2010). However, the applications of synthetic conduits for VTE are severely limited in smaller-diameter vessels because of the increased incidence of thrombosis, infection, and graft failure (Naito et al., 2011; Cleary et al., 2012; Seifu et al., 2013).

4.4 NANOBIOPOLYMERS FOR CARTILAGE AND LIGAMENT TE

4.4.1 CARTILAGE TE

Cartilage, a predominantly avascular, alymphatic and aneural tissue is represented by chondroblasts embedded within a dense ECM. Cartilage chondrocytes consist of type II collagen fibers incorporating proteoglycan macromolecules. Negatively charged, strongly hydrated cartilage proteoglycans can handle mechanical stress. Cartilage damage especially occurs in osteoarthritis, rheumatoid arthritis, and different traumas, with important clinical consequences because of the limited intrinsic potential for healing (Tuli et al., 2003; Kuo et al., 2006; Kim and Fisher, 2007; Chung and Burdick, 2008). Surgical procedures include chondrocyte transplantation and total joint replacement autografts, allografts, xenografts, or artificial prostheses. Also, autologous chondrocyte implantation and natural nanobiomaterials, such as biocompatible and biodegradable type II collagen and collagen–hyaluronan scaffolds, are commonly used for cartilage TE (Kim et al., 2012; Makris et al., 2015; Li and Hu, 2015).

Cartilage TE applications are based mainly on natural polymers, such as carbohydrates (agarose, alginate, cellulose, chitin, chitosan, HA) and proteins (collagen, gelatin, fibrin): self-assembling peptide hydrogel fosters chondrocyte ECM production and cell division (Kisiday et al., 2002; Kopesky et al., 2010); electrospun type II collagen scaffold as suitable environment for chondrocyte growth, for the development of articular cartilage repair (Shields et al., 2004; Kessler and Grande, 2008; Kessler et al., 2008); chondrogenic differentiation of human adipose-derived adult stem cells in agarose, alginate, and porous gelatin scaffolds (Awad et al., 2004); *in vitro* cartilage regeneration using 3D porous aqueous-derived silk scaffolds and MSCs or silk hydrogels (Wang et al., 2005; Chao et al., 2010); chondrogenic differentiation of bovine bone-marrow-derived MSCs in different hydrogels—influence of collagen type II ECM on MSC chondrogenesis (Bosnakovski et al., 2006; Lu et al., 2010); electrospun hyaluronic acid nanofibers for articular cartilage regeneration (Lee et al., 2009); self-assembled rosette nanotubes (RNts)−hydrogel composites, more accurate self-assembled nanotubes from DNA base pairs, alginate/agarose hydrogels, fibroblast-like type-B synoviocytes (SFB cells), and chondrocytes, promoting cell adhesion, growth, and viability (Chen et al., 2010); supramolecular design of self-assembling PA nanofibers for articular cartilage regeneration in a full-thickness chondral defect treated with microfracture in a rabbit model with or even without the addition of exogenous growth factor (TGF-β1) (Shah and Shah, 2010).

Different biocompatible and biodegradable semisynthetic polymers are also used for cartilage TE: photo-cross-linkable hyaluronan (HA-MA) as a scaffold for articular cartilage repair, accelerating healing in an *in vivo* osteochondral defect model (Nettles et al., 2004); electrospun chitosan−PEO nanofibers providing good chondrocyte biocompatibility for potential applications in cartilage repair (Subramanian et al., 2005); variations in matrix composition and GAG fine structure among scaffolds for cartilage TE—bovine articular chondrocytes seeded into agarose, alginate, collagen I, fibrin, and PGA constructs (Mouw et al., 2005); tissue-engineered cartilage using fibrin−hyaluronan (HA) composite gel and its *in vivo* implantation (Park et al., 2005); collagen nanofiber-covered porous biodegradable carboxymethyl-chitosan microcarriers for chondrocyte growth and development (Lu et al., 2008); RGD (Arg-Gly-Asp)-conjugated thermosensitive chitosan−Pluronic (CP) hydrogel as a cell-supported scaffold for articular cartilage regeneration (Park et al., 2008); injectable *in situ* forming biodegradable chitosan−hyaluronic-acid-based hydrogels (*N*-succinyl-chitosan (S-CS) and aldehyde hyaluronic acid (A-HA)), supporting cell survival and retaining bovine articular chondrocytic morphology (Tan et al., 2009); influence of 3D hyaluronic acid microenvironments on MSC chondrogenesis (Chung and Burdick, 2009); cartilage repair using hyaluronan hydrogel-encapsulated hESC-derived chondrogenic cells (Toh et al., 2010); electrospun PCL−collagen membrane for the resurfacing of cartilage defects, as a novel alternative to the conventional periosteal graft in autologous chondrocyte implantation (Ho et al., 2010; Zhang et al., 2005a); chemically cross-linked chitosan derivative (CML) hydrogel loaded with gelatin for chondrocyte encapsulation (Hu et al., 2011).

In recent decades, synthetic polymers (PLA, PGA, PEO, PEG) are increasingly required for cartilage TE: transdermal photopolymerization of poly(ethylene oxide) (PEO)-based injectable hydrogels for tissue-engineered cartilage—semi-interpenetrating networks of varying proportions of PEO-dimethacrylate and PEO and primary bovine articular chondrocytes were implanted in athymic mice (Elisseeff et al., 1999); effect of PEG molecular weight on tensile and swelling properties of oligo[PEG–fumarate] hydrogels for cartilage TE (Temenoff et al., 2002); electrospun PLGA nanofiber scaffolds for articular cartilage reconstruction, exhibiting mechanical stability, degradation, and cellular responses under mechanical stimulation *in vitro* (Shin et al., 2006); designing 3D photopolymer PEG hydrogels to regulate biomechanical cues and tissue growth for cartilage TE (Bryant et al., 2008, 2004); *in vitro* and *in vivo* test of PEG/PCL-based hydrogel scaffold for cell delivery application (rabbit chondrocytes for the formation of neocartilage) (Park et al., 2007); chondrogenic and osteogenic differentiations of multipotent human bone-marrow-derived mesenchymal stem cells (hMSCs) on a highly porous PLLA nanofibrous scaffold with designed pore network, for osteochondral defect repair (Hu et al., 2009); transplantation of poly(*N*-isopropylacrylamide-*co*-vinyl-imidazole) (p(NiPAAm-*co*-VI)) hydrogel constructs composed of rabbit chondrocytes and growth-factor-loaded nanoparticles for neocartilage formation (Park et al., 2009c; Ahmed and Hincke, 2010); electrospun PCL nanofiber meshes and adult bone-marrow-derived MSCs (Li et al., 2005; Alves da Silva et al., 2010); injectable biodegradable PEG–RGD peptide hybrid hydrogels for *in vitro* chondrogenesis of hMSCs – tetrahydroxyl PEG was functionalized with acrylate, and then reacted with thiol-containing RGD peptide (Liu et al., 2010); surface modification of electrospun PLLA nanofibers by plasma treatment and cationized gelatin immobilization (Chen and Su, 2011); semidegradable hydrogels based on poly(vinyl alcohol) (PVA) and PLGA for cartilage repair (Spiller et al., 2011); porous PVA–hydrogel matrix-engineered biosynthetic cartilage (Bichara et al., 2011).

4.4.2 LIGAMENT TISSUE ENGINEERING

Ligaments are bone–bone connective tissues with reduced cell density, very important for the mechanical transfer of forces within the musculoskeletal system, requiring small amounts of oxygen and nutrients (Vunjak-Novakovic et al., 2004; Woo et al., 2006). Compared to other human body ligaments, the anterior cruciate ligament (ACL) exhibits poor healing potential and limited vascularization (Lu et al., 2005). Consequently, ligament tissue engineering (LTE) is focused mainly on ACL repair/regeneration, through biologic tissue grafts, growth factors, gene transfer and gene therapy, cell therapy (stem cells), mechanical factors, and custom-designed natural or synthetic biodegradable scaffolds (West and Harner, 2005; Laurencin and Freeman, 2005; Petrigliano et al., 2006; Murray et al., 2006, 2010; Nau and Teuschl, 2015).

Biocompatible and biodegradable natural polymers are extensively used for LTE application, such as: "ligament analogs" produced from high-strength resorbable collagen fiber scaffolds, enhancing *in vitro* and *in vivo* rabbit fibroblast proliferation (Dunn et al., 1995; Bellincampi et al., 1998); silkworm silk-nanofibrous matrix for tissue-engineered ACLs, exhibiting adequate fatigue performance and supporting the attachment, expansion, and differentiation of adult human progenitor bone marrow stromal cells (BMSCs) (Altman et al., 2002); human BMSCs and ligament fibroblast responses on RGD-modified silk fibers (Chen et al., 2003); ACL regeneration using a knitted silk scaffold combined with collagen sponge (Chen et al., 2008); alginate and chitosan polyion complex hybrid nanofibers for scaffolds for LTE and tendon tissue engineering (alginate with 0.05% or 0.1% chitosan) (Majima et al., 2005); MSCs grown on a 3D-specific HA-based prototype ligament scaffold (HYAFF 11), producing collagen type I, type III, LN, FN, and actin (Cristino et al., 2005); collagen–platelet-rich plasma (PRP) hydrogel scaffold enhancing primary repair of the porcine ACL (Murray et al., 2007b; Everts et al., 2006); enhanced histological repair in central wound of ACL canine knees with a collagen–PRP scaffold (Murray et al., 2007a; Fallouh et al., 2010); protein-based nanofibers as scaffold materials for ACL regeneration (Kuo et al., 2010); fibrin scaffolds affect ACL fibroblast proliferation and collagen synthesis (Vavken et al., 2011; Harrison et al., 2011; Illingworth et al., 2010); local administration of vascular endothelial growth factor (VEGF) improved mechanical characteristics of the semitendinosus tendon graft after ACL reconstruction in sheep (Yoshikawa et al., 2006). Some semisynthetic polymers are also available for LTE applications, e.g., PLGA–collagen hybrid mesh for 3D culture of canine ACL cells (Chen et al., 2004).

Nowadays, modern researches highlighted the increasingly importance of synthetic polymers for LTE: ACL regeneration using braided biodegradable scaffolds, *in vitro* optimization studies for three compositions of poly-α-hydroxyester fibers, namely PGA, PLLA, and polylactic-*co*-glycolic acid 82:18 (PLAGA) (Lu et al., 2005); biodegradable nano-microfibrous polymer scaffold produced by electrospinning PLGA nanofibers onto a knitted PLGA scaffold, promoting cell proliferation, function, and differentiation for potential application in tendon/LTE (Sahoo et al., 2006); improved biological characteristics of PLLA electrospun membrane by incorporation of MWCNTs–hydroxyapatite nanoparticles (Mei et al., 2007); 0.5, 1, and 2.5 wt.% oxidized multiwalled carbon nanotubes (MWCNT–COOHs) as effective reinforcement and thermal stability agents of PLA ligaments (Chrissafis et al., 2010; Mackle et al., 2011); biodegradable PLA–PCL nanofibers for ACL regeneration (Vieira et al., 2011); PLA-poloxamer/poloxamine multiblock copolymers for LTE, macromolecular design for degradable scaffolds, and mesenchymal stem cell (MSC) differentiation (Leroy et al., 2015).

4.5 NANOBIOPOLYMERS FOR SKIN TE

Complete wound closure and the restoration of the normal functions of dermal tissue are the main objectives for skin TE. Nanobiopolymers must mimic human skin, acting as a hemostatic barrier against bacteria, absorbing exudates and maintaining a moist environment, easily removable, painless for the patient, readily transplanted in large amounts, and without significant scarring (Böttcher-Haberzeth et al., 2010; Shevchenko et al., 2010; Groeber et al., 2011). At the skin level, biocompatible and biodegradable polymeric nanofibrous membranes, such as dermo-epidermal 3D substitutes/scaffolds manufactured by electrospinning, phase separation or self-assembly techniques, attract fibroblasts that secrete ECM components (collagen, cytokines—growth factors, angiogenic factors) to rebuild damaged tissues (Zhong et al., 2010; Sundaramurthi et al., 2014; Mohd Hilmi and Halim, 2015).

Natural polymers for skin TE include different nanobiomaterials exhibiting wound-healing properties: collagen and fibrin encapsulating growth factors widely used as active wound dressings (AWDs) for diabetic skin injuries (Zahedi et al., 2010); photo-cross-linkable chitosan hydrogel containing fibroblast growth factor-2 for wound healing of full-thickness skin incisions on the back of healing-impaired diabetic (db/db) mice (Obara et al., 2003); accelerated wound closure of pressure ulcers in aged mice by chitosan scaffolds with or without bFGF contained in gelatin microparticles (Park et al., 2009a); releasing of bFGF from a cross-linked GAG (chondroitin sulfate–heparin) hydrogel promoting the healing of chronic wounds (Liu et al., 2007); *in vitro* constitution and *in vivo* implantation of engineered skin constructs with sweat glands for skin regeneration/wound closure—sweat gland cells (SGCs) were cultured on gelatin microspheres containing epidermal growth factor (EGF) as multifunctional vehicles, then SGC–microsphere complexes (SMCs) were delivered into the engineered skin construct created *in vitro* by culturing human keratinocytes on top of a fibroblast-embedded collagen-based matrix, in an organotypic co-culture model (Huang et al., 2010); self-assembling elastin-like peptides–keratinocyte growth factor (KGF) chimeric nanoparticles for the treatment of chronic wounds (Koria et al., 2011); silk fibroin–human hair keratin-based 3D biocompatibile and biodegradable scaffolds applied as highly vascular dermal tissue-engineered skin substitutes (Bhardwaj et al., 2015).

PCL–collagen-coated nanofibers and collagen–PGA hybrid matrix are the main semisynthetic polymers applied as dermal substitutes for skin regeneration: PCL nanofiber membranes coated with collagen exhibited good cell adhesion, proliferation, and migration of fibroblasts into the nanofibrous matrix (Venugopal and Ramakrishna, 2005a); collagen–PGA hybrid matrix with bFGF accelerated angiogenesis and granulation tissue formation of full-thickness skin defects on the back of type 2 diabetic Lepr(db) mice (Nagato et al., 2006).

Synthetic polymers include different scaffolds (PLGA, PLLA, PCL, PEG) used for wound healing and growth factor encapsulation: electrospun-nanofibrous polymeric bandages highlighting AWD effects against diabetic skin ulcers (Zahedi et al., 2010); *in vivo* wound healing of diabetic ulcers using PCL/PEG electrospun nanofibers immobilized with human EGF, increasing proliferation and phenotypic expression of keratinocytes (Choi et al., 2008); promotion of skin regeneration in diabetic rats by electrospun cyclodextrin/PEG–PLLA core-sheath fibers loaded with bFGF, enhancing cell adhesion, proliferation, and secretion of ECM (Yang et al., 2011); biocompatible and bioactive EGF-loaded PLGA nanofibrous scaffold obtained through emulsion electrospinning technique, for skin TE applications (Norouzi et al., 2015).

4.6 CONCLUSIONS AND FUTURE PERSPECTIVES

TE, an interdisciplinary area linking chemistry, engineering, biology, and medicine, aims to reconstruct damaged tissues or organs starting from natural and synthetic nanobiomaterials. Due to modern fabrication techniques (molecular self-assembly, phase separation, electrospinning), biocompatible and biodegradable polymeric nanomaterials have many advantages, such as synthetic versatility and precise control of the size, shape, surface geometry, mechanical strength, composition, and physicochemical stability. Also, nanopolymeric scaffolds can mimic ECM, thus interacting with natural tissues and better supporting tissue regeneration. Nanotechnology, TE, and RM are highly topical scientific fields in which future researches are mandatory, focused on improving the biocompatibility and decreasing the toxicity of nanobiomaterials.

ACKNOWLEDGMENTS

This paper was partially supported by the Sectoral Operational Programme Human Resources Development, financed from the European Social Fund and by the Romanian Government under the contract number POSDRU/89/1.5/S/64153.

REFERENCES

Abruzzo, A., Fiorica, C., Palumbo, V.D., Altomare, R., Damiano, G., Gioviale, M.C., et al., 2014. Using polymeric scaffolds for vascular tissue engineering. Int. J. Polym. Sci. 2014, 689390.

Ahmed, T.A., Hincke, M.T., 2010. Strategies for articular cartilage lesion repair and functional restoration. Tissue Eng. B Rev. 16 (3), 305–329.

Ai, J., Kiasat-Dolatabadi, A., Ebrahimi-Barough, S., Ai, A., Lotfibakhshaiesh, N., Norouzi-Javidan, A., et al., 2014. Polymeric scaffolds in neural tissue engineering: a review. Arch. Neurosci. 1 (1), 15–20.

Altman, G.H., Horan, R.L., Lu, H.H., Moreau, J., Martin, I., Richmond, J.C., et al., 2002. Silk matrix for tissue engineered anterior cruciate ligaments. Biomaterials 23 (20), 4131–4141.

Altman, G.H., Diaz, F., Jakuba, C., Calabro, T., Horan, R.L., Chen, J., et al., 2003. Silk-based biomaterials. Biomaterials 24 (3), 401–416.

Alves da Silva, M.L., Martins, A., Costa-Pinto, A.R., Costa, P., Faria, S., Gomes, M., et al., 2010. Cartilage tissue engineering using electrospun PCL nanofiber meshes and MSCs. Biomacromolecules 11 (12), 3228–3236.

Angeloni, N.L., Bond, C.W., Tang, Y., Harrington, D.A., Zhang, S., Stupp, S.I., et al., 2011. Regeneration of the cavernous nerve by Sonic hedgehog using aligned peptide amphiphile nanofibers. Biomaterials 32 (4), 1091–1101.

Aubin, H., Nichol, J.W., Hutson, C.B., Bae, H., Sieminski, A.L., Cropek, D.M., et al., 2010. Directed 3D cell alignment and elongation in microengineered hydrogels. Biomaterials 31 (27), 6941–6951.

Awad, H.A., Wickham, M.Q., Leddy, H.A., Gimble, J.M., Guilak, F., 2004. Chondrogenic differentiation of adipose-derived adult stem cells in agarose, alginate, and gelatin scaffolds. Biomaterials 25 (16), 3211–3222.

Bellincampi, L.D., Closkey, R.F., Prasad, R., Zawadsky, J.P., Dunn, M.G., 1998. Viability of fibroblast-seeded ligament analogs after autogenous implantation. J. Orthop. Res. 16 (4), 414–420.

Berthiaume, F., Maguire, T.J., Yarmush, M.L., 2011. Tissue engineering and regenerative medicine: history, progress, and challenges. Annu. Rev. Chem. Biomol. Eng. 2, 403–430.

Bhardwaj, N., Sow, W.T., Devi, D., Ng, K.W., Mandal, B.B., Cho, N.J., 2015. Silk fibroin-keratin based 3D scaffolds as a dermal substitute for skin tissue engineering. Integr. Biol. (Camb) 7 (1), 53–63.

Biazar, E., Khorasani, M.T., Montazeri, N., Pourshamsian, K., Daliri, M., Rezaei, M., et al., 2010. Types of neural guides and using nanotechnology for peripheral nerve reconstruction. Int. J. Nanomed. 5, 839–852.

Bichara, D.A., Zhao, X., Bodugoz-Senturk, H., Ballyns, F.P., Oral, E., Randolph, M.A., et al., 2011. Porous poly(vinyl alcohol)-hydrogel matrix-engineered biosynthetic cartilage. Tissue Eng. A 17 (3–4), 301–309.

Bini, T.B., Gao, S., Tan, T.C., Wang, S., Lim, A., Hai, L.B., et al., 2004. Electrospun poly (L-lactide-*co*-glycolide) biodegradable polymer nanofibre tubes for peripheral nerve regeneration. Nanotechnology 15 (11), 1459.

Boffito, M., Sartori, S., Ciardelli, G., 2014. Polymeric scaffolds for cardiac tissue engineering: requirements and fabrication technologies. Polym. Int. 63 (1), 2–11.

Bonnans, C., Chou, J., Werb, Z., 2014. Remodelling the extracellular matrix in development and disease. Nat. Rev. Mol. Cell Biol. 15 (12), 786–801.

Bosnakovski, D., Mizuno, M., Kim, G., Takagi, S., Okumura, M., Fujinaga, T., 2006. Chondrogenic differentiation of bovine bone marrow mesenchymal stem cells (MSCs) in different hydrogels: influence of collagen type II extracellular matrix on MSC chondrogenesis. Biotechnol. Bioeng. 93 (6), 1152–1163.

Böttcher-Haberzeth, S., Biedermann, T., Reichmann, E., 2010. Tissue engineering of skin. Burns 36 (4), 450–460.

Briggs, T., Arinzeh, T.L., 2011. Growth factor delivery from electrospun materials. J. Biomater. Tissue Eng. 1 (2), 129–138.

Briggs, T., Arinzeh, T.L., 2014. Examining the formulation of emulsion electrospinning for improving the release of bioactive proteins from electrospun fibers. J. Biomed. Mater. Res. A 102 (3), 674–684.

Bryant, S.J., Bender, R.J., Durand, K.L., Anseth, K.S., 2004. Encapsulating chondrocytes in degrading PEG hydrogels with high modulus: engineering gel structural changes to facilitate cartilaginous tissue production. Biotechnol. Bioeng. 86 (7), 747–755.

Bryant, S.J., Nicodemus, G.D., Villanueva, I., 2008. Designing 3D photopolymer hydrogels to regulate biomechanical cues and tissue growth for cartilage tissue engineering. Pharm. Res. 25 (10), 2379–2386.

Burdick, J.A., Ward, M., Liang, E., Young, M.J., Langer, R., 2006. Stimulation of neurite outgrowth by neurotrophins delivered from degradable hydrogels. Biomaterials 27 (3), 452–459.

Catto, V., Farè, S., Freddi, G., Tanzi, M.C., 2014. Vascular tissue engineering: recent advances in small diameter blood vessel regeneration. ISRN Vasc. Med. 2014, 923030.

Chan, J.M., Zhang, L., Tong, R., Ghosh, D., Gao, W., Liao, G., et al., 2010. Spatiotemporal controlled delivery of nanoparticles to injured vasculature. Proc. Natl. Acad. Sci. U.S.A. 107 (5), 2213–2218.

Chang, W.C., Kliot, M., Sretavan, D.W., 2008. Microtechnology and nanotechnology in nerve repair. Neurol. Res. 30 (10), 1053–1062.

Chao, P.H.G., Yodmuang, S., Wang, X., Sun, L., Kaplan, D.L., Vunjak-Novakovic, G., 2010. Silk hydrogel for cartilage tissue engineering. J. Biomed. Mater. Res. B Appl. Biomater. 95 (1), 84–90.

Chen, G., Sato, T., Sakane, M., Ohgushi, H., Ushida, T., Tanaka, J., et al., 2004. Application of PLGA-collagen hybrid mesh for three-dimensional culture of canine anterior cruciate ligament cells. Mater. Sci. Eng. C 24 (6–8), 861–866.

Chen, J., Altman, G.H., Karageorgiou, V., Horan, R., Collette, A., Volloch, V., et al., 2003. Human bone marrow stromal cell and ligament fibroblast responses on RGD-modified silk fibers. J. Biomed. Mater. Res. A 67 (2), 559–570.

Chen, X., Qi, Y.Y., Wang, L.L., Yin, Z., Yin, G.L., Zou, X.H., et al., 2008. Ligament regeneration using a knitted silk scaffold combined with collagen matrix. Biomaterials 29 (27), 3683–3692.

Chen, Y., Bilgen, B., Pareta, R.A., Myles, A.J., Fenniri, H., Ciombor, D.M., et al., 2010. Self-assembled rosette nanotube/hydrogel composites for cartilage tissue engineering. Tissue Eng., Part C 16 (6), 1233–1243.

Chen, J.P., Su, C.H., 2011. Surface modification of electrospun PLLA nanofibers by plasma treatment and cationized gelatin immobilization for cartilage tissue engineering. Acta Biomater. 7 (1), 234–243.

Chen, Q.Z., Harding, S.E., Ali, N.N., Lyon, A.R., Boccaccini, A.R., 2008. Biomaterials in cardiac tissue engineering: ten years of research survey. Mater. Sci. Eng. R Rep. 59 (1–6), 1–37.

Chew, S.Y., Mi, R., Hoke, A., Leong, K.W., 2007. Aligned protein–polymer composite fibers enhance nerve regeneration: a potential tissue-engineering platform. Adv. Funct. Mater. 17 (8), 1288–1296.

Chiu, L.L.Y., Radisic, M., 2013. Cardiac tissue engineering. Curr. Opin. Chem. Eng. 2 (1), 41–52.

Choi, J.S., Leong, K.W., Yoo, H.S., 2008. *In vivo* wound healing of diabetic ulcers using electrospun nanofibers immobilized with human epidermal growth factor (EGF). Biomaterials 29 (5), 587–596.

Chrissafis, K., Paraskevopoulos, K.M., Jannakoudakis, A., Beslikas, T., Bikiaris, D., 2010. Oxidized multiwalled carbon nanotubes as effective reinforcement and thermal stability agents of poly(lactic acid) ligaments. J. Appl. Polym. Sci. 118 (5), 2712–2721.

Chung, C., Burdick, J.A., 2008. Engineering cartilage tissue. Adv. Drug Deliv. Rev. 60 (2), 243–262.

Chung, C., Burdick, J.A., 2009. Influence of three-dimensional hyaluronic acid microenvironments on mesenchymal stem cell chondrogenesis. Tissue Eng. A 15 (2), 243–254.

Cleary, M.A., Geiger, E., Grady, C., Best, C., Naito, Y., Breuer, C., 2012. Vascular tissue engineering: the next generation. Trends Mol. Med. 18 (7), 394–404.

Cleland, J.L., Duenas, E.T., Park, A., Daugherty, A., Kahn, J., Kowalski, J., et al., 2001. Development of poly-(D,L-lactide-*co*-glycolide) microsphere formulations containing recombinant human vascular endothelial growth factor to promote local angiogenesis. J. Controlled Release 72 (1–3), 13–24.

Corey, J.M., Gertz, C.C., Wang, B.S., Birrell, L.K., Johnson, S.L., Martin, D.C., et al., 2008. The design of electrospun PLLA nanofiber scaffolds compatible with serum-free growth of primary motor and sensory neurons. Acta Biomater. 4 (4), 863–875.

Cristino, S., Grassi, F., Toneguzzi, S., Piacentini, A., Grigolo, B., Santi, S., et al., 2005. Analysis of mesenchymal stem cells grown on a three-dimensional HYAFF 11-based prototype ligament scaffold. J. Biomed. Mater. Res. A 73 (3), 275–283.

Cui, W., Zhou, Y., Chang, J., 2010. Electrospun nanofibrous materials for tissue engineering and drug delivery. Sci. Technol. Adv. Mater. 11 (1), 014108.

Cunha, C., Panseri, S., Antonini, S., 2011. Emerging nanotechnology approaches in tissue engineering for peripheral nerve regeneration. Nanomedicine 7 (1), 50–59.

Ding, T., Lu, W.W., Zheng, Y., Li, Z.Y., Pan, H.B., Luo, Z., 2011. Rapid repair of rat sciatic nerve injury using a nanosilver-embedded collagen scaffold coated with laminin and fibronectin. Regen. Med. 6 (4), 437–447.

Dunn, M.G., Liesch, J.B., Tiku, M.L., Zawadsky, J.P., 1995. Development of fibroblast-seeded ligament analogs for ACL reconstruction. J. Biomed. Mater. Res. 29 (11), 1363–1371.

Dvir, T., Timko, B.P., Brigham, M.D., Naik, S.R., Karajanagi, S.S., Levy, O., et al., 2011. Nanowired three-dimensional cardiac patches. Nat. Nanotechnol. 6 (11), 720–725.

Elisseeff, J., Anseth, K., Sims, D., McIntosh, W., Randolph, M., Yaremchuk, M., et al., 1999. Transdermal photopolymerization of poly(ethylene oxide)-based injectable hydrogels for tissue-engineered cartilage. Plast. Reconstr. Surg. 104 (4), 1014–1022.

Everts, P.A., Knape, J.T., Weibrich, G., Schönberger, J.P., Hoffmann, J., Overdevest, E.P., et al., 2006. Platelet-rich plasma and platelet gel: a review. J. Extra-Corpor. Technol. 38 (2), 174–187.

Fallouh, L., Nakagawa, K., Sasho, T., Arai, M., Kitahara, S., Wada, Y., et al., 2010. Effects of autologous platelet-rich plasma on cell viability and collagen synthesis in injured human anterior cruciate ligament. J. Bone Jt. Surg., Am. Vol. 92 (18), 2909–2916.

Fernandes, H., Moroni, L., van Blitterswijk, C., de Boer, J., 2009. Extracellular matrix and tissue engineering applications. J. Mater. Chem. 19 (31), 5474–5484.

Fisher, M.B., Mauck, R.L., 2013. Tissue engineering and regenerative medicine: recent innovations and the transition to translation. Tissue Eng. B Rev. 19 (1), 1–13.

Gelain, F., Bottai, D., Vescovi, A., Zhang, S., 2006. Designer self-assembling peptide nanofiber scaffolds for adult mouse neural stem cell 3-dimensional cultures. PLoS One 1, e119.

Georgiadis, V., Knight, R.A., Jayasinghe, S.N., Stephanou, A., 2014. Cardiac tissue engineering: renewing the arsenal for the battle against heart disease. Integr. Biol. (Camb) 6 (2), 111–126.

Ghasemi-Mobarakeh, L., Prabhakaran, M.P., Morshed, M., Nasr-Esfahani, M.H., Ramakrishna, S., 2008. Electrospun poly(ε-caprolactone)/gelatin nanofibrous scaffolds for nerve tissue engineering. Biomaterials 29 (34), 4532–4539.

Goldberg, M., Langer, R., Jia, X., 2007. Nanostructured materials for applications in drug delivery and tissue engineering. J. Biomater. Sci. Polym. Ed. 18 (3), 241–268.

Gonçalves, N.P., Oliveira, H., Pêgo, A.P., Saraiva, M.J., 2012. A novel nanoparticle delivery system for *in vivo* targeting of the sciatic nerve: impact on regeneration. Nanomedicine (Lond) 7 (8), 1167–1180.

Groeber, F., Holeiter, M., Hampel, M., Hinderer, S., Schenke-Layland, K., 2011. Skin tissue engineering—*in vivo* and *in vitro* applications. Adv. Drug Deliv. Rev. 63 (4–5), 352–366.

Gui, L., Niklason, L.E., 2014. Vascular tissue engineering: building perfusable vasculature for implantation. Curr. Opin. Chem. Eng. 3, 68–74.

Guo, J., Su, H., Zeng, Y., Liang, Y.X., Wong, W.M., Ellis-Behnke, R.G., et al., 2007. Reknitting the injured spinal cord by self-assembling peptide nanofiber scaffold. Nanomedicine 3 (4), 311–321.

Harrison, R.H., St-Pierre, J.P., Stevens, M.M., 2014. Tissue engineering and regenerative medicine: a year in review. Tissue. Eng. B Rev. 20 (1), 1–16.

Harrison, S.L., Vavken, P., Murray, M.M., 2011. Erythrocytes inhibit ligament fibroblast proliferation in a collagen scaffold. J. Orthop. Res. 29 (9), 1361–1366.

Hasirci, V., Vrana, E., Zorlutuna, P., Ndreu, A., Yilgor, P., Basmanav, F.B., et al., 2006. Nanobiomaterials: a review of the existing science and technology and new approaches. J. Biomater. Sci. Polym. Ed. 17 (11), 1241–1268.

Hirt, M.N., Hansen, A., Eschenhagen, T., 2014. Cardiac tissue engineering: state of the art. Circ. Res. 114 (2), 354–367.

Ho, S.T.B., Ekaputra, A.K., Hui, J.H., Hutmacher, D.W., 2010. An electrospun polycaprolactone–collagen membrane for the resurfacing of cartilage defects. Polym. Int. 59 (6), 808–817.

Holmes, T.C., de Lacalle, S., Su, X., Liu, G., Rich, A., Zhang, S., 2000. Extensive neurite outgrowth and active synapse formation on self-assembling peptide scaffolds. Proc. Natl. Acad. Sci. U.S.A. 97 (12), 6728–6733.

Houweling, D.A., Lankhorst, A.J., Gispen, W.H., Bär, P.R., Joosten, E.A.J., 1998. Collagen containing neurotrophin-3 (NT-3) attracts regrowing injured corticospinal axons in the adult rat spinal cord and promotes partial functional recovery. Exp. Neurol. 153 (1), 49–59.

Hu, A., Zuo, B., Zhang, F., Lan, Q., Zhang, H., 2012. Electrospun silk fibroin nanofibers promote Schwann cell adhesion, growth and proliferation. Neural. Regen. Res. 7 (15), 1171–1178.

Hu, J., Feng, K., Liu, X., Ma, P.X., 2009. Chondrogenic and osteogenic differentiations of human bone marrow-derived mesenchymal stem cells on a nanofibrous scaffold with designed pore network. Biomaterials 30 (28), 5061–5067.

Hu, X., Li, D., Gao, C., 2011. Chemically cross-linked chitosan hydrogel loaded with gelatin for chondrocyte encapsulation. Biotechnol. J. 6 (11), 1388–1396.

Huang, S., Xu, Y., Wu, C., Sha, D., Fu, X., 2010. *In vitro* constitution and *in vivo* implantation of engineered skin constructs with sweat glands. Biomaterials 31 (21), 5520–5525.

Hubmacher, D., Apte, S.S., 2013. The biology of the extracellular matrix: novel insights. Curr. Opin. Rheumatol. 25 (1), 65–70.

Huyer, L.D., Montgomery, M., Zhao, Y., Xiao, Y., Conant, G., Korolj, A., et al., 2015. Biomaterial based cardiac tissue engineering and its applications. Biomed. Mater. 10 (3), 034004.

Iannotti, C., Li, H., Yan, P., Lu, X., Wirthlin, L., Xu, X.M., 2003. Glial cell line-derived neurotrophic factor-enriched bridging transplants promote propriospinal axonal regeneration and enhance myelination after spinal cord injury. Exp. Neurol. 183 (2), 379–393.

Illingworth, K.D., Musahl, V., Lorenz, S.G.F., Fu, F.H., 2010. Use of fibrin clot in the knee. Oper. Tech. Orthop. 20 (2), 90–97.

Jin, G.Z., Kim, M., Shin, U.S., Kim, H.W., 2011. Neurite outgrowth of dorsal root ganglia neurons is enhanced on aligned nanofibrous biopolymer scaffold with carbon nanotube coating. Neurosci. Lett. 501 (1), 10–14.

Ju, Y.M., Choi, J.S., Atala, A., Yoo, J.J., Lee, S.J., 2010. Bilayered scaffold for engineering cellularized blood vessels. Biomaterials 31 (15), 4313–4321.

Kakinoki, S., Uchida, S., Ehashi, T., Murakami, A., Yamaoka, T., 2011. Surface modification of poly(L-lactic acid) nanofiber with oligo(D-lactic acid) bioactive-peptide conjugates for peripheral nerve regeneration. Polymers 3 (2), 820–832.

Kessler, M.W., Grande, D.A., 2008. Tissue engineering and cartilage. Organogenesis 4 (1), 28–32.

Kessler, M.W., Ackerman, G., Dines, J.S., Grande, D., 2008. Emerging technologies and fourth generation issues in cartilage repair. Sports Med. Arthrosc. 16 (4), 246–254.

Khademhosseini, A., Langer, R., 2006. Nanobiotechnology. Drug delivery and tissue engineering. Chem. Eng. Prog. 102 (2), 38–42.

Khaing, Z.Z., Schmidt, C.E., 2012. Advances in natural biomaterials for nerve tissue repair. Neurosci. Lett. 519 (2), 103–114.

Kijeńska, E., Prabhakaran, M.P., Swieszkowski, W., Kurzydlowski, K.J., Ramakrishna, S., 2012. Electrospun bio-composite P(LLA-CL)/collagen I/collagen III scaffolds for nerve tissue engineering. J. Biomed. Mater. Res. B Appl. Biomater. 100 (4), 1093–1102.

Kim, K., Fisher, J.P., 2007. Nanoparticle technology in bone tissue engineering. J. Drug Target 15 (4), 241–252.

Kim, S.H., Park, D.Y., Min, B.H., 2012. A new era of cartilage repair using cell therapy and tissue engineering: turning current clinical limitations into new ideas. Tissue Eng. Regen. Med. 9 (5), 240–248.

Kisiday, J., Jin, M., Kurz, B., Hung, H., Semino, C., Zhang, S., et al., 2002. Self-assembling peptide hydrogel fosters chondrocyte extracellular matrix production and cell division: implications for cartilage tissue repair. Proc. Natl. Acad. Sci. U.S.A. 99 (15), 9996–10001.

Kokai, L.E., Ghaznavi, A.M., Marra, K.G., 2010. Incorporation of double-walled microspheres into polymer nerve guides for the sustained delivery of glial cell line-derived neurotrophic factor. Biomaterials 31 (8), 2313–2322.

Kopesky, P.W., Vanderploeg, E.J., Sandy, J.S., Kurz, B., Grodzinsky, A.J., 2010. Self-assembling peptide hydrogels modulate *in vitro* chondrogenesis of bovine bone marrow stromal cells. Tissue Eng. A 16 (2), 465–477.

Koria, P., Yagi, H., Kitagawa, Y., Megeed, Z., Nahmias, Y., Sheridan, R., et al., 2011. Self-assembling elastin-like peptides growth factor chimeric nanoparticles for the treatment of chronic wounds. Proc. Natl. Acad. Sci. U.S.A. 18 (3), 1034–1039.

Kuo, C.K., Li, W.J., Mauck, R.L., Tuan, R.S., 2006. Cartilage tissue engineering: its potential and uses. Curr. Opin. Rheumatol. 18 (1), 64–73.

Kuo, C.K., Marturano, J.E., Tuan, R.S., 2010. Novel strategies in tendon and ligament tissue engineering: advanced biomaterials and regeneration motifs. Sports Med. Arthrosc. Rehabil. Ther. Technol. 2, 20.

Kurakhmaeva, K.B., Voronina, T.A., Kapica, I.G., Kreuter, J., Nerobkova, L.N., Seredenin, S.B., et al., 2008. Antiparkinsonian effect of nerve growth factor adsorbed on polybutylcyanoacrylate nanoparticles coated with polysorbate-80. Bull. Exp. Biol. Med. 145 (2), 259–262.

Langer, R., Vacanti, J.P., 1993. Tissue engineering. Science 260 (5110), 920–926.

Laurencin, C.T., Freeman, J.W., 2005. Ligament tissue engineering: an evolutionary materials science approach. Biomaterials 26 (36), 7530–7536.

Leach, M.K., Feng, Z.Q., Gertz, C.C., Tuck, S.J., Regan, T.M., Naim, Y., et al., 2011. The culture of primary motor and sensory neurons in defined media on electrospun poly-L-lactide nanofiber scaffolds. J. Vis. Exp. 48, e2389.

Lee, A.C., Yu, V.M., Lowe III, J.B., Brenner, M.J., Hunter, D.A., Mackinnon, S.E., et al., 2003. Controlled release of nerve growth factor enhances sciatic nerve regeneration. Exp. Neurol. 184 (1), 295–303.

Lee, J.Y., Bashur, C.A., Goldstein, A.S., Schmidt, C.E., 2009. Polypyrrole-coated electrospun PLGA nanofibers for neural tissue applications. Biomaterials 30 (26), 4325–4335.

Lee, K.Y., Jeong, L., Kang, Y.O., Lee, S.J., Park, W.H., 2009. Electrospinning of polysaccharides for regenerative medicine. Adv. Drug Deliv. Rev. 61 (12), 1020–1032.

Leroy, A., Nottelet, B., Bony, C., Pinese, C., Charlot, B., Garric, X., et al., 2015. PLA-poloxamer/poloxamine copolymers for ligament tissue engineering: sound macromolecular design for degradable scaffolds and MSC differentiation. Biomater. Sci. 3 (4), 617–626.

Li, K.C., Hu, Y.C., 2015. Cartilage tissue engineering: recent advances and perspectives from gene regulation/therapy. Adv. Healthcare Mater. 4 (7), 948–968.

Li, S., Wu, H., Hu, X.D., Tu, C.Q., Pei, F.X., Wang, G.L., et al., 2012. Preparation of electrospun PLGA-silk fibroin nanofibers-based nerve conduits and evaluation *in vivo*. Artif. Cells Blood Substit. Immobil. Biotechnol. 40 (1–2), 171–178.

Li, S., Sengupta, D., Chien, S., 2014. Vascular tissue engineering: from *in vitro* to *in situ*. Wiley Interdiscip Rev. Syst. Biol. Med. 6 (1), 61–76.

Li, W.J., Tuli, R., Okafor, C., Derfoul, A., Danielson, K.G., Hall, D.J., et al., 2005. A three-dimensional nanofibrous scaffold for cartilage tissue engineering using human mesenchymal stem cells. Biomaterials 26 (6), 599–609.

Liu, H., Ding, X., Zhou, G., Li, P., Wei, X., Fan, Y., 2013. Electrospinning of nanofibers for tissue engineering applications. J. Nanomater. 2013, 495708.

Liu, T., Teng, W.K., Chan, B.P., Chew, S.Y., 2010. Photochemical cross-linked electrospun collagen nanofibers: synthesis, characterization and neural stem cell interactions. J. Biomed. Mater. Res. A 95 (1), 276–282.

Liu, T., Xu, J., Chan, B.P., Chew, S.Y., 2012. Sustained release of neurotrophin-3 and chondroitinase ABC from electrospun collagen nanofiber scaffold for spinal cord injury repair. J. Biomed. Mater. Res. A 100 (1), 236–242.

Liu, Y., Cai, S., Shu, X.Z., Shelby, J., Prestwich, G.D., 2007. Release of basic fibroblast growth factor from a crosslinked glycosaminoglycan hydrogel promotes wound healing. Wound Repair Regen. 15 (2), 245–251.

Liu, S.Q., Tian, Q., Wang, L., Hedrick, J.L., Hui, J.H., Yang, Y.Y., et al., 2010. Injectable biodegradable poly(ethylene glycol)/RGD peptide hybrid hydrogels for *in vitro* chondrogenesis of human mesenchymal stem cells. Macromol. Rapid Commun. 31 (13), 1148–1154.

Lu, G., Sheng, B., Wei, Y., Wang, G., Zhang, L., Ao, Q., et al., 2008. Collagen nanofiber-covered porous biodegradable carboxymethyl chitosan microcarriers for tissue engineering cartilage. Eur. Polym. J. 44 (9), 2820–2829.

Lu, H., Feng, Z., Gu, Z., Liu, C., 2009. Growth of outgrowth endothelial cells on aligned PLLA nanofibrous scaffolds. J. Mater. Sci. Mater. Med. 20 (9), 1937–1944.

Lu, Z., Doulabi, B.Z., Huang, C., Bank, R.A., Helder, M.N., 2010. Collagen type II enhances chondrogenesis in adipose tissue-derived stem cells by affecting cell shape. Tissue Eng. A 16 (1), 81–90.

Lu, H.H., Cooper Jr., J.A., Manuel, S., Freeman, J.W., Attawia, M.A., Ko, F.K., et al., 2005. Anterior cruciate ligament regeneration using braided biodegradable scaffolds: *in vitro* optimization studies. Biomaterials 26 (23), 4805–4816.

Ma, Z., Kotaki, M., Yong, T., He, W., Ramakrishna, S., 2005. Surface engineering of electrospun polyethylene terephthalate (PET) nanofibers towards development of a new material for blood vessel engineering. Biomaterials 26 (15), 2527–2536.

Mackle, J.N., Blond, D.J., Mooney, E., McDonnell, C., Blau, W.J., Shaw, G., et al., 2011. *In vitro* characterization of an electroactive carbon-nanotube-based nanofiber scaffold for tissue engineering. Macromol. Biosci. 11 (9), 1272–1282.

Madden, L.R., Mortisen, D.J., Sussman, E.M., Dupras, S.K., Fugate, J.A., Cuy, J.L., et al., 2010. Proangiogenic scaffolds as functional templates for cardiac tissue engineering. Proc. Natl. Acad. Sci. U.S.A. 107 (34), 15211–15216.

Majima, T., Funakosi, T., Iwasaki, N., Yamane, S.T., Harada, K., Nonaka, S., et al., 2005. Alginate and chitosan polyion complex hybrid fibers for scaffolds in ligament and tendon tissue engineering. J. Orthop. Sci. 10 (3), 302–307.

Makris, E.A., Gomoll, A.H., Malizos, K.N., Hu, J.C., Athanasiou, K.A., 2015. Repair and tissue engineering techniques for articular cartilage. Nat. Rev. Rheumatol. 11 (1), 21–34.

Mammadov, B., Mammadov, R., Guler, M.O., Tekinay, A.B., 2012. Cooperative effect of heparan sulfate and laminin mimetic peptide nanofibers on the promotion of neurite outgrowth. Acta Biomater. 8 (6), 2077–2086.

Martins, A.M., Eng, G., Caridade, S.G., Mano, J.F., Reis, R.L., Vunjak-Novakovic, G., 2014. Electrically conductive chitosan/carbon scaffolds for cardiac tissue engineering. Biomacromolecules 15 (2), 635–643.

Mei, F., Zhong, J., Yang, X., Ouyang, X., Zhang, S., Hu, X., et al., 2007. Improved biological characteristics of poly(L-lactic acid) electrospun membrane by incorporation of multiwalled carbon nanotubes/hydroxyapatite nanoparticles. Biomacromolecules 8 (12), 3729–3735.

Mi, F.L., Shyu, S.S., Wu, Y.B., Lee, S.T., Shyong, J.Y., Huang, R.N., 2001. Fabrication and characterization of a sponge-like asymmetric chitosan membrane as a wound dressing. Biomaterials 22 (2), 165–173.

Mittnacht, U., Hartmann, H., Hein, S., Oliveira, H., Dong, M., Pêgo, A.P., et al., 2010. Chitosan/siRNA nanoparticles biofunctionalize nerve implants and enable neurite outgrowth. Nano Lett. 10 (10), 3933–3939.

Mo, X., Weber, H.J., 2004. Electrospinning P (LLA-CL) nanofiber: a tubular scaffold fabrication with circumferential alignment. Special Issue: Contributions from 6th Austrian Polymer Meeting. Macromol. Symp. 217 (1), 413–416.

Mohd Hilmi, A.B., Halim, A.S., 2015. Vital roles of stem cells and biomaterials in skin tissue engineering. World J. Stem Cells 7 (2), 428–436.

Mouw, J.K., Case, N.D., Guldberg, R.E., Plaas, A.H., Levenston, M.E., 2005. Variations in matrix composition and GAG fine structure among scaffolds for cartilage tissue engineering. Osteoarthritis Cartilage 13 (9), 828–836.

Mukhatyar, V.J., Salmerón-Sánchez, M., Rudra, S., Mukhopadaya, S., Barker, T.H., García, A.J., et al., 2011. Role of fibronectin in topographical guidance of neurite extension on electrospun fibers. Biomaterials 32 (16), 3958–3968.

Murray, M.M., Spindler, K.P., Devin, C., Snyder, B.S., Muller, J., Takahashi, M., et al., 2006. Use of a collagen-platelet rich plasma scaffold to stimulate healing of a central defect in the canine ACL. J. Orthop. Res. 24 (4), 820–830.

Murray, M.M., Spindler, K.P., Ballard, P., Welch, T.P., Zurakowski, D., Nanney, L.B., 2007a. Enhanced histologic repair in a central wound in the anterior cruciate ligament with a collagen-platelet-rich plasma scaffold. J. Orthop. Res. 25 (8), 1007–1017.

Murray, M.M., Spindler, K.P., Abreu, E., Muller, J.A., Nedder, A., Kelly, M., et al., 2007b. Collagen-platelet rich plasma hydrogel enhances primary repair of the porcine anterior cruciate ligament. J. Orthop. Res. 25 (1), 81–91.

Murray, M.M., Magarian, E., Zurakowski, D., Fleming, B.C., 2010. Bone-to-bone fixation enhances functional healing of the porcine anterior cruciate ligament using a collagen-platelet composite. Arthroscopy 26 (9 Suppl.), S49–S57.

Nagato, H., Umebayashi, Y., Wako, M., Tabata, Y., Manabe, M., 2006. Collagen-poly glycolic acid hybrid matrix with basic fibroblast growth factor accelerated angiogenesis and granulation tissue formation in diabetic mice. J. Dermatol. 33 (10), 670–675.

Naito, Y., Shinoka, T., Duncan, D., Hibino, N., Solomon, D., Cleary, M., et al., 2011. Vascular tissue engineering: towards the next generation vascular grafts. Adv. Drug Deliv. Rev. 63 (4–5), 312–323.

Nau, T., Teuschl, A., 2015. Regeneration of the anterior cruciate ligament: current strategies in tissue engineering. World J. Orthop. 6 (1), 127–136.

Nettles, D.L., Vail, T.P., Morgan, M.T., Grinstaff, M.W., Setton, L.A., 2004. Photocrosslinkable hyaluronan as a scaffold for articular cartilage repair. Ann. Biomed. Eng. 32 (3), 391–397.

Nichol, J.W., Koshy, S.T., Bae, H., Hwang, C.M., Yamanlar, S., Khademhosseini, A., 2010. Cell-laden microengineered gelatin methacrylate hydrogels. Biomaterials 31 (21), 5536–5544.

Norouzi, M., Shabani, I., Atyabi, F., Soleimani, M., 2015. EGF-loaded nanofibrous scaffold for skin tissue engineering applications. Fibers Polym. 16 (4), 782–787.

Obara, K., Ishihara, M., Ishizuka, T., Fujita, M., Ozeki, Y., Maehara, T., et al., 2003. Photocrosslinkable chitosan hydrogel containing fibroblast growth factor-2 stimulates wound healing in healing-impaired db/db mice. Biomaterials 24 (20), 3437–3444.

Orlova, Y., Magome, N., Liu, L., Chen, Y., Agladze, K., 2011. Electrospun nanofibers as a tool for architecture control in engineered cardiac tissue. Biomaterials 32 (24), 5615–5624.

Panseri, S., Cunha, C., Lowery, J., Del Carro, U., Taraballi, F., Amadio, S., et al., 2008. Electrospun micro- and nanofiber tubes for functional nervous regeneration in sciatic nerve transections. BMC Biotechnology 8, 39.

Park, J.S., Woo, D.G., Sun, B.K., Chung, H.M., Im, S.J., Choi, Y.M., et al., 2007. *In vitro* and *in vivo* test of PEG/PCL-based hydrogel scaffold for cell delivery application. J. Control. Release 124 (1–2), 51–59.

Park, C.J., Clark, S.G., Lichtensteiger, C.A., Jamison, R.D., Johnson, A.J.W., 2009a. Accelerated wound closure of pressure ulcers in aged mice by chitosan scaffolds with and without bFGF. Acta Biomater. 5 (6), 1926–1936.

Park, K.H., Kim, H., Na, K., 2009b. Neuronal differentiation of PC12 cells cultured on growth factor-loaded nanoparticles coated on PLGA microspheres. J. Microbiol. Biotechnol. 19 (11), 1490–1495.

Park, K.H., Lee, D.H., Na, K., 2009c. Transplantation of poly(*N*-isopropylacrylamide-*co*-vinylimidazole) hydrogel constructs composed of rabbit chondrocytes and growth factor-loaded nanoparticles for neocartilage formation. Biotechnol. Lett. 31 (3), 337–346.

Park, K.M., Joung, Y.K., Park, K.D., Lee, S.Y., Lee, M.C., 2008. RGD-conjugated chitosan-pluronic hydrogels as a cell supported scaffold for articular cartilage regeneration. Macromol. Res. 16 (6), 517–523.

Park, S.H., Park, S.R., Chung, S.I., Pai, K.S., Min, B.H., 2005. Tissue-engineered cartilage using fibrin/hyaluronan composite gel and its *in vivo* implantation. Artif. Organs 29 (10), 838–845.

Petrigliano, F.A., McAllister, D.R., Wu, B.M., 2006. Tissue engineering for anterior cruciate ligament reconstruction: a review of current strategies. Arthroscopy 22 (4), 441–451.

Prabhakaran, M.P., Ghasemi-Mobarakeh, L., Jin, G., Ramakrishna, S., 2011. Electrospun conducting polymer nanofibers and electrical stimulation of nerve stem cells. J. Biosci. Bioeng. 112 (5), 501–507.

Pradhan, S., Farach-Carson, M.C., 2010. Mining the extracellular matrix for tissue engineering applications. Regen. Med. 5 (6), 961–970.

Radisic, M., Christman, K.L., 2013. Materials science and tissue engineering: repairing the heart. Mayo Clin. Proc. 88 (8), 884–898.

Raghavan, S., Nelson, C.M., Baranski, J.D., Lim, E., Chen, C.S., 2010. Geometrically controlled endothelial tubulogenesis in micropatterned gels. Tissue Eng. A 16 (7), 2255–2263.

Ravi, S., Chaikof, E.L., 2010. Biomaterials for vascular tissue engineering. Regen. Med. 5 (1), 107–120.

Ren, X., Feng, Y., Guo, J., Wang, H., Li, Q., Yang, J., et al., 2015. Surface modification and endothelialization of biomaterials as potential scaffolds for vascular tissue engineering applications. Chem. Soc. Rev. 44 (15), 5680–5742.

Rim, N.G., Shin, C.S., Shin, H., 2013. Current approaches to electrospun nanofibers for tissue engineering. Biomed. Mater. 8 (1), 014102.

Rosso, F., Giordano, A., Barbarisi, M., Barbarisi, A., 2004. From cell-ECM interactions to tissue engineering. J. Cell. Physiol. 199 (2), 174–180.

Sahoo, S., Ouyang, H., Goh, J.C., Tay, T.E., Toh, S.L., 2006. Characterization of a novel polymeric scaffold for potential application in tendon/ligament tissue engineering. Tissue Eng. 12 (1), 91–99.

Sakai, T., Kuno, N., Takamatsu, F., Kimura, E., Kohno, H., Okano, K., et al., 2007. Prolonged protective effect of basic fibroblast growth factor-impregnated nanoparticles in Royal College of Surgeons rats. Invest. Ophthalmol. Vis. Sci. 48 (7), 3381–3387.

Santos, M.I., Tuzlakoglu, K., Fuchs, S., Gomes, M.E., Peters, K., Unger, R.E., et al., 2008. Endothelial cell colonization and angiogenic potential of combined nano- and microfibrous scaffolds for bone tissue engineering. Biomaterials 29 (32), 4306–4313.

Santos, M.I., Unger, R.E., Sousa, R.A., Reis, R.L., Kirkpatrick, C.J., 2009. Crosstalk between osteoblasts and endothelial cells co-cultured on a polycaprolactone-starch scaffold and the *in vitro* development of vascularization. Biomaterials 30 (26), 4407–4415.

Sapir, Y., Kryukov, O., Cohen, S., 2011. Integration of multiple cell-matrix interactions into alginate scaffolds for promoting cardiac tissue regeneration. Biomaterials 32 (7), 1838–1847.

Sapir, Y., Cohen, S., Friedman, G., Polyak, B., 2012. The promotion of *in vitro* vessel-like organization of endothelial cells in magnetically responsive alginate scaffolds. Biomaterials 33 (16), 4100–4109.

Saracino, G.A., Cigognini, D., Silva, D., Caprini, A., Gelain, F., 2013. Nanomaterials design and tests for neural tissue engineering. Chem. Soc. Rev. 42 (1), 225–262.

Schmidt, C.E., Leach, J.B., 2003. Neural tissue engineering: strategies for repair and regeneration. Annu. Rev. Biomed. Eng. 5, 293–347.

Seifu, D.G., Purnama, A., Mequanint, K., Mantovani, D., 2013. Small-diameter vascular tissue engineering. Nat. Rev. Cardiol. 10 (7), 410–421.

Semino, C.E., Kasahara, J., Hayashi, Y., Zhang, S., 2004. Entrapment of migrating hippocampal neural cells in three-dimensional peptide nanofiber scaffold. Tissue Eng. 10 (3–4), 643–655.

Serbo, J.V., Gerecht, S., 2013. Vascular tissue engineering: biodegradable scaffold platforms to promote angiogenesis. Stem Cell Res. Ther. 4 (1), 8.

Shachar, M., Tsur-Gang, O., Dvir, T., Leor, J., Cohen, S., 2011. The effect of immobilized RGD peptide in alginate scaffolds on cardiac tissue engineering. Acta Biomater. 7 (1), 152–162.

Shah, R.N., Shah, N.A., Del Rosario Lim, M.M., Hsieh, C., Nuber, G., Stupp, S.I., 2010. Supramolecular design of self-assembling nanofibers for cartilage regeneration. Proc. Natl. Acad. Sci. U.S.A. 107 (8), 3293–3298.

Shevchenko, R.V., James, S.L., James, S.E., 2010. A review of tissue-engineered skin bioconstructs available for skin reconstruction. J. R. Soc. Interface 7 (43), 229–258.

Shields, K.J., Beckman, M.J., Bowlin, G.L., Wayne, J.S., 2004. Mechanical properties and cellular proliferation of electrospun collagen type II. Tissue Eng. 10 (9–10), 1510–1517.

Shin, H., Jo, S., Mikos, A.G., 2003. Biomimetic materials for tissue engineering. Biomaterials 24 (24), 4353–4364.

Shin, H.J., Lee, C.H., Cho, I.H., Kim, Y.J., Lee, Y.J., Kim, I.A., et al., 2006. Electrospun PLGA nanofiber scaffolds for articular cartilage reconstruction: mechanical stability, degradation and cellular responses under mechanical stimulation *in vitro*. J. Biomater. Sci. Polym. Ed. 17 (1–2), 103–119.

Silva, E.A., Mooney, D.J., 2007. Spatiotemporal control of vascular endothelial growth factor delivery from injectable hydrogels enhances angiogenesis. J. Thromb. Haemost. 5 (3), 590–598.

Silva, G.A., Czeisler, C., Niece, K.L., Beniash, E., Harrington, D.A., Kessler, J.A., et al., 2004. Selective differentiation of neural progenitor cells by high-epitope density nanofibers. Science 303 (5662), 1352–1355.

Spiller, K.L., Holloway, J.L., Gribb, M.E., Lowman, A.M., 2011. Design of semi-degradable hydrogels based on poly(vinyl alcohol) and poly(lactic-*co*-glycolic acid) for cartilage tissue engineering. J. Tissue Eng. Regen. Med. 5 (8), 636–647.

Subramanian, A., Vu, D., Larsen, G.F., Lin, H.Y., 2005. Preparation and evaluation of the electrospun chitosan/PEO fibers for potential applications in cartilage tissue engineering. J. Biomater. Sci. Polym. Ed. 16 (7), 861–873.

Subramanian, A., Krishnan, U.M., Sethuraman, S., 2011. Fabrication of uniaxially aligned 3D electrospun scaffolds for neural regeneration. Biomed. Mater. 6 (2), 025004.

Sun, K.H., Liu, Z., Liu, C.J., Yu, T., Shang, T., Huang, C., et al., 2015. Alginate hydrogel conglutinate cells on the surface of polycaprolactone vascular scaffolds fabricated by electrospinning. J. Biomater. Tissue Eng. 5 (1), 64–70.

Sundaramurthi, D., Krishnan, U.M., Sethuraman, S., 2014. Electrospun nanofibers as scaffolds for skin tissue engineering. Polym. Rev. 54 (2), 348–376.

Sur, S., Pashuck, E.T., Guler, M.O., Ito, M., Stupp, S.I., Launey, T., 2012. A hybrid nanofiber matrix to control the survival and maturation of brain neurons. Biomaterials 33 (2), 545–555.

Tan, H., Chu, C.R., Payne, K.A., Marra, K.G., 2009. Injectable *in situ* forming biodegradable chitosan-hyaluronic acid based hydrogels for cartilage tissue engineering. Biomaterials 30 (13), 2499–2506.

Tan, G.N., Gundogan, A., Farhatnia, B., Nayyer, Y., Mahdibeiraghdar, L., Rajadas, S., et al., 2015. Tissue engineering vascular grafts a fortiori: looking back and going forward. Expert Opin. Biol. Ther. 15 (2), 231–244.

Taylor, S.J., McDonald III, J.W., Sakiyama-Elbert, S.E., 2004. Controlled release of neurotrophin-3 from fibrin gels for spinal cord injury. J. Control. Release 98 (2), 281–294.

Temenoff, J.S., Athanasiou, K.A., LeBaron, R.G., Mikos, A.G., 2002. Effect of poly (ethylene glycol) molecular weight on tensile and swelling properties of oligo[poly(ethylene glycol) fumarate] hydrogels for cartilage tissue engineering. J. Biomed. Mater. Res. 59 (3), 429–437.

Tillman, B.W., Yazdani, S.K., Lee, S.J., Geary, R.L., Atala, A., Yoo, J.J., 2009. The *in vivo* stability of electrospun polycaprolactone-collagen scaffolds in vascular reconstruction. Biomaterials 30 (4), 583–588.

Timnak, A., Gharebaghi, F.Y., Shariati, R.P., Bahrami, S.H., Javadian, S., Emami, S.H., et al., 2011. Fabrication of nano-structured electrospun collagen scaffold intended for nerve tissue engineering. J. Mater. Sci. Mater. Med. 22 (6), 1555–1567.

Toh, W.S., Lee, E.H., Guo, X.M., Chan, J.K., Yeow, C.H., Choo, A.B., et al., 2010. Cartilage repair using hyaluronan hydrogel-encapsulated human embryonic stem cell-derived chondrogenic cells. Biomaterials 31 (27), 6968–6980.

Tsur-Gang, O., Ruvinov, E., Landa, N., Holbova, R., Feinberg, M.S., Leor, J., et al., 2009. The effects of peptide-based modification of alginate on left ventricular remodeling and function after myocardial infarction. Biomaterials 30 (2), 189–195.

Tuli, R., Li, W.J., Tuan, R.S., 2003. Current state of cartilage tissue engineering. Arthritis Res. Ther. 5 (5), 235–238.

Vavken, P., Joshi, S.M., Murray, M.M., 2011. Fibrin concentration affects ACL fibroblast proliferation and collagen synthesis. Knee 18 (1), 42–46.

Venugopal, J., Ramakrishna, S., 2005a. Biocompatible nanofiber matrices for the engineering of a dermal substitute for skin regeneration. Tissue Eng. 11 (5–6), 847–854.

Venugopal, J., Ramakrishna, S., 2005b. Applications of polymer nanofibers in biomedicine and biotechnology. Appl. Biochem. Biotechnol. 125 (3), 147–158.

Venugopal, J., Prabhakaran, M.P., Low, S., Choon, A.T., Zhang, Y.Z., Deepika, G., et al., 2008a. Nanotechnology for nanomedicine and delivery of drugs. Curr. Pharm. Des. 14 (22), 2184–2200.

Venugopal, J., Low, S., Choon, A.T., Ramakrishna, S., 2008b. Interaction of cells and nanofiber scaffolds in tissue engineering. J. Biomed. Mater. Res. B. Appl. Biomater. 84 (1), 34–48.

Vieira, A.C., Vieira, J.C., Ferra, J.M., Magalhães, F.D., Guedes, R.M., Marques, A.T., 2011. Mechanical study of PLA-PCL fibers during *in vitro* degradation. J. Mech. Behav. Biomed. Mater. 4 (3), 451–460.

Vunjak-Novakovic, G., Altman, G., Horan, R., Kaplan, D.L., 2004. Tissue engineering of ligaments. Annu. Rev. Biomed. Eng. 6, 131–156.

Vunjak-Novakovic, G., Tandon, N., Godier, A., Maidhof, R., Marsano, A., Martens, T.P., et al., 2010. Challenges in cardiac tissue engineering. Tissue Eng. B Rev. 16 (2), 169–187.

Vunjak-Novakovic, G., Eschenhagen, T., Mummery, C., 2014. Myocardial tissue engineering: *in vitro* models. Cold Spring Harb. Perspect. Med. 4 (3), a014076.

Wang, C., Wang, M., 2014. Electrospun multifunctional tissue engineering scaffolds. Front. Mater. Sci. 8 (1), 3–19.

Wang, W., Itoh, S., Matsuda, A., Ichinose, S., Shinomiya, K., Hata, Y., et al., 2008. Influences of mechanical properties and permeability on chitosan nano/microfiber mesh tubes as a scaffold for nerve regeneration. J. Biomed. Mater. Res. A 84 (2), 557–566.

Wang, W., Itoh, S., Yamamoto, N., Okawa, A., Nagai, A., Yamashita, K., 2010. Enhancement of nerve regeneration along a chitosan nanofiber mesh tube on which electrically polarized β-tricalcium phosphate particles are immobilized. Acta Biomater. 6 (10), 4027–4033.

Wang, X., Ding, B., Li, B., 2013. Biomimetic electrospun nanofibrous structures for tissue engineering. Mater. Today (Kidlington) 16 (6), 229–241.

Wang, Y., Kim, U.J., Blasioli, D.J., Kim, H.J., Kaplan, D.L., 2005. *In vitro* cartilage tissue engineering with 3D porous aqueous-derived silk scaffolds and mesenchymal stem cells. Biomaterials 26 (34), 7082–7094.

Wang, Y., Yao, M., Zhou, J., Zheng, W., Zhou, C., Dong, D., et al., 2011a. The promotion of neural progenitor cells proliferation by aligned and randomly oriented collagen nanofibers through $\beta 1$ integrin/MAPK signaling pathway. Biomaterials 32 (28), 6737–6744.

Wang, Y., Zhao, Z., Zhao, B., Qi, H.X., Peng, J., Zhang, L., et al., 2011b. Biocompatibility evaluation of electrospun aligned poly(propylene carbonate) nanofibrous scaffolds with peripheral nerve tissues and cells *in vitro*. Chin. Med. J. (Engl) 124 (15), 2361–2366.

Wang, C.Y., Zhang, K.H., Fan, C.Y., Mo, X.M., Ruan, H.J., Li, F.F., 2011c. Aligned natural-synthetic polyblend nanofibers for peripheral nerve regeneration. Acta Biomater. 7 (2), 634–643.

Wang, H.B., Mullins, M.E., Cregg, J.M., Hurtado, A., Oudega, M., Trombley, M.T., et al., 2009. Creation of highly aligned electrospun poly-L-lactic acid fibers for nerve regeneration applications. J. Neural. Eng. 6 (1), 016001.

Wang, T.Y., Forsythe, J.S., Parish, C.L., Nisbet, D.R., 2012. Biofunctionalisation of polymeric scaffolds for neural tissue engineering. J. Biomater. Appl. 27 (4), 369–390.

Wells, M.R., Kraus, K., Batter, D.K., Blunt, D.G., Weremowitz, J., Lynch, S.E., et al., 1997. Gel matrix vehicles for growth factor application in nerve gap injuries repaired with tubes: a comparison of biomatrix, collagen, and methylcellulose. Exp. Neurol. 146 (2), 395–402.

West, R.V., Harner, C.D., 2005. Graft selection in anterior cruciate ligament reconstruction. J. Am. Acad. Orthop. Surg. 13 (3), 197–207.

Willerth, S.M., Sakiyama-Elbert, S.E., 2007. Approaches to neural tissue engineering using scaffolds for drug delivery. Adv. Drug Deliv. Rev. 59 (4–5), 325–338.

Woo, S.L.Y., Abramowitch, S.D., Kilger, R., Liang, R., 2006. Biomechanics of knee ligaments: injury, healing, and repair. J. Biomech. 39 (1), 1–20.

Xie, Y., Ye, L., Zhang, X., Cui, W., Lou, J., Nagai, T., et al., 2005. Transport of nerve growth factor encapsulated into liposomes across the blood–brain barrier: *in vitro* and *in vivo* studies. J. Control. Release 105 (1–2), 106–119.

Xu, X., Yee, W.C., Hwang, P.Y.K., Yu, H., Wan, A.C.A., Gao, S., et al., 2003. Peripheral nerve regeneration with sustained release of poly(phosphoester) microencapsulated nerve growth factor within nerve guide conduits. Biomaterials 24 (13), 2405–2412.

Xu, C.Y., Inai, R., Kotaki, M., Ramakrishna, S., 2004. Aligned biodegradable nanofibrous structure: a potential scaffold for blood vessel engineering. Biomaterials 25 (5), 877–886.

Xu, X.Y., Li, X.T., Peng, S.W., Xiao, J.F., Liu, C., Fang, G., et al., 2010. The behaviour of neural stem cells on polyhydroxyalkanoate nanofiber scaffolds. Biomaterials 31 (14), 3967–3975.

Yang, F., Murugan, R., Wang, S., Ramakrishna, S., 2005. Electrospinning of nano/micro scale poly (L-lactic acid) aligned fibers and their potential in neural tissue engineering. Biomaterials 26 (15), 2603–2610.

Yang, Y., Xia, T., Zhi, W., Wei, L., Weng, J., Zhang, C., et al., 2011. Promotion of skin regeneration in diabetic rats by electrospun core-sheath fibers loaded with basic fibroblast growth factor. Biomaterials 32 (18), 4243–4254.

Yim, E.K., Reano, R.M., Pang, S.W., Yee, A.F., Chen, C.S., Leong, K.W., 2005. Nanopattern-induced changes in morphology and motility of smooth muscle cells. Biomaterials 26 (26), 5405–5413.

Yoshikawa, T., Tohyama, H., Katsura, T., Kondo, E., Kotani, Y., Matsumoto, H., et al., 2006. Effects of local administration of vascular endothelial growth factor on mechanical characteristics of the semitendinosus tendon graft after anterior cruciate ligament reconstruction in sheep. Am. J. Sports Med. 34 (12), 1918–1925.

You, J.O., Rafat, M., Ye, G.J., Auguste, D.T., 2011. Nanoengineering the heart: conductive scaffolds enhance connexin 43 expression. Nano Lett. 11 (9), 3643–3648.

Zahedi, P., Rezaeian, I., Ranaei-Siadat, S.O., Jafari, S.H., Supaphol, P., 2010. A review on wound dressings with an emphasis on electrospun nanofibrous polymeric bandages. Polym. Adv. Technol. 21 (2), 77–95.

Zhang, B., Xiao, Y., Hsieh, A., Thavandiran, N., Radisic, M., 2011. Micro- and nanotechnology in cardiovascular tissue engineering. Nanotechnology 22 (49), 494003.

Zhang, S., Uludağ, H., 2009. Nanoparticulate systems for growth factor delivery. Pharm. Res. 26 (7), 1561–1580.

Zhang, Y., Lim, C.T., Ramakrishna, S., Huang, Z.M., 2005a. Recent development of polymer nanofibers for biomedical and biotechnological applications. J. Mater. Sci. Mater. Med. 16 (10), 933–946.

Zhang, Y., Ouyang, H., Lim, C.T., Ramakrishna, S., Huang, Z.M., 2005b. Electrospinning of gelatin fibers and gelatin/PCL composite fibrous scaffolds. J. Biomed. Mater. Res. B Appl. Biomater. 72 (1), 156–165.

Zheng, Y., Chen, J., Craven, M., Choi, N.W., Totorica, S., Diaz-Santana, A., et al., 2012. *In vitro* microvessels for the study of angiogenesis and thrombosis. Proc. Natl. Acad. Sci. U.S.A. 109 (24), 9342–9347.

Zhong, S.P., Zhang, Y.Z., Lim, C.T., 2010. Tissue scaffolds for skin wound healing and dermal reconstruction. Wiley Interdiscip. Rev. Nanomed. Nanobiotechnol. 2 (5), 510–525.

Zhou, J., Zhao, Y., Wang, J., Zhang, S., Liu, Z., Zhen, M., et al., 2012. Therapeutic angiogenesis using basic fibroblast growth factor in combination with a collagen matrix in chronic hindlimb ischemia. Sci. World J. 2012, 652794.

CHAPTER

Machine design for multimaterial processing

5

Carmelo De Maria[1,2], Aurora De Acutis[1], Michele Carrabba[1], Giuseppe Criscenti[1] and Giovanni Vozzi[1,2]

[1]Research Center E. Piaggio, University of Pisa, Pisa, Italy [2]Department of Ingegneria dell'Informazione, University of Pisa, Pisa, Italy

5.1 INTRODUCTION

The construction of an engineered tissue, according to the principles of tissue engineering (TE), starts with the design and construction of bioinspired scaffolds. Scaffolds are biocompatible and bioabsorbable structures that are capable of mimicking the extracellular matrix (ECM) and transmitting the appropriate biochemical and mechanical stimuli to guide the regeneration of a three-dimensional (3D) living tissue (Lanza et al., 2007; Ortinau et al., 2010; Singh et al., 2008; Lo et al., 2000).

A biological tissue can be described as a composite material with an architecture and spatial organization characterized by a hierarchical structure from the nanometer up to the millimeter scale, closely related to the functions of the tissue.

For this reason, many studies are focused on fabricating multimaterial scaffolds processed at multiple scales with adequate structural and mechanical properties that provide optimal conditions for cell response. At the nanometer level, these scaffolds have to show a large surface area for the distribution of ligands to promote the adhesion and development of the phenotypic expression for the regeneration of a specific tissue (Stevens and George, 2005); instead, at the micrometric level, scaffolds have to exhibit a structure with a completely interconnected pore network to allow adequate perfusion of nutrients, removal of waste products of cellular metabolism, and the development of a capillary network (Darling et al., 2005; Zhang et al., 2009).

In this field of research polymeric and bioceramic materials have been tested. Polymeric materials of natural origin, such as collagen, hyaluronic acid, alginate, and agarose, are not immunogenic and they mimic the ECM, offering signals which promote cell adhesion, differentiation, and proliferation.

However, their use for scaffold fabrication is limited by their weak mechanical performance and their high cost. To overcome these problems, synthetic polymers, such as PLLA, PLGA, and PLA, find a great application in TE, in fact they

Nanobiomaterials in Soft Tissue Engineering. DOI: http://dx.doi.org/10.1016/B978-0-323-42865-1.00005-2

can be produced in large quantities, with uniform and controlled mechanical properties. Natural and synthetic polymers are often used in the form of hydrogels.

In bone TE, even bioceramic materials, such as hydroxyapatite (HA) and tricalcium phosphate (TCP), are commonly used thanks to their good biocompatibility, corrosion resistance, and high compression resistance. However, despite many advantages, they are also characterized by difficult processing, a lack of resilience, and a slow degradation rate.

In recent years, a successful and rational strategy has been proposed to combine the biological performance of natural polymer with the optimal mechanical performance of synthetic and bioceramic material to obtain multimaterial structures with good 3D cell guidance.

In this regard, an extensive example of composite bioinspired structures is hydrogel-based scaffolds, with a lower stiffness than the tissue that has to be regenerated, reinforced with the incorporation of nanoparticles or nanotubes in order to combine good mechanical and biological properties.

The final structural, mechanical and physical properties of a scaffold depend on the choice of both building materials and microfabrication techniques.

Additive manufacturing (AM), also known as also rapid prototyping (RP), techniques are quite promising in TE, in fact they allow the processing of many different materials (Hutmacher, 2001) and control of pore volume and architecture in a CAD/CAM manner with a micrometric resolution to customize scaffolds for the regeneration of a specific tissue.

Many materials, such as ceramic or thermoplastic materials, can be involved in the RP process for TE, also hydrogels seem suitable to be processed by RP techniques using many different and cell-friendly approaches (Hutmacher et al., 2004).

Also, RP techniques can be integrated, or hybridized, with others to introduce nanoscale features and improve scaffold bioactivity (Moroni et al., 2008a,b). For example, a scaffold can be functionalized through the incorporation of a network of nano-microfibers that can provide the high surface/volume ratio that is necessary to promote cell adhesion (Ma and Zhang, 1999). To date, electrospinning is one of the most used technologies for the production of nanofibers (Centola et al., 2010).

Many research groups have successfully obtained multimaterial or multiscale scaffolds using hybrid microfabrication processes; in most cases these are sequential processes that use independent systems for the application of the selected techniques of micro- or nanofabrication (Moroni et al., 2008a,b). These are long and delicate processes that can damage the structure under construction. For this reason the goal of this research is the design of a machine, based on the Maryland manipulator architecture, which can combine three different biofabrication technologies: piston-driven extrusion, pressure-driven extrusion, and electrospinning system. The piston-driven extrusion tool allows the deposition of high-viscosity solutions following precise spatial patterns; conversely, the pressure-driven extrusion tool is suited to dispose of low-viscosity solutions.

Electrospinning exploits the action of electrostatic forces to create polymeric fibers at micrometric and nanometric scales. All these tools can be integrated on the Maryland's end-effector to fabricate bioinspired structures at different scales, with different materials, through a simple change of tool.

The design work was structured into the following phases:

- Defining the design specifications
- Geometric and dynamic dimensioning
- CAD modeling of the manipulator and of related tools for microfabrication
- Creation of the prototype and validation tests.

Then multifunctional hydrogel-based scaffolds were fabricated as a demonstration of the validity of the developed device and also with the aim of identifying novel strategies to biofabricate hydrogel-based scaffolds able to maintaining their shape and at the same time give guidance to cells.

5.2 THE ROLE OF THE SCAFFOLDS IN TE: DESIGN FEATURES

The construction of an engineered tissue starts with the design and the fabrication of a scaffold tailored for the tissue which has to be regenerated (Vozzi et al., 2004). Typically these structures consist of a polymer matrix that mimics the ECM for adhesion and cell proliferation. These scaffolds, besides having a suitable superficial topography to promote cell adhesion, proliferation, and differentiation, should be highly porous, with a fully interconnected pore network, for cell growth as well as to allow optimal cell migration and at the same time ensure sufficient transport of nutrients and the removal of metabolic wastes (Malda et al., 2004).

The scaffold should operate as a temporary mechanical support for 3D organization of cells and its degradation rate should coincide as much as possible with that of the tissue formation; this means that while the seeded cells synthesize the matrix around itself, the scaffold should be able to provide structural integrity to leave enough space for the neo-tissue regeneration.

The aim of recent studies is to manufacture multifunctional structures that should give mechanical support and at the same time stimulate tissue regeneration. For this reason, the design process, which is behind the fabrication of a scaffold for TE, needs a plan that considers the necessity of a compromise between different and important material properties as biological and mechanical cues. Therefore, from the point of view of the materials and structural properties and in the perspective of an *in vivo* remodeling process, a bioinspired scaffold for TE applications should possess the following features:

- Scaffolds should be manufactured with materials that have appropriate mechanical properties to emulate those of the specific tissue, and to provide

the right mechanical stimuli for neo-tissue formation: this is currently possible through the fabrication of composite or multimaterial scaffolds.
- Scaffolds should be characterized by a functional and easily reproducible architecture, from nano- up to microscale, with a porosity and interconnection to guarantee an adequate ratio to promote cell adhesion and proliferation on the structure. To date, it is possible to get these features fabricating a bioinspired 3D scaffold with a defined multiscale architecture.

5.2.1 MULTIMATERIAL SCAFFOLD

Over recent years, the role of TE in the current science world has been considerably strengthened due to the great development of new materials that interact with the biological environment; these materials are known as biomaterials.

Research on the design and construction of 3D scaffolds is focused prevalently on polymeric biomaterials. Polymeric materials from natural sources (such as collagen, elastin, chitosan, hyaluronic acid, or alginate and agarose) offer the advantage of mimicking the role of ECM, giving optimal biological recognition. However, such materials are taken from human or animal tissues and, therefore, are not always available in large quantities. In addition, materials of natural origin can be carriers of pathogens and, in addition, also differ considerably independently depending on the body from which they are taken. Moreover, these materials have limited versatility in the construction of scaffolds with specific properties, in particular in terms of mechanical strength. However, the complex management of their stimuli and their scarce mechanical performance have moved the attention of the world of biofabrication to synthetic polymers. The use of synthetic materials, such as PLA, PLLA, PCL, and PLGA, has become common due to two important reasons: because they are industrially reproducible on a large scale and they can be synthesized with a great deal of control over mechanical and chemical properties to customize performance in terms of tissue. The main disadvantage of synthetic materials is in the absence of specific signals for cell recognition.

Overall, synthetic polymers offer more advantages than natural materials, as they are designed to cover a wide range of properties and furthermore they are also free from the risk of immunogenicity. For both classes of materials, the ideal polymers to use in a specific application should be designed to have some particular characteristics:

- Have mechanical properties that match up with the application
- Have the capability to be fabricated easily
- Do not induce inflammation or a toxic response
- Can be metabolized by biological tissues at the end of the task
- Have areasonable lifespan
- Can be easily sterilized.

Synthetic and natural polymers can also be used in the form of hydrogels, a class of highly hydrated polymeric material that is used in the biomedical field, including the fabrication of scaffolds. Hydrogel-based scaffolds are typically biodegradable, with mechanical properties more similar to many tissues, such as high permeability for oxygen, nutrients, and other water-soluble metabolites. Unlike from hydrogels based on natural polymer, hydrogels based on synthetic polymer are less suitable to be used in this area due to their cytotoxicity and because they do not provide any binding site to promote cell viability.

Also, bioceramic materials are appreciated in TE, especially in bone TE, due to their good compatibility, corrosion resistance, and compression. However, they are hardly used as a building material in bioinspiration scaffolds because of their low rate of degradation and high density and fragility.

Because none of the above-discussed materials shows the ideal characteristics requested from TE, an innovative approach is to fabricate a multimaterial scaffold combining the adequate biological features of natural polymers and the controllable mechanical features of synthetic polymers to regenerate a specific tissue. Otherwise it is possible to combine biodegradable polymeric materials with bioactive inorganic particles, like bioceramic particles, to achieve optimal mechanical performance. In fact, polymers are generally flexible, with a lack of mechanical rigidity, while ceramics are known to be too rigid and fragile; the combination of the two leads to composite materials with improved mechanical properties due to the intrinsic rigidity and higher resistance of the inorganic material. However, the addition of the bioceramic material alters the degradation rate of the polymer.

In the literature there are numerous examples of combinations of natural and synthetic polymers with bioceramic materials in order to integrate the best features of each component. One of the methods used to form a composite scaffold for TE is the random incorporation of synthetic polymer fibers or of inorganic nanoparticles in an ordered hydrogel-based structure or in an organic polymeric bulk. The main advantage of this approach is that the fibers, or the nanoparticles, provide reinforcement of the structure, improving its mechanical performance.

For example, Chen et al. developed scaffolds to engineer cartilage tissue, made up of a PGL network and collagen in the form of a microsponge; the collagen filled the pores of the PGL network to promote cell adhesion and therefore the formation of new tissue (Chen et al., 2003). Instead, Sargeant et al. synthesized an injectable hydrogel for TE made of collagen and PEG where the collagen had the function of activating cell adhesion while the PEG adjusted the mechanical properties (Sargeant et al., 2012).

The bioceramic materials, however, are used in composite scaffolds to reproduce the mechanical properties of bone matrix; as a demonstration of this application, Zhao et al. produced porous HA-based scaffolds coated with PCL characterized by mechanical properties and a bioactivity that promoted osteoinduction (Zhao et al., 2008). With the main objective of improving the rate of degradation of scaffold containing bioceramic material, Peter et al. fabricated scaffolds made of chitosan and microspheres of HA using the coprecipitation method (Peter et al., 2010). Finally, Vozzi et al. developed a multimaterial microfabrication technique known as Pressure-Activated Microsyringe2 (PAM2).

In this work, a parallel manipulator with multiple-dispensing tools capable of deposition of multiple materials has been developed to fabricate multifunctional scaffolds for TE.

5.2.2 MULTISCALE SCAFFOLDS

A biological tissue presents a precise architecture constituted by two main structures:

- Cells, organized into functional units
- The ECM.

Regarding the ECM, it is now established that it provides cells and the adequate spatial organization and chemical support containing biochemical information to regulate all their functions including adhesion, proliferation, survival, and differentiation (Moroni et al., 2008a,b).

The ECM presents a precise and dynamic hierarchical organization of the architecture from the nanoscale up to the micrometric scale. The nanoscale structure of the native ECM consists of a network of proteins and polysaccharides that drive cell behavior. In fact, the 3D environment *in vivo* strongly influences the changes in the shape of cells, which in turn influences the process of differentiation and other cellular activities (Puppi et al., 2014). It is likely that the cells *in vitro* require the entire context of the 3D matrix to maintain their phenotypic shape and to establish patterns of natural behavior. Therefore, many research groups are investigating the structural characteristics that scaffolds for TE should have, at the micro and nano levels, to create a biomimetic environment with the same details as the tissue that has to be generated (Kumbar et al., 2008). For this reason, the scaffold should have at a microscopic level, a highly porous structure, with a fully interconnected geometry, that provides a large surface area to promote cell growth, uniform cell distribution, and that facilitates the neovascularization of the constructs.

In the last year it has been shown that highly porous materials are preferable for the construction of bioinspired scaffolds to facilitate the diffusion of nutrients and the removal of waste substances. The ratio of area/volume offered by porous materials depends on the density and the average pore diameter; the minimum size of the pores depends on the cell type that will be seed on the structure. Experiments show that the optimal size of the pores is 5 μm for neovascularization and 200–350 μm for osteoinduction. Also, the interconnectivity of pores is a critical feature, in fact it should be such as to ensure that all cells are 200 μm from the blood flow to have optimal oxygen and nutrient transport.

The most important components of ECM are collagen and proteoglycans, which together form a structure with a certain mechanical stability. The collagen is organized in a 3D structure composed of nano- and microfibers, which supply an available surface for cell adhesion. Therefore, many studies have demonstrated that the biocompatibility of a scaffold depends on the presence of elements on the same scale as those in natural ECM. Fibers, with a diameter of tens of nanometers up to hundreds of micrometers, provide an ample surface area useful for the absorption of proteins and for the exhibition of sites for cell membrane receptors favoring cell adhesion (Karageorgiou and Kaplan, 2005). However, as a result, combining micro/nanofibers it is possible to obtain a 3D structure that is also characterized by nutrient and cell mass transport.

To date, several approaches have been developed to fabricate structures bioinspired with a multiscale topology for TE; recent studies have demonstrated that an excellent approach is the combination of RP techniques and the micro- or nanofabrication techniques. For example, exploiting the combination of RP techniques and electrospinning it is possible to fabricate nanofibrous scaffold with a microporous structure.

5.3 RP OF 3D SCAFFOLDS

It is widely known that the final properties of a scaffold can be determined by the microfabrication process. To manufacture 3D scaffolds different microfabrication techniques have been used, from the more traditional techniques such as the textile techniques or molding processes, to the most recent RP techniques. The most discriminant factor to select the appropriate process of microfabrication is the building materials, especially for their chemical or physical properties that often cannot fit with the principles of operation of the production processes, as well as the rheological and mechanical properties of the biomaterials.

As discussed above, there is a close relationship between the structure and function of a biologic tissue, in fact, the cells tend to organize themselves spatially to correctly exert their function and make the tissue/organ a functional system. The necessity of controlling the architecture of a scaffold in terms of size, shape, geometry, mechanical properties, porosity, and pore interconnectivity has led to the use of microfabrication techniques based on RP technologies.

The term RP indicates a group of technologies that allows the automatic realization of a physical model based on the design data using a computer (Xu et al., 2006).

RP processes belong to the generative (or additive) production processes. Generative production processes is the generic term (seldom used in practice) to indicate an additive production process. More common are expressions such as "AM" (Melchels et al., 2012) or "solid freeform fabrication" (Sachlos and Czernuszka, 2003), which emphasize the ability to produce framed solids by means of freeform surfaces.

In RP processes the final object is formed by joining volume elements, in which each two-dimensional layer is built in the *XY* plane and the third dimension of the structure is obtained with the layer-by-layer approach; this approach applied to TE is called "bioprinting" (Lam et al., 2002), defined as the use of computer-aided transfer processes for patterning and assembling living and non-living materials with prescribed 2D or 3D organization in order to produce bio-engineered structures serving in regenerative medicine, pharmacokinetics, and basic cell biology studies.

Bioprinting is included in the wider field of "computer-aided tissue engineering" (CATE), the application of advanced computer technologies to TE and regenerative medicine problems. In summary, the 3D scaffold is designed using a computer (computer-aided design (CAD) phase), which then sends the machine instructions to get the desired shape (computer-aided manufacturing (CAM) phase), building it layer by layer. Sometimes the geometry is extrapolated from tomographic scans of a specific part of the human body, using dedicated segmentation algorithms, in order to obtain structures customized for a specific patient.

In the context of TE, different microfabrication technologies are currently available to implement the RP principles. These different microfabrication techniques can be classified as a function of the physical nature or on the basis of the material processed; in this chapter, however, classification based on their operating principle is adopted:

- RP technologies based on the extrusion process
- Ink-jet printing
- RP technologies based on the light-curing process
- Hybrid RP technologies.

Each technique is characterized by its own resolution and fabrication speed, and requires specific features as regards the rheological properties or the curing rate of the different materials.

Recently it has been has demonstrated that one of the great challenges in the bioprinting field centers around the generation of human 3D functional organs in laboratory environment through the deposition of a bio-ink with the same approach as the RP technologies (Derby, 2012); the bio-ink is usually made up of biochemical, biological materials and living cells, and it is prepared for building of a specific target tissue that has to be regenerated.

A bioprinter dispensed the bio-ink in a layer-by-layer approach suitable for the specific application. During the bioprinting process the bio-ink is printed with a predefined pattern on a hydrogel substrate that acts as a support material, or as a sacrificial material to reproduce the multiscale network of channels typical of the native ones. Exploiting the bioprinting process it is possible to manufacture tissues from microscale tissues up to larger structures (Organovo, 2014; Laboratory Equipment, 2014). The printing of complex and vital organs might be technically feasible in the future; the flexibility of bioprinting technology allows the targeting of many different tissues for the development of a human tissue model for research study and drug discovery applications, or for preclinical testing and drug discovery research as well as to fulfill the vision of building human tissues for surgical therapy and transplantation. Other immediate benefits of bioprinting reside in helping researchers to improve the process of drug discovery (Toffenetti and Royaee, 2014); in fact a short-term goal for bioprinting might be the printing of small sections of functional tissue that can be used to verify the patient-specific response to the drugs or printing miniature of organs and blood vessels that will be connected with a substitute of blood to study the native tissue biology and anatomy. These systems have the potential to accelerate the development of new drugs and replace animal testing, which are too slow, expensive, and not always accurate. This new technology raises a fundamental question from the point of the patenting of the printed part: can a human organ or human tissue fabricated with 3D printing from human cells be patented, or it is simply a product of nature and therefore cannot be patented?

5.3.1 RP TECHNOLOGIES BASED ON EXTRUSION PROCESSES

These RP technologies, also known as directed writing techniques, can generally perform the deposition of material following a piston-drive, screw-driven, or pneumatic-driven approach.

This class of RP technologies allows to make use of a wide variety of biomaterials (in the form of filaments or drops) as hotmelt polymers, hydrogels, pastes, or a polymeric solution. In all these techniques, the thickness of the deposited material can be modulated by varying the deposition rate, the nozzle diameter, or the applied pressure.

An example of a pneumatic-driven microfabrication technology is the pressure-activated microsyringe (PAM), developed by Vozzi and coworkers (Mariani et al., 2006), which provides the deposition of polymeric solutions with a resolution of up to 5 mm. This technique uses a motorized system along $x-y-z$ axes for movement in the $x-y$ plane of the deposition plane and along the z-axis of a syringe in controlled pressure for the extrusion of the material in the liquid state. This system has been designed for the extrusion of polymeric materials in solution with a highly volatile solvent using microneedles of glass. With this system, 2D and 3D structures were fabricated using PLLA, PCL, and blends of PLLA and PCL.

The second version of the PAM system, known as PAM2, is also equipped with a piston-driven syringe tool to deposit hydrogel materials with higher viscosity (Tirella et al., 2008); in this case the viscosity is a necessary feature to fabricate structures characterized by high shape fidelity.

Fused deposition modeling (FDM) is another important representative of this class of RP technology; the layer-by-layer fabrication of a bioinspired scaffold with a common FDM 3D printer is based on the heating of a polymeric filament until bringing it to a semiliquid state and finally expelling it through a special nozzle. Using this RP technology Zein et al. fabricated PCL-based scaffolds, while Samar and coworkers have successfully produced a composite and porous scaffold with characteristics comparable to those of natural bone (Zein et al., 2002; Kalita et al., 2003).

The disadvantages of the FDM technique include the need to make the biomaterial available in filament form, with the result that the FDM has a limited range of working materials, with almost complete exclusion of natural polymers. Furthermore, the deposited material solidifies, preventing the formation of microporosity, a key element for the vascularization process and cell adhesion. Finally the resolution of FDM is relatively low, about 250 μm, and the operating temperature of the system is too high to incorporate biomolecules in the structure, thus limiting the biomimetic aspects. These limitations have promoted the emergence of novel techniques, such as 3D fiber deposition and the 3D Bioplotter. Three-dimensional fiber deposition makes use of a material in the form of pellets or granules which can be poured directly into a heated chamber and then extruded from a syringe applying pressure (Moroni et al., 2006). Woodfield et al., with this RP technology, fabricated a PEGT-PBT-based scaffold; while Moroni et al., exploiting the same technique, studied the mechanical properties of scaffolds made up of a thermoplastic polymer, PEOT-PBT, which combined good mechanical performance and easy workability (Woodfield et al., 2004).

Another variant of the FDM process is the 3D Bioplotter; this was developed by Landers and Mülhaupt especially for processing hydrogels. The material can be deposited in a continuous or discontinuous way from a pneumatic or piston extruder. The key features of this process are the ability to print viscous materials into a liquid medium with a corresponding density and the ability to process thermally sensitive biocomponents, even cells. Benefiting from the advantages of a 3D Bioplotter, Landers et al. realized hydrogel-based scaffolds with interconnected pores with a diameter of 200–400 μm and a smooth surface which is not suitable for good cell adhesion (Landers and Mulhaupt, 2000) Therefore, recently, Kim and Son modified the system for the 3D Bioplotter by adding a piezoelectric PZT to generate vibrations during printing and fabricating scaffold with a rougher surface (Kim and Son, 2009).

5.3.2 INK-JET PRINTING

This class includes those RP techniques that implement ink-jet technology to fabricate bioinspired structures ejecting a small volume of bio-ink from the nozzles of a printhead on a substrate following a layer-by-layer approach. Most of these machines are drop-on demand systems as the expulsion of material occurs by receiving a signal from a computer. The ink-jet printing is used for the controlled deposition of low-viscosity materials, for easy ejection from the nozzles, such as PBS, cell culture media, or a liquid precursor of hydrogels. In the latter case, the ejected precursor should have low viscosity, it should cross-link only after its ejection, and finally the cross-linked hydrogel should have remarkable mechanical properties to maintain the 3D structure.

For example, Boland et al. developed an ink-jet printer for the fabrication of biodegradable scaffolds (Boland et al., 2006). This research group printed 3D scaffolds depositing a cross-linker solution of $CaCl_2$ (0.25 M) on a substrate of alginic acid to 2% (w/v). When a layer is totally cross-linked, the deposition platform is lowered to cover the cross-linked layer and to provide a new interface for the next layer. This is also a kind of ink-jet printer called the Model Maker II; this system uses a single jet to deposit the building material and supporting material; Taboas et al. produced PLLA-based structures with a specific micro- and macroporosity to engineer the bone tissue; the macroporosity (500 μm) was computationally designed, while the local pores (50–100 μm) were achieved through a porogen agent. Xu et al. used this technology for fabricating structures made from fibrin gels to engineer neural tissue (Xu et al., 2006). There fibrin was obtained using the enzymatic polymerization of fibrinogen by addition of thrombin and $CaCl_2$. Instead, to demonstrate the great potential of this technology, Nakamura et al. built a piezoelectric ink-jet printer and successfully manufactured 3D structures from the direct printing of cells (Nakamura et al., 2010).

The final 3D printing technology uses ink-jet technology to print a liquid binder on a bed of powder material; a 3D structure is built in a layer-by-layer fashion, without the use of supporting material as it is the unlinked powder that performs this function. Using this technique it is possible to fabricate porous structures with controlled macroporosity and microporosity; in fact the microporosity depends on the size of the grain of powder, while the macroporosity can be controlled mixing a pore agent in the building powder. The work conducted by Lam et al. showed the possibility of using this technique with natural biopolymers and deionized water as a binder, eliminating the problem of biocompatibility relating to organic solvents (Lam et al., 2002). However, these structures were soluble in water and required a post-processing step to make them waterproof.

5.3.3 RP TECHNOLOGIES BASED ON LIGHT-CURING PROCESSES

The RP technologies which belong to this class use photocurable polymers or light-sintering powders to fabricate rapid prototypes for TE. One of these techniques is stereolithography SLA which is based on the use of a UV laser (or similar power source) spot to transform a liquid polymeric material into a solid material, building the different sections in which the prototype is divided until the complete creation of complex 3D geometry.

The process of laser curing can occur in two different configurations: the first approach provides a spot laser which scans the surface curing the photosensitive material, while the second approach processes one layer at a time, in which a DLP (digital light projection) technology uses a DMD (digital mirror device) to selectively solidify one 2D layer at a time. Cooke et al. fabricated polypropylene fumarate-based scaffolds as a demonstration of the possibility of using SLA technology in the TE field. Similarly, Sodian et al. using data obtained from

CT scans, built customized scaffold for a heart valve made up of thermoplastic elastomers such as PHOH and P4HB (Sodian et al., 2002).

The SLA technology was applied to fabricate hydrogel-based porous scaffolds; Yu et al. fabricated 3D scaffold made of hydroxyethyl methacrylate followed by a drying process and subsequent rehydration to allow cell adhesion (Yu et al., 2002). Many other research groups also selected PEG-DA (polyethylene glycol diacrylate) as the starting material to fabricate structures. In addition to synthetic polymers, hyaluronic-acid-based photopolymers were processed with the technology in question (Khademhosseini et al., 2006).

Another technology that exploits a photoreactive resin is known as solid ground curing (SGS); this is based on the exposure of a photopolymer resin to a UV lamp using specific masks to print each layer of a 3D structure. In TE, the SGC technology is used to process polymers opportunely modified for the photochemistry cross-linking process (Nguyen and West, 2002); in this case, the UV lamp serves to convert a liquid monomer into a hydrogel by radical easily controllable polymerization, even in physiological conditions (Vail et al., 1999).

In this category of RP, there are technologies that can be classified as selective laser sintering (SLS). SLS is an AM technique very similar to SLA, however, it uses a spot laser to sinter a powder following a predefined pattern. This technology is preferably used in TE for the fabrication of porous scaffold for the regeneration of bone. Vail et al. sintered a mixture of PEEK-HA-obtained scaffolds characterized by a good compromise between mechanical properties and bioactivity (Matsuda and Magoshi, 2002). Among all these technologies, which dispense energy following a specific pattern, SLS is the only one that is not suitable for processing hydrogels.

5.3.4 HYBRID RP TECHNOLOGIES

It is now established that ECM provides cells with a physical and chemical support containing critical biochemical information to regulate all their functions including adhesion, proliferation, survival, and differentiation. For these reasons, the biocompatibility of a scaffold can be classified in surface biocompatibility, which depends on the material, and in structural biocompatibility which depends on its topology and architecture. The dimensions of the building elements are important factors for the regulation of cell activities; in fact, previous studies have shown that the cell response is influenced by the architectural and hierarchical organization of the scaffold. The previous paragraphs have underlined the importance of the RP technologies in TE. All these techniques allow the design of scaffold architecture in a CAD/CAM-controlled way to cover the requirements of specific tissue, resulting in a modulation of the mechanical properties and in the chance to obtain structures with a completely interconnected porosity. They also allow the fabrication of multifunctional scaffolds, which consist of different materials and also of gradients of porosity.

However, RP scaffolds do not have adequate surface features, and the resolution of their pores is still limited in terms of efficiency of cell adhesion. The pore size of the scaffold RP is relatively large if compared to the cell size and therefore a high number of cells is required to obtain a sufficient number of adherent cells that produce sufficient ECM to functionalize the construct. This eventually results in high costs for the cell isolation, for the processes of cell expansion, and for the cell culture, which can create an obstacle to the clinical relevance of these 3D structures. As many research studies have recognized the importance of nanostructured architecture in TE applications, the introduction of a network of fibers on a nano- or microscale is the optimal solution to improve the structural biocompatibility of RP scaffolds. This network of fibers provides a very high surface/volume ratio to promote cell response and support at the nanoscale level and appropriate biochemical cues. To recreate multifunctional structures for TE, different approaches have been developed. Many research groups proposed the application of hybrid technologies that combine RP systems and an electrospinning process to produce 3D structures with the aim of recreating the complexity of the biological environment through a multiscale architecture.

The electrospinning process consists of the use of a high-voltage electrostatic field to produce an electrically charged jet from a polymer solution, which by drying during evaporation, leads to the formation of nanofibers. The traditional electrospinning machine is composed of a syringe pump to hold the polymer solution, two electrodes and a DC voltage supply in the kV range. Electrospinning can also involve molten polymer as the drawing fluid. Unlike a conventional drawing method where there is an external mechanical force that pushes the solution, electrospinning makes use of charges that are applied to the fluid to provide a stretching force to a collector where there is a potential gradient. During the electrospinning process a solution is contained in a syringe (a few ml) and an electrode is connected to the needle of the syringe, in order to charge the solution and at a certain distance from the needle is positioned in a grounded deposition plan.

After setting the flow rate in output from the syringe and the desired voltage (usually between 10 and 50 kV), a drop of the solution out of the tip of the needle due to the charge surface acquired can overcome the surface tension and take on the shape known as cone of Taylor. From the Taylor cone, only one nanofiber has its origin and moves to the collector, forming a mat of unwoven fibers. This mat consists of a single nanofiber with nanometric diameter, completely randomly arranged on the deposition plane. There is also the possibility of finding some collectors, specifically designed, to make the fibers deposit on them in an organized pattern. It is recommended to choose the solvent, the distance between the needle and the collector, and the temperature, such as to ensure that the spun fiber is completely dry when it reaches the collector. Furthermore, since research studies demonstrated that the morphology and size of the fibers influence the rate of cell proliferation, it is possible to electrospin fibers of different diameter and surface area, varying the flow rate or the intensity of the electric field, and the concentration of the polymer solution.

In the literature there are many examples of RP technology combined with the electrospinning technique; for example, Moroni et al. (2008a,b) successfully integrated of 3D fiber deposition with electrospinning techniques to fabricate a new set of multiscale scaffolds for cartilage regeneration. They fabricated PEOT- and PET-based scaffolds that were characterized by a periodic alternation between an RP network and electrospun fibers. To vary the fiber density in the scaffolds, the electrospinning process was performed for every two layers deposited by means of 3D fiber deposition for 15 s or 2 min, keeping constant the parameters relative to the applied voltage and the syringe flow rate. Park et al. (2008) instead adopted a hybrid process to fabricate 3D scaffolds combining the FMD process and an electrospinning one. In this case a PCL-based filament was extruded through FDM nozzles to obtain an architecture with appropriate mechanical properties, while a PCL solution was electrospun to provide additional surface area and improve the cell adhesion phenomena. The hybrid process consisted of two phases that were repeated sequentially until completion of the scaffold: deposition of a layer with FDM system according to a precise pattern and a subsequent deposition of electrospun microfibers.

5.4 DEVICE DESIGN

5.4.1 MARYLAND MANIPULATOR AND DESIGN SPECIFICATION

Many research groups successfully fabricated multifunctional ECM-like scaffold exploiting novel strategies that involve hybrid manufacturing processes. These manufacturing processes are focused on the combination and integration of different scaffold fabrication technologies; in most cases they are sequential processes which use independent systems for the application of different techniques of micro- or nanofabrication. This is not the optimal solution, because the passage of the structure under construction from one system to the other is executed manually by an operator, making the process complex and time-consuming. In other cases robotic systems were designed, mostly Cartesian manipulators, which provide a change of the tool of microfabrication, instead of the displacement of the structure. Following this approach, this work is focused on the design of a robotic system with a parallel architecture for the fabrication of multiscale and multimaterial scaffolds.

The great interest for parallel manipulators arises from their kinematic structure which offers many advantages compared to serial structures (Laribi et al., 2008): e.g., the high loading capacity, which derives from the possibility of subdividing the external forces between all the legs that support the end-effector. Parallel manipulators also offer the possibility to place the actuators on the frame for having low moving masses and, as a result, of obtaining high accelerations for the end-effector. The accuracy is very high, for the dynamic characteristics discussed above, and because the errors on the various axes do not add up to each other as happens to serial structures. A drawback is that they have limited workspace and are characterized by complex kinematic equations (Merlet, 2000; Tsai, 1999). In the literature, many parallel robots are described: the first attempt is attributed to Gough and Stewart, another widely known example was designed by Clavel, generally referred to as the Delta robot (Clavel, 1988). The architecture presented in this paper is the Maryland manipulator (Tsai et al., 1996a,b).

In the Maryland manipulator, three identical limbs connect the base and the end-effector (also referred to as platform). Each limb is made up of a lower arm and an upper arm connected by revolute joints. The upper limb is a simple bar and the lower limb is made up of a planar four-bar mechanism which constrains the movement of the platform only to translational degrees of freedom. The lower and upper arms are connected to the base and platform with revolute joints, respectively. The design is very similar to that of the Delta robot, but here only revolute joints are used to define the structure; this design choice makes the structure stiffer and more economically feasible (CuikSuite, 2014a,b).

In the simplest possible version of this mechanism, the platform parameters are the lengths of the limbs and the anchoring points of the legs at the base/platform. The axis of the revolute joints connecting the base and the legs can be taken as tangent to the circumference inscribing the triangle formed by the anchoring points.

As guidelines for the design of the parallel manipulator, the following specifications were defined:

1. A workspace with a cubic volume with a side of 200 mm was estimated useful for the required application
2. A payload of 60 N was defined as taking into account the contribution of the platform and tools
3. A maximum speed of 600 mm/s, typical of this category of manipulators, was defined as further specification
4. Finally, as the system will have to be immersed in an electric field, the building materials have to show insulating properties.

5.4.2 TOOL'S DESIGN

There are many methods for controlling the fluid flow during the layer-by-layer deposition of material, as a linear motor driving the syringe piston, or constant air pressure on the material in a reservoir with a controlled outlet valve.

In this work, a dispensing system with valves was used to control the deposition of a low-viscosity solution with high precision. The valve of the Series 752 V (Nordson) was selected to provide the extrusion process. For this tool, an appropriate holder was designed so that it could be attached to the end-effector of the machine.

The design of the piston-based tool, for processing high-viscosity materials, was inspired by the 2-Syringe Tool mounted on the Fab@Home 3D-printer

(Fab@home, 2014). This tool is equipped with two stepper motors and two syringes to build up objects with multiple materials. For this work the tool was also modified to permit the deposition of two separated materials (the building material and the support material) or two mixed materials.

For integrating the electrospinning module, the parallel manipulator was introduced into a commercially available electrospinning system. As the Maryland structure does not possess a high displacement in the vertical direction, this system was also equipped with an additional axis which guaranteed the motion of the deposition plane in the vertical direction to adjust the distance between the needle and the collector.

5.5 DIMENSIONAL ANALYSIS OF THE MARYLAND MANIPULATOR FOR A GIVEN WORKSPACE

The structural design of the device was made on the basis of design specifications about the workspace (Merlet, 1997).

Cuiksuite, an open-source set of tools to analyze configuration spaces defined by systems of kinematic equations (CuikeSuite, 2014) was used to determine the optimal length of the upper (l_u) and lower leg (l_l) of each arm, and the length of the off-set link (l_o) of each parallelogram (Figure 5.1).

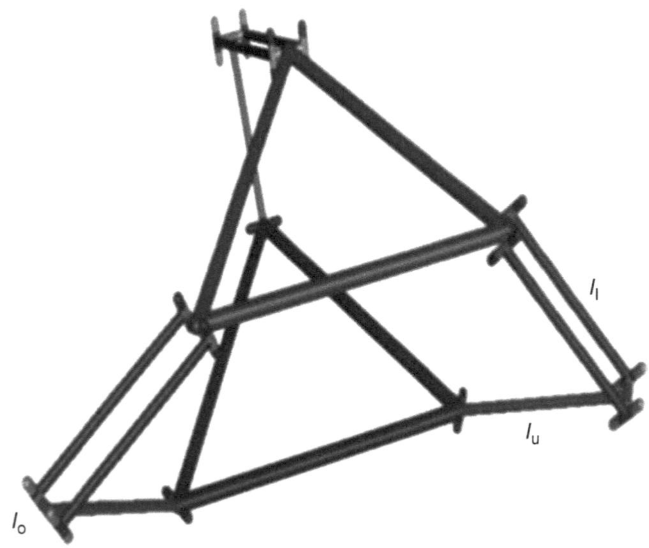

FIGURE 5.1

Result obtained by structural sizing with Cuiksuite.

Therefore, after setting the geometry of the platform and base as equilateral triangles of sides 350 and 200 mm, respectively, and the motion ranges of each actuated joint algorithm of the Cuiksuite toolbox were solved for various combinations of the three lengths and fixing the pose for the platform at various points on the edge of the workspace. In this way, $l_u = 150$ mm, $l_l = 300$ mm, and $l_o = 130$ mm were defined as the optimal lengths to guarantee the necessary workspace with more relaxed joints.

After the choice of lengths, a preliminary static analysis under a payload of 60 N was necessary to estimate the functional cross-section of the link in each limb.

5.6 INVERSE KINEMATIC MODEL OF THE MARYLAND MANIPULATOR

An inverse kinematics model was developed to determine the vector of the nine joint angles (θ_{1i}, θ_{2i}, θ_{3i} for $i = 1, 2, 3$) for a known position of the center of the end-effector P in a fixed-frame $\{S\}$, whose origin is at the center of the base. The problem was solved using a vectorial approach, fixing a local frame $\{S_i\}$ for each limb at the same origin as the frame $\{S\}$ but at a rotation of $\Phi_1 = 0°$, $\Phi_2 = 120°$, and $\Phi_3 = 240°$ (Tsai et al., 1996a,b). Finally, exploiting the symmetry of the system, the kinematic model was calculated applying the loop-closure equation (Eqn 5.1; Traslosheros et al., 2010) to each limb schematized as in Figure 5.2.

$$\overline{A_iPb_i} + \overline{Pb_iPc_i} = \overline{O_{xyz}P} + \overline{PPc_i} - \overline{O_{xyz}A_i} \tag{5.1}$$

The loop-closure equation (Eqn 5.1) imposed that the point C_i has to remain rigidly connected to the same point of the end-effector. Exploiting Eqn (5.1), the position of each point Pc_i was determinated in each local frame $\{S_i\}$ as shown in Eqn (5.2):

$$\begin{bmatrix} Pc_{ix} \\ Pc_{iy} \\ Pc_{iz} \end{bmatrix} = \begin{bmatrix} l_a\cos(\theta_{1i}) + l_b\sin(\theta_{1i})\cos(\theta_{1i} + \theta_{2i}) \\ l_b\cos(\theta_{3i}) \\ l_a\sin(\theta_{1i}) + l_b\cos(\theta_{3i})\sin(\theta_{1i} + \theta_{2i}) \end{bmatrix} \tag{5.2}$$

The points P and P_{ci} were related, as shown in Eqn (5.3), where starting from the coordinates of P_{ci} in local coordinates, allowed to get in the center of the platform in the global frame.

$$\begin{bmatrix} P_x \\ P_y \\ P_z \end{bmatrix} = \begin{bmatrix} \cos(\Phi_i) & \sin(\Phi_i) & 0 \\ -\sin(\Phi_i) & \cos(\Phi_i) & 0 \\ 0 & 0 & 1 \end{bmatrix} \left[\begin{bmatrix} Pc_{ix} \\ Pc_{iy} \\ Pc_{iz} \end{bmatrix} + \begin{bmatrix} H_i - h_i \\ 0 \\ 0 \end{bmatrix} \right] \tag{5.3}$$

Thus, knowing the position of the platform in the global frame, exploiting Eqn (5.3), it was possible to determine the coordinates of Pc_i in the local frame.

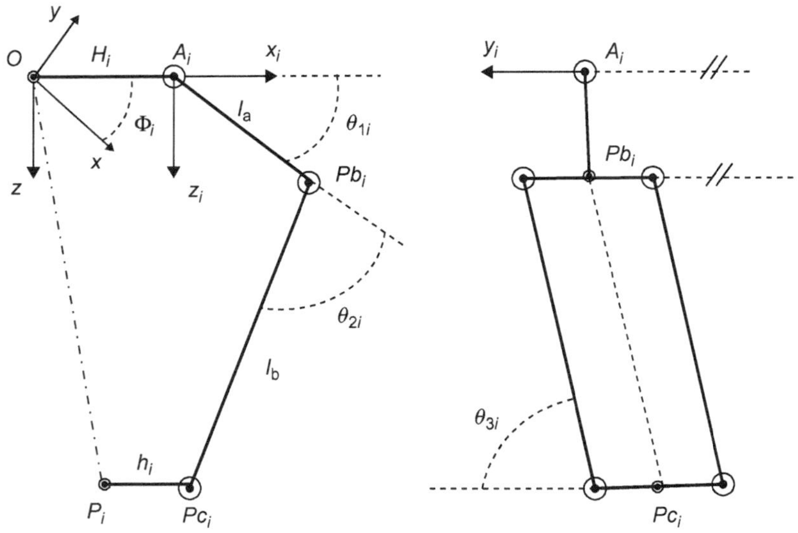

FIGURE 5.2

Simplified model for the kinematics and dynamics study of the manipulator.

After that, the nine joint angles (θ_{1i}, θ_{2i}, θ_{3i} for $i = 1, 2, 3$) were derived from Eqn (5.2) by a few simple algebraic steps.

For each position of the center of the end-effector, two solutions for θ_{2i} and θ_{3i} were produced. Solutions for θ_{2i} are independent from those of θ_{3i}, this resulted in four solution sets for θ_{3i}, but for each of the four solution sets there was a single value for θ_{1i}. To confirm the validity of the model, the nine joint variables were identified and plotted, varying the platform position along the z-axis. It was expected that the three joints variables for each limb had the same behavior; it was also verified that the platform has a limited range of translation along the z-axis complying with the specification of the workspace.

5.7 JACOBIAN MATRIX GENERATION

The Jacobian matrix allowed mapping of the velocities of the active joints (θ_{1i}) in joint space with the velocities of the center of the end-effector in Cartesian space. The Jacobian matrix for the Maryland manipulator was derived from a set of loop-closure equations (Eqn 5.4) that linked the Cartesian space variables to the joint space variables (Codourey, 1998).

$$||Pc_iPb_i||_2^2 - l_b^2 = 0 \tag{5.4}$$

The Jacobian matrix was derived by differentiating Eqn (5.4) for each limb and rearranging the results in a matrix form to obtaining the following expression:

$$\begin{pmatrix} \dot{P}_x \\ \dot{P}_y \\ \dot{P}_z \end{pmatrix} = J(\theta_{1i}, P) \cdot \begin{pmatrix} \dot{\theta}_{11} \\ \dot{\theta}_{12} \\ \dot{\theta}_{13} \end{pmatrix} \tag{5.5}$$

where $\dot{P} = \left(\dot{P}_x \dot{P}_y \dot{P}_z\right)^{\mathrm{T}}$ is the twist of the platform, and $\dot{\theta} = \left(\dot{\theta}_{11} \dot{\theta}_{12} \dot{\theta}_{13}\right)^{\mathrm{T}}$ is the vector of the joint velocities. The Jacobian matrix ($J \in R^{3\times 3}$) is a function of θ_{1i} and of the end-effector position. The results from Eqn (5.4) were derived with respect to the time to map the acceleration in Cartesian space with acceleration in joint space.

5.8 DYNAMICS MODELING WITH PRINCIPLE OF VIRTUAL WORKS

The key issue in dynamic analysis for a parallel manipulator is to establish an inverse dynamic model so that the required actuator forces and/or torques can be computed when a desired trajectory of the mobile platform is given.

In this case, the complexity of the dynamic model derives from the presence of the articulated quadrilateral in each lower limb. To simplify the dynamic analysis, since the connecting rods of the arms can be built with low-density materials and neglecting the rotational inertia of lower limb, the mass of each lower limb was split into two parts: two-thirds were placed at its upper extremity (the end of upper link) and the other third at its lower extremity. In this way, the manipulator was reduced into four bodies: the traveling plate (end-effector) and the three upper arms (Li and Xu, 2005a,b).

Applying the principle of virtual work (Eqn 5.6), neglecting the friction forces and assuming no application of external forces, the gravitational and inertial contribution forces were calculated from the end-effector and from each upper limb to the actuated joints (Li and Xu, 2005a,b):

$$\tau^{\mathrm{T}} \cdot \delta\theta = F^{\mathrm{T}} \cdot \delta P \tag{5.6}$$

In Eqn (5.6), τ is the force/torque vector corresponding to joint space virtual displacement $\delta\theta$ and F is the force/torque acting on the traveling plate corresponding to the virtual displacement δP in Cartesian space.

Introducing the relationship between joint velocity and Cartesian velocity, the above equation can be used to transform the forces/torques acting in Cartesian space to joint space as:

$$\tau = J^{\mathrm{T}} \cdot F \tag{5.7}$$

The vector of actuator torques was determined according to the d'Alembert principle obtaining the following expression (Eqn 5.8):

$$\tau = \tau_b + \tau_n - (\tau_{g\_n} + \tau_{g\_b}) \tag{5.8}$$

where τ_n and τ_{g_n} are the contribution of inertial force and gravity force acting on the traveling platform in joint space, while τ_b and τ_{g_b} are the contribution of inertial force and gravity force from the upper limb.

In particular, starting from the masses calculated as described above (Eqn 5.9):

$$\tau_n = J^T \cdot m_t \cdot \ddot{P} \tag{5.9}$$

where m_t is the mass of traveling platform with the addition of the one-third of each lower limb,

$$\tau_{g\_n} = J^T \cdot m_t \cdot ((0 \quad 0 \quad -g))^T \tag{5.10}$$

$$\tau_b = I_b \cdot \ddot{\theta} \tag{5.11}$$

where I_b the inertia matrix of upper limbs.

Finally:

$$\tau_{g\_b} = r_{g\_b} \cdot G \cdot (\cos\theta_{1i}\cos\theta_{2i}\cos\theta_{3i}) \tag{5.12}$$

where r_{g_b} is the center of mass of each upper limb (m_{ul}) and G was defined as shown in Eqn (5.13)

$$G = m_{ul} * g \tag{5.13}$$

Starting from the masses calculated as described above and design specifications (velocity 600 mm/s, acceleration 6×10^4 mm/s^2), Equation (5.6) allows us to select a servomotor with brake and characterized by a nominal torque of 7.16 Nm and a velocity of 2000 rpm.

5.9 RESULTS OF DEVICE DESIGN

On the basis of the results obtained from the studies of structural and dynamic design two different prototypes were designed: a technical prototype and a validation prototype.

The CAD model of a technical prototype was designed using the CAD software Inventor® (Autodesk Inc.). This is shown in Figure 5.3 in which it is possible to recognize the typical elements of the Maryland architecture: a fixed base, a mobile platform, and three legs with an identical kinematic structure. The manipulator was characterized by the geometric parameters that make it structurally suitable to ensure the working space required by specific design with an adequate

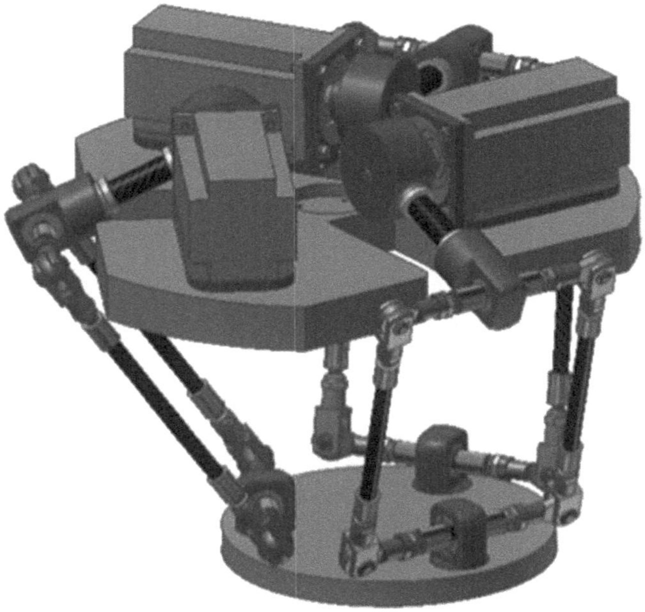

FIGURE 5.3

CAD model of the Maryland manipulator.

dexterity and the minimum encumbrance. Materials, including Macor, carbon fiber, and Derlin, were selected as building materials for their insulating properties.

Macor is a glass-ceramic that can be machined in a quick, accurate and economic way; the carbon fiber provides good mechanical properties and good resistance to temperature and chemical agents; finally, the Derlin can be processed in various shapes and provides a satisfactory combination of mechanical and chemical properties. Some components were commercially available, others were custom-fabricated.

The validation prototype was designed and assembled to check the implemented model of the inverse kinematics, to test the biofabrication tool, to verify if components were difficult to assemble, and whether it could be considered in the stages of assembly.

The validation prototype, as shown in Figure 5.4, is structurally identical to the technical model, the only difference being that the various components are made of wood or of PLA printed with an ordinary PrusaI3 FDM printer. The actuators selected for this system were servo motors SG5010; it was controlled with an electronic open source (Arduino) according to the kinematic implemented model using a proper GUI designed with Matlab® as shown in Figure 5.5.

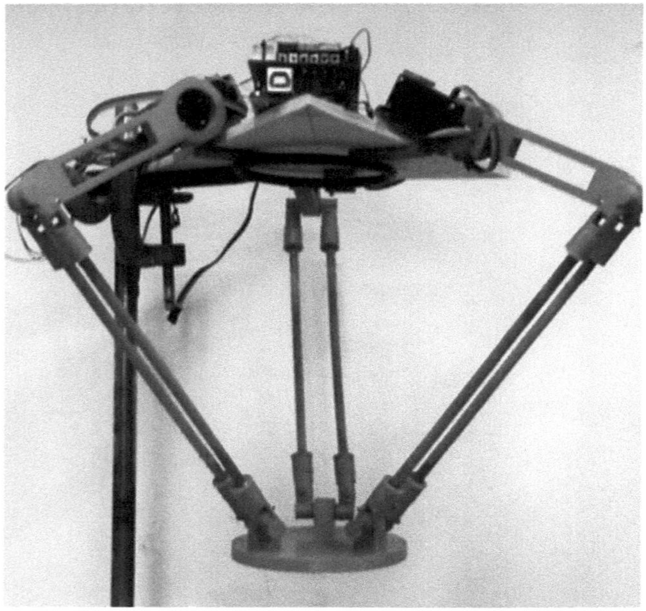

FIGURE 5.4

Validation prototype of the Maryland manipulator.

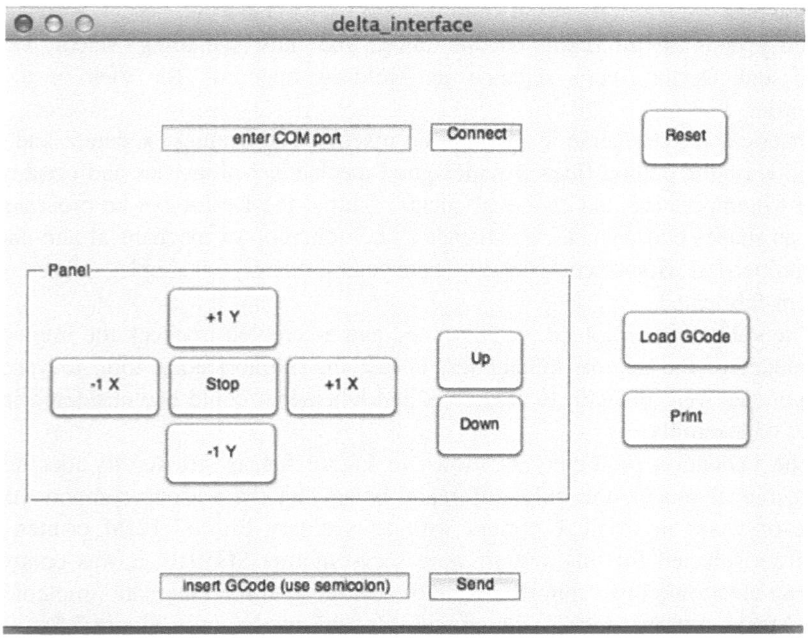

FIGURE 5.5

Graphical user interface developed in Matlab®.

The Arduino firmware was based on an open source project, and the protocol of communication based on the GCode allowed easy communication between the firmware and the GUI.

The firmware Arduino was based on an available open source project, whose structure, shown in Figure 5.6, provided for an arm class that described the various links that made up each kinematic chain, and a joint structure that determined the kinematic constraints; within these structures were the three vector structures which defined the coordinates of the end-effector in space. The inverse kinematics of the manipulator was determined by suitably combining the arm structure.

The GUI was equipped with a button to connect the system, one to activate the COM port, one to load the GCode file, and finally one to activate the platform for the deposition of materials following a precise pattern. Moreover, the user could insert a single line of GCode in the proper space, this may be the best choice for calibrating the machine; this information could be transmitted to Arduino through the proper button.

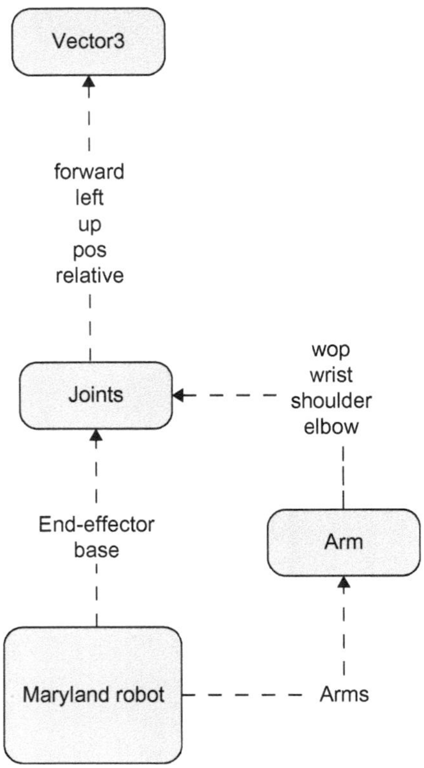

FIGURE 5.6

Structure of the open-source firmware.

5.10 SCAFFOLD FABRICATION

To demonstrate the validity of the proposed fabrication system, hydrogel-based scaffolds were designed and built using the piston-based extrusion tool shown in Figure 5.7. Pure hydrogels or hydrogels loaded with nanoparticles

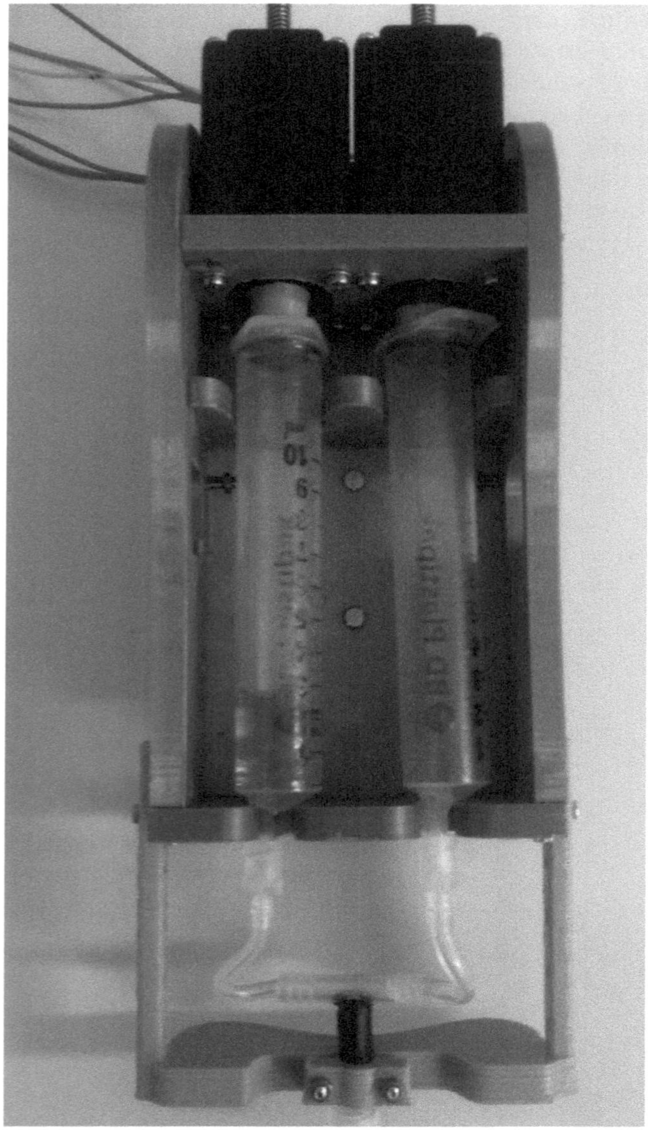

FIGURE 5.7

Piston-driven extrusion tool.

were deposited in various 3D shapes, with features that ranged from micrometric to millimetric. The nanometric features were obtained thanks to embedded nanoparticles.

5.10.1 MATERIAL PREPARATION

Vinyl-pyrrolidone/Vinyl-alcohol copolymer was purchased from Lodovico Martelli (Florence, Italy) and used at it was, or colored with food coloring to distinguish the complex structures and demonstrate the two-material fabrication procedure.

Alginic acid (Sigma Aldrich, Italy) solution 5% (w/v) was prepared by dissolving the powder in milliQ water. After extrusion, the gel was physically cross-linked by dipping the scaffold into a solution of $CaCl_2$.

Alginate hydrogel was reinforced with the introduction of both a solution of nanoparticles of TiO_2 (6% w/v) and nanohydroxyapatite (Sigma Aldrich, Italy) at various percentages.

5.10.2 SCAFFOLD FABRICATION

The scaffold fabrication started with drawing the CAD model of the structure with the desiderated architecture. Then the CAD file (.STL) was imported into the model using a slicing software, which translates the sliced coordinate information in GCode controls which manage the movement of the tool in 3D and the dispensing of biomaterials for each layer. In this work, various shapes were designed using the CAD software Inventor® (Autodesk Inc.), and the GCode was produced with Cura (Ultimaker Inc.), varying parameters such as shape, fill density, and line thickness.

A 21G cylindrical metallic needle, with a flat end, and two commercial 10-ml syringes were used to print the scaffold. The material was deposited onto a glass slide.

The piston extrusion tool suitably modified for the deposition of mixed materials was used for the printing of multimaterial scaffolds; this modification prevented the inoperative needle from taking away the material deposited by the working needle.

In this case, to obtain the deposition of two distinct materials it was necessary to set appropriately the amount of material per layer in the wipe&prime tower (in the slicing software) deposited near of the structures under construction.

As shown in Figure 5.8, PVA-based hydrogels, with high viscosity, were obtained in two different colorations with a good shape fidelity; in particular, these figures show the capabilities of the system of printing structures characterized by a different porosity. The control of the porosity was possible by adjusting

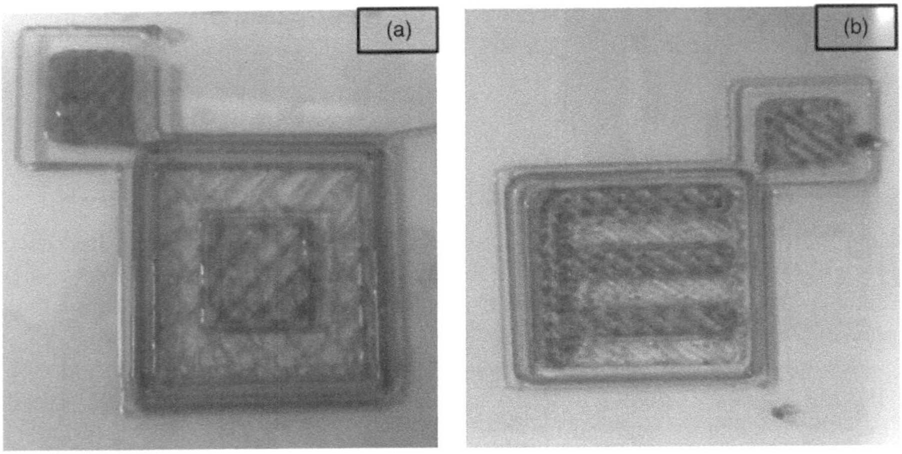

FIGURE 5.8

Examples of PVA hydrogel-based structures.

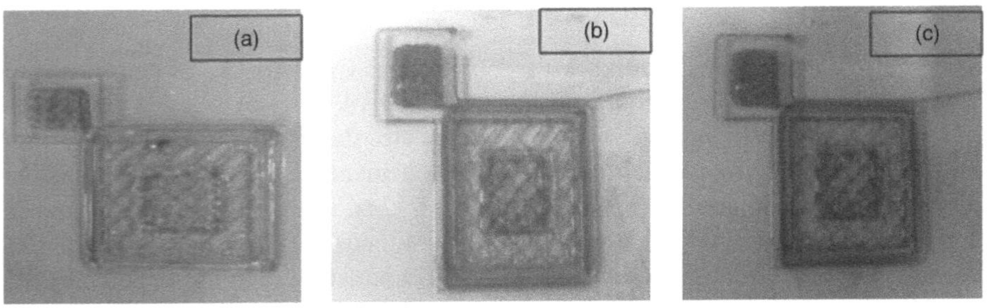

FIGURE 5.9

Three different structures printed with different amount of wipe&prime volume per layer.

the percentage of fill density when the CAD files were imported in the slicing software to generate the GCode. Figure 5.9 shows three identical structures obtained with different amounts of wipe&prime volume per layer; as shown in Figure 5.9c, with 25 mm^3 of wipe&prime volume per layer it was possible to extrude two completely distinct materials.

The alginate-based scaffolds are shown in Figure 5.10. This figure highlights the capacity of the system to process composite material with different viscosity without losing resolution and accuracy.

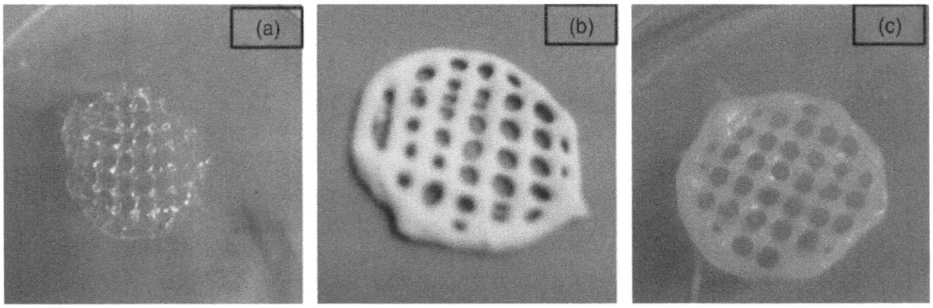

FIGURE 5.10

Example of alginate hydrogel-based structure (a), example of alginate with nanoparticles of TIO_2 hydrogel-based structure (b), example of alginate with nanohydroxyapatite hydrogel-based structure (c).

5.11 CONCLUSIONS

In this research a Maryland manipulator was designed for multiscale and multi-material microfabrication of scaffold through a combination of pressure extrusion, syringe extrusion, and electrospinning. Starting from appropriate specifications, the design was focused on the structural and actuator sizing, thanks to the kinematic and dynamic models implemented ad hoc for the Maryland architecture. Starting from the CAD model, a scale prototype was printed to validate the implemented kinematic model. As a demonstration of the validity of the design, the syringe extrusion tool was used to fabricate composite hydrogel structures for TE applications.

REFERENCES

Boland, T., Xu, T., Damon, B., Cui, X., 2006. Application of inkjet printing to tissue engineering. Biotechnol. J. 1 (9), 910–917.

Centola, M., Rainer, A., Spadaccio, C., De Porcellinis, S., Genovese, J.A., Trombetta, M., 2010. Combining electrospinning and fused deposition modeling for the fabrication of a hybrid vascular graft. Biofabrication 2 (1), 014–102.

Chen, G., Sato, T., Ushida, T., Hirochika, R., Shirasaki, Y., 2003. The use of a novel PLGA fiber/collagen composite web as a scaffold for engineering of articular cartilage tissue with adjustable thickness. J. Biomed. Mater. Res. A 67 (4), 1170–1180.

Clavel, R., 1988. Delta, a fast robot with parallel geometry. In: Proc. IEEE International Symposium on Industrial Robot, pp. 91–100.

Codourey, A., 1998. Dynamic modeling of parallel robots for computed-torque control implementation. Int. J. Robotics Res. 17 (12), 1325–1336.

CuikSuite, 2014a. [Online] Available from: http://www-iri.upc.es/people/porta/Soft/CuikSuite-Doc/html/index.html.

CuikeSuite, 2014b. [Online] Avaible from: http://www.iri.upc.edu/people/porta/Soft/CuikSuite2-Doc/html/.

Darling, A., Shor, L., Khalil, S., Mondrinos, M., Lelkes, P., Guceri, S., et al., 2005. Multimaterial scaffolds for tissue engineering. Macromol. Symp. 227 (1), 345–356.

Derby, B., 2012. Printing and prototyping of tissues and Scaffolds. Science 338, 921–926.

Fab@home, 2014. [Online] Available from: http://www.fabathome.org/.

Hutmacher, D.W., 2001. Scaffold design and fabrication technologies for engineering tissues-state of the art and future perspectives. J. Biomater. Sci. Polym. Ed. 12 (1), 107–124.

Hutmacher, D.W., Sittinger, M., Risbud, M.V., 2004. Scaffold-based tissue engineering: rationale for computer-aided design and solid free-form fabrication systems. Trends Biotechnol. 22 (7), 354–362.

Kalita, S.J., Bose, S., Hosick, H.L., Bandyopadhyay, A., 2003. Development of controlled porosity polymerceramic composite scaffolds via fused deposition modeling. Mater. Sci. Eng. C23, 611–620.

Karageorgiou, V., Kaplan, D., 2005. Porosity of 3D biomaterial scaffolds and osteogenesis. Biomaterials 26 (27), 5474–5491.

Khademhosseini, A., Eng, G., Yeh, J., Fukuda, J., Blumling, J., Langer, R., et al., 2006. Micromolding of photocross-linkable hyaluronic acid for cell encapsulation and entrapment. J. Biomed. Mater. Res. A 79A, 522–532.

Kim, G.H., Son, J.T., 2009. 3D polycaprolactone (PCL) scaffold with hierarchical structure fabricated by a piezoelectric transducer (PZT)-assisted bioplotter. Appl. Phys. 94, 781–785.

Kumbar, S.G., James, R., Nukavarapu, S.P., Laurencin, C.T., 2008. Electrospun nanofiber scaffolds: engineering soft tissues. Biomed. Mater. 3 (3), 034002.

Laboratory Equipment, 2014. [Online] Available from: http://digital.laboratoryequipment.com/labequipment/august_2013?pg=10.

Lam, C.X.F., Mo, X.M., Teoh, S.H., 2002. Scaffold development using 3D printing with a starch-based polymer. Mater. Sci. Eng. C 20, 49–56.

Landers, R., Mulhaupt, R., 2000. Desktop manufacturing of complex objects, prototypes and biomedical scaffolds by means of computer-assisted design combined with computer-guided 3D plotting of polymers and reactive oligomers. Macromol. Mater. Eng. 282, 17–21.

Lanza, R., Langer, R., Vacanti, J., 2007. Principles of Tissue Engineering. Academic Press, San Diego, CA, USA.

Laribi, M.A., Romdhane, L., Zeghloul, S., 2008. Advanced synthesis of the DELTA parallel robot for a specified workspace. In: Huapeng, W. (Ed.), Parallel Manipulators, Towards New Applications. InTech, Rijeka, Croatia, ISBN: 978-3-902613-40-0.

Li, Y., Xu, Q., 2005a. Dynamic analysis of a modified DELTA parallel robot for cardiopulmonary resuscitation. In: Proc. in IEEE/RSJ International Conference of Intelligent Robots and Systems, pp. 3371–3376.

Li, Y., Xu, Q., 2005b. Kinematics and inverse dynamics analysis for a general 3-PRS spatial parallel mechanism. Robotica 23, 219–229.

Lo, C.M., Wang, H.B., Dembo, M., Wang, Y.L., 2000. Cell movement is guided by the rigidity of the substrate. Biophys. J. 79 (1), 144–152.

Ma, P.X., Zhang, R., 1999. Synthetic nano-scale fibrous extracellular matrix. J. Biomed. Mater. Res. 46 (1), 60–72.

Malda, J., Woodfield, T.B., Van Der Vloodt, F., Kooy, F.K., Martens, D.E., Tramper, J., et al., 2004. The effect of PEGT/PBT scaffold architecture on oxygen gradients in tissue engineered cartilaginous constructs. Biomaterials 25 (26), 5773–5780.

Mariani, M., Rosatini, F., Vozzi, G., Previti, A., Ahluwalia, A., 2006. Characterization of tissue-engineered scaffolds microfabricated with PAM. Tissue Eng. 12 (3), 547–557.

Matsuda, T., Magoshi, T., 2002. Preparation of vinylated polysaccharidesand photofabrication of tubular scaffolds as potential use in tissue engineering. Biomacromolecules 3, 942–950.

Melchels, F.P.W., Domingos, M.A.N., Klein, T.J., Malda, J., Bartolo, P.J., Hutmacher, D., 2012. Additive manufacturing of tissues and organs. Prog. Polym. Sci. 37 (31), 1079–1104.

Merlet, J.P., 1997. Designing a parallel manipulator for a specific workspace. Int. J. Robotics Res. 16 (4), 545–556.

Merlet, J.P. (Ed.), 2000. Parallel Robot. Kluwer, Dordrecht.

Moroni, L., de Wijna, J.R., van Blitterswijk, C.A., 2006. 3D fiber-deposited scaffolds fortissue engineering: influence of pores geometry and architecture on dynamic mechanical properties. Biomaterials 27, 974–985.

Moroni, L., de Wijn, J.R., van Blitterswijk, C.A., 2008a. Integrating novel technologies to fabricate smart scaffold. J. Biomater. Sci. Polym. Ed. 19, 543–572.

Moroni, L., Schotel, R., Hamann, D., De Wijn, J. R., Van Blitterswijk, C.A., 2008b. 3D fiber-deposited electrospun integrated scaffolds enhance cartilage tissue formation. Adv. Funct. Mater. 18, 53–60.

Nakamura, M., Iwanaga, S., Henmi, C., Arai, K., Nishiyama, Y., 2010. Biomatrices and biomaterials for future developments of bioprinting and biofabrication. Biofabrication 2 (1), 014110.

Nguyen, K.T., West, J.L., 2002. Photopolymerizable hydrogels for tissue engineering applications. Biomaterials 23, 4307–4314.

Organovo, 2014. [Online] Available from: http://www.organovo.com/science-technology/bioprinting-process.

Ortinau, S., Schmich, J., Block, S., Liedmann, A., Jonas, L., Weiss, D., et al., 2010. Effect of 3D-scaffold formation on differentiation and survival in human neural progenitor cells. Biomed. Eng. OnLine 9, 70.

Park, S.H., Kim, T.G., Kim, H.C., Yang, D.Y., Park, T.G., 2008. Development of dual scale scaffolds via direct polymermelt deposition and electrospinning for applications in tissue regeneration. Acta Biomater. 4, 1198–1207.

Peter, M., Ganesh, N., Selvamurugan, N., Nair, S.V., Furuike, T., Tamura, H., et al., 2010. Preparation and characterization of chitosan-gelatinnano-hydroxyapatite composite scaffolds for tissue engineering applications. Carbohyd. Polym. 80 (3), 687–694.

Puppi, D., Zhang, X., Yang, L., Chiellini, F., Sun, X., Chiellini, E., 2014. Nano/microfibrous polymeric constructs loaded with bioactive agents and designed for tissue engineering applications: a review. J. Biomed. Mater. Res. Part B 102, 1562–1579.

Sachlos, E., Czernuszka, J.T., 2003. Making tissue engineering scaffolds work. Review on the application of solid freeform fabrication technology to the production of tissue e ngineering scaffolds. Eur. Cells Mater. 5, 29–40.

Sargeant, T.D., Desai, A.P., Banerjee, S., Agawu, A., Stopek, J.B., 2012. An *in situ* forming collagen-PEG hydrogel for tissue regeneration. Acta Biomaterialia 8 (1), 124–132.

Singh, M., Berkland, C., Detamore, M.S., 2008. Strategies and applications for incorporating physical and chemical signal gradients in tissue engineering. Tissue Eng. Part B Rev. 14 (4), 341–366.

Sodian, R., Loebe, M., Hein, A., Martin, D.P., Hoerstrup, S., Hausmann, H., et al., 2002. Application of Stereolithography for scaffold fabrication for tissue engineered heart valves. ASAIO J. 48, 12–16.

Stevens, M.M., George, J.H., 2005. Exploring and engineering the cell surface interface. Science 310, 1135–1138.

Tirella, A., Vozzi, G., Ahluwalia, A., 2008. Biomimicry of PAM microfabricated hydrogel scaffold. In: Nip24/Digital Fabrication 2008: 24th International Conference on Digital Printing Technologies. Tech. Program Proc.; pp. 496–500.

Toffenetti, J.L., Royaee, A.R., 2014. Patentability of 3D-printed organs. Genet. Eng. Biotechol. News [Online] Available from: http://www.genengnews.com/insight-and-intelligence/patentability-of-3d-printed-organs/77900129/.

Traslosheros, A., Angel, L., Sebastian, J.L., Roberti, F., Carelli, R., Vaca, R., 2010. New visual servoing control strategies in tracking tasks using a PKM. In: Milella, A., Di Paola, D., Cicirelli, G. (Eds.), Mechatronic Systems Simulation Modeling and Control. InTech, Rijeka, Croatia, ISBN: 978-953-307-041-4.

Tsai, L.W., 1999. Robot Analysis: The Mechanics of Serial and Parallel Manipulators. Wiley-IEEE, Seattle, WA, USA.

Tsai, L.W., Walsh, G.C., Stamper, E.R., 1996a. Kinematics of a Novel Three DOF Translational. In: Proc. IEEE Internaltional Conf. on Robotics and Automation, vol. 1, pp. 345–350.

Tsai, L.W., Walsh, G.C., Stamper, R.E., 1996b. Kinematics of novel three DOF translation platform, In: Proc. IEEE International Conference on Robotics and Automation, vol. 4, pp. 3446–3451.

Vail, N.K., Swain, L.D., Fox, W.C., et al., 1999. Materials for biomedical applications. Mater. Des. 20, 123–132.

Vozzi, G., Previti, A., Ciaravella, G., Ahluwalia, A., 2004. Microfabricated fractal branching networks. J. Biomed. Mater. Res. A 71 (2), 326–333.

Woodfield, T.B., Malda, J., de Wijn, J., Péter, F., van Blitterswijk, C.A., 2004. Design of porous scaffolds for cartilage tissue engineering using a three-dimensional fiber-deposition technique. Biomaterials 25 (18), 4149–4161.

Xu, T., Gregory, C.A., Molnar, P., Cui, X., Jalota, S., Bhaduri, S.B., et al., 2006. Viability and electrophysiology of neural cell structures generated by the inkjet printing method. Biomaterials 27 (9), 3580–3588.

Yu, T., Chiellini, F., Schmaljohan, D., Solaro, R., Ober, C., 2002. Microfabrication of hydrogels for biomedical applications. In: Fedynyshyn, T.H. (Ed.), Advances in Resist Technology and Processing. Bellingham, Washington, DC, pp. 854–860.

Zein, I., Hutmacher, D., Tan, K.K., Theo, S.H., 2002. Fused deposition modeling of novel scaffold architectures for tissue engineering applications. Biomaterials 23, 1169–1185.

Zhang, K., Wang, X., Jing, D., Yang, Y., Zhu, M., 2009. Bionic electrospun ultrafine fibrous poly(L-lactic acid) scaffolds with a multi-scale structure. Biomed. Mater. 4, 035004.

Zhao, J., Guo, L.Y., Yang, X.B., Weng, J., 2008. Preparation of bioactive porous HA/PCL composite scaffolds. Appl. Surf. Sci. 255, 2942–2946.

CHAPTER

Advanced nanobiomaterials in tissue engineering: synthesis, properties, and applications

6

Mustafa Abu Ghalia and Yaser Dahman

Department of Chemical Engineering, Ryerson University, Toronto, Canada

6.1 INTRODUCTION

Tissue engineering has been defined as a novel regenerative medicine in the treatment of malfunctioning or lost organs. Applying bionanocomposite materials in tissue engineering is the most recent innovative domain where biodegradable materials provide unique surfaces that promote the regeneration and reconstruction of human organs. The constant effort of cell biologists, materials scientists, and engineers is creating a bright future for biodegradable polymer as biomaterials (Smith et al., 2009). Various types of natural and synthetic biodegradable polymers have been investigated for medical and pharmaceutical applications, as an example of natural polymers; cellulose and starches are still commonly used in biomedical research in addition to synthetic biodegradable polymers such as polylactic acid (PLA), poly-glycolic acid (PGA), and poly-caprolactone (PCL) as well as their copolymers which are now generally used in biomedical devices because of their excellent biocompatibility. In particular, PLA is widely used in biomedical applications due to its bioresorbability and biocompatible properties in the human body. The main reported examples on medical or biomedical products are fracture devices like screws, sutures, delivery systems, microtitration plates, and materials for tissue engineering. In tissue engineering, cells can be grown in a PLA scaffold that is inserted at the site of the organ defect (Doi and Steinbuchel, 2002). Therefore, Huan et al. (2011) have investigated interactions between PLA/CDHA [carbonated calcium-deficient hydroxyapatite (HAP)] for tissue engineering approaches to tissue substitutes to enhance biocompatibility. Biodegradable polymers such as PLA and PGA have been conventionally used as tissue engineering scaffolds due to their biocompatibility and biodegradability (Majola et al., 1991).

Nanobiomaterials in Soft Tissue Engineering. DOI: http://dx.doi.org/10.1016/B978-0-323-42865-1.00006-4

However, their limits in mechanical properties compared to bone and lack of osteoconductivity have been a reason for reinforcement with inorganic materials. Bioceramics such as hydroxyapatite (nHAP) are a class of material used for bone repair. These materials are similar to the mineral components of bone and show good osteoconductivity. They are inherently brittle and difficult to process into tissue engineering materials. Hence, the development of nanobiocomposite materials is one strategy that Michael et al. (1997) have used to study the osteoconductivity of collagen–PLA nanocomposite by fabricated embedding parallel collagen fibers within a PLA to improve biocompatibility and processability of biodegradable polymers. Another new class of synthetic polymer is bacterial cellulose (BC)–collagen nanocomposite that can be used as an alternative biomaterial for vascular tissue engineering (Saska et al., 2012). Carbon nanotubes (CNTs) applied in the creation of tissue engineering scaffolds because of potential advantages in their high strength and low weight, despite the biocompatibility and cytotoxicity of CNTs, are not yet clear (Mahshid et al., 2011). In recent years, more attention has turned toward understanding and manipulating the unique physical properties of polymer nanocomposites. This increasing interest can be ascribed to a growing recognition that moves beyond formulating polymers with nanoparticles, and toward efficiently engineered, designed, and functional nanocomposites (Yan et al., 2001). In this chapter (Figure 6.1), we describe the main stages of the literature reviews into creating bionanocomposite materials for applications in bone tissue regenerative.

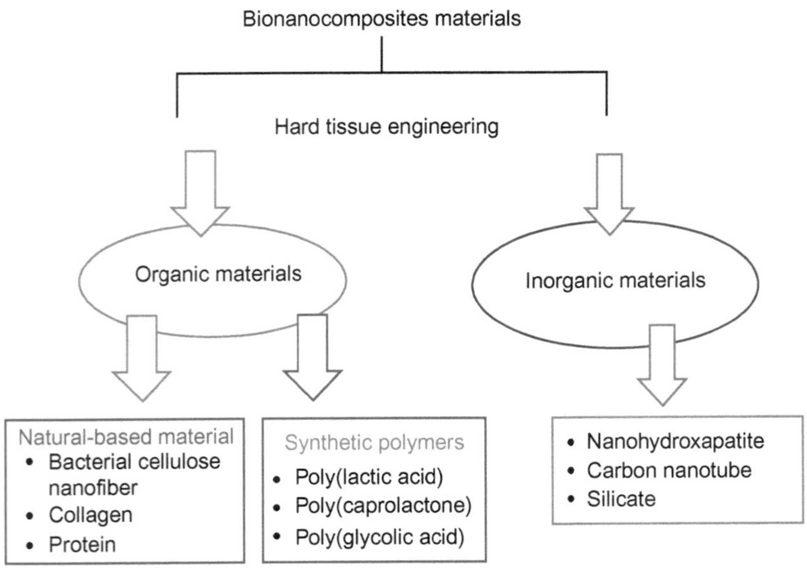

FIGURE 6.1

Diagram of bionanocomposite materials in tissue engineering applications.

6.2 NATURAL AND SYNTHETIC BIOPOLYMERS FOR TISSUE ENGINEERING

In recent times, polymers have been the most fascinating materials selected as a scaffold design in terms of applications in tissue engineering and drug-delivery materials. In particular, biodegradable polymerics have been widely employed and categorized as natural and synthetic biopolymers. Preferable classes of synthetic biodegradable polymers that offer superior mechanical strength due to it can be manipulated during synthesis to control the rate of biodegradability and biocompatibility. However, due to their hydrophobicity and their lower cell affinity they encourage natural-derived polymer *in situ* copolymerization with synthetic biodegradable polymers to gain a high potential advantage for enhancing cell adhesion and biological structure. However, they have poor mechanical properties with limitations of sufficient supply and source variation. Therefore, biopolymer nanocomposites play an important role in mimicking the composite nature of real bone combining the toughness of the polymer phase with the compressive strength of an inorganic one to generate bioactive materials with improved mechanical properties (Lu et al., 2003; Zhang and Sun, 2005; Woodard et al., 2007).

6.2.1 BIODEGRADABLE POLYMERS

As shown in Figure 6.2, an attempt has been made to classify the biodegradable polymers into two groups and four different families. The main groups are (i) the

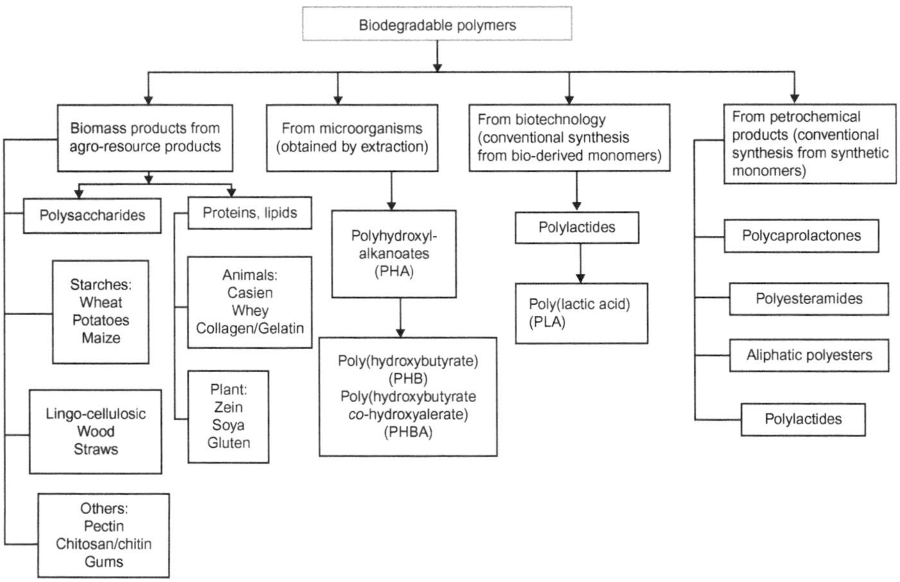

FIGURE 6.2

Classification of the biodegradable polymers (Averous, 2004).

agropolymers (polysaccharides, proteins, etc.) and (ii) the biopolyesters (biodegradable polyesters) such as PLA, polyhydroxyalkanoate, and aromatic and aliphatic copolyesters (Zhang and Sun, 2005). Biodegradable polymers show a large range of properties and can now compete with nonbiodegradable thermoplastics in different fields (packaging, textile, and biomedical applications). Aliphatic polyesters, such as poly (lactic acid) (PLA), poly (glycolic acid) (PGA), poly (3-caprolactone) (PCL), have attracted wide attention for their biodegradability and biocompatibility in the human body. A logical consequence has been the introduction of organic and inorganic nanofillers into biodegradable polymers to produce nanocomposites based on HA, metal nanoparticles, or carbon nanostructures, in order to prepare new biomaterials with enhanced properties. Consequently, the improvement in interfacial adhesion between the polymer and the nanostructures has become the key technique in the nanocomposite process. There is no single biodegradable polymer that can meet all the requirements for biomedical scaffolds. Consequently, the design and preparation of multicomponent polymer systems presents a viable strategy in order to develop innovative multifunctional biomaterials (Averous, 2004).

6.2.2 BC FOR TISSUE ENGINEERING

BC has been the most extensively investigated nanocellulose biomaterial for tissue engineering (Petersen and Gatenholm, 2011). BC is chemically composed of glucose monomers as shown in Figure 6.3. Cellulose is a linear polysaccharide homopolymer of D-glucose with a disaccharide repeat unit consisting of two glucose residues joined by a β(1−4) glycosidic bond (Bielecki et al., 2002). Its chemical formula is $(C_6H_{10}O_5)_n$. The number of glucose units in native cellulose (cellulose made by living organisms) depends on the source, such as primary or secondary cell walls. Primary cell wall cellulose polymers have about 8000 glucose units per chain (degree of polymerization of 8000). Secondary wall cellulose has a higher degree of polymerization that is up to 15,000. BC is highly advantageous over cellulose from plant sources because it has a higher water retention capacity, and a higher permeability to oxygen, among many others (Dahman, 2009). Its high surface-to-volume ratio, combined with its unique properties such

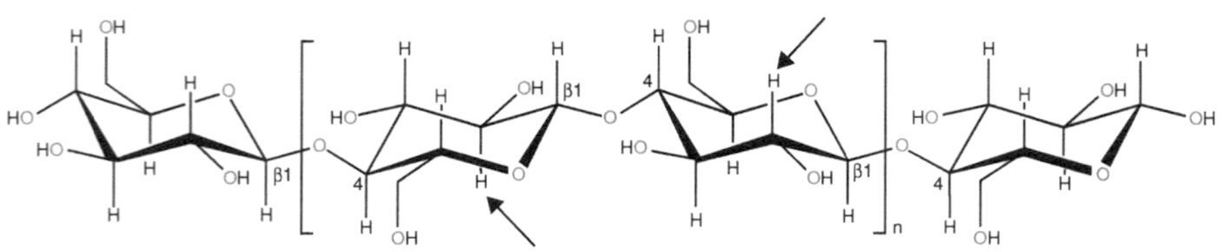

FIGURE 6.3

Structural formula of cellulose. The arrows point to the basic repeat unit, which is a cellobiose molecule (Klemm et al., 2001).

as polyfunctionality, hydrophilicity, and biocompatibility, make it an important material for different green biomedical fields. Signficant studies by Wahib and Dahman (2013) were performed to synthesize green biocellulose nanofibers (BCNs) of wheat straw as widely available agricultural residues by two different fermentation methods: separate hydrolysis fermentation (SHF) and saccharification fermentation (SSF) under different acidic and enzymatic conditions. BCN production achieved by Dahman et al. (2010) was ~9.7 g/L in SHF and 10.89 g/L in SSF.

BC is usually prepared by static suspension culture of *Gluconacetobacter xylinus* (*Acetobacter xylinum*) in a liquid medium. Under such conditions, a gelatinous material (termed a pellicle) is deposited at the air–medium interface with thickness increasing over time. The pellicle consists of nanofibers with diameters of less than 100 nm and a total water content of approximately 99%. Much of the interest in BC is due to the purity of the cellulose compared to plant-derived cellulose, as well as the long fiber length, high degree of crystallinity, web-like structure of the secreted material, and nanoscale fibril dimensions. However, the potential interest in BC for medical applications is increasing due to its unique combination of mechanical properties (high wet strength), interconnected porosity, biocompatibility, and ability to absorb and hold large quantities of water. All of these properties are required for vascular tissue engineering and are found in a unique combination in BC with different types of synthetic polymers (Czaja et al., 2007). Therefore, BC is becoming a promising biopolymer for several biomedical processes (Klemm et al., 2001; Pochan et al., 2003) (e.g., wound dressings, artificial skin, and scaffolds for soft tissue replacement).

6.2.2.1 BC-based nanocomposites

The advantages of BC nanocomposite materials when compared to conventional composites are that they are superior in thermal, mechanical, and barrier properties at low reinforcement levels (e.g., BC 5 wt%), as well as their better recyclability, transparency, and low weight. Biodegradable polymers may require improvements in terms of brittleness, low thermal stability, and poor barrier properties (Czaja et al., 2007). A number of researchers have therefore explored the concept of fully bio-derived nanocomposites as a route to development of bioplastics or bioresins with better properties. Recently, a new generation of resorbable materials has been developed for tissue regeneration purposes including BC, which has shown possible osteoconduction properties. From recent studies published in the literature on the application of BC to tissue engineering, most progress has been made in vascular tissue engineering. The first study by Jarcho (1981) described a proprietary material scaffold that consisted of BC formed *in situ* into a tubular form during biosynthesis. The author cited the remarkable wet strength, high water absorption, and low roughness of the lumen surface as favorable properties of the biomaterial. The device was evaluated as a microvascular "endoprosthesis" to replace a section of carotid artery several millimeters long in a rat model. After 4 weeks the implanted device was surrounded by vascularized connective tissue and the lumen had been re-endothelialized by oriented cells. No significant immunological response was observed and a high level of patency (ability to functionally withstand blood pressure) was noted (Klemm et al., 2001). In addition, several studies (Bielecki et al., 2002; Petersen and Gatenholm, 2011; Saska et al., 2012) have sought to modify BC scaffolds in a variety of ways in order to improve their bioactive properties. Moreover, Fang et al. (2004) modified BC by biomimetic mineralization of HA to produce BC–HA composite scaffolds. When compared to unmodified BC, the BC–HA scaffolds supported increased adhesion and proliferation of human bone marrow-derived mesenchymal stem cells and induced an increased osteogenic differentiation, both spontaneously and under osteoinduction conditions.

6.2.2.2 BC–HA nanocomposites

HAs are drawing a great deal of attention for used as bioactive materials due to their resemblance to natural bone mineral in addition to their superior biocompatibility and osteocondutivity. HA has been enhanced by reduction of its particle size to its interaction propensity for attracting osteoblasts, whereas it possesses a low rate of resorption *in vivo* and is brittle, particularly in highly porous structures. Therefore, the main approach to overcome these drawbacks is through utilization of BC nanocomposites for bone tissue regeneration based on fabricating both natural and synthetic polymers under certain varying compositions. In addition, there is another favorable method to synthesize BC-based nanocomposites which depends on the polymerization of monomers in the presence of the BC nanofiber network (Barnes et al., 2007). BC nanocomposites from nHAP have been confirmed by introducing BC culture media and then the nHAP was introduced and remained suspended in the culture medium throughout the formation of BC nanofibers. In a relevant study, Fang et al. (2004) presented HA for incorporation into several natural and synthetic polymers, including PLA, PGA, polyamide, and PCL to synthesize nanocomposite scaffolds. The high potential of incorporating HA particles with synthetic polymers results in improved control of biomaterial design properties, such as porosity, rate of degradation, and mechanical properties, when compared to pure HA scaffolds. Sometimes porosities greater than 90% are possible, while pure HA scaffold porosity is typically less than 70%. The use of highly reactive nanocrystalline HA particles in natural polymer scaffolds has been proved to improve the mechanical properties compared with only synthesized polymer control scaffolds and the high HA loading results in potentially decreased adverse impacts associated with the degradation behavior of synthetic polymers. The significant methods for fabricating polymer/HA nanocomposite scaffolds is classified into two categories: incorporation during processing and biomimetically, raising the apatite onto a designed polymer scaffold (Smith et al., 2006) uses a unique technique for fabricating nanocomposite scaffolds based on incorporating HA particles directly into the polymer solution prior to solidification. Another study was conducted by Wei and Ma (2004), who developed a novel technique to reinforce monocrystalline HA into

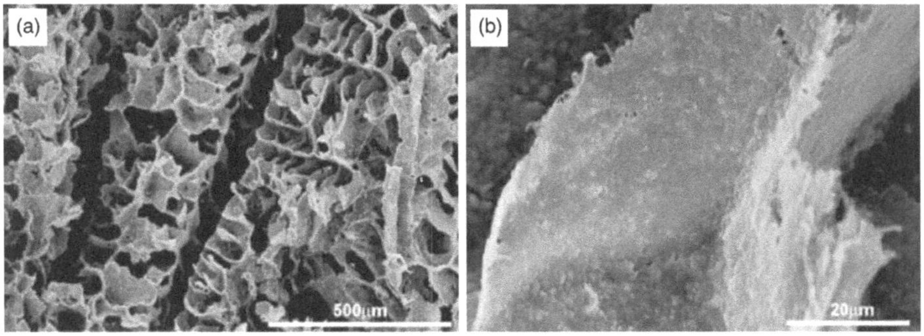

FIGURE 6.4

SEM micrographs of nanoHA/PLLA 50:50 scaffold, ×100, ×1000. Adapted from Wei and Ma (2004). Copyright 2004, Elsevier.

PLA matrices. Their significant results demonstrated nanocomposite scaffolds with porosities as high as 95%. As an example of this polymer scaffold technique is shown in Figure 6.4.

The porosity and pore morphology are the most important properties related to the design of a typical scaffold and they can be manipulated and controlled in two methods. The first method is using different solvents, such as pure dioxane, pure benzene, and various mixtures of dioxane/water. The second method is by controlling particle size under a certain varying of HA particles, specifically in nanoscale instead of micron-scale particles. These techniques are likely to be most effective at low-volume fractions of HA powders in poly (l-lactic acid) (PLLA) matrices and a small quantity of reinforced HA particles stayed locked in the scaffold structure (He et al., 2009; Smith et al., 2009).

6.3 POLY-LACTIC ACID

PLA shows great potential in the biomedical field. The properties of PLA are excellent biocompatibility, biodegradability, less toxicity, mechanical properties and it is also easily molded into different shapes making it a very suitable material for biomedical applications (Majola et al., 1991; Iwatake et al., 2008). Thermal processing of PLA is much easier compared to other biopolymers and it requires less energy for the production of PLA. However, PLA possesses some demerits like poor toughness (it is very brittle and possesses very poor tensile strength), slow biodegradability, hydrophobicity, and lack of reactive side chains. There are multiple factors that affect the biodegradability of PLA, which generally takes place by hydrolysis of an ester group. Some of these factors are diffusion of water on PLA, homogeneity of weight distribution, and isomeric content (Figure 6.5). There are many ways to improve the properties of PLA, the

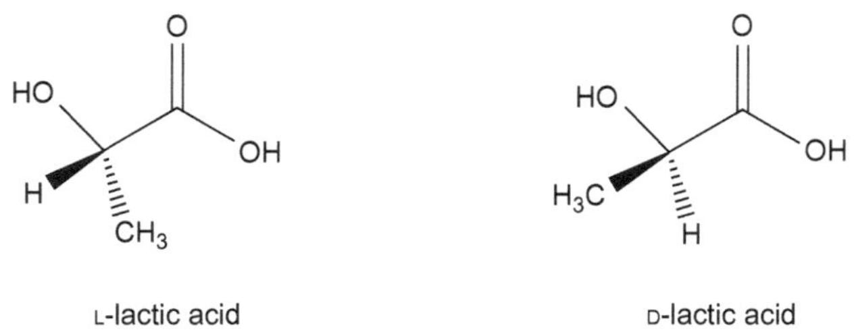

FIGURE 6.5

The stereoisomers of lactic acid.

most common way is to blend PLA with other materials to enhance its properties. PLA is produced from lactic acid monomer. There are various ways that lactic acid can be polymerized to obtain PLA. The most common of those methods is by ring-opening polymerization in the presence of stannous octate or $Sn^{(II)}$-based catalyst. Various researches and studies are being carried out around the world on PLA, and it has proven itself to be a very promising material in the field of bone fixation, drug-delivery carrier, tissue engineering, scaffold, and various other biomedical applications (Savioli et al., 2012).

6.3.1 PLA-BASED NANOCOMPOSITES

The natural resource of PLA has an advantage of providing the required high-purity lactic acid that is suitable for reinforcing with several natural materials such as cellulose nanofibers. Iwatake et al. (2008) have sufficiently studied the reinforcement of PLA by using a casting film technique to fabricate microfibrillated cellulose (MFC). Their significant aim was to investigate the potential of MFC reinforcement by a nanofiber into PLA chains and to approach a green nanocomposite by used a low quantity of organic solvent to achieve uniform dispersion of MFC in PLA matrices, the characterizations of the film that was prepared by hot-pressing were investigated, and the mechanical and thermomechanical properties of the film after hot-pressing were also studied and different aspect ratios of fillers [Needle-leaf Bleached Kraft Pulp (NBKP) and refiner-treated NBKP] were employed to examine the impact of fillers on the morphology. Their results demonstrated that MFC increased both Young's modulus and tensile strength of PLA by 40% and 25%, respectively, without significant effect of yield strain at 10% fiber loading. In contrast, NBKP decreased the yield strain by 30% and strength by 15% at a specific fiber 5 wt% content. Furthermore, the storage modulus of the nanocomposites was kept constantly above the glass transition temperature of matrix polymer. MFC is a promising reinforcement for PLA composites (Figure 6.6; Du et al., 1998; Dang et al., 2001; Chen et al., 2002; Singh and Ray, 2007; Astrid et al., 2012).

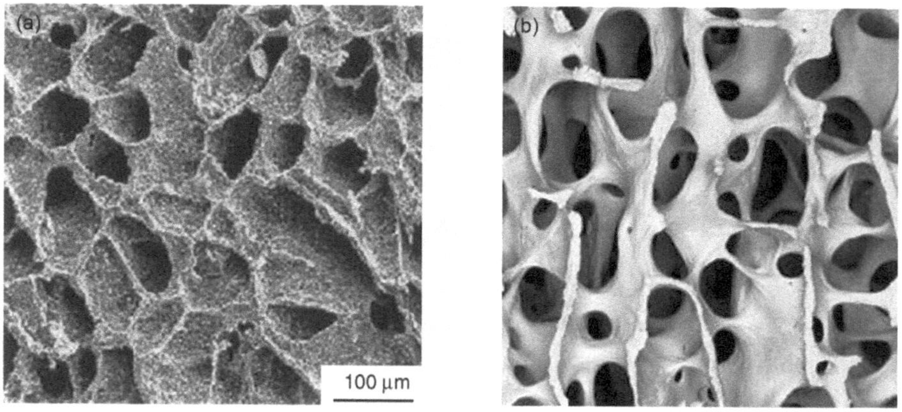

FIGURE 6.6

Similarities between the structure of PLA scaffold and human bone. (a) Microscopic structure of PLA scaffold; (b) microscopic structure of human bone (Gibson, 1985; Roshan et al., 2011).

Table 6.1 Nanocomposites of PLA and Their Enhanced Properties

Composite of PLA	Enhancement	Reference
nHA/PLA	Porosity, protein adhesion, bioactivity	Kothapalli et al. (2005)
Sol-gel bioactive glass/PLA	Hydrophobicity, retention of mechanical properties for longer duration	Sepulveda et al. (2001)
PLA/CDHA	Biodegradability, cell adhesion, and growth capability	Huan et al. (2011)
PLLA/PLA	Lower crystallinity, faster hydrolysis, and degradation	Carrubba et al. (2008)
SR-PDLLA/PLLA	Mechanical strength, retention of strength for longer duration	Majola et al. (1992)
Collagen/PLA	Tensile strength, fibrous tissue ingrowths	Fang et al. (2004)
PLA/starch	Young's modulus, water absorption	Averous (2004)
PLLA/layered silicate nanocomposite	Storage modulus, crystallinity, miscibility of the surfactants	Klemm et al. (2001)
PLA/modified TiO_2	Improves crystallinity, improves mechanical properties, reduces complex viscosity during molding	Mahshid et al. (2011)
PLA/organo-montmorillonite	Thermal properties were greatly enhanced	Depan et al. (2009)

Nanocomposite formed with different components enhances different properties of PLA. Therefore, the different nanocomposites are formed in accordance with the purpose of their application. Some of the PLA nanocomposites and enhancement induced by different techniques are discussed in Table 6.1.

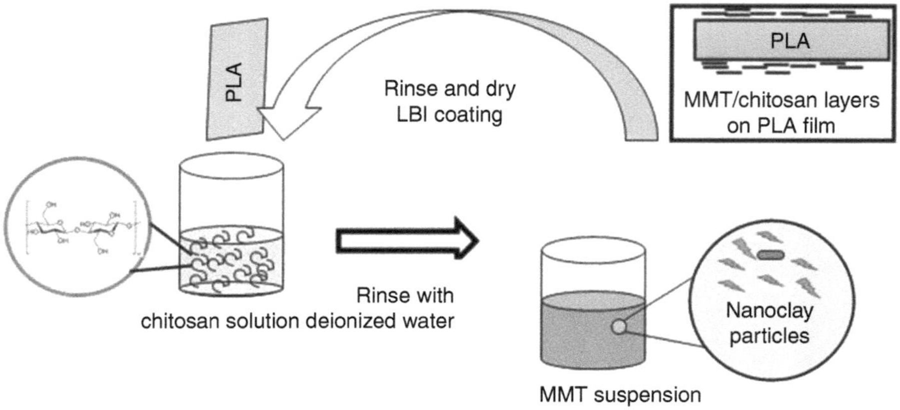

FIGURE 6.7

Multilayer deposition process on PLA films (where drying was only employed once per deposition cycle).

6.3.2 PLA/SILICATE NANOCOMPOSITES

There are a number of researches dedicated to PLA-based nanocomposites in the presence of layered silicates to target highly exfoliated structures. Ray and Okamoto (2003) reported the main routes for preparation of PLA/layered silicate nanocomposites.

Extruded PLA films were prepared by simple layer-by-layer processing steps (Figure 6.7). Compared to neat PLA, PLA films were coated with 70 bilayers of montmorillonite/chitosan (CS). Moreover, three main structures were achieved based on: (1) intercalation, (2) melt-intercalation, and (3) *in situ* intercalation (Figure 6.8). When the affinity between silicate layers and polymeric matrices was low, the polymer was not intercalated within the clay layers. A microcomposite was obtained where the properties of resulting materials were scarcely improved, and even diminished after addition of layered silicates. An intercalated nanocomposite was obtained when polymer chains were partially intercalated between the silicate layers, accompanying an increase of the inter layer distance (Mittal, 2009).

6.3.3 CARBON NANOTUBE/BIODEGRADABLE POLYMER NANOCOMPOSITES

Excellent mechanical properties, high specific surface area, and low density of CNTs makes them ideal for fabrication of tissue engineering scaffolds with high strength and low weight. Although the biocompatibility and cytotoxicity of CNTs are not clear, many researchers have found that biofunctionalized CNTs are water-soluble and can be cleared from the systemic blood circulation through the

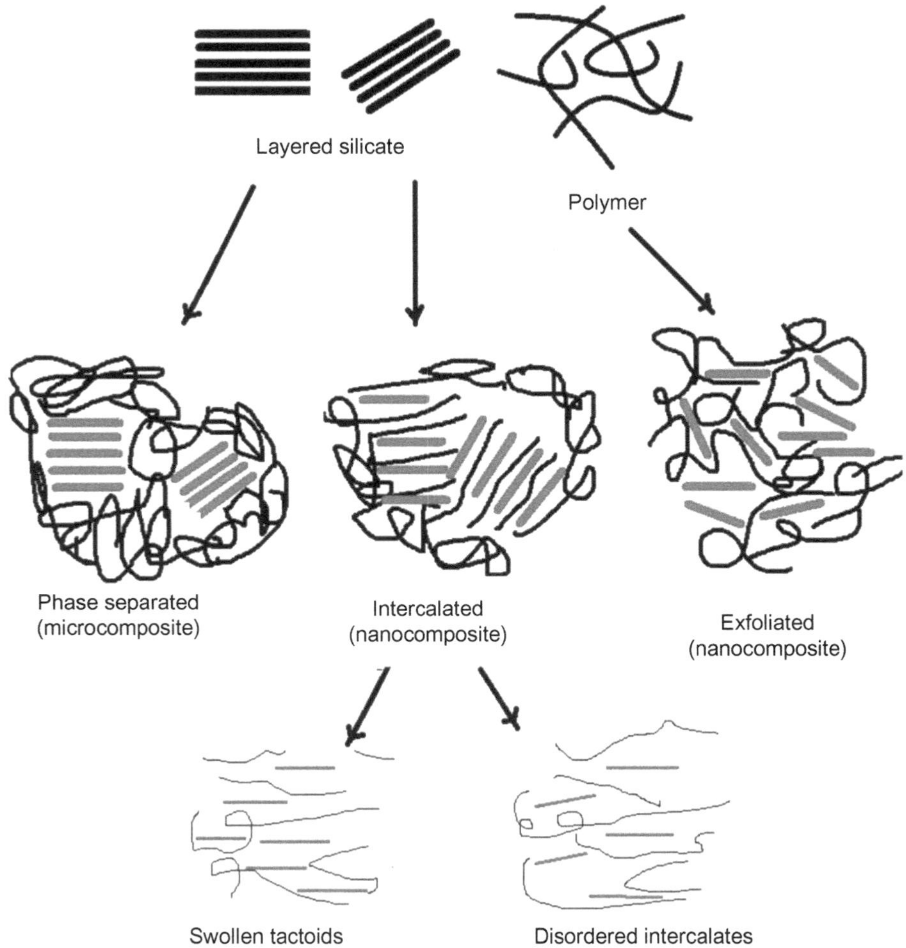

FIGURE 6.8

Different structures of layered silicate/polymer nanocomposites.

renal excretion route, indicating that biofunctionalized CNTs are safe for biomedical applications. Recently, the application of CNT/biopolymer nanocomposites to tissue engineering has attracted increased attention. CNTs have been incorporated into different polymer matrices such as PCL, CS, and poly-lactide-*co*-glycolide (PLGA) to synthesize polymer scaffolds for employment in bone tissue engineering (Lee et al., 2003; Erisken et al., 2008; Pan et al., 2012), both of which were fabricated with multiwalled carbon nanotube (MWCNT)/PCL nanocomposites by using a solution casting and evaporation technique. Their resulted confirmed that both the tensile and compressive moduli were dramatically enhanced as a function of specific addition of MWCNT content. Meanwhile, the compressive modulus of nanocomposites reinforced under 0.5, 1, and 2 wt% MWCNTs were increased significantly by 37.2%, 38.8%, and 54.5%, respectively, compared with pure PCL. Furthermore, the advantage of addition of MWCNTs to PCL was useful in terms of facilitated cell growth and promoted cell attachment. In the cell adhesion assays, the rat bone marrow-derived stroma cells covered the whole surface of the nanocomposite scaffold, but only 60% of the surface of the pure PCL scaffold, suggesting better cellular compatibility of the MWCNT/PCL scaffold, which may result from rough nanoscale surface topography of the nanocomposite scaffold. It was found that the nanocomposite scaffold containing 0.5 wt% MWCNT exhibited the best enhancement of the proliferation and differentiation of bone marrow-derived stroma cells, while a content of MWCNTs above 2 wt% could lead to a reduced effect on cell growth. Mattioli-Belmonte et al. (2012) also fabricated a bone-like structure scaffold based on MWCNT/PCL nanocomposites by solution mixing. The elastic modulus of nanocomposites increased to 75 MPa with 11 wt% MWCNT, which is much higher than that of pure PCL (10 MPa). The colorimetric methyl tetrazolium (MTT) assay showed that the nanocomposites could sustain osteoblast proliferation and osteoblast viability depending on the intrinsic rigidity of the substrate, as well as the architecture and morphology of the substrate.

6.4 DESIGN AND FABRICATION OF SCAFFOLDS

Bone is a natural composite of collagen and hydroxycarbonate apatite with a 10–30% porous hard outer layer (i.e., cortical bone) and a 30–90% porous interior (i.e., cancellous bone). For achievement of appropriate bone tissue scaffold, the mechanical properties of polymer scaffolds should mimic human bone and be tailored with a wide range of soft tissue (cancellous) to hard tissue (cortical bone) by adjusting processing parameters, whereas one of the hindrances to creating an ideal scaffold design is related to the control aspect ratios of the scaffold associated with types of scaffold techniques that are consequently used (Table 6.2). The specific properties that desire to achieve suitable scaffolds for bone tissue engineering are described in the following:

1. Macroporous size should be $>100\ \mu m$ and pore size $<20\ \mu m$.
2. Adequate interconnected open porosity for *in vivo* tissue in-growth.
3. Appropriate mechanical strength and control of rate of degradation.

6.4.1 PROPERTIES FOR DESIGNING SOFT TISSUE SCAFFOLD

Assessments of the biomechanical properties of scaffold polymers that mimic human tissues are difficult to provide. Therefore, an ideal scaffold should have the following properties to bring about the desired biological response.

Table 6.2 Physical and Mechanical Properties of Bone Scaffolds

Scaffold Composition	Porosity (%)	Pore Size	Compressive Strength (MPa)	Reference
80 ± 3% + 20 ± 3% β-TCP	70	400	Not available	Tarafder et al. (2013)
HA	41	250–350	34.4 ± 2.2	Roohani-Esfahani et al. (2010)
β-TCP + 0.5% SiO_2 + 0.25 ZnO	32.16	300 ± 8.26	10.21 ± 0.11	Xue et al. (2009)
33% HA + 67% Si-β tcp + BMSC	60	301 ± 2.3		Depan et al. (2009)
(40% HA + 60% β-TCP) coated with HA/PCL	90.8	550	2.1	Erisken et al. (2008)
TCP scaffold coated with 5% PCL	70	300–800	2.41	Lei et al. (2007)
Bioactive glass (Ca/p/Si = 15/5/80 molar ratio)	0.30 cm^3/gm	300–500		Couto et al. (2009)
PGA:β-TCP = 1:3	88.4 ± 0.7	483.3 ± 113.6		Mittal (2009)
HA:PU = 1:5	90 ± 2	200 ± 16		Pan et al. (2012)

Note: TCP, tricalcium phosphate.

6.4.1.1 Biocompatibility

Biocompatibility is one of the most significant properties that should be taken into account when designing hard and soft tissue scaffolds. The biocompatibility of a scaffold is designated to replace part of a living system and support normal cellular activity, associate with molecular signaling systems by not being toxic and causing immunological rejection of the host tissue (Adani et al., 2011). A typical scaffold has the ability to be osteoconductive and the scaffold permits the cells to adhere, proliferate, and create extracellular matrix (ECM) on its surface and pores. The scaffold has the capability to generate new tissue formation by biomolecular signals and recruiting progenitor cells. The typical polymer scaffold is successful in forming blood vessels on the implant within a short time of implantation for active support of nutrient, oxygen, and waste transport (Rickert et al., 2006).

6.4.1.2 Mechanical properties

The design of polymer scaffolds should be tailored, with a wide range of mechanical properties and matching host tissue properties. As an example of Young's modulus in cortical bone, the range is between 1520 GPa (hard tissues) and 0.1–2 GPa for cancellous bone (soft tissues). In addition, the compressive strength for cortical bone varies between 100–200 MPa and 2–20 MPa for cancellous bone. However, large variations in mechanical properties and scaffold design dimensions make it difficult to optimize a typical tissue scaffold (Gomes et al., 2002).

6.4.1.3 Pore size

The pore size is defined as one of the scaffold properties that is linked to the interconnected porosity to favor tissue integration, and pore size should be at least 100 μm in diameter for complete diffusion of the nutrients and oxygen in cell survivability (Zhou and Wu, 2012). In addition to the study conducted by Loh and Chong (2013), who investigated the role of three-dimensional scaffolds for pore size and porosity, their results showed that the pore sizes in tissues should be in the range of 200–350 μm. Furthermore, O'Brien et al. (2007) studied the effect of pore size on permeability and cell attachment in collagen scaffolds and their result concluded that multiscale porous scaffolds linking both micro- and macroporosity can be a better achievement than only macroporous scaffolds. However, the reduction in compressive and tensile properties was one of the drawbacks of increasing porosity; various porous scaffolds using polymers, ceramic, composites, and metals have been investigated. In particular, the mechanical properties of bioceramic materials are similar to cortical bone. Moreover, synthesis polymer scaffolds, in terms of pore size, porosity and biodegradation, can be adequately tailored to the requirements for cancellous bone. Blends with varying quantities of ceramic/polymer nanocomposite scaffolds are potentially advantageous to meet the specific requirements of bone tissue. On the other hand, porous metallic scaffolds are appropriate for mechanical properties, whereas they are still unsuccessful in providing essential implant–tissue integration (Rezwan et al., 2006).

6.4.1.4 Biodegradability

Biodegradability is an essential property for design scaffolds in tissue regeneration. In spite of this, a typical scaffold should have similar mechanical properties to the host tissue. However, the rate of biodegradation is another factor that requires *in vivo* study. The control of biodegradation in polymer scaffolds is dependent on properties such as molecular weight and the biodegradation time of the implanted scaffold can be varied from months to years, based on its amorphous or crystalline and hydrophilic/hydrophobic behaviors. Future researches that emphasize a number of parameters including polymerization conditions, composition, and scaffold techniques, in the synthesis of polymer scaffolds may be able to optimize and control desired applications for tissue engineering (Jenck et al., 2004; Tarafder et al., 2013). Table 6.3 provides information about the physical properties of human tissues as a reference for the selection of polymer materials.

Polymers remain the most commonly used biomaterials for scaffold fabrication, because of their mechanical properties and degradation rates, which closely match those of proteins in tissues. They are good candidates for the development of synthetic tissues and vascular scaffolds. The primary focus is on the main properties of biopolymers and synthetic polymers, namely, biocompatibility, biodegradability, and mechanical performance, and their applications as scaffolds for soft and vascular tissue engineering. These major polymeric scaffold requirements and a summary of their main characteristics, with respect to bone and vascular tissue engineering, are depicted in Figure 6.9.

6.4.2 TISSUE ENGINEERING SCAFFOLDS

A hard tissue like bone exhibits a hierarchical structure with structural units that range from the microscale to the nanoscale (Sosnowski et al., 1996; Garlotta, 2001;

Table 6.3 Mechanical Property of Human Bone Tissue (Majola et al., 1992; Jenck, 2004)

Human Bone Tissue	Tensile Strength (MPa)	Compressive Strength (MPa)	Young's Modulus (GPa)	Fracture Toughness (MPa ml/2)
Cancellous bone	7.4	4–12	0.02–0.05	N/A
Cortical bone	60–160	130–180	3–30	2–12
Cartilages	3.7–10.5		0.7–15.3	N/A
Ligament	13–46	N/A	0.065–0.541	N/A
Tendon	24–112	N/A	0.143–2.31	N/A

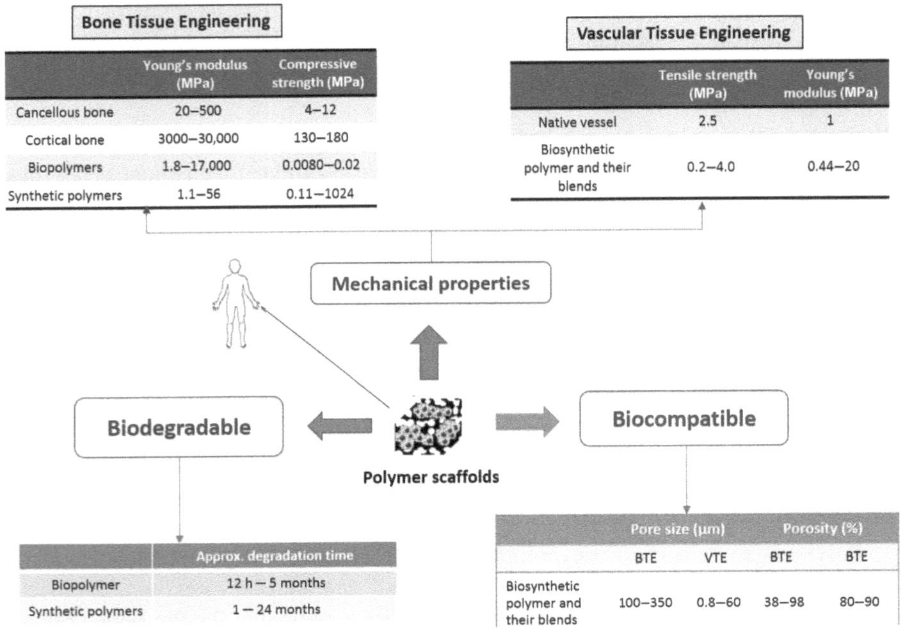

FIGURE 6.9

Major scaffold requirement (BTE, bone tissue engineering, VTE, vascular tissue engineering) (Nowsheen et al., 2013).

Nowsheen et al., 2013). In addition, bone consists of cells that reside in an ECM that consists of structural (collagen and elastin) and adhesive (fibronectin and vitronectin) protein fibers, in the nanometer range. An environment that consists of nanoscale features is more conducive for initial cell attachment and proliferation due to the increased sensitivity of the cells via the filopodia (Ralph and Müller, 2009). This type of cellular behavior has also been attributed to an increase in the number of atoms and crystal grains, along with an increase in surface area in the case of nanostructures (Zhou et al., 2014). It has also been shown that the interaction of proteins (such as fibronectin, vitronectin, laminin, and collagen) that affect the behavior of osteoblasts occurs to a greater extent on nanoscale materials. Cells that belong to the osteogenic lineage (e.g., osteoblasts, osteocytes, osteoclasts), in addition to scaffold and growth factors, represent the key components for bone tissue engineering (Figure 6.9) that are used to mimic the *in vivo* environment for bone tissue regeneration in order to cure bone defects (although it should be noted that osteoblasts, osteocytes, and osteoclasts may also be derived from stem cells). As noted above, the scaffold serves as one of the key components of bone tissue engineering, and should be designed to mimic the hierarchical structure of the ECM in order to replicate the intracellular and

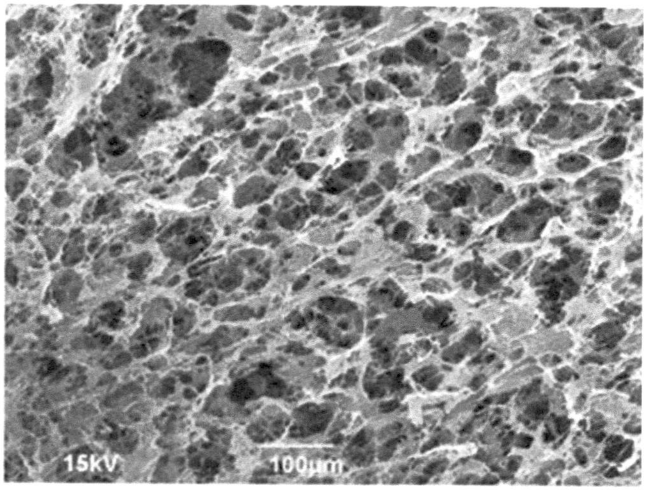

FIGURE 6.10

Scanning electron microscopy image of a bone tissue engineering scaffold structure (Averous, 2004).

intercellular responses required in cell differentiation and proliferation (Chandrahasa et al., 2011). Scaffolds are porous structures (see Figure 6.10) that support cell growth, proliferation, and differentiation. The cell surface receptors react to the mechanical properties of the ECM by converting mechanical signals to chemical signals. These receptors also interact with chemical ligands present in nanostructured ECM, thus affecting the cell behavior, while the nanofibrous structure of the ECM is also responsible for the clustering of chemical ligands that affect cell behavior. Consequently, it is possible to modulate cell behavior via both the mechanical and chemical properties of the surrounding three-dimensional (3D) environment with such modulation being both space- and time-dependent. The cells will be influenced by the spatial arrangement of the surrounding environment, and by the time-dependent changes in the molecules involved in adhesion between the cell and the ECM (Chen et al., 2002; Zhao et al., 2013).

6.5 PROCESSING METHODS FOR NANOCOMPOSITES IN TISSUE ENGINEERING

The nanoscale designs have a significant effect on cell behavior, emphasizing the importance of nanocomposites in tissue engineering. In order to obtain appropriate nanoscale features or nanostructures in the final nanocomposite, it is necessary to use appropriate processing methods (Figure 6.11). Today, a number of

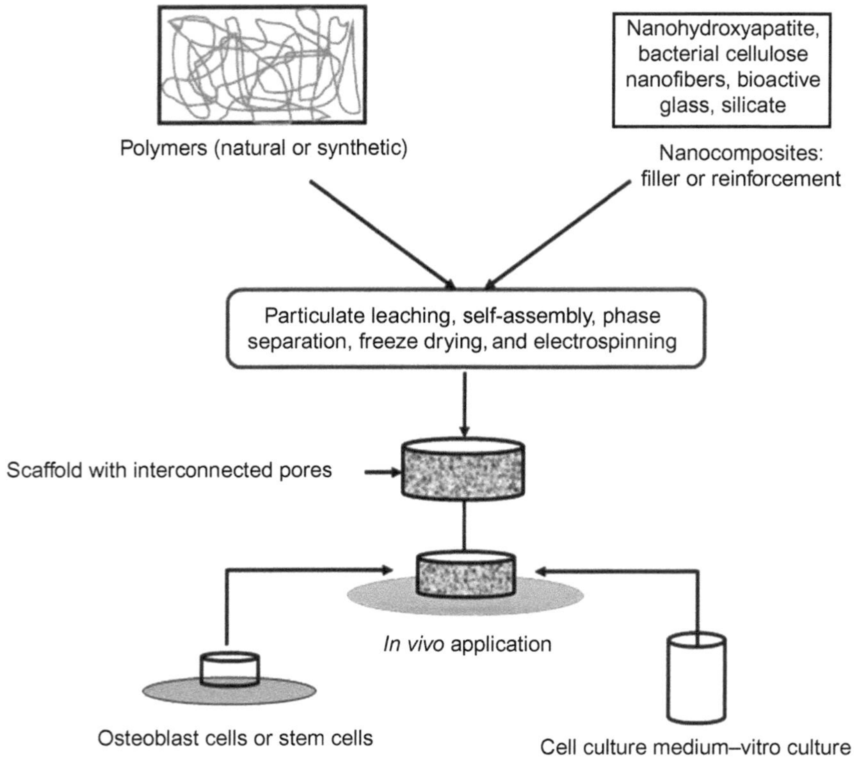

FIGURE 6.11

Preparation methods to produce tissue engineering.

challenges are associated with the preparation of these nanocomposites, one of which is the need to conserve the intrinsic properties of the materials used. The processing method used might affect the conformation of the polymer chains in the case of polymers, or the distribution of nanosized inorganic materials in the form of particles while preparing nanocomposites (Goldberg et al., 2007). The changes in conformation of the polymer chains in the case of natural polymers may affect the available biomolecule sequences and cell behavior. In addition, the properties of polymeric materials, such as melting point T_g, viscosity, and resistance to the solvents used during processing may also limit the number of routes by which such processing can be affected. In the case of bone regeneration, it is necessary first to develop nanocomposites with structural features that mimic, or at least resemble, the structural traits of the ECM. In this literature review, there are several methods available for the development of nanocomposites for bone tissue engineering. These routes are discussed in the following sections (Salgado et al., 2004; Boccaccini and Blaker, 2005; Stevens and George, 2005).

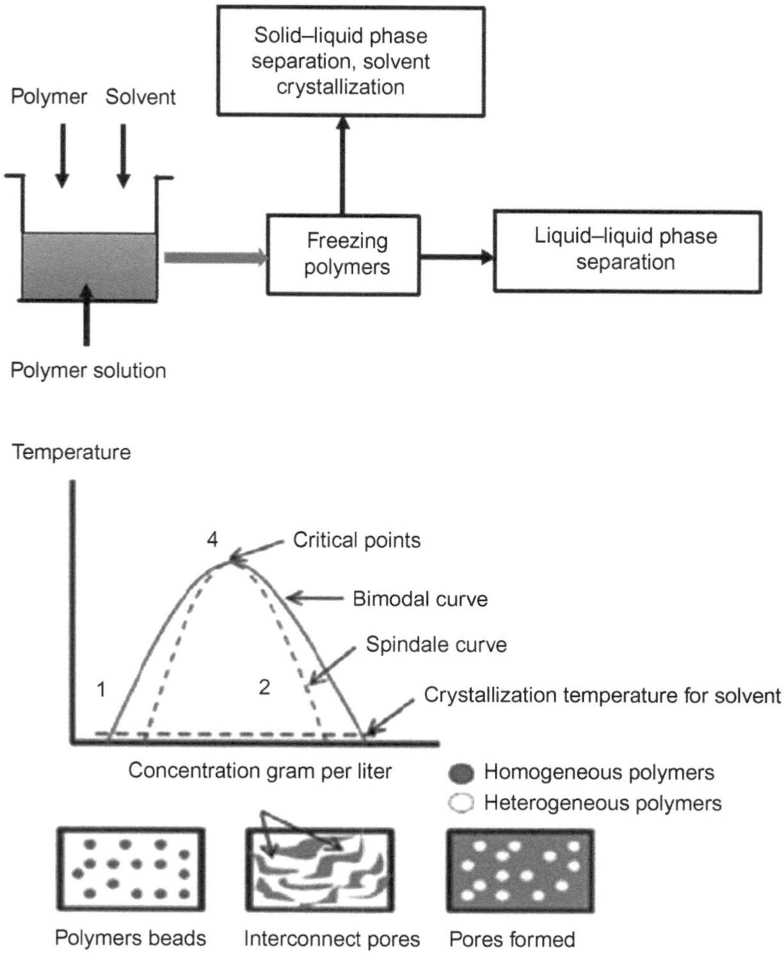

FIGURE 6.12

Scheme of the phase separation process (Kalpana et al., 2012).

6.5.1 PHASE SEPARATION

Phase separation as shown in Figure 6.12 is fundamentally based on a thermodynamic process which is used for preparing interwoven, nanofibrous scaffolds in tissue engineering. Whilst the thermally induced phase separation (TIPS) method is most often used for phase separation, it is also possible to use with absence of solvent for the polymer in order to induce phase separation. This process is shown schematically in Figure 6.12. TIPS is of two types, namely, "solid–liquid phase separation" and "liquid–liquid phase separation," depending on the crystallization temperature (freezing point) of the solvent used. In the case of solid–liquid phase separation, the crystallization temperature of the solvent used is higher than the liquid–liquid phase separation temperature; this causes the solvent to crystallize and the polymer to separate when the temperature of the polymer solution is lowered. The crystallized solvent is further removed by freeze-drying (sublimation), which leaves behind pores with a morphology similar to that of the solvent crystallites. Thus, it is possible to control the pore structure and type of phase separation by using solvents with different crystallization (freezing) properties (Lu et al., 2003; Maquet et al., 2004; Kong et al., 2006; He et al., 2009; Chen et al., 2013).

The advantage of the phase separation technique is that the morphology of the scaffold can be controlled by changing parameters such as polymer type and concentration, freezing temperature, and use of different types of porogen. This method can also be useful for preparing scaffolds of different shapes according to requirements, and for maintaining batch-to-batch consistency. In spite of being a simple technique, phase separation remains a laboratory-scale procedure that is limited to a few polymers. The phase separation technique has been used to prepare scaffolds based on polymer systems such as PEG/PLLA (Kim et al., 2004), PLA–dextran blend (Taboas et al., 2003; Devendra et al., 2009), HAP/CS–gelatin (Fang et al., 2002; Kong et al., 2006), PLGA (Hua et al., 2003; Hirenkumar et al., 2011), PLLA (Budyanto et al., 2009), and HAP/poly (hydroxybutyrate-*co*-hydroxyvalerate) (Jing et al., 2008).

6.5.2 FREEZE-DRYING

Freeze-drying is a process typically used to remove residual solvent from a material to produce a dry powder that can be easily loaded into a cell. The material is dissolved in solvent and frozen in a dry-ice bath. The solvent sublimates and is removed by vacuum, leaving a dry powder. During freeze-drying, the temperature is maintained sufficiently low that any remixing of the phase-separated polymer solution is prevented. The freeze-drying technique, shown schematically in Figure 6.13, has been used in several studies related to tissue regeneration, for developing scaffolds based on polymers such as PLLA (Sultana and Wang, 2012), CS (Madihally and Matthew, 1999; Tarun et al., 2012), gelatin (Wu et al., 2010), carboxymethylcellulose (CMC) (Fasai and Somchai, 2011), poly(ether ester) (Deschamps et al., 2002), and silk fibroin/hyaluronan (Nopporn et al., 2014). Other studies have also involved the use of nanocomposite scaffolds prepared through the phase separation technique for tissue engineering applications. Typical examples of polymer nanocomposite scaffolds fabricated via freeze-drying include PLA/nHAP (Chengde et al., 2014), collagen/HAP (Yunoki et al., 2007), CS/HAP (Kong et al., 2006), gelatin/HAP (Landi et al., 2008; Liu et al., 2009; Wu et al., 2010), and PLA foam/bioglass (Blaker et al., 2003; Blaker et al., 2005). Polyelectrolyte complex fibrous scaffolds for tissue engineering have also been synthesized, and scaffolds fabricated via freeze-drying method (Devendra et al., 2009). Typically, the design parameters to be optimized are the temperature ranges and time, as well as the concentrations of the polymer solutions.

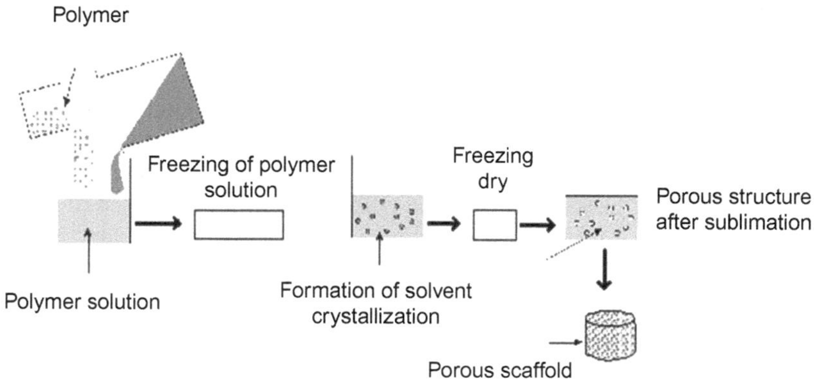

FIGURE 6.13

Schematic of the freeze-drying process (Kalpana et al., 2012).

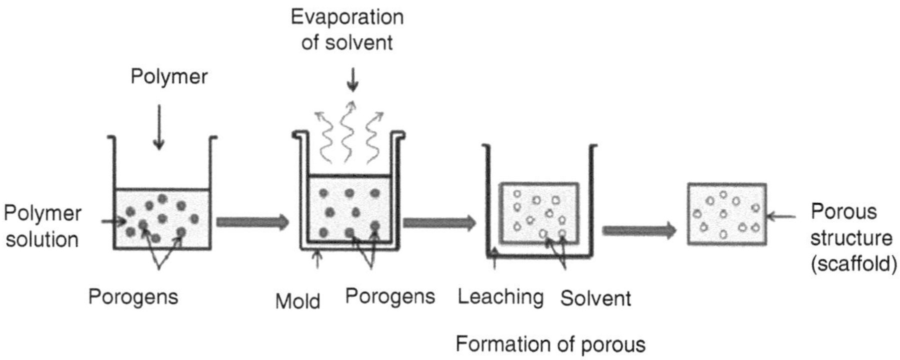

FIGURE 6.14

Stages of the particulate leaching process.

6.5.3 PARTICULATE LEACHING

Particulate leaching is a comparatively simple technique that is used to prepare porous scaffolds by using porogens that are soluble in water or nontoxic solvents; typical examples include sugar, sodium chloride- and saccharide. A polymer solution into which the porogens are dispersed is cast into a mold; the solvent is then removed by evaporation, after which leaching of the porogen produces a porous scaffold. The process is schematically represented in Figure 6.14. The main advantage of particulate leaching is that it provides effective control of pore size and porosity, simply by varying the size and amount of the porogens. However, it has certain limitations: (i) that the solvent removal by evaporation may be incomplete; (ii) that there may be a lack of interconnectivity and open-pore structure in scaffolds requiring a low porosity (due to too few contact points between the porogens), and (iii) it is more suited to producing thin scaffolds. Despite particulate leaching having been used in combination with other techniques, the lack of interconnectivity represents the major limitation. When Liu et al. (2009) prepared gelatin/apatite nanofibrous scaffolds by combining TIPS and particulate (porogen) leaching techniques, the mold was preheated to develop interconnectivity between the particulates (and thus between the scaffold pores), which in turn helped to distribute the cells throughout the scaffold. Several studies related to tissue generation have been conducted using scaffolds prepared via particulate leaching, with recent trends seeking to further improve this method (Wei and Ma, 2004; Gong et al., 2007).

6.5.4 SELF-ASSEMBLY

The self-assembly technique, which is useful for preparing nanofibrous scaffolds, is present everywhere in nature, from microscopic to macroscopic levels, and is "the spontaneous association and organization of numerous individual entities into coherent and well-defined structures without external intervention" (Thomas et al., 2014). Molecular self-assembly involves diffusion followed by the association of molecules through noncovalent interactions, such as hydrogen bonding, ionic bonding, hydrophobic interactions, and van der Waals interactions. These interactions, although weak, are capable of forming the higher-ordered structures seen in biomacromolecules, because of their large numbers (Kong et al., 2006; Lei et al., 2004; Ding et al., 2014).

6.5.5 ELECTROSPINNING

As shown in Figure 6.15, the fiber formation and structure are affected by three general types of variables: solution properties (concentration, viscosity, conductivity, and surface tension), process factors (applied potential, collection distance, emitting electrode polarity, and feed rate), and environmental parameters (temperature, relative humidity, and velocity of the surrounding air in the spinning chamber) (Deitzel et al., 2002; Murugan et al., 2007; Sill and Recum, 2008; Prabaharan et al., 2011; Table 6.4).

For comparison, the mechanical properties of human cortical and cancellous bones, as example of hard and soft tissues, are listed. Representative morphologies of the fabricated scaffolds are illustrated in Figure 6.16, taken from Rezwan et al. (2006).

Blaker et al. (2005) developed highly porous PDLLA/bioglasss composite scaffolds prepared by TIPS with bimodal and anisotropic pore structures composed of tubular macropores of 100 mm, interconnected with micropores of 10–50 mm in diameter, as shown in Figure 6.16a. The pore volume was shown to decrease from 9.5 to 5.7 cm^3/g after including 40 wt% bioglasss, with little change observed in the overall pore morphology (Pereira and Hench, 1996;

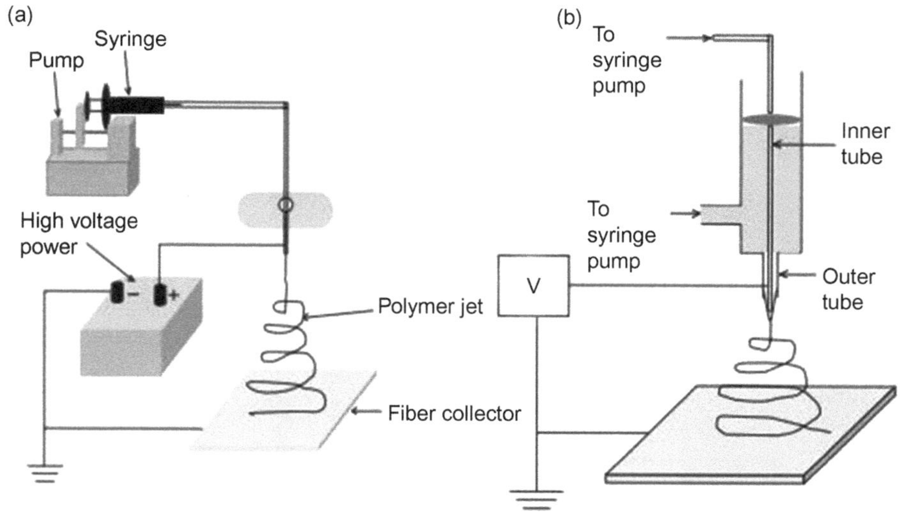

FIGURE 6.15

(a) Typical electrospinning setup using a grounded static collector. (b) Configuration of the coaxial electrospinning setup used for preparing core-shell structured nanofibers (Chen et al., 2013).

Carrubba et al., 2008; Mandal and Kundu, 2009). A 3D structure of controlled porosity is formed based on this method, combined with particle leaching and microsphere packing. Figure 6.16b illustrates a typical pore morphology obtained by this technique. The method shares similar advantages and disadvantages with the solvent casting technique. Superconducting flux flow transistors (SFFTs), such as fused deposition modeling, have been employed to fabricate highly reproducible scaffolds with fully interconnected porous networks as shown in Figure 6.16c. Using digital data produced by an imaging source, such as computer tomography or magnetic resonance imaging, enables accurate design of the scaffold structure (Yunoki et al., 2007; Chen et al., 2013). Solid freeform (SFF) manufacturing coupled with foam scaffold fabrication procedures (phase separation, emulsion-solvent diffusion, or porogen leaching) may be used to develop scaffolds with controlled micro- and macroporous structures. Maquet et al. (2004) reported the effect of bioglass content on the polymer/bioglass structure using varying of bioglass content. The uniform of the particles dispersion was found to be effective at 10 wt % of bioglass contents. A superior qualitative interaction provided between the polymer matrix and bioglass particles as shown in Figure 6.16d. Bioceramic-coated porous scaffolds have been produced either as foams, fibrous bodies, or meshes (Oliveira et al., 2006) by slurry dipping or electrophoretic deposition.

Table 6.4 Fabrication Routes for 3D Composite Scaffolds with High Pore Interconnectivity and Their Advantages and Disadvantages

Technique Route	Advantages	Disadvantages
TIPS (Kim et al., 2005; Carrubba et al., 2008)	High porosities ($\sim$90%)	Long time to sublime solvent (48 h)
	Highly interconnected pore structure	Shrinkage tissues
	Anisotropic and tubular pore possible control of structure and pore size	Small-scale production
		Use of organic solvents
Freeze-drying (Wu et al., 2010; Ding et al., 2014)	Porous structure can be tailored to host tissue protein and cell encapsulation, good interface	Resolution needs to be improved to the microscale, some methods use organic solvents
Solvent casting/particles leaching (Kong et al., 2006)	Controlled porosity	Structures generally isotropic
	Controlled interconnectivity (if particles are sintered)	Use of organic solvents
Self-assembly (Zhai et al., 2002; Wu et al., 2010)	Easy to get fiber diameter on lowest scale. Great control over 3D shape	Low yield. Complex process
		Little control over fiber dimension and orientation
		Only short fiber can be obtained. Limited to a few polymers
Electrospinning (Murugan et al., 2007; Prabaharan et al., 2011)	Well-established and characterized technique. Long continuous fiber with diameter from microscale down to nanoscale	Difficult to fabricate 3D shape
	Control over fiber diameter and orientation. Tailorable mechanical properties. Plethora of polymers may be used	Difficult to control pore size and shape

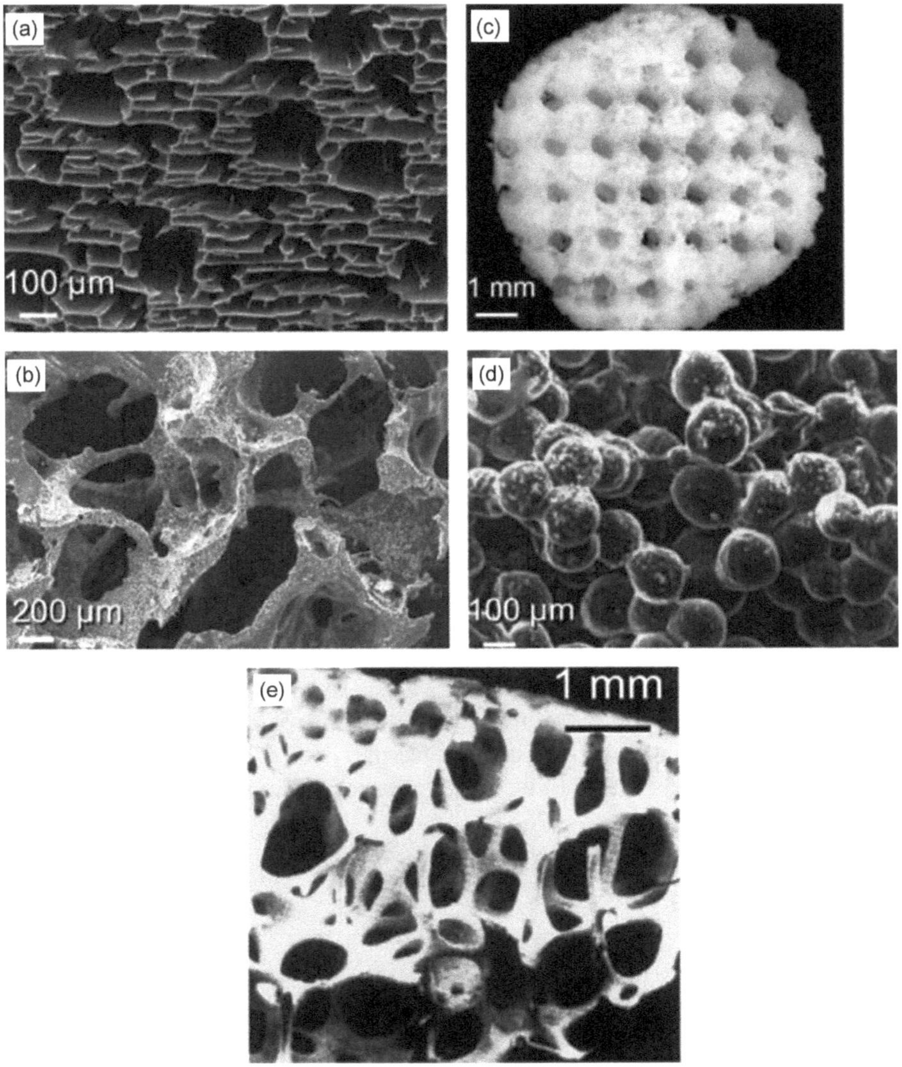

FIGURE 6.16

Typical morphologies of porous polymer foams produced by different techniques and structure of cancellous bone. (a) TIPS (adapted from Boccaccini and Blaker, 2005), (b) solvent casting and particle leaching (Weng et al., 2002), (c) SFF fabrication technique (Taboas et al., 2003), (d) microsphere sintering (Lu et al., 2003), and (e) cancellous bone (Gibson, 1985).

6.6 CONCLUSIONS

Synthetic or natural polymer matrices offer a wide range of mechanical properties and exhibit different biodegradation features, whereas various inorganic nanoparticles provide the indispensable bioactivity. Furthermore, their integration makes it possible to fabricate materials that mimic the structural and morphological organization of native tissues. There is great potential for improvement of current biomaterials and development of advanced nanocomposite scaffolds for tissue regeneration. However, complex interactions between nanocomposites and tissues still remain to be discovered. In addition, the following disadvantages of polymer nanocomposites still exist: somehow uncertain biocompatibility, component stability, and structural integrity in long-term service, and the related mechanical strength, especially the fatigue limit. Basically, we are convinced that there is great feedback to utilizing nanocomposites in tissue regeneration. However, much more research is needed to understand the mechanism of nanocomposite tissue interactions and to optimize the composition, structure, and properties of different polymer nanocomposites, in order to finally achieve the full potential of nanocomposites in soft tissue regeneration. Meanwhile, the future development of inorganic nanoparticles, such as nHA, and natural materials, like bacterial cellulose nanofibers, for medical applications are hard to completely predict from the small number of studies already published. In terms of tissue engineering, nevertheless, it seems likely that the high aspect ratio of inorganic nanoparticles will be applied to engineering structurally oriented tissues, such as skeletal muscle, tendons, ligaments, and nerves, in order to produce 3D scaffolds. In addition, further studies concerning the potential cell targeting and delivery of molecules such as drugs and probes using biodegradable polymers with friendly inorganic nanoparticles need to be investigated in more detail.

REFERENCES

Adani, F., Papa, G., Schievano, A., Cardinale, G., D'Imporzano, G., Tambone, F., 2011. Nanoscale structure of the cell wall protecting cellulose from enzyme attack. Environ. Sci. Technol. 45, 1107–1113.

Astrid, J.R.L., Guillermo, R., Betânia, H.L., André, L.J., Filho, R.M., 2012. Poly-lactic acid synthesis for application in biomedical devices—a review. Biotechnol. Adv. 30, 321–328.

Averous, L., 2004. Biodegradable multiphase system based on plasticized starch. A review. J. Macromole. Sci. C C44, 231–274.

Barnes, C.P., Sell, S.A., Boland, E.D., Simpson, D.G., Bowlin, G.L., 2007. Nanofiber technology: designing the next generation of tissue engineering scaffolds. Adv. Drug Deliv. Rev. 59, 1413–1433.

Bielecki, S., Krystynowicz, A., Turkiewicz, M., Kalinowska, H., 2002. Bacterial cellulose. In: Vandamme, J., Baets, S.D., Steinbüchel, A. (Eds.), Biopolymers (Polysaccharides I: Polysaccharides from Prokaryotes), 5. Wiley-VCH, Verlag, Wein, pp. 37–90.

Blaker, J., Gough, J.E., Maque, V., Notingher, I., Boccaccini, A., 2003. *In vitro* evaluation of novel bioactive composites based on Bioglass-filled polylactide foams for bone tissue engineering scaffolds. J. Biomed. Mater. Res. A. 67, 1401–1411.

Blaker, A., Maquet, V., Boccaccini, A.R., 2005. Mechanical properties of highly porous PDLLA/bioglass composite foams as scaffolds for bone tissue engineering. Acta Biomater. 1, 643–652.

Boccaccini, A.R., Blaker, J., 2005. Bioactive composite materials for tissue engineering scaffolds. Expert Opin. Med. Devices 2, 303–317.

Budyanto, L., Goh, Y.Q., Qoi, C.P., 2009. Fabrication of porous poly (L-lactide) (PLLA) scaffolds for tissue engineering using liquid-liquid phase separation and freeze extraction. J. Mater. Sci. Mater. Med. 20, 105–111.

Carrubba, V., Carfi Pavia, F., Brucato, V., Piccarolo, S., 2008. PLLA/PLA scaffolds prepared via Thermally Induced Phase Separation (TIPS): tuning of properties and biodegradability. Int. J. Mater. 1 (Supp l), 619–622.

Chandrahasa, S., Murray, P.E., Namerow, K.N., 2011. Proliferation of mature *ex vivo* human dental pulp using tissue engineering scaffolds. J. Endod. 37, 1236–1239.

Chen, G., Ushida, T., Tateishi, T., 2002. Scaffold design for tissue engineering. Macromol. Biosci. 2, 67–77.

Chen, H., Truckenmuller, R., Van, C., and Moron, L., 2013. Fabrication of nanofibrous scaffolds fir tissue engineering applications. Woodhead Pub. Lim. Available from: http://dx.doi.org10.1533/9780857097231.1.158.

Chengde, G., Youwen, D., Pei, F., Zhongzheng, M., 2014. Current progress in bioactive ceramic scaffolds for bone repair and regeneration. Int. J. Mol. Sci. 15, 4714–4732.

Couto, D.S., Hong, Z., Mano, J.F., 2009. Development of bioactive and biodegradable chitosan-based injectable systems containing bioactive glass nanoparticles. Acta Biomater. 5, 115–123.

Czaja, W., Young, D.J., Kawecki, M., Brown, M., 2007. The future prospects of microbial cellulose in biomedical applications. J. Biomacromol. 8, 1–12.

Dahman, Y., 2009. Production and utilization of bacterial cellulose nanofibres, Encyclopedia of Nanoscience and Nanotechnology, Ch. 298, sixth ed., vol. 21, pp. 459–479.

Dahman, Y., Kithsiri, E., Magdalina, K., 2010. Potential of biocellulose nanofibers production from agricultural renewable resources: preliminary study. Appl. Biochem. Biotechnol. 162, 1647–1659.

Dang, X., Hao, J., Wang, C., 2001. Preparation and mechanical properties of nanocomposites of poly (D, L-lactide) with Ca-deficient hydroxyapatite nanocrystals. J. Biomater. 22, 2867–2873.

Deitzel, J., Kosik, W., McKnight, S., Beck Tan, N., Desimone, J., Crette, S., 2002. Electrospinning of polymer nanofibers with specific surface chemistry. J. Polym. 43, 1025–1029.

Depan, D., Kumar, A.P., Singh, R.P., 2009. Cell proliferation and controlled drug release studies of nanohybrids based on chitosan-g-lactic acid and montmorillonite. Acta Biomater. 5, 93–100.

Deschamps, A.A., Claase, M.B., Sleijster, W., de Briijn, J.D., Griipma, D.W., Fejjen, J., 2002. Design of segmented poly (ether ester) materials and structures for the tissue engineering of bone. J. Control. Release 17, 175–186.

Devendra, V., Katti, K.S., Katti, D.R., 2009. Polyelectrolyte-complex nanostructured fibrous scaffolds for tissue engineering. J. Mater. Sci. Eng. C 29, 2079–2084.

Ding, X., Janjanam, J., Tiwari, A., Thompson, M., Heiden, P.A., 2014. Peptide-directed self-assembly of functionalized polymeric nanoparticles part I: design and self-assembly of peptide-copolymer conjugates into nanoparticle fibers and 3D scaffolds. Macromol. Biosci. 14, 853–871.

Doi, Y., Steinbuchel, A., 2002. Biopolymers, Applications and Commercial Products, vol. 4. Wiley-VCH Verlag GmbH, Weinhein, pp. 129–177.

Du, C., Cui, F., Feng, Q., Zhu, X., Groot, K., 1998. Tissue response to nano-hydroxapatite/collagen composite implants in marrow cavity. J. Biomed. Mater. Res. 42, 540–548.

Erisken, C., Kalyon, D.M., Wang, H.J., 2008. Functionally graded electrospun polycaprolactone and beta-tricalcium phosphate nanocomposites for tissue engineering applications. J. Biomater. 29, 4065–4073.

Fang, Z., Yuji, Y., William, W., Lu, J., Chiyan, L., Wenyi, Z., et al., 2002. Preparation and histological evaluation of biomimetic three-dimensional hydroxyapatite/chitosan-gelatin network composite scaffolds. J. Biomater. 23, 3227–3234.

Fang, Z., Lair, S., Cui, W., Zhang, Q., Feng, L., 2004. Hierarchically biomimetic bone scaffold materials: nano-HA/collagen/PLA composite. J. Biomed. Mater. Res. B Appl. Biomater. 15, 158–165.

Fasai, W., Somchai, P., 2011. Influence of blending carboxymethylcellulose with gelatin scaffold on mechanical properties. In: The Second TSME International Conference on Mechanical Engineering, pp. 19–21.

Garlotta, D., 2001. A literature review of poly (lactic acid). J. Polym. Environ. 9, 63–84.

Gibson, L.J., 1985. The mechanical behaviour of cancellous bone. J. Biomech. 18, 317–328.

Goldberg, M., Langer, R., Jia, X.Q., 2007. Nanostructured materials for applications in drug delivery and tissue engineering. J. Biomater. Sci. Polym. Ed. 18, 241–268.

Gomes, M.E., Godinho, J.S., Tchalamov, D., Cunha, A.M., Reis, R.L., 2002. Alternative tissue engineering scaffolds based on starch: processing methodologies, morphology, degradation and mechanical properties. Mater. Sci. Eng. C 20, 19–26.

Gong, Y., Zhou, Q., Gao, C., Shen, J., 2007. *In vitro* and *in vivo* degradability and cyto-compatibility of poly (L-lactic acid) scaffold fabricated by a gelatin particle leaching method. Acta Biomater. 3, 531–540.

He, L., Zhang, Y., Zeng, X., Quan, D., Liao, S., Zeng, Y., 2009. Fabrication and characterization of poly (L-lactic acid) 3D nanofibrous scaffolds with controlled architecture by liquid-liquid phase separation from a ternary polymer-solvent system. J. Polym. 50, 4128–4138.

Hirenkumar, K., Makadia, K., Steven, J., 2011. Poly lactic-co-glycolic acid (PLGA) as biodegradable controlled drug delivery carrier. J. Polym. (Basel) 3, 1377–1397.

Hua, F.J., Park, T.G., Lee, D.S., 2003. A facile preparation of highly interconnected macroporous poly (L-lactic acid-co-glycolic acid) (PLGA) scaffolds by liquid-liquid phase separation of a PLGA-dioxane-water ternary system. J. Polym. 44, 1911–1920.

Huan, Z., Ahmed, H., Touny, M., Sarit, B., 2011. Fabrication of novel PLA/CDHA bionanocomposite fibers for tissue engineering applications via electrospinning. J. Mater. Sci. Mater. Med. 22, 1183–1193.

Iwatake, A., Nogi, M., Yano, H., 2008. Cellulose nanofiber-reinforced polylactic acid. Comp. Sci. Tech. 68, 2103–2106.

Jarcho, M., 1981. Calcium phosphate ceramics as hard tissue prosthetics. Clin. Orthop. Relat. Res. 157, 259–278.

Jenck, J.F., Agterberg, F., Droescher, M.J., 2004. Products and processes for a sustainable chemical industry: a review of achievements and prospects. Green Chem. 6, 544–556.

Jing, Xi, Ling, Z., Zhenhu, A., Guogiang, C., Yandao, G., Nanming, Z., Xiufang, Z., 2008. Preparation and evaluation of porous poly (3-hydroxybutyrate-co-3-hydroxyhexanoate) hydroxyapatite composite scaffolds. J. Biomater. Appl. 22, 293–307.

Kalpana, S.K., Katti, D.R., Avinas, H., 2012. Nanocomposites for Bone Tissue Engineering. Wiley-VCH Verlag GmbH & Co. KGaA. Available from: http://dx.doi.org/10.1002/9783527610419.ntls0226.

Kim, H.D., Bae, E., Kwon, I., Pal, R., Nam, J., Lee, D., 2004. Effect of PEG-PLLA diblock copolymer on macroporous PLLA scaffolds by thermally induced phase separation. J. Biomater. 25, 2319–2329.

Kim, H.W., Kim, H.E., Salih, V., 2005. Stimulation of osteoblast responses to biomimetic nanocomposites of gelatin-hydroxyapatite for tissue engineering scaffolds. J. Biomater. 26, 5221–5230.

Klemm, D., Schumann, D., Udhardt, U., Marsch, S., 2001. Bacterial synthesized cellulose—artificial blood vessels for microsurgery. Prog. Polym. Sci. 26, 1561–1603.

Kong, L., Gao, Y., Lu, G., Gong, Y., Zhao, N., Zhang, X., 2006. A study on the bioactivity of chitosan/nano-hydroxyapatite composite scaffolds for bone tissue engineering. Eur. Polym. J. 42, 3171–3179.

Kothapalli, C.R., Shaw, M.T., Wei, M., 2005. Biodegradable HA-PLA 3-D porous scaffolds: effect of nano-sized filler content on scaffold properties. Acta Biomater. 1, 653–662.

Landi, E., Valentini, F., Tampieri, A., 2008. Porous hydroxyapatite/gelatin scaffolds with ice-designed channel-like porosity for biomedical applications. Acta Biomater. 4, 1620–1626.

Lee, K., Kim, H., Khil, M., Ra, Y., Lee, D., 2003. Characterization of nano-structured poly (ε-caprolactone) nonwoven mats via electrospinning. J. Polym. 44, 1287–1294.

Lei, Z., Sheng, H., Gregoire, C., Engin, B., Gido, P., 2004. Polymer nanocomposites through controlled self-assembly of cubic silsesquioxane scaffolds. J. Macromol. 37, 8606–8611.

Lei, Y., Rai, B., Ho, K.H., Teoh, S.H., 2007. *In vitro* degradation of novel bioactive polycaprolactone–20% tricalcium phosphate composite scaffolds for bone engineering. Mater. Sci. Eng. C 27, 293–298.

Liu, X., Smith, L.A., Hu, J., Ma, P.X., 2009. Biomimetic nanofibrous gelatin/apatite composite scaffolds for bone tissue engineering. J. Biomater. 30, 2252–2258.

Loh, Q.L., Chong, C., 2013. Three-dimensional scaffolds for tissue engineering applications: role of porosity and pore size. Tissue Eng. B. Rev. 19, 485–502.

Lu, H.H., El-Amin, S.F., Scott, K.D., Laurencin, C.T., 2003. Three-dimensional, bioactive, biodegradable, polymer-bioactive glass composite scaffolds with improved mechanical properties support collagen synthesis and mineralization of human osteoblast-like cells *in vitro*. J. Biomed. Mater. Res. A. 64A, 465–474.

Madihally, S.V., Matthew, H.W., 1999. Porous chitosan scaffolds for tissue engineering. J. Biomater. 20, 1133–1142.

Mahshid, S., Luo, S., Yang, L., Mahshid, S.S., Askari, M., Dolati, A., et al., 2011. Carbon-Pt nanoparticles modified TiO_2 nanotubes for simultaneous detection of dopamine and uric acid. J. Nanosci. Nanotechnol. 11, 6668–6675.

Majola, A., Vainionpa, S., Vihtonen, K., Mero, M., Vasenius, J., Yormala, P., 1991. Absorption, biocompatibility and fixation properties of polylactic acid in bone tissue: an experimental study in rate. Clin. Orthop. Relat. Res. 268, 260–269.

Majola, S., Vainionpää, P., Rokkanen, H., Mikkola, P., 1992. Absorbable self-reinforced polylactide (SR-PLA) composite rods for fracture fixation: strength and strength retention in the bone and subcutaneous tissue of rabbits. J. Mater. Sci. Mater. Med. 3, 43–47.

Mandal, B.B., Kundu, S.C., 2009. Cell proliferation and migration in silk fibroin 3D scaffolds. J. Biomater. 30, 2956–2965.

Maquet, V., Boccaccini, A.R., Pravata, L., Notingher, I., Jérôme, R., 2004. Porous poly (α-hydroxyacid)/Bioglass® composite scaffolds for bone tissue engineering. I: Preparation and *in vitro* characterization. J. Biomater. 25, 4185–4194.

Mattioli-Belmonte, M., Vozzi, G., Whulanzac, M., Valentina, F., Giovanna, O., Arti, A., 2012. Tuning polycaprolactone–carbon nanotube composites for bone tissue engineering scaffolds. Mater. Sci. Eng. C 32, 152–159.

Michael, G., Dunn, L., Bellincampi, D., Alfred, J., Tria, I.R., Joseph, P.Z., 1997. Preliminary development of a collagen-PLA composite for ACL reconstruction. J. Polym. Appl. Sci. 63, 1423–1428.

Mittal, V., 2009. Polymer layered silicate nanocomposites: a review. J. Mater. 2, 992–1057.

Murugan, R., Huang, Z.M., Yang, F., Ramakrishna, S., 2007. Nanofibrous scaffold engineering using electrospinning. J. Nanosci. Nanotech. 7, 4595–4603.

Nopporn, S., Teerasak, D., Wilairat, L., Jearanaikoon, T., 2014. Fabrication and characterization of silk fibroin–gelatin/chondroitin sulfate/hyaluronic acid scaffold for biomedical applications. Mater. Lett. 126, 207–210.

Nowsheen, G., Archana, B.-L., Gary, L., Dhanjay, J., 2013. An assessment of biopolymer-and synthetic polymer-based scaffolds for bone and vascular tissue engineering. Polym. Int. 62, 523–533.

O'Brien, F.J., Harley, B.A., Waller, M.A., Yannas, I.V., Gibson, L.J., Prendergast, P.J., 2007. The effect of pore size on permeability and cell attachment in collagen scaffolds for tissue engineering. Technol. Health Care 15, 3–17.

Oliveira, J.M., Rodrigues, M.T., Silva, S.S., Malafaya, P.B., Gomes, M.E., Viegas, C.A., 2006. Novel hydroxyapatite/chitosan bilayered scaffold for osteochondral tissue engineering applications: scaffold design and its performance. J. Biomater. 27, 6123–6137.

Pan, L., Pei, X., He, R., Wan, Q., Wang, J., 2012. Multiwall carbon nanotubes/polycaprolactone composites for bone tissue engineering application. Colloids Surf. B Biointerfaces 93, 226–234.

Pereira, M.M., Hench, L.L., 1996. Mechanisms of hydroxyapatite formation on porous gel-silica substrates. J. Sol.-Gel. Sci. Technol. 7, 59–68.

Petersen, N., Gatenholm, P., 2011. Bacterial cellulose-based materials and medical devices: current state and perspectives. Appl. Microbiol. Biotechnol. 91, 1277–1286.

Pochan, J., Krikorian, V., Darrin, M., 2003. Poly(l-lactic acid)/layered silicate nanocomposite: fabrication characterization, and properties. Chem. Mater. 15, 4317–4324.

Prabaharan, M., Jayakumar, R., Nair, S., 2011. Electrospun nanofibrous scaffolds-current status and prospects in drug delivery. Adv. Polym. Mater. Sci. 246, 241–262.

Ralph, M., Müller, R., 2009. Hierarchical microimaging of bone structure and function. Nat. Rev. Rheumatol. 5, 373–381.

Ray, S., Okamoto, M., 2003. Polymer/layered silicate nanocomposites: a review from preparation to processing. Prog. Polym. Sci. 28, 1539–1641.

Rezwan, K., Chen, Q.Z., Blaker, J.J., Boccaccini, A.R., 2006. Biodegradable and bioactive porous polymer/inorganic composite scaffolds for bone tissue engineering. J. Biomater. 27, 3413–3431.

Rickert, D., Lendlein, A., Peters, I., Moses, M., Franke, R., 2006. Biocompatibility testing of novel multifunctional polymeric biomaterials for tissue engineering applications in head and neck surgery: an overview. Eur. Arch. Otorhinolaryngol. 263, 215–222.

Roohani-Esfahani, S.I., Nouri-Khorasani, S., Lu, Z., Appleyard, R., Zreiqat, H., 2010. The influence hydroxyapatite nanoparticle shape and size on the properties of biphasic calcium phosphate scaffolds coated with hydroxyapatite-PCL composites. J. Biomater. 31, 5498–5509.

Roshan, J., Meng, D., Cato, T.L., Sangamesh, G., 2011. Nanocomposites and bone regeneration. Front. Mater. Sci. 5, 342–357.

Salgado, A.J., Coutinho, O.P., Reis, R.L., 2004. Bone tissue engineering: state of the art and future trends. J. Macromol. Biosci. 4, 743–765.

Saska, S., Barud, H., Gaspar, M., Marchetto, R., Ribeiro, L., Messaddeq, Y., 2012. Bacterial cellulose-hydroxyapatite nanocomposites for bone regeneration. J. Mater. Chem. 22, 22102–22112.

Savioli, L.M., Jardini, A., Maciel, L., Filho, R., 2012. Poly (lactic acid) production for tissue engineering applications. J. Proc. Eng. 42, 1402–1413.

Sepulveda, P., Jones, J.R., Hench, L.L., 2001. Characterization of melt-derived 45S5 and sol-gel-derived 58S bioactive glasses. J. Biomed. Mater. Res. 58, 734–740.

Sill, T.J., Recum, V., 2008. Electrospinning: applications in drug delivery and tissue engineering. J. Biomater. 29, 1989–2006.

Singh, S., Ray, S.S., 2007. Polylactide based nanostructured biomaterials and their applications. J. Nanosci. Nanotechnol. 7, 2596–2615.

Smith, I.O., McCabe, L.R., Baumann, M.J., 2006. MC3T3-E1 osteoblast attachment and proliferation on porous hydroxyapatite scaffolds fabricated with nanophases powder. Int. J. Nanomed. 1, 189–194.

Smith, I.O., Liu, X.H., Smith, A., 2009. Nanostructured polymer scaffolds for tissue engineering and regenerative medicine. J. Nanomed. Nanobiotechnol. 1, 226–236.

Sosnowski, S., Gadzinowski, M., Slowkowski, S., 1996. Poly (l,l-lactide) microspheres by ring-opening polymerization. J. Macromol. 29, 4556–4564.

Stevens, M.M., George, J.H., 2005. Exploring and engineering the cell surface interface. J. Sci. 310, 1135–1138.

Sultana, N., Wang, M., 2012. PHBV/PLLA-based composite scaffolds fabricated using an emulsion freezing/freeze-drying technique for bone tissue engineering: surface modification and *in vitro* biological evaluation. J. Biofabricat. 4, 015004.

Taboas, J., Maddox, R., Krebsbach, P., Hollister, J., 2003. Indirect solid free form fabrication of local and global porous, biomimetic and composite 3D polymer-ceramic scaffolds. J. Biomater. 24, 181–194.

Tarafder, S., Balla, V.K., Davies, N.M., Bandyopadhyay, A., Bose, S., 2013. Microwave-sintered 3D printed tricalcium phosphate scaffolds for bone tissue engineering. J. Tissue Eng. Regen. Med. 7, 631–641.

Tarun, G., Arsh, C., Ravi, J., 2012. Preparation of chitosan scaffolds for tissue engineering using freeze drying technology. IOSR J. Pharm. 2, 072–073.

Thomas, P., Natalia, F., Natalia, V., Katja, U., Claus, D., Dmitry, V., 2014. Microporous polymeric 3D scaffolds template by the layer-by-layer self-assembly. Macromol. Rapid Commun. 35, 1408–1413.

Wahib, A., Dahman, Y., 2013. Production of green biocellulose nanofibers by *Gluconacetobacter xylinus* through utilizing the renewable resources of agriculture residues. Bioprocess Biosyst. Eng. 36, 1735–1743.

Wei, G., Ma, P., 2004. Structure and properties of nano-hydroxyapatite/polymer composite scaffolds for bone tissue engineering. J. Biomater. 25, 4749–4757.

Weng, J., Wang, M., Chen, J., 2002. Plasma-sprayed calcium phosphate particles with high bioactivity and their use in bioactive scaffolds. J. Biomater. 23, 2623–2629.

Woodard, J.R., Hilldore, A.J., Lan, S., Park, C., Morgan, A., Eurell, J., et al., 2007. The mechanical properties and osteoconductivity of hydroxyapatite bone scaffolds with multi-scale porosity. J. Biomater. 28, 45–54.

Wu, X., Liu, Y., Li, X., Wen, P., Zhang, Y., Long, Y., 2010. Preparation of aligned porous gelatin scaffolds by unidirectional freeze-drying method. Acta Biomater. 6, 1167–1177.

Xue, W., Bandyopadhyay, A., Bose, S., 2009. Polycaprolactone coated porous tricalcium phosphate scaffolds for controlled release of protein for tissue engineering. J. Biomed. Mater. Res. B Appl. Biomater. 91, 831–838.

Yan, Z., Wan, Y.L., Wang, Q.Y., Li, X., 2001. Influence of surface treatment of Carbone fibers on interfacial adhesion strength and mechanical properties of PLA-based composites. J. Appl. Polym. Sci. 80, 367–376.

Yunoki, S., Marukawa, E., Ikoma, T., Sotome, S., Fan, H., Zhang, S., 2007. Effect of collagen fibril formation on bioresorbability of hydroxyapatite/ collagen composites. J. Mater. Sci. Mater. Med. 18, 2179–2183.

Zhang, F., Sun, X., 2005. Poly (lactic acid) based bioplastics. In: Smith, R. (Ed.), Biodegradable Polymers for Industrial Applications. CRC Pub Limted, Cambridge, pp. 251–288.

Zhao, C., Tan, A., Pastorin, G., Ho, H., 2013. Nanomaterial scaffolds for stem cell proliferation and differentiation in tissue engineering. Biotechnol. Adv. 31, 654–668.

Zhou, C.J., Wu, Q.J., 2012. Recent development in applications of cellulose nanocrystals for advanced polymer-based nanocomposites by novel fabrication strategies. In: Neralla, S. (Ed.), Nanocrystals – Synthesis, Characterization and Applications. In Tech, Rijeka, pp. 103–120.

Zhou, Ye, Fan, Y., Ma, L., Tan, Y., Qing, F., Zhang, X., 2014. Biomimetic fabrication of a three-level hierarchical calcium phosphate/collagen/hydroxyapatite scaffold for bone tissue engineering. J. Biofabricat. 6, 035013.

CHAPTER

Collagen-based nanobiomaterials: challenges in soft tissue engineering

7

Gabriela Purcel[1], Daniela Meliţă[1], Ecaterina Andronescu[2] and Alexandru Mihai Grumezescu[2]

[1]Department of Science and Engineering of Oxide Materials and Nanomaterials, University Politehnica of Bucharest, Bucharest, Romania [2]Department of Science and Engineering of Oxide Materials and Nanomaterials, Faculty of Applied Chemistry and Materials Science, University Politehnica of Bucharest, Bucharest, Romania

7.1 INTRODUCTION

Collagen is the main structural protein of mammalian fibrous tissues, being found in tendons, ligaments, and skin. It also constitutes about 1.5% of the muscular tissue and is abundant in cornea, blood vessels, and cartilage. Collagen occurred early in phylogeny, being present in primeval marine animals, like jellyfishes, corals, and anemones. It is synthesized by fibroblasts arising from pluripotential adventitial cells or reticulum cells (Selestina and Vanja, 2011; Lee et al., 2001).

To date, 29 collagen types have been discovered and described, however, the main collagen type from the body is type I collagen which can be found in bones, skin, ligatures, and even organs. Even though type I collagen occupies over 90% of the collagen in the human body, when it comes to the formation of scar tissue because of age or as a cause of injuries, an interchange between types I and III occurs (Selestina and Vanja, 2011).

Collagen has a particular and uncommon structure, consisting of three polypeptide chains twisted together as in a three-stranded rope, each one with its individual twist in the opposite direction. It has a repetitive sequence of which every third residue of collagen molecule is glycine and the whole sequence of the polypeptide chain can be described as X−Y−glycine, where X and Y are proline and hydroxyproline (Lee et al., 2001).

Regarding the biomedical applications of collagen, due to its excellent structural, physical, immunological, and chemical properties, more exactly biodegradability, biocompatibility, and the capability to support cellular growth, it has been

Nanobiomaterials in Soft Tissue Engineering. DOI: http://dx.doi.org/10.1016/B978-0-323-42865-1.00007-6

used for tissue engineering, wound repair, heart valves, vascular grafts and blood vessels, ocular surfaces, tendon repair, nerve regeneration, and muscular engineering (Lee et al., 2001; Parenteau-Bareil et al., 2010).

The purpose of this chapter is to give a brief description of the collagen molecule, taking into account its structure, origin, and the functions of various types of collagen, followed by the main methods of extraction, and, ultimately, the main applications and developments in collagen-based soft tissue engineering biomaterials will be discussed.

7.2 GENERAL DESCRIPTION AND ORIGIN

In order to select starting materials (one of the most important steps in biomaterial development) we must keep in mind that they must mimic a biological tissue. From the biomimetic materials group, collagen can be used since it is a constituent part of the body. Tissues and organs are characterized by their three-dimensional extracellular matrix structure (Davidenko et al., 2012). The extracellular matrix of connective tissues contains mainly fibrous proteins and glycosaminoglycans which provide structural integrity and a variety of other physiological functions (Gelse et al., 2003).

Collagen is one of the key fibrous proteins within the extracellular matrix and represents up to 30% of the whole-body mammalian protein content. The role of collagen in the extracellular matrix is to provide tensile strength, regulate cell adhesion, and direct tissue development (Frantz et al., 2010).

Collagen is synthesized by fibroblasts and due to their properties, such as tensile strength and elasticity, is mostly found in fibrous tissues—skin, tendons, and ligaments—but is also found in bones, cartilage, corneas, and blood vessels (Notbohm et al., 2005).

The use of collagen in the biomedical field dates from 1881 when Joseph Lister and William Macewen created a suture called “catgut”; this is a biodegradable collagen-rich biomaterial prepared from the small intestine of a sheep. It has provided a springboard for the many inventions that followed (Chattopadhyay and Raines, 2014).

7.3 COLLAGEN STRUCTURE

The first proposal about the structure of the collagen molecule was made by Astbury and Bell, in 1940, who considered that the molecule has a single polypeptide chain in extended form with *cis* conformation amide bonds. Next, in 1951, a new structure was proposed by Pauling and Corey for collagen. This structure consisted of three polypeptide strands fasten by hydrogen bonds in a helical conformation. Later, in the 1950s, two other researchers proposed an advanced model for collagen structure, one of a triple helix using fiber diffraction data and after 5 years this structure was refined to the triple helix structure accepted today (Shoulders and Raines, 2009).

In the structure of collagen three parallel polypeptide chains, each with a conformation of left-handed polyproline type II (PPII) helical conformation, are twisted and held together in order to form a right-handed triple helix. This triple helix represents a quaternary structure stabilized by hydrogen bonds, intramolecular van der Waals interactions and covalent bonds, linked into microfibrils and fibrils and comprised of collagen fibers (Selestina and Vanja, 2011). The right-handed helix, formed by the three chains, has 18 amino acids per turn (Shoulders and Raines, 2009). Each chain consists of about 1000 amino acids residues and has a length of about 300 nm and a diameter of 1.4 nm.

Collagen has a special characteristic represented by a regular arrangement of amino acids in each subunit. Within the helix, glycine (Gly) occupies every third residue place, while in the repeating three amino acids sequence, the first two residues can be any amino acid (Shoulders and Raines, 2009; Selestina and Vanja, 2011; Gelse et al., 2003). Despite the fact that all 28 types of collagen have this repetition of Gly structure, in non-fibrillar collagens the repeat is interrupted at certain points within the helix. Amino acids occupying the first two positions are represented by (2*S*)-proline (Pro, 28%) and (2*S*,4*R*)-4-hydroxyproline (Hyp, 38%). These two amino acids constitute about a sixth of the total sequence and can participate in different interactions, more precisely in intramolecular stabilization due to their steric repulsion (Shoulders and Raines, 2009; Selestina and Vanja, 2011). The triplet ProHypGly is the most common in the structure of collagen (Gelse et al., 2003). The telopeptides (short non-helical domains with 9–26 amino acids) contribute to collagen fibril formation and natural crosslinking, as well as in coupling with other structures from the surrounding matrix (Selestina and Vanja, 2011).

Other components which play an important role in the formation of triple helical structure are C- and N-propeptides. Thus, C-propeptides contribute to the initiation of triple helix formation, while N-propeptides are implicated in the adjustment of primary fibrils diameters (Frantz et al., 2010).

The twisted structure of collagen is stabilized by the bonds created between Gly and Pro and by the water network. Also, the content of 4-hydroxyproline is important for the formation of hydrogen bonds and therefore the stability of triple helical conformation. The Gly repeat structure defines the collagenous domain of all collagens. All glycine residues are placed in the center of the helix due to the way the chains assemble around the central axis. This type of arrangement allows close bundling along the central axis (Selestina and Vanja, 2011).

Collagens can be separated based on their organization into different categories as follows: fibril-associated collagens with interrupted triple helices (FACITs), membrane-associated collagens with interrupted triple helices (MACITs), multiple triple helix domains and interruptions (MULTIPLEXINs), fibril-forming collagens, network-forming collagens, and others with different functions (Shoulders and Raines, 2009; Gelse et al., 2003).

FACIT collagens have their triple helix interrupted by non-collagenous domains which can act as joints. Furthermore, these non-collagenous domains, characterized by structural and functional diversity, can be involved in network formation and aggregation (Gelse et al., 2003; Gordon and Hahn, 2009). These interruptions are useful because they allow proteolytic cleavage of the structure overcoming the resistance to proteases of native triple helices (Gelse et al., 2003).

Collagen types are different, with a structure characterized by diversity and complexity. Also, they can be differentiated by the presence of additional non-collagenous domains (non-Gly), their assembly, and functions (Gordon and Hahn, 2009). The most common family of collagen, more precisely fibril-forming collagens, contains about 90% of the total collagen. Even though the collagen types are different in terms of structure, all collagens have a characteristic feature represented by a right-handed triple helix made of three α-chains (Figure 7.1) (Gelse et al., 2003). The three identical chains of collagen structure are named homotrimers and can be found in collagens II, III, VII, VIII, and X. When two or more chains are different, they are called heterotrimers and can be found in collagens I, IV, V, VI, IX, and XI (Gelse et al., 2003).

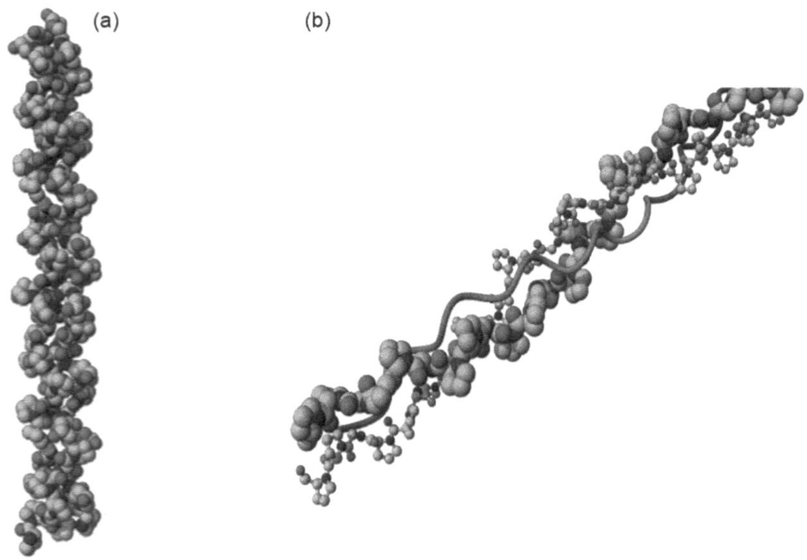

FIGURE 7.1

Overview of collagen triple helix. (a) Collagen structure (Protein Data Bank id: 1cag, YASARA image). (b) Collagen triple helix with the three chains illustrated in ball and sticks, balls and ribbon (Protein Data Bank id: 1k6f, YASARA image).

7.4 COLLAGEN TYPES

To date 29 types of collagen have been identified, 90% of these are type I collagen. By structure, there are several classes of collagen which are illustrated in Table 7.1.

Figure 7.2 shows the way that collagen molecules are formed and assemble into fibrils.

7.4.1 FIBRILLAR COLLAGEN FAMILY

The fibrillar collagen family includes types I, II, III, V, XI, and more recently this family was increased with two others added, XXIV and XXVII, respectively.

Fibrillar collagen type I represents the most important component of extracellular matrix and one of the most abundant mammalian proteins. It is usually found in ligamentous and tendinous tissues where it provides tensile strength, but serves as a scaffold for cells. Collagen I fibrils are formed in a hierarchical self-assembly process and start with triple helical monomeric tropocollagen monomers (1.5 nm thick, 300 nm long), through microfibrillar units of 4–5 nm in diameter.

Collagen type I has the periodicity of D-banding of 67 resulting from the collagen chains during fibrillogenesis. This band helps at optimal electrostatic pairing between neighboring monomers and also in maximizing contact between hydrophobic domain regions (Stamov et al., 2015). A single molecule contains three amino acid chains that form a triple helix (there are two $\alpha 1$ chains and one $\alpha 2$ chain), but each chain consists of just over 1000 amino acids. The molecule is characterized by three domains: N-telopeptide domain at the beginning located at the N-terminal, a triple helical domain, and a C-telopeptide domain at the end located at the C-terminal, and shows hook conformation which helps in the formation of enzymatic covalent crosslinks and so ensures structural integrity, strength, and stiffness to collagenous tissues (Kwansa et al., 2014).

Type II collagen is a homotrimer composed of three collagen $\alpha 1$(II) chains. Each α-chain contains 1014 amino acids, including glycine, proline, and hydroxyproline (Kannu et al., 2011). Collagen type II is the primary component of the cartilage extracellular matrix and its synthesis is provided by chondrocyte cells. Collagen type II ensures the development of cartilage anlagen and is essential for endochondral bone formation. It is also found in the vitreous humor and the inner ear (Kannu et al., 2011; Kuo et al., 2013; Tekari et al., 2014).

Collagen type III is homotrimer fibril-forming composed of three $\alpha 1$(III) chains and is found in many connective tissues. It is present in skin and blood vessels and is involved in the healing process of bone, tendon, ligament, and skin (Miedel et al., 2015).

Collagen type V is regulatory fibril-forming and intervenes in the developing stage of tendon and bone, but it was also identified in cornea. This influences the

Table 7.1 Collagen Types

Group	Type	Molecular Composition	Genes	Tissue Distribution
Fibrillar	I	[a1(I)]2a2(I)	COL1A1 (17q21.31–q22)	Bone, dermis, tendon, ligaments, cornea, skin, vascular ligature, organs, dentin, interstitial tissues
	II	[a1(II)]3	COL2A1 (12q13.11–q13.2)	Cartilage, vitreous humor, nucleus pulposus
	III	[a1(III)]3	COL3A1 (2q31)	Skin, blood vessels, reticular fibers of most tissues (lungs, liver, spleen, etc.)
	V	a1(V), a2(V), a3(V)	COL5A1 (9q34.2–q34.3) COL5A2 (2q31) COL5A3 (19p13.2)	Lung, cornea, bone, placenta, together with type I collagen, teeth, smooth muscle, skin, cell surfaces
	XI	a1(XI)a2(XI)a3(XI)	COL11A1 (1p21) COL11A2 (6p21.3) COL11A3 = COL2A1	Cartilage, vitreous body
	XXIV			Eye, ear, lung
	XXVII			Cartilage
Fibril-associated	IX	a1(IX)a2(IX)a3(IX)	COL9A1 (6q13) COL9A2 (1p33–p32.2)	Cartilage, vitreous humor, cornea
	XII	[a1(XII)]3	COL12A1 (6q12–q13)	Perichondrium, ligaments, tendon
	XIV	[a1(XIV)]3	COL9A1 (8q23)	Dermis, tendon, vessel wall, placenta, lungs, liver
	XVI	[a1(XVI)]3	COL16A1 (1p34)	Fibroblasts, amnion, keratinocytes
	XIX	[a1(XIX)]3	COL19A1 (6q12–q14)	Human rhabdomyosarcoma
	XX	[a1(XX)]3		Corneal epithelium, embryonic skin, sternal cartilage, tendon
	XXI	[a1(XXI)]3	COL21A1 (6p12.3–11.2)	Blood vessel wall
	XXII			Cell junction
	XXVI			Testis and ovary
Anchoring fibrils	VII	[a1(VII)]3	COL7A1 (3p21.3)	Skin, dermal–epidermal junctions; oral mucosa, cervix
Network forming	VI	a1(VI),a2(VI),a3(VI)	COL6A1 (21q22.3) COL6A2 (21q22.3)	Widespread: dermis, cartilage, placenta, lungs, vessel wall, intervertebral disk, interstitial tissues

			COL6A3 (2q37)	
	IV	[a1(IV)]2a2(IV); a1–a6	COL4A1 (13q34)	Basement membranes
			COL4A2 (13q34)	
			COL4A3 (2q36–q37)	
			COL4A4 (2q36–q37)	
			COL4A5 (Xq22.3)	
			COL4A6 (Xp22.3)	
	VIII	[a1(VIII)]2a2(VIII)	COL8A1 (3q12–q13.1)	Endothelial cells, Descemet's membrane, brain, heart, kidney
			COL8A2 (1p34.3–p32.3)	
	X	[a3(X)]3	COL10A1 (6q21–q22.3)	Hypertrophic cartilage
	XXIII			Retina, heart
Transmembrane	XIII	[a1(XIII)]3	COL13A1 (10q22)	Epidermis, hair follicle, endomysium, intestine, chondrocytes, lungs, liver, eye, heart
	XVII	[a1(XVII)]3	COL17A1 (10q24.3)	Dermal–epidermal junctions
	XXV			Nerve cells, heart, testis
Multiplexins	XV	[a1(XV)]3	COL15A1 (9q21–q22)	Fibroblasts, smooth muscle cells, kidney, pancreas
	XVIII	[a1(XVIII)]3)	COL18A1 (21q22.3)	Lungs, liver
Others	XXVIII	–	–	Sciatic nerve, dermis

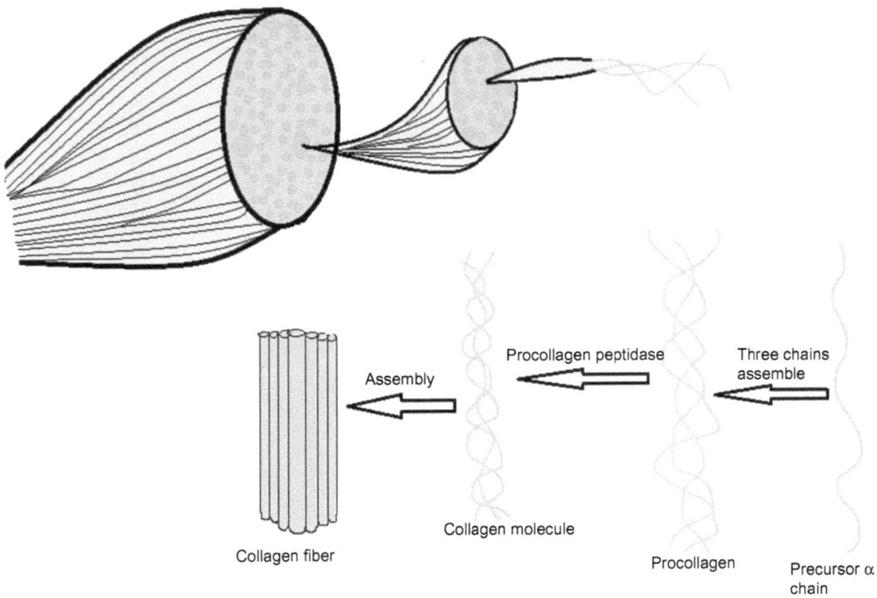

FIGURE 7.2

Assembly of α-chains into trimeric collagen molecules and then of molecules into fibrils.

total collagen content by regulating the diameter of the collagen type I fibril. At present, the structural fibril of collagen V has not been reported (Wang et al., 2012; Berchtold et al., 2015).

Collagen type XI is heterotrimer collagen molecule and serves to regulate type II fibril diameters in cartilage. In cartilage, types II and XI copolymerize with type IX to form a heteropolymeric fibrillar framework to ensure the tensile strength of cartilage (McAlinden et al., 2014). During mesenchymal stem cell chondrogenic differentiation, this type is the first cartilage collagen deposited by these cells (Shanmugasundaram et al., 2011). In structural terms these are characterized by small chains which contain some non-helical domains (Selestina and Vanja, 2011).

Collagen types XXIV and XXVII differ from other fibrillar collagens in that they show a triple helix slightly shorter with 997 amino acids (Exposito et al., 2010). This group also presents a short imperfection in the triple helix—two successive glycine substitutions and one glycine–proline–hydroxyproline imperfection. It is supposed that type XXIV intervenes in regulating collagen type I fibrillogenesis during fetal development (Koch et al., 2003). Collagen type XXIV is found predominantly in bone tissue, but it may intervene in organogenesis due to expression in lower levels in brain and the eye.

7.4.2 FIBRIL-ASSOCIATED COLLAGEN FAMILY

Collagens types IX, XII, XIV, XIX, XX, XXI, XXII, and XXVI belong to the class called "FACITs" (fibril-associated collagens with interrupted triple helices), presenting an alternation of triple helical domains with short non-triple helical domains (Rest and Garrone, 1991).

Collagen type IX is a heterotrimeric protein located at the interior of collagen II and XI fibril and serves to stabilize the fibrillar and proteoglycan networks together with them. Another function of this collagen consists of regulating the diameter of collagen fibrils (Krug et al., 2013; Imagawa et al., 2014).

Collagen type XII is a homotrimer of $\alpha1$ chains and is characterized by three non-collagenous domains and two collagenous domains (Izu et al., 2011). The embryo collagen type XII is involved in bone developing, ligaments, tendons, fibrocartilage, smooth muscle, and skin. After birth, it is found in certain dense connective tissues (cornea, periodontal ligament, and dermis around hair follicles) (Chiquet et al., 2014).

Collagen type XIV is a homotrimer of three $\alpha1$ chains and is strongly expressed in native human bone marrow (Klein et al., 1998). It presents 10 collagenous domains which are flanked by non-collagenous domains (Hsu et al., 2013). It has been shown that it is highly expressed in areas with high mechanical stress. Its main function consist of interactions with collagen type I to promote fiber assembly (Tao et al., 2012).

Collagen type XVI is a FACIT collagen which plays an important role in anchoring microfibrils to basement membranes. It is produced by dermal fibroblasts, dermal dendrocytes, articular and costal chondrocytes, smooth muscle cells, oral keratinocytes, neurons, and astrocytoma cells (Bedal et al., 2014).

Collagen type XIX is a minor collagen which is found in basement membrane, together with types IV, XV, and XVIII (Ramont et al., 2007). It is a homotrimer of three $\alpha1$ chains; each α-chain is composed of 1142 amino acids—6 non-collagenous domains and 5 collagenous domains. Usually it is found in the basement membrane of vascular, neuronal, mesenchymal and epithelial tissues. During embryogenesis it participates in extracellular matrix assembly (Khaleduzzaman et al., 1997; Oudart et al., 2013).

Collagen type XX was included in the FACIT family thanks to sequence similarity to types XII and XIV. At present, its structure has not yet been elucidated (Koch et al., 2001).

Collagen type XXI is a protein which contains 957 amino acids and is found in blood vessel walls (Li et al., 2005).

Collagen type XXII is deposited in the basement membrane of the myotendinous junction from muscle, tendons, the heart, articular cartilage, and skin (Rest and Garrone, 1991; Misawa et al., 2014).

Collagen type XXVI is expressed in testis and ovaries during development. It is a small molecule and contain only 438 amino acids (Blum and Ruggiero, 2005).

7.4.3 ANCHORING FIBRILS COLLAGEN

Collagen type VII belongs to this category and represents the major component of anchoring fibrils, being shown to merge into the banded collagen fibrils of the dermis, suggesting that collagen type VII plays an important role in maintaining epidermal–dermal adherence (Rest and Garrone, 1991; Chen et al., 1997). It is a homotrimeric molecule composed of three α-chains.

7.4.4 NETWORK-FORMING COLLAGENS

This family includes collagen types IV, VI, VIII, and X, which form different networks.

Collagen type IV is a principal constituent of the basement membrane, providing tensile strength in different tissues, represents a scaffold for ECM constituents, and interacts with growth factors to establish signaling gradients (Sand et al., 2013; McCall et al., 2014; Fang et al., 2013).

Collagen type VI is an important constituent of the extracellular matrix of many connective tissues (Vanegas et al., 2001; Koudouna et al., 2014). It is a heterotrimeric protein which consists of three different chains α1, α2, and α3. Its main function is to bind to cells and interact with the other components of the extracellular matrix. It forms a microfilamentous network in the pericellular region and currently its physiological role is not exactly known, but it has been implicated in various cellular interactions (cell adhesion, migration, and apoptosis). It has also been found in cartilaginous matrix and fetal bone (Izu et al., 2012).

Collagen type VIII is a non-fibrillar protein included in the short-chain collagen family, it is a heterodimer composed of two chains α1 and α2. Its main function is to control atherosclerosis, being present in very low amounts in normal arteries, but its concentration increases in atherosclerotic lesion and in aged vessels. Following injury, its expression is simulated by cytokinase, oxidase lipids, and several growth factors depositing near sublumenal support smooth muscle cell which helps intimal thickening (Loeffler et al., 2012; Lopes et al., 2013; Adiguzel et al., 2013).

Collagen type X represents a major hypertrophic cartilage matrix protein implicated in endochondral ossification. Type X collagen is a homotrimer because it contains only one α-chain (Sweeney et al., 2013).

Collagen type XXIII was found in prostatic cancer tissues, but is also expressed in a high proportion of tissue and urine samples taken from patients with non-small-cell lung cancer (Banyard et al., 2003).

7.4.5 TRANSMEMBRANOUS COLLAGENS

This family is formed by collagen types XIII, XVII, and XXV, which are transmembrane molecules.

Collagen type XIII is expressed in mesenchymal tissues. It is involved in the development, differentiation, and maturation of musculoskeletal tissues, vessels, and periosteum (Heikkinen et al., 2012), but in mature adult tissues its expression is very low (Väisänen, 2005).

Collagen type XVII is a homotrimer of three α-chains (Has et al., 2013) and represents a structural component of hemidesmosomes that mediate adhesion of keratinocytes to the epidermal basement membrane. Recent studies have revealed that this type is involved in both congenital and subepidermal autoimmune diseases (Natsuga et al., 2012; Ettinger et al., 2012).

Collagen type XXV encodes a type II transmembrane protein and is expressed only in neurons where it is a component of the amyloid β (Aβ) who is responsible for Alzheimer disease, and is probably involved in the development of brain degeneration (Li et al., 2012; Parmar et al., 2012).

7.4.6 MULTIPLEXINS COLLAGENS

The multiplexins collagen family includes types XV and XVIII. Collagen types XV and XVIII represent a molecule of the basement membranes (Momota et al., 2013, 2011).

Collagen XV is a chondroitin-sulfate-modified glycoprotein which plays a critical role in the structural integrity of ECM. Usually, it is found in skeletal and cardiac muscle. Loss of collagen type XV leads to basement membrane invasion and metastasis in aggressive forms of cancer. It is known that collagen type XV is a dose-dependent suppressor of tumorigenicity (Clementz et al., 2012, 2013; Clementz and Harris, 2013; Mutolo et al., 2012).

Collagen type XVIII is a heparan sulfate proteoglycan which is expressed in subepithelial and subendothelial basement membranes, but represents a prominent ECM component in the liver. Its expression increases in profibrotic stages of fibrosis, cirrhosis, and various cancers of the liver. It has been shown that in physiological conditions, collagen type XVIII is mostly needed in eye development (Duncan et al., 2013; Seppinen and Pihlajaniemi 2011; Aikio et al., 2014).

7.4.7 OTHERS COLLAGENS

Collagen type XXVIII is expressed by dorsal root ganglia and peripheral nerves. This was detected in adult sciatic nerve which means a long half-life for the molecule (Veit et al., 2006).

7.5 COLLAGEN EXTRACTION METHODS

Collagen used for biomedical applications is extracted from tissues. In the process of extraction very often collagen structure is degraded. The three major methods of collagen extraction are: extraction with neutral salt, acid isolation, and enzymatic solution. The development of a standard method of extraction for all types of collagen is difficult due to high dissimilarity between tissues and collagen types. The biochemical properties and thermal stability of collagen extracted by the methods presented above might be different because of reaction conditions (Mocan et al., 2011).

Collagen can also be isolated by pepsin digestion. This method consists of a depolymerization process in order to remove the amino and carboxyl terminal telopeptides and leads to properties similar to those of the commercial collagen (Selestina and Vanja, 2011).

Regardless of the extraction method, the isolated collagen presents poor thermal stability and mechanical strength due to the destruction of the natural assembly structure during extraction process. In order to correct these limitations, to increase their properties, and preserve their stability, collagen constructs are stabilized using crosslinking agents. Also, the process of crosslinking allows a reduction in collagen antigenicity (Selestina and Vanja, 2011).

7.6 COLLAGEN SOURCES

Various sources can be used for collagen extraction, from every living animal, including alligators and kangaroos, to humans. Nowadays, common sources from which collagen can be extracted in order to be used in soft tissue applications include bovine skin and tendons, porcine skin, and rat tail. Also, collagen can be isolated from marine species, especially from sponges, jellyfish, or other fishes. Despite the fact that these types of collagen are less utilized in the clinical environment, they are worth investigating because their properties differ from one animal to another. One more source for collagen is represented by humans. The rationale behind using human collagen is provided by the fact that human collagen is less immunogenic than animal sources and identical in composition. A cellular collagen from decellularized extracellular matrix produced from human or porcine dermis, swine intestine, or bladder submucosa can also be used, but the use of this collagen type is restricted due to immunological issues (Parenteau-Bareil et al., 2010).

7.7 BIOMEDICAL APPLICATIONS OF COLLAGEN IN SOFT TISSUE ENGINEERING

Collagen, one of the major components of extracellular matrix, is intensively studied for use in soft tissue engineering. Being a natural biomaterial, collagen is characterized by low mechanical strength and antigenicity and excellent biocompatibility and biodegradability. It can be used in both crude and processed forms like sponges, sheets, and gels. Also, collagen can be crosslinked with other materials or substances in order to become stronger or to modify the degradation profile. The use of collagen-based biomaterials in peripheral nerve regeneration, spinal cord formation, tendon regeneration, skeletal muscle engineering, and corneal tissue engineering has been reported in various studies (Mohamed and Xing, 2012).

An important reason for the efficiency of collagen in biomedical applications is the fact that collagen can form strong and stable fibers due to its self-aggregation and crosslinking process. Collagen can be used as bioengineered tissue such as blood vessels and heart valves due to its hemostatic properties.

Fifteen years ago, an extracellular support made from type I collagen was created. This support was able to organize cells into a 3D structure *in vitro*. Earlier, a graft made from bovine collagen was used as a scaffold for remodeling into a functional blood vessel. It was demonstrated that three-dimensional biodegradable collagen scaffolds provide a larger surface area for the attachment of cells and the support vascularization process, which recommends the use of collagen as artificial blood vessels and heart valves (Lee et al., 2001).

Considering the advantages of collagen, especially its low antigenicity and the ability to integrate with surrounding tissues, the researchers used collagen for abdominal wall repair. New generations of collagen tissues can be remodeled due to its simple configuration, uniformity, and availability.

A new type of surgical adhesive made from porcine collagen and polyglutamic acid presents the above-mentioned characteristics and is developed for prevention of air loss from the lungs. Also, the absorption rate of this adhesive can be controlled by collagen concentration (Lee et al., 2001).

Various applications involve different collagen formulations (Table 7.2).

7.7.1 CARDIOVASCULAR DISEASES AND VASCULAR TISSUE ENGINEERING

Cardiovascular disease is a major cause of death. One big problem for cardiovascular tissue engineering is that the tissues must be able to function immediately and with accuracy in conditions of a continuously beating heart. The implanted biomaterials suffer from degradation due to the body's response, thus losing their strength and integrity. Thus, to improve the treatment of peripheral and cardiovascular disease, it is necessarily to develop new tissue engineering approaches capable of producing functional vascular networks (Critser et al., 2010).

One mechanism to improve cardiovascular disease treatment is represented by the use of biomaterial carriers capable of promoting the differentiation and vessel formation. *In vitro* and *in vivo* studies performed by Critser et al. (2010) have shown that fibril density and stiffness of collagen matrices can influence vessel formation. More precisely, varied collagen fibril density and matrix stiffness, due to collagen concentration modification, affects endothelial colony-forming cell (ECFC) vessel density, the proportion of ECFC to host vessels, and blood

Table 7.2 Biomedical Applications of Collagen

Composition	Biomaterial Form	Application
Collagen	Gel	Cosmetic skin defects
		Drug delivery
		Vitreous replacement
		Surgical coating of bioprostheses
	Sponge	2D cell culture
		Wound dressing
		Hemostatic agent
		Skin replacement
	Hollow fiber tubing	Cell culture
		Nerve regeneration
	Sphere	Microcarrier for cell culture
		Drug delivery
	Membrane	Wound dressing dialysis
		Tissue regeneration
		Corneal shield
		Skin patches
Collagen + GAGs	Rigid form	Bone repair
Collagen + hydroxyapatite	Powder sponge	Bond-filling and repair drug delivery (BMP)

vascular areas. Also, the researchers found that the use of increased collagen concentrations to form cellularized matrices determined a diminishing of vessel density and an increase average vessel area and total vascular area, whereas low collagen concentration was conducted to increased densities of smaller area vessels. It can be concluded that physical properties are responsible for the vascularization mediated by ECFC, thus representing an important standard for cell delivery systems (Critser et al., 2010).

Another strategy for vascular tissue engineering is represented by the local delivery of a fibroblast growth factor with bovine type I collagen scaffold as a delivery vehicle to smooth muscle cells. Pang et al. demonstrated in their study a great retention of growth factor by collagen scaffold and almost complete distribution. Also, they suggested that the incorporated growth factor would have a biological effect on smooth muscle cells throughout the collagen, thus representing an important step in blood vessel engineering. Although the results are optimistic, further research is necessary in order to understand whether the cause for the negligible effect on the proliferative activity of smooth muscle cells demonstrated by the collagen-binding growth factor linked to collagen matrix is the blocking of the diffusion of the growth factor into the scaffold produced by the large volume of collagen (Pang et al., 2010).

7.7.2 SKELETAL MUSCLE TISSUE ENGINEERING

The main obstacle for tissue engineering of skeletal muscle is represented by the finding of a proper matrix. Such applications require the fulfillment of major requirements in terms of biocompatibility, fabrication in three-dimensional form, and suitable balance of elasticity, stability, and degradation profile. Over time, different materials such as gels, sponges, and most recently electrospun nanofibers have been studied and tested (Beier et al., 2009).

Collagen is a promising material for skeletal muscle tissue engineering because it mimics the natural extracellular matrix, thereby contributing to myoblast proliferation and differentiation. Beier et al. (2009) developed a collagen sponge with different combinations of collagens for skeletal muscle tissue engineering. Also, based on the possibility of processing parallel aligned muscle cells and myotubes, they developed electrospun collagen I nanofibers as a potential matrix for skeletal muscle. The first has recently been introduced in tissue engineering. The results of the performed tests showed that the cells adhered to the collagen nanofiber matrix within 2–6 h and after 10 days the matrix was completely overgrown by cells. In the case of collagen sponges no lysis was observed after 4 weeks of incubation. Also, using phase contrast microscopy showed that the myoblasts adopted a parallel configuration on oriented collagen I nanofibers.

Based on the fact that electrospinning of collagen with additives conducts the damaging and thinning of fibers, Beier et al. showed that the use of nanofiber matrix made of pure type I collagen conducts satisfactory cell proliferation and preservation of myogenic phenotype. Also, the fact that the cells adhered quickly to the matrix demonstrated the good biocompatibility of the material. Another observation was the parallel alignment of cell proliferation which is produced by the orientation of the matrix fibers in accordance with the contact guidance phenomenon. The obtaining of parallel alignment of myoblasts is one of the most important properties of a suitable matrix for skeletal muscle tissue engineering. Considering this statement, they concluded that orientated nanofibers made of type I collagen may be the most promising matrix at the moment (Beier et al., 2009).

7.7.3 CORNEAL TISSUE ENGINEERING

Corneal disease is the second cause of vision loss and affects millions of people worldwide, followed by trachoma and corneal injury. The correction of these affections mainly consists of the use of donor corneal grafts. Although the potential of cornea grafts is recognized, there are still difficulties associated with the obtaining of quality graft material. Donor grafts are different in quality, being subject to failure due to immunological rejection or endothelial decompensation resulting in a failure rate of about 18% for initial grafts. Considering these facts, the development of a satisfactory replacement for donor graft material is important. Cornea have an avascular, thin and multilaminar structure. To realize a cornea by tissue engineering methods, it is necessary to provide compatible and suitable media for culture of all cell types, more precisely for epithelial cells, fibroblasts or keratocytes, and endothelial cells. Also, the functions of corneal tissue are realized by a complex stromal extracellular matrix (Ruberti and Zieske, 2008).

In terms of the corneal epithelium *ex vivo* culture, since 1994, several researchers (Ruberti and Zieske, 2008) have seeded human corneal epithelial cells onto collagen substrates with acceptable success. Thus, the first attempt was made with primary cells cultured on collagen gels, followed years later by the immortalization of cells on glutaraldehyde-fixed collage/chondroitin sulfate gels and the seeding of primary limbal epithelial cells onto collagen populated with keratocytes. One year later, researchers (Ruberti and Zieske, 2008) used primary epithelial cells on dehydrothermally crosslinked collagen sponges populated with keratocytes and in the presence of endothelial cells and demonstrated that primary human keratocytes migrated into the collagen sponges and proliferated and also synthesized collagen. Research has shown that the location of cell seeding is very important due to the spatial differences between the proliferative capacities of human cells.

Another study (Ruberti and Zieske, 2008) demonstrated that the contact guidance phenomenon leads to an alignment of fibroblasts in the direction of the fibrils when in contact with shear-aligned collagen gels.

Classical tissue engineering of the human corneal stroma consists of seeding human corneal cells onto scaffolds made of type I collagen derived from bovine skin or rat tail tendon. Although the gels are native-looking type I collagen fibrils, it is not known if they are stable *in vivo* or *in vitro* without crosslinking (Ruberti and Zieske, 2008).

7.7.4 PERIPHERAL NERVE REGENERATION

Injuries to the peripheral nervous system resulted from trauma, such as explosive injury and automobile accidents, leading to a decreased quality of life and most of the time needing reconstruction through complicated surgical interventions. Although nerve autografting is the gold standard for peripheral nerve reconstruction, the use of sensory nerves from the patient tissue is not the optimal choice as it leads to loss of function of the donor site and requires a new surgical intervention (Alberti et al., 2014).

In the last 10 years, several alternatives have been used for peripheral nerve repair, including nerve guidance conduits. This conduit objective is to build a pathway along which the ends of a sectioned nerve can regrow toward each other. The reconstruction of the nerve includes stages like infiltration of fluid, fibrin matrix formation, and migration of specific cells. A greater nerve guidance construct must have properties like controllable degradation rate, suitable permeability, and stiffness (Alberti et al., 2014).

One alternative for peripheral nerve engineering is represented by nerve guidance matrices fabricated from tendon-derived collagen which preserves the native collagen fiber structure. This nerve guidance construct consists of several layers of fibers with different orientation, with an interior layer made of collagen nanofibers parallel to the length of construct and the exterior layers in alternate directions. The fiber orientation assures the contact of the cell with the fibers from the center, while the outer fibers provide strength and sustain the suturing and prevent the breakage of sutures (Alberti et al., 2014).

Researchers (Alberti et al., 2014) observed an increased proliferation of Schwann cells on poly-D-lysine-coated tendon-derived collagen constructs as a result of increased initial adhesion and by reason of poly-D-lysine properties. Also, they studied the alignment and morphology of the Schwann cells and observed that collagen construction leads to a defined alignment of Schwann cells parallel to the collagen fibers. The alignment is very important because it increases the markers of myelination and decreases the neurotrophin and neurotrophic receptors responsible for immature Schwann cell phenotype. Also, Alberti et al. affirmed that the increased degree of alignment observed on tendon-derived collagen may be beneficial for nerve repair and connection formation. Finally, they concluded that the nanofibrous collagen found in tendon has the ability to guide and support neuronal cell growth, while the alignment produced by collagen fibers may result in a more mature phenotype and may encourage the formation of the correct connections between the ends of the sectioned nerve (Alberti et al., 2014).

7.7.5 NERVE CONDUITS FOR SPINAL CORD REPAIR

Spinal cord injuries lead to functional damage at the site of injuries due to loss of axon connections and limited neuronal regeneration. Although tissue-engineered scaffolds can be regarded as a potential treatment method, the results are still limited as a result of the complex inhibitory microenvironment at the injury site. An ideal construct for spinal cord injuries treatment should be able to support the regeneration of axons across the wound, reduce glial scar formation, and restore functional connection. Thus, Liu et al. used plain electrospun collagen nanofibers to support neurite outgrowth. Also, using a contact guidance phenomenon, they tried to organize and orientate the regenerated axons according to nanofiber alignment (Liu et al., 2012).

The *in vitro* studies showed that fiber diameter influences axonal outgrowth, thus larger-diameter fibers (about 1.3 μm) excited longer neurite growth and smaller-diameter fibers (about 290 nm) resulted in smaller neurite growth. Moreover, linear axon regeneration was observed inside aligned collagen conduits. It has been observed that a significant cell penetration into collagen scaffolds as well as a reduction in acute inflammatory response which leads to the idea that electrospun collagen scaffolds not only induced and supported tissue regeneration by providing an extracellular matrix, but they were biocompatible, diminishing astrocyte accumulation at the injury site and providing a suitable environment for neural fiber grow (Liu et al., 2012).

7.7.6 NASAL CARTILAGE REPAIR

Trauma, tumor resection, or congenital defects can cause the deterioration of cartilaginous facial structures. Such defects can lead to inadaptability in the social environment, functional and medical complications, a severe sense of rejection, and other psychosocial problems. In order to overcome the limitations of self-repair capacity of cartilage, in is necessary to use transplants, especially the transplant of autologous cartilage. Although this is the gold standard in nasal cartilage repair, the use of this type of implant often results in infection of the graft. Thus, soft tissue engineering is a promising alternative for nose reconstruction (Bermueller et al., 2013).

Cartilage reconstruction scaffold should respond to several demands, especially in terms of design. The architecture of the construct should mimic the shape of the native tissue and support the attachment, proliferation, and differentiation of specific cells. Also, it must be able to stabilize the reconstructed cartilage until the new one is formed and capable of reaching full mechanical stability and functionality.

The study performed by Bermueller et al. evaluated the utility of marine collagen, more precisely homotrimer collagen extracted by lyophilization of a jellyfish, as a scaffold for nasal cartilage reconstruction in a rat model and demonstrated that this type of scaffold is suitable for clinical cartilage tissue engineering (Bermueller et al., 2013). Marine collagen matrices revealed high porosity and interconnectivity, which lead to the idea that this scaffold permits the diffusion of nutrients, oxygen, and serum and interconnectivity allows the migration of chondrocytes through the collagen matrix. Also, marine collagen scaffolds provide an appropriate background for homogeneous production of cartilaginous extracellular matrix. From the comparison between type I and II collagen matrices, researchers (Bermueller et al., 2013) observed that type II collagen scaffolds provide a better environment for hyaline chondrocytes that collagen type I matrices. As a conclusion, they affirmed that marine collagen provide a safe medium, with excellent biocompatibility and reduced local inflammatory reactions, suitable for chondrocyte migration and proliferation and, thus, nasal cartilage engineering (Bermueller et al., 2013).

7.7.7 SKIN REGENERATION

The skin represents a natural barrier between the internal organism and external environment and represents the largest organ of our body.

Skin integrity may be affected by burn injuries, chronic wounds, surgical procedures, and limited blood circulation. Epidermal, superficial, and partial-thickness skin defects can regenerate by self-healing, but full-thickness skin wounds are more severe and need skin grafting. Currently, there are three types of grafts: autografts (limited availability), allografts (risk of rejection by the body), and xenografts. Their use is limited by the donor sites, risk of infection, slow healing, and association with the formation of scar (Uzunalan et al., 2013). To remedy these shortcomings the researchers turned to biomedical scaffolds. Based on the principle of tissue engineering, biomedical skin substitutes represent an important therapeutic option for the treatment of skin loss (Liu et al., 2013; Yildirimer et al., 2012; Seifert et al., 2012). The scaffold should serve as a template for tissue regeneration, for cellular adhesion and differentiation and as guide to development of new functional tissues (Liu et al., 2013). The main materials used in skin tissue engineering are: collagen, hyaluronan, amnion, polyactide, polyglycolide, and polybutylene terephthalate (Shokrgozar et al., 2012).

Collagen-based scaffolds are characterized by good biocompatibility, biodegradability, and low immunogenicity, but their applications are limited by their poor mechanical properties. It has been shown that artificial polymers such as poly(ε-caprolactone) (PCL), poly(lactic acid), poly(glycolic acid), and their copolymer poly(lactic-*co*-glycolic acid) (PLGA) are characterized by excellent mechanical properties (Wang et al., 2013).

Collagen–chitosan scaffolds are the most commonly used in skin regeneration. *In vivo* tests suggest that this scaffold was filled with fibroblasts when it was crosslinked with GA, highlighting the biostability and biocompatibility (Ma et al., 2003b). This scaffold may be able to support and accelerate fibroblast infiltration and proliferation (Ma et al., 2003a).

Collagen–chitosan porous membrane combined with fibrin glue prepared using a "two-step shaping" method showed an ideal environment for cell growth and differentiation. Therefore, fibroblast cells adhere to the scaffold surface and increased secretion of ECM suggested a good growth of fibroblasts, which means excellent biocompatibility of scaffold (Han et al., 2010).

To ensure the stability of the collagen scaffolds, it has been proposed to reinforce this scaffold with nanofibers. Reinforced hybrid scaffold collagen–chitosan with PLGA knitted mesh inhabited the wound contraction and there was a good repair of the full-thickness mouse skin defects (Wang et al., 2013).

PLGA knitted mesh does not affect the microstructure of the scaffold and it improved the mechanical strength to levels close to those of the dermis (Wang et al., 2013).

Development of PCL/gelatin/collagen type I composite nanofibrous scaffold by electrospinning technique provides a high viability and proliferation rate of L929 mouse fibroblast cells on the scaffold surface. Scaffold seeded with fibroblasts on the surface may be a promising candidate for skin tissue engineering (Gautam et al., 2014).

Collagen gels and hydrogels were considered promising candidates for skin replacement but unfortunately their dramatic contraction after being mixed with cells and their poor mechanical properties represent a major disadvantage toward their utilization as skin graft. By plastic compression of the gel a decrease in contraction of the collagen gel, and thus am improvement of its mechanical strength, have been shown. Seeded dermal fibroblasts and epidermal cells survived well in this gel and, moreover, epidermal cells gradually developed an epidermal layer, suggesting its use in skin engineering (Hu et al., 2010).

On the other hand, it was demonstrated that increasing collagen concentrations by 3 mg/ml determined a smaller contraction, is easy to handle, and favors cell growth and neovascularization. After *in vivo* implantation it was found that this gel can be rapidly integrated into the organism, and if it is seeded with fibroblasts these could grow and restore the function of the dermis (Helary et al., 2010).

7.7.8 TENDON REPAIR

Tendons are unidirectional fiber-reinforced composites and represent unique forms of connective tissue; their main function is to connect and transmit forces from muscle to bone. Tendons are stronger than muscle and their tensile strength is comparable with that of bone (Docheva et al., 2015; Shepherd and Screen 2013). Tendons must withstand the high tensile forces that locomotion depends on. The ECM of a tendon is composed of collagen type I which represents the fibrous phase reinforcing a matrix of hydrated proteoglycan matrix.

Because the tendon's function is to transmit muscle-generated forces into skeletal motion, it is subjected to high mechanical stress and repeated loading and can lead to injury. If damage occurs it forms scar tissue which affects the ECM composition and organization and decreases mechanical properties (Glass et al., 2014).

There have been various proposals for repairing partial injuries based on a number of surgical techniques and fixation strategies, but regeneration of severe injuries remains a big problem in the orthopedic field. At present, the main ways of repairing the tendon is the use of lengthening, grafting, two-stage reconstruction, or tenoplasty and tendon transfers (Cerovac and Miranda, 2013; Kew et al., 2012). However, autografting, allografting, and synthetic grafting are limited by donor site morbidity, immunoreaction, spread of infective diseases, and fatigue tearing. These problems can be resolved by developing a bioresorbable scaffold capable of withstanding load and able to progressively regenerate native tissue (Cerovac et al., 2013; Kew et al., 2012, 2011; Enea et al., 2012).

Scaffold development with microfibers is based on a variety of natural polymers, such as collagen and silk, and also synthetic polymers, such as poly-L-lactic acid (PLLA), polylactide-*co*-glycolide (PLGA), and polyurethane. Collagen scaffolds have been widely studied for tendon and ligament tissue reconstruction due to their high percentage of mimicry with the ECM. Collagen nanofibers can be fabricated with a variety of techniques, such as drawing, template synthesis, temperature-induced phase separation, molecular self-assembly, and electrospinning (Zhang et al., 2012).

The combination of collagen scaffolds with growth factors represents a significant opportunity to achieve tendon or ligament regeneration (Kew et al., 2011).

Coupling cylindrical collagen–glycosaminoglycan (CG) scaffold, characterized by aligned tracks of ellipsoidal pores, with growth factors (PDGF-BB and IGF-1) led to enhanced tendon motility, cell viability, and metabolic activity in dose-dependent manners which means it can be considered a 3D material system for tendon tissue engineering (Caliari et al., 2011). In other studies, it was demonstrated that soluble factors PDGF-BB, IGF-1, bFGF, SDF-1α, and GDF-5 have some influence on tenocyte migration, viability, collagen synthesis, and gene expression within anisotropic CG scaffolds: it has been shown that only pairing proliferative (IGF-1) and phenotypic (GDF-5) factors can support significantly increased tenocyte proliferation and soluble collagen synthesis, which means that combining these factors with CG scaffold may lead to tendon regeneration (Caliari and Harley, 2013).

It was also demonstrated that increasing the degree of GAG sulfating in CG scaffold contributes to decreasing the amount of growth factors, keeping the same effects (Hortensius and Harley, 2013).

Tendon regeneration has been achieved by seeding scaffolds with stem cells. It has been shown that directly loading platelet-derived growth factors containing PLGA and PEG nanoparticles into aligned collagen fiber biomaterials led to enhancing the proliferation and tenogenic differentiation of adipose-derived stem cells, which means that these materials are promising for tendon repair and regeneration (Cheng et al., 2014). In other studies, the efficacy of tendon-derived stem cells was measured in a poly(L-lactide-*co*-ε-caprolactone)/collagen (P(LLA-CL)/Col) scaffold under mechanical stimulation. *In vitro* tests showed good proliferation of TDSC, and *in vivo* experiments suggest that mechanical stimulation can promote neo-tendon tissues formation in mice (Xu et al., 2014).

By incorporation of human embryonic stem-cell-derived mesenchymal stem cells (hESC-MSCs) within a knitted silk–collagen sponge scaffold, after *in vitro* mechanical stimulation, hESC-MSCs can differentiate into the tenocyte-lineage. This biomaterial was implanted in a rat's Achilles tendon with induced injury and it has been shown that mechanical stimulation has led to the more regularly aligned cells and larger collagen fibers that may represent an alternative for future clinical applications (Chen et al., 2010).

7.8 CONCLUSIONS AND PERSPECTIVES

Collagen represents the most abundant protein in the body (up to 30%) and possesses a fibrillar structure. Collagen is involved in the biomechanical functions of the body, particularly at the level of connective tissues. Also, collagen represents the main element of the extracellular matrix and at this level it exhibits important functions involved in the storage and release of growth factors. In terms of collagen sources, it can be extracted from every living animal. The main sources of collagen are bovine skin and tendons, porcine skin, and rat tail, but it can also be isolated from marine species, especially from sponges, jellyfish, or other fish. Due to their properties, such as biodegradability, low immunogenicity, biocompatibility, and renewable sources, collagens drew the attention of researchers for widespread use in medicine, cosmetics, pharmaceuticals, and the food industry. Many collagen biomaterials, including gels, hydrogels, sponges, membranes, spheres, and powder sponges, have been developed.

Nowadays, researchers are focused on the development of collagen-based implants for skin graft, tendon regeneration and repair, cardiac and blood vessels, cartilage, and bone tissue. The present challenges consist of finding ways to improve the collagen scaffolds' mechanical properties by reinforcement with synthetic polymers or with collagen nanofibers. Also, the development of collagen/CNT bionanocomposites as a substrate to study the electrical stimulation of cells and as a transducer for future biosensors is envisaged.

REFERENCES

Adiguzel, E., Hou, G., Sabatini, P., Bendeck, M., 2013. Type VIII collagen signals via β1 integrin and RhoA to regulate MMP-2 expression and smooth muscle cell migration. Matrix Biol. 32 (6), 332–341.

Aikio, M., Elamaa, H., Vicente, D., Izzi, V., Kaur, I., Seppinen, L., et al., 2014. Specific collagen XVIII isoforms promote adipose tissue accrual via mechanisms determining adipocyte number and affect fat deposition. Proc. Natl. Acad. Sci. 111 (30), E3043–E3052.

Alberti, K., Hopkins, A., Tang-Schomer, M., Kaplan, D., Xu, Q., 2014. The behavior of neuronal cells on tendon-derived collagen sheets as potential substrates for nerve regeneration. Biomaterials 35 (11), 3551–3557.

Banyard, J., Bao, L., Zetter, B., 2003. Type XXIII collagen, a new transmembrane collagen identified in metastatic tumor cells. J. Biol. Chem. 278 (23), 20989–20994.

Bedal, K., Grässel, S., Oefner, P., Reinders, J., Reichert, T., Bauer, R., 2014. Collagen XVI induces expression of MMP9 via modulation of AP-1 transcription factors and facilitates invasion of oral squamous cell carcinoma. PLoS One 9 (1), e86777.

Beier, J., Klumpp, D., Rudisile, M., Dersch, R., Wendorff, J., Bleiziffer, O., et al., 2009. Collagen matrices from sponge to nano: new perspectives for tissue engineering of skeletal muscle. BMC Biotechnol. 9 (1), 34.

Berchtold, S., Grünwald, B., Krüger, A., Reithmeier, A., Hähl, T., Cheng, T., et al., 2015. Collagen type V promotes the malignant phenotype of pancreatic ductal adenocarcinoma. Cancer Lett. 356 (2), 721–732.

Bermueller, C., Schwarz, S., Elsaesser, A., Sewing, J., Baur, N., von Bomhard, A., et al., 2013. Marine collagen scaffolds for nasal cartilage repair: prevention of nasal septal perforations in a new orthotopic rat model using tissue engineering techniques. Tissue Eng. A 19 (19–20), 2201–2214.

Brinckmann, J., Müller, P., Notbohm, H., 2005. Collagen. Springer-Verlag, Berlin, Heidelberg, the Netherlands.

Caliari, S., Harley, B., 2011. The effect of anisotropic collagen–GAG scaffolds and growth factor supplementation on tendon cell recruitment, alignment, and metabolic activity. Biomaterials 32 (23), 5330–5340.

Caliari, S., Harley, B., 2013. Composite growth factor supplementation strategies to enhance tenocyte bioactivity in aligned collagen–gag scaffolds. Tissue Eng. A 19 (9–10), 1100–1112.

Camacho Vanegas, O., Bertini, E., Zhang, R., Petrini, S., Minosse, C., Sabatelli, P., et al., 2001. Ullrich scleroatonic muscular dystrophy is caused by recessive mutations in collagen type VI. Proc. Natl. Acad. Sci. 98 (13), 7516–7521.

Cerovac, S., Miranda, B.H., 2013. Tendon "turnover lengthening" technique. J. Plast. Reconstr. Aesthet. Surg. 66 (11), 1587–1590.

Chattopadhyay, S., Raines, R., 2014. Review collagen-based biomaterials for wound healing. Biopolymers 101 (8), 821–833.

Chen, J., Yin, Z., Shen, W., Chen, X., Heng, B., Zou, X., et al., 2010. Efficacy of hESC-MSCs in knitted silk-collagen scaffold for tendon tissue engineering and their roles. Biomaterials 31 (36), 9438–9451.

Chen, M., Marinkovich, M.P., Veis, A., Cai, X., Rao, C.N., O'Toole, E.A., et al., 1997. Interactions of the amino-terminal noncollagenous (NC1) domain of type VII collagen with extracellular matrix components. A potential role in epidermal-dermal adherence in human skin. J. Biol. Chem. 272 (23), 14516–14522.

Cheng, X., Tsao, C., Sylvia, V., Cornet, D., Nicolella, D., Bredbenner, T., et al., 2014. Platelet-derived growth-factor-releasing aligned collagen–nanoparticle fibers promote the proliferation and tenogenic differentiation of adipose-derived stem cells. Acta Biomater. 10 (3), 1360–1369.

Chiquet, M., Birk, D., Bönnemann, C., Koch, M., 2014. Collagen XII: protecting bone and muscle integrity by organizing collagen fibrils. Int. J. Biochem. Cell Biol. 53, 51–54.

Clementz, A., Harris, A., 2013. Collagen XV: exploring its structure and role within the tumor microenvironment. Mol. Cancer Res. 11 (12), 1481–1486.

Clementz, A., Mutolo, M., Harris, A., 2012. Abstract 5174: novel signaling interactions of type XV collagen: implications for tumor suppression. Cancer Res. 72 (8 Suppl.), p. 5174.

Clementz, A., Mutolo, M., Harris, A., 2013. Abstract 1626: The impact on tumor-stromal interactions of loss of collagen XV from the basement membrane zone. Cancer Res. 73 (8 Suppl.), p. 1626.

Critser, P., Kreger, S., Voytik-Harbin, S., Yoder, M., 2010. Collagen matrix physical properties modulate endothelial colony forming cell-derived vessels *in vivo*. Microvasc. Res. 80 (1), 23–30.

Davidenko, N., Gibb, T., Schuster, C., Best, S., Campbell, J., Watson, C., et al., 2012. Biomimetic collagen scaffolds with anisotropic pore architecture. Acta Biomater. 8 (2), 667–676.

Docheva, D., Müller, S., Majewski, M., Evans, C., 2015. Biologics for tendon repair. Adv. Drug Deliv. Rev. 84, 222–239.

Duncan, M., Yang, C., Tanjore, H., Boyle, P., Keskin, D., Sugimoto, H., et al., 2013. Type XVIII collagen is essential for survival during acute liver injury in mice. Dis. Model. Mech. 6 (4), 942–951.

Enea, D., Gwynne, J., Kew, S., Arumugam, M., Shepherd, J., Brooks, R., et al., 2012. Collagen fibre implant for tendon and ligament biological augmentation. *In vivo* study in an ovine model. Knee Surg. Sports Traumatol. Arthrosc. 21 (8), 1783–1793.

Ettinger, M., Gratz, I., Gruber, C., Hauser-Kronberger, C., Johnson, T., Mahnke, K., et al., 2012. Targeting of the hNC16A collagen domain to dendritic cells induces tolerance to human type XVII collagen. Exp. Dermatol. 21 (5), 395–398.

Exposito, J., Valcourt, U., Cluzel, C., Lethias, C., 2010. The fibrillar collagen family. IJMS 11 (2), 407–426.

Fang, M., Yuan, J., Peng, C., Pang, D., Li, Y., 2013. Quantum dots-based in situ molecular imaging of dynamic changes of collagen IV during cancer invasion. Biomaterials 34 (34), 8708–8717.

Frantz, C., Stewart, K., Weaver, V., 2010. The extracellular matrix at a glance. J. Cell Sci. 123 (24), 4195–4200.

Gautam, S., Chou, C., Dinda, A., Potdar, P., Mishra, N., 2014. Surface modification of nanofibrous polycaprolactone/gelatin composite scaffold by collagen type I grafting for skin tissue engineering. Mater. Sci. Eng. C 34, 402–409.

Gelse, K., Pöschl, E., Aigner, T., 2003. Collagens—structure, function, and biosynthesis. Adv. Drug Deliv. Rev. 55 (12), 1531–1546.

Glass, Z., Schiele, N., Kuo, C., 2014. Informing tendon tissue engineering with embryonic development. J. Biomech. 47 (9), 1964–1968.

Gordon, M., Hahn, R., 2009. Collagens. Cell Tissue Res. 339 (1), 247–257.

Han, C., Zhang, L., Sun, J., Shi, H., Zhou, J., Gao, C., 2010. Application of collagen-chitosan/fibrin glue asymmetric scaffolds in skin tissue engineering. J. Zhejiang Univ. Sci. B 11 (7), 524–530.

Has, C., Kiritsi, D., Mellerio, J., Franzke, C., Wedgeworth, E., Tantcheva-Poor, I., et al., 2013. The missense mutation p.R1303Q in type XVII collagen underlies junctional epidermolysis bullosa resembling kindler syndrome. J. Invest. Dermatol. 134 (3), 845–849.

Heikkinen, A., Tu, H., Pihlajaniemi, T., 2012. Collagen XIII: a type II transmembrane protein with relevance to musculoskeletal tissues, microvessels and inflammation. Int. J. Biochem. Cell Biol. 44 (5), 714–717.

Helary, C., Bataille, I., Abed, A., Illoul, C., Anglo, A., Louedec, L., et al., 2010. Concentrated collagen hydrogels as dermal substitutes. Biomaterials 31 (3), 481–490.

Hortensius, R., Harley, B., 2013. The use of bioinspired alterations in the glycosaminoglycan content of collagen–GAG scaffolds to regulate cell activity. Biomaterials 34 (31), 7645–7652.

Hsu, H., Murasawa, Y., Qi, P., Nishimura, Y., Wang, P., 2013. Type V collagen fibrils in mouse metanephroi. Biochem. Biophys. Res. Commun. 441 (3), 649–654.

Hu, K., Shi, H., Zhu, J., Deng, D., Zhou, G., Zhang, W., et al., 2010. Compressed collagen gel as the scaffold for skin engineering. Biomed. Microdevices 12 (4), 627–635.

Imagawa, K., de Andrés, M., Hashimoto, K., Itoi, E., Otero, M., Roach, H., et al., 2014. Association of reduced type ix collagen gene expression in human osteoarthritic chondrocytes with epigenetic silencing by DNA hypermethylation. Arthritis Rheumatol. 66 (11), 3040–3051.

Izu, Y., Sun, M., Zwolanek, D., Veit, G., Williams, V., Cha, B., et al., 2011. Type XII collagen regulates osteoblast polarity and communication during bone formation. J. Cell Biol. 193 (6), 1115–1130.

Izu, Y., Ezura, Y., Mizoguchi, F., Kawamata, A., Nakamoto, T., Nakashima, K., et al., 2012. Type VI collagen deficiency induces osteopenia with distortion of osteoblastic cell morphology. Tissue Cell 44 (1), 1–6.

Kannu, P., Bateman, J., Savarirayan, R., 2011. Clinical phenotypes associated with type II collagen mutations. J. Paediatr. Child Health 48 (2), E38–E43.

Kew, S., Gwynne, J., Enea, D., Abu-Rub, M., Pandit, A., Zeugolis, D., et al., 2011. Regeneration and repair of tendon and ligament tissue using collagen fibre biomaterials. Acta Biomater. 7 (9), 3237–3247.

Kew, S., Gwynne, J., Enea, D., Brookes, R., Rushton, N., Best, S., et al., 2012. Synthetic collagen fascicles for the regeneration of tendon tissue. Acta Biomater. 8 (10), 3723–3731.

Khaleduzzaman, M., Sumiyoshi, H., Ueki, Y., Inoguchi, K., Ninomiya, Y., Yoshioka, H., 1997. Structure of the Human Type XIX collagen (COL19A1) gene, which Suggests it has arisen from an ancestor gene of the facit family. Genomics 45 (2), 304–312.

Klein, G., Kibler, C., Schermutzki, F., Brown, J., Müller, C., Timpl, R., 1998. Cell binding properties of collagen type XIV for human hematopoietic cells. Matrix Biol. 16 (6), 307–317.

Koch, M., Foley, J., Hahn, R., Zhou, P., Burgeson, R., Gerecke, D., et al., 2001. 1(XX) collagen, a new member of the collagen subfamily, fibril-associated collagens with interrupted triple helices. J. Biol. Chem. 276 (25), 23120–23126.

Koch, M., Laub, F., Zhou, P., Hahn, R., Tanaka, S., Burgeson, R., et al., 2003. Collagen XXIV, a vertebrate fibrillar collagen with structural features of invertebrate collagens: selective expression in developing cornea and bone. J. Biol. Chem. 278 (44), 43236–43244.

Koudouna, E., Young, R.D., Ueno, M., Kinoshita, S., Quantock, A.J., Knupp, C., 2014. Three-dimensional architecture of collagen type VI in the human trabecular meshwork. Mol. Vis. 20, 638–648.

Krug, D., Klinger, M., Haller, R., Hargus, G., Büning, J., Rohwedel, J., et al., 2013. Minor cartilage collagens type IX and XI are expressed during embryonic stem cell-derived *in vitro* chondrogenesis. Ann. Anat. Anat. Anz. 195 (1), 88–97.

Kuo, S., Chiang, M., Lan, C., Niu, G., Chang, S., 2013. Evaluation of nanoarchitectured collagen type II molecules on cartilage engineering. J. Biomed. Mater. Res. A 101A (2), 368–377.

Kwansa, A., De Vita, R., Freeman, J., 2014. Mechanical recruitment of N- and C-crosslinks in collagen type I. Matrix Biol. 34, 161–169.

Lee, C., Singla, A., Lee, Y., 2001. Biomedical applications of collagen. Int. J. Pharm. 221 (1–2), 1–22.

Li, D., Zhao, H., Kranzler, H., Oslin, D., Anton, R., Farrer, L., et al., 2012. Association of COL25A1 with comorbid antisocial personality disorder and substance dependence. Biol. Psychiatr. 71 (8), 733–740.

Li, H., Huang, C., Chen, S., Chou, M., 2005. Assembly of homotrimeric type XXI minicollagen by coexpression of prolyl 4-hydroxylase in stably transfected *Drosophila melanogaster* S2 cells. Biochem. Biophys. Res. Commun. 336 (2), 375–385.

Liu, T., Houle, J., Xu, J., Chan, B., Chew, S., 2012. Nanofibrous collagen nerve conduits for spinal cord repair. Tissue Eng. A 18 (9–10), 1057–1066.

Liu, X., Ma, L., Gao, C., 2013. RNAi functionalized scaffold for scarless skin regeneration. Organogenesis 9 (2), 76–78.

Loeffler, I., Liebisch, M., Wolf, G., 2012. Collagen VIII influences epithelial phenotypic changes in experimental diabetic nephropathy. AJP Renal Physiol. 303 (5), F733–F745.

Lopes, J., Adiguzel, E., Gu, S., Liu, S., Hou, G., Heximer, S., et al., 2013. Type VIII collagen mediates vessel wall remodeling after arterial injury and fibrous cap formation in atherosclerosis. Am. J. Pathol. 182 (6), 2241–2253.

Ma, L., Gao, C., Mao, Z., Zhou, J., Shen, J., Hu, X., et al., 2003a. Collagen/chitosan porous scaffolds with improved biostability for skin tissue engineering. Biomaterials 24 (26), 4833–4841.

Ma, L., Gao, C., Mao, Z., Shen, J., Hu, X., Han, C., 2003b. Thermal dehydration treatment and glutaraldehyde cross-linking to increase the biostability of collagen–chitosan porous scaffolds used as dermal equivalent. J. Biomater. Sci. Polym. Ed. 14 (8), 861–874.

McAlinden, A., Traeger, G., Hansen, U., Weis, M., Ravindran, S., Wirthlin, L., et al., 2014. Molecular properties and fibril ultrastructure of types II and XI collagens in cartilage of mice expressing exclusively the α1(IIA) collagen isoform. Matrix Biol. 34, 105–113.

McCall, A., Cummings, C., Bhave, G., Vanacore, R., Page-McCaw, A., Hudson, B., 2014. Bromine is an essential trace element for assembly of collagen iv scaffolds in tissue development and architecture. Cell 157 (6), 1380–1392.

Miedel, E., Brisson, B., Hamilton, T., Gleason, H., Swain, G., Lopas, L., et al., 2015. Type III collagen modulates fracture callus bone formation and early remodeling. J. Orthop. Res. 33 (5), 675–684.

Misawa, K., Kanazawa, T., Imai, A., Endo, S., Mochizuki, D., Fukushima, H., et al., 2014. Prognostic value of type XXII and XXIV collagen mRNA expression in head and neck cancer patients. Mol. Clin. Oncol. 2 (2), 285–291.

Mocan, E., Tagadiuc, O., Nacu, V., 2011. Aspects of collagen isolation procedure. Clin. Res. Stud. 2, 3–5.

Mohamed, A., Xing, M.M., 2012. Nanomaterials and nanotechnology for skin tissue engineering. Int. J. Burns Trauma 2 (1), 29.

Momota, R., Naito, I., Ninomiya, Y., Ohtsuka, A., 2011. Drosophila type XV/XVIII collagen, Mp, is involved in wingless distribution. Matrix Biol. 30 (4), 258–266.

Momota, R., Narasaki, M., Komiyama, T., Naito, I., Ninomiya, Y., Ohtsuka, A., 2013. Drosophila type XV/XVIII collagen mutants manifest integrin mediated mitochondrial dysfunction, which is improved by cyclosporin A and losartan. Int. J. Biochem. Cell Biol. 45 (5), 1003–1011.

Mutolo, M., Morris, K., Leir, S., Caffrey, T., Lewandowska, M., Hollingsworth, M., et al., 2012. Tumor suppression by collagen XV is independent of the restin domain. Matrix Biol. 31 (5), 285–289.

Natsuga, K., Nishie, W., Shinkuma, S., Ujiie, H., Nishimura, M., Sawamura, D., et al., 2012. Antibodies to pathogenic epitopes on type XVII collagen cause skin fragility in a complement-dependent and -independent manner. J. Immunol. 188 (11), 5792–5799.

Oudart, J., Brassart-Pasco, S., Luczka, E., Dupont-Deshorgue, A., Bellon, G., Boudko, S., et al., 2013. Analytical methods for measuring collagen XIX in human cell cultures, tissue extracts, and biological fluids. Anal. Biochem. 437 (2), 111–117.

Pang, Y., Wang, X., Ucuzian, A., Brey, E., Burgess, W., Jones, K., et al., 2010. Local delivery of a collagen-binding FGF-1 chimera to smooth muscle cells in collagen scaffolds for vascular tissue engineering. Biomaterials 31 (5), 878–885.

Parenteau-Bareil, R., Gauvin, R., Berthod, F., 2010. Collagen-based biomaterials for tissue engineering applications. Materials 3 (3), 1863–1887.

Parmar, A., Nunes, A., Baum, J., Brodsky, B., 2012. A peptide study of the relationship between the collagen triple-helix, amyloid. Biopolymers 97 (10), 795–806.

Ramont, L., Brassart-Pasco, S., Thevenard, J., Deshorgue, A., Venteo, L., Laronze, J., et al., 2007. The NC1 domain of type XIX collagen inhibits *in vivo* melanoma growth. Mol. Cancer Ther. 6 (2), 506–514.

Ricard-Blum, S., Ruggiero, F., 2005. The collagen superfamily: from the extracellular matrix to the cell membrane. Pathol. Biol. 53 (7), 430–442.

Ruberti, J., Zieske, J., 2008. Prelude to corneal tissue engineering—gaining control collagen organization. Prog. Retin. Eye Res. 27 (5), 549–577.

Sand, J.M., Martinez, F.J., Hogaboam, C.M., Han, M., Karsdal, M., Leeming, D.J., et al., 2013. Type IV collagen degradation is elevated in serum of COPD, Ipf patients. Am. J. Respir. Crit. Care Med. 187, A3371.

Seifert, A., Monaghan, J., Voss, S., Maden, M., 2012. Skin regeneration in adult axolotls: a blueprint for scar-free healing in vertebrates. PLoS One 7 (4), e32875.

Selestina, G., Vanja, K., 2011. Collagen- vs. gelatine-based biomaterials and their biocompatibility: review and perspectives. In: Pignatello, R. (Ed.), Biomaterials Applications for Nanomedicine. InTech, ISBN: 978-953-307-661-4. Available from: http://dx.doi.org/10.5772/24118. Available from: http://www.intechopen.com/books/biomaterials-applications-for-nanomedicine/collagen-vs-gelatine-based-biomaterials-and-their-biocompatibility-review-and-perspectives.

Seppinen, L., Pihlajaniemi, T., 2011. The multiple functions of collagen XVIII in development and disease. Matrix Biol. 30 (2), 83–92.

Shanmugasundaram, S., Logan-Mauney, S., Burgos, K., Nurminskaya, M., 2011. Tissue transglutaminase regulates chondrogenesis in mesenchymal stem cells on collagen type XI matrices. Amino Acids 42 (2–3), 1045–1053.

Shepherd, J., Screen, H., 2013. Fatigue loading of tendon. Int. J. Exp. Pathol. 94 (4), 260–270.

Shokrgozar, M.A., Fattahi, M., Bonakdar, S., Kashani, I.R., Majidi, M., Haghighipour, N., et al., 2012. Healing potential of mesenchymal stem cells cultured on a collagen-based scaffold for skin regeneration. Iran Biomed. J. 16 (2), 68.

Shoulders, M., Raines, R., 2009. Collagen structure and stability. Ann. Rev. Biochem. 78 (1), 929–958.

Stamov, D., Stock, E., Franz, C., Jähnke, T., Haschke, H., 2015. Imaging collagen type I fibrillogenesis with high spatiotemporal resolution. Ultramicroscopy 149, 86–94.

Sweeney, E., Roberts, D., Lin, A., Guldberg, R., Jacenko, O., 2013. Defective endochondral ossification-derived matrix and bone cells alter the lymphopoietic niche in collagen X mouse models. Stem Cells Dev. 22 (19), 2581–2595.

Tao, G., Levay, A., Peacock, J., Huk, D., Both, S., Purcell, N., et al., 2012. Collagen XIV is important for growth and structural integrity of the myocardium. J. Mol. Cell. Cardiol. 53 (5), 626–638.

Tekari, A., Luginbuehl, R., Hofstetter, W., Egli, R., 2014. Chondrocytes expressing intracellular collagen type II enter the cell cycle and co-express collagen type I in monolayer culture. J. Orthop. Res. 32 (11), 1503–1511.

Uzunalan, G., Ozturk, M., Dincer, S., Tuzlakoglu, K., 2013. A newly designed collagen-based bilayered scaffold for skin tissue regeneration. J. Composites Biodegradable Polym. 1 (1), 8–15.

Väisänen, T., Väisänen, M., Autio-Harmainen, H., Pihlajaniemi, T., 2005. Type XIII collagen expression is induced during malignant transformation in various epithelial and mesenchymal tumours. J. Pathol. 207 (3), 324–335.

Van der Rest, M., Garrone, R., 1991. Collagen family of proteins. FASEB J. 5 (13), 2814–2823.

Veit, G., Kobbe, B., Keene, D., Paulsson, M., Koch, M., Wagener, R., 2006. Collagen XXVIII, a novel von willebrand factor a domain-containing protein with many imperfections in the collagenous domain. J. Biol. Chem. 281 (6), 3494–3504.

Wang, X., Li, Q., Hu, X., Ma, L., You, C., Zheng, Y., et al., 2012. Fabrication and characterization of poly(L-lactide-*co*-glycolide) knitted mesh-reinforced collagen–chitosan hybrid scaffolds for dermal tissue engineering. J. Mech. Behav. Biomed. Mater. 8, 204–215.

Wang, X., You, C., Hu, X., Zheng, Y., Li, Q., Feng, Z., et al., 2013. The roles of knitted mesh-reinforced collagen–chitosan hybrid scaffold in the one-step repair of full-thickness skin defects in rats. Acta Biomater. 9 (8), 7822–7832.

Xu, Y., Dong, S., Zhou, Q., Mo, X., Song, L., Hou, T., et al., 2014. The effect of mechanical stimulation on the maturation of TDSCs-poly(L-lactide-*co*-e-caprolactone)/collagen scaffold constructs for tendon tissue engineering. Biomaterials 35 (9), 2760–2772.

Yildirimer, L., Thanh, N., Seifalian, A., 2012. Skin regeneration scaffolds: a multimodal bottom-up approach. Trends Biotechnol. 30 (12), 638–648.

Zhang, X., Bogdanowicz, D., Erisken, C., Lee, N., Lu, H., 2012. Biomimetic scaffold design for functional and integrative tendon repair. J. Shoulder Elbow Surg. 21 (2), 266–277.

CHAPTER

8 Micro/nanofiber-based scaffolds for soft tissue engineering applications: potential and current challenges

Pablo R. Cortez Tornello, Florencia Montini Ballarin, Pablo C. Caracciolo and Gustavo A. Abraham

Research Institute for Materials Science and Technology, INTEMA (UNMdP-CONICET), Mar del Plata, Argentina

8.1 INTRODUCTION

The broad interest in nanobiomaterials is leading to the creation of a huge variety of nanostructured systems, including nanoparticles, nanocapsules, nanogels, nanofibers, nanotubes, and dendrimers, among other systems (Goldberg et al., 2007; Kumari et al., 2010; Duncan, 2011). Electrospun nanofibers have served as a highly versatile platform for a broad range of applications in widely different areas, such as catalysis, nanofluidics, sensors, medicine, energy, environmental engineering, biotechnology, defense and security, and healthcare (Ramakrishna et al., 2006; Fang et al., 2008).

The development of biomimetic highly porous scaffolds is essential for successful tissue engineering, since it provides a structural support for cell accommodation and nutrient transportation, and guides cell growth in three-dimensional space into a specific tissue (Xie et al., 2008). In this way, biomimetic electrospun matrices facilitate cell attachment and regulate cell differentiation in order to regenerate functional tissues (Liao et al., 2006; Ramalingam and Ramakrishna, 2006).

Recent efforts have addressed control over cell behavior and tissue formation. Thus, the native extracellular matrix (ECM) is mimicked by nanoscale topography (Sell et al., 2007; Venugopal et al., 2008), and cell orientation and tissue growth behavior can be influenced by fiber orientation (Ramalingam and Ramakrishna, 2007). The dispersion, solubilization, and release of bioactive agents from nanofibrous structures is also a focus of attention, since it can greatly improve the

Nanobiomaterials in Soft Tissue Engineering. DOI: http://dx.doi.org/10.1016/B978-0-323-42865-1.00008-8

performance of tissue-engineered matrices (Beachley and Wen, 2010; Cortez Tornello et al., 2012; Zhang et al., 2012).

This chapter summarizes the research advances made in electrospun scaffolds for soft tissue engineering applications, focusing on wound dressing, cartilage, muscle, cardiovascular, nerve, and skin tissues. Finally, a vision of the challenges and future directions is presented.

8.2 ELECTROSPINNING AS A VERSATILE PROCESSING TECHNIQUE FOR SCAFFOLDING

Processing techniques to produce polymeric nanofibers include phase separation, self-assembly, and electrospinning (Dahlin et al., 2011). Phase separation does not require specialized equipment, needs several steps to produce nanofibers of a limited number of polymers, and scaling-up is difficult to achieve. Self-assembly can also be used for nanofiber fabrication. Intermolecular forces assemble small molecules, peptides, proteins, and nucleic acids into fibers. Thus, this process is limited to a few polymers and only creates short fibers of several micrometers. Electrospinning emerges as a versatile processing technique with great potential in numerous innovative and attractive research areas (Sill and von Recum, 2008). Non-woven micro/nanofibrous structures, made from polymers, ceramics, and metals, are possible to obtain with a wide range of morphologies and functionalities by this technique. Polymeric fibers are in the diameter range of a few nanometers to several micrometers (usually between 3 nm and 5 μm). Electrospun meshes form three-dimensional scaffolds with high porosity, interconnected pore structure, and high surface-area-to-volume ratio. The advantages of electrospinning include a relatively inexpensive setup, and the possibility to create different fiber architectures for use in many technological fields. Although the major attraction of electrospinning is its simplicity, the process is governed by a number of parameters that greatly affect fiber formation and structure. In order to produce defect-free nanofibers with controlled fiber diameter distribution and orientation, these parameters must be precisely controlled. Studies of processing parameters and their influence on the electrospinning process can be found in the literature (Pham et al., 2006; Sill and von Recum, 2008), whereas a number of excellent reviews resume aspects of this technology (Greiner and Wendorff, 2007; Bhardwaj and Kundu, 2010). The great interest in electrospinning is evidenced by the large number of scientific articles and patents reported in recent years (Greiner and Wendorff, 2007; Kumbar et al., 2008a,b).

8.3 ELECTROSPUN STRUCTURES FOR TISSUE ENGINEERING APPLICATIONS

Electrospun scaffolds are ideal for biomedical applications, especially for controlled release of bioactive agents and tissue engineering. Tissue engineering has recently been defined as "the creation (or formation) of new tissue for the therapeutic reconstruction of the human body, by the deliberate and controlled stimulation of selected target cells through a systematic combination of molecular and mechanical signals" (Williams, 2009). Although there is no mention of a biomaterial, a scaffold biomaterial is usually employed to support cell growth and provide shape to the developing tissue-engineered construct, as well as to facilitate the delivery of molecular and mechanical signals. Current challenges lie in the election/design of natural, synthetic or composite biocompatible and bioresorbable materials to produce functional scaffolds that mimic the biological functions of natural ECM (Ma, 2008). The ECM is a three-dimensional network in which collagen embedded in proteoglycans organizes in nanometer-scale multifibrils. The structure and morphology of the ECM also greatly contribute to the properties and functions of each organ. Hence, the development of nanostructured porous scaffolds with interconnected pores, wide pore size distributions, large surface areas, and adequate mechanical properties also constitutes a dare. Together with the election of appropriate materials, these parameters affect not only cell survival, signaling, adhesion, proliferation, and reorganization, but also their gene expression and the preservation, or not, of their phenotype, or their differentiation in the case of stem cells. Moreover, the ideal scaffold should also present seeded cells uniformly distributed throughout the entire matrix. Therefore, another challenge to be overcome by tissue engineering is the maintenance of cell viability after implantation. A functional vasculature is fundamental for the delivery of nutrients and removal of metabolites from cells, otherwise cell survival is not possible. The support of this vasculature is mainly dependent on the surface and pore size characteristics of the scaffold, which control the adhesion and organization of the vascular endothelial cells into blood vessels (Araujo et al., 2008).

Up to date, a wide variety of materials and processing methods have been proposed for the design of scaffolds to regenerate human tissues. Bone, cartilage, skin, cardiovascular and neural tissues, spinal cord, blood vessels, tendons, ligaments, and organ tissue regeneration show promise for a large portion of individuals with special needs. In this context, electrospinning has recently emerged as a promising technology for the generation of micro/nanofiber-based scaffolds, which not only mimic the fibrous structure of natural ECM but also its spatial organization on the mesoscopic scale (control over fiber orientation and spatial placement). Matrices with appropriate fiber diameters, topology, texture, pore size, chemical compatibility, and mechanical properties adequate for specific target tissues can be obtained. Thus, electrospun matrices constitute an interesting approach/option for soft tissue engineering (Lannutti et al., 2007; Lim and Mao, 2009).

In certain cases, an efficient cellular infiltration can be hindered due to the low fiber diameter intrinsic to the electrospinning process (Nam et al., 2007). In recent years, the preparation of electrospun scaffolds with controllable macroscopic porosity by several techniques, such as electrospinning with salt leaching and salt leaching/gas foaming, auxiliary electrodes and chemical blowing agents, cryogenic electrospinning, and tailored collectors, have been reported.

Nanofibers can be functionalized through encapsulation, grafting, coating, or blending of biologically active compounds such as proteins, enzymes, and growth factors. Moreover, by manipulating the nanofiber alignment, stacking, or folding, a variety of nanofibrous arrays or architectures can be produce.

The production of individual fibers, random non-wovens, or highly aligned non-wovens can be achieved by an appropriate selection of electrode arrays or collector configurations (Xie et al., 2008). The orientation of nanofibers is interesting for many tissue engineering applications where a distinct growth direction for the cells is required (Wan and Xu, 2009; Díaz-Gómez et al., 2014). Furthermore, the basic setup can be modified to prepare core-shell micro- and nanofibers, increasing the possibilities and potential areas of application (Yarin, 2011).

8.4 SOFT TISSUE ENGINEERING APPLICATIONS

Electrospinning has been used for the fabrication of nanofibrous scaffolds from numerous bioresorbable synthetic and natural polymers, blends, and composites (Greiner and Wendorff, 2007). Figure 8.1 illustrates different applications of nanofibrous structures in this field.

Natural polymers such as collagen, elastin, gelatin, and fibrinogen make up much of the body's native ECM, and were explored as platforms for tissue-engineered constructs. Moreover, polysaccharides, such as chitosan (CS), starch, alginate, dextran, and many others were also electrospun for these purposes. The ability of the electrospinning technique to utilize natural polymers to create tissue engineering scaffolds has yielded promising results, both *in vitro* and *in vivo*, due in part to the enhanced bioactivity afforded by materials normally found within the human body (Sell et al., 2010).

Classical synthetic polyesters can provide the necessary strength for structural stability, and their electrospun scaffolds have been explored for the regeneration of musculoskeletal tissue, myocardial tissue grafts, and blood vessel substitutes. However, they are relatively stiff, non-elastic materials and not ideally suited for engineering of soft flexible tissues such as cardiovascular, urological, or gastrointestinal tissues.

The development of soft tissue engineering needs bioresorbable materials exhibiting elastomeric properties. Elastomeric polyurethane (PU) scaffolds can withstand the action of stress and load and undergo an elastic recovery with little or no hysteresis. In recent years, biocompatible and biodegradable segmented polyurethanes (SPU) have been investigated for applications in the tissue engineering field, such as cardiovascular tissue engineering, musculoskeletal applications (anterior cruciate ligament, knee joint meniscus, smooth muscle cell constructs for contractile muscle), and nerve regeneration. Their highly variable chemistry allows the preparation of biocompatible materials with controlled

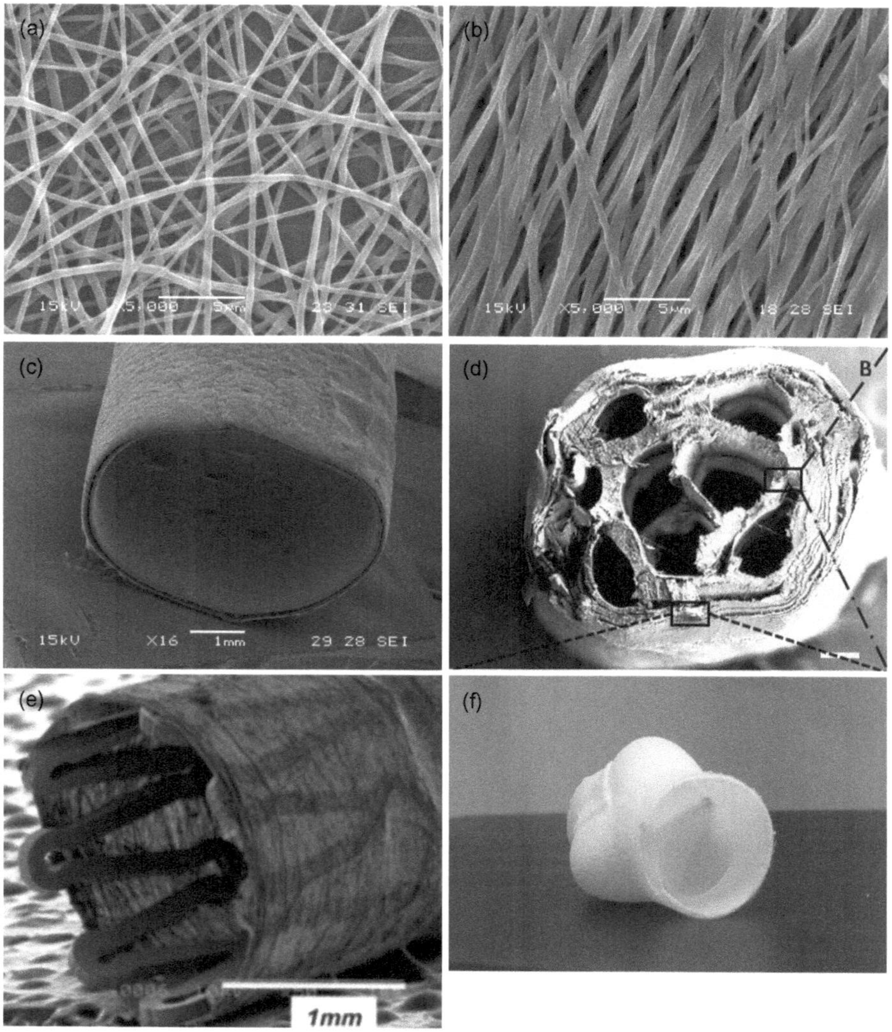

FIGURE 8.1

Examples of soft tissue-engineered electrospun scaffolds: (a) random non-woven scaffold for skin tissue engineering and hernia mesh (Montini Ballarin, unpublished work), (b) aligned nanofibrous scaffold for nerve tissue engineering (Montini Ballarin, unpublished work), (c) tubular structure for small-diameter vascular graft tissue engineering (Montini Ballarin, unpublished work), (d) tube with intraluminal guidance channel for nerve tissue engineering (Dinis et al., 2015), (e) device coating, i.e., stent coating (Kuraishi et al., 2009), (f) 3D scaffold for heart valve tissue engineering.

Courtesy of M. Simonet.

physicochemical, mechanical, and biodegradation properties that can be achieved through the appropriate selection of monomers and the manipulation of hard and soft content. Biodegradation into non toxic components can be promoted by the use of aliphatic diisocyanates. Bioresorbable polyester soft segments are commonly used to provide hydrolytically labile linkages, whereas chain extenders containing easily hydrolyzable bonds increase the SPU degradation rate (Moore, 2005).

Surprisingly, SPU and segmented poly(urethane urea) (SPUU) have been infrequently used for the fabrication of electrospun scaffolds. So far, only limited studies on nanofibrous PU have been reported as tissue-engineered scaffolds (Kidoaki et al., 2006). Our group reported the preparation, characterization, and properties of novel electrospun elastomeric PU scaffolds, employing bioresorbable SPU and SPUU, based on poly(ε-caprolactone) (PCL), hexamethylene diisocyanate, and new chain extenders with urea groups or ester groups derived from desaminotyrosine (Caracciolo et al., 2009a). These polymers were chosen because of the combination of mechanical properties and promising *in vitro* biological properties (Caracciolo et al., 2008, 2009b). The optimization of the processing parameters led to defect-free SPU and SPUU fibers with controlled diameters after an exhaustive exploration. The strong hydrogen-bonding interactions present in the polymeric structures make it difficult to achieve the electrospinning conditions. Moreover, the degradation rate depended on the chemical structure of the chain extenders, as well as the morphology and crystallinity of the materials (Caracciolo et al., 2011).

8.4.1 CARTILAGE TISSUE ENGINEERING

Articular cartilage protects the bones conforming articulating joints. This tissue has a complex structure and lacks autorepair ability. Therefore, when injuries or lesions are produced they may lead to painful osteoarthritic joint degeneration. Biomaterial-based tissue engineering emerges as a promising treatment, which helps guide and promote chondrocyte regeneration. Different approaches were studied to develop grafts or patches that enable healing of chondral and osteochondral lesions. These advances in the field made it possible to take on the challenge of regenerating extensive joint injuries in, for example, osteoarthritis (Johnstone et al., 2013).

The biomaterials used have evolved from the initial porous biodegradable polyesters (Freed et al., 1993, 1998), and non-biodegradable and inert hydrogels (alginate, agarose, and PEG networks) (Buschmann et al., 1992; Elisseeff et al., 2000; Chang et al., 2001) toward advanced scaffolds made of natural and synthetic materials (Lutolf et al., 2003; Burdick et al., 2005; Lutolf and Hubbell, 2005).

The nanofibrous morphology present in cartilage native ECM converts electrospun scaffolds as ideal matrices for cartilage tissue engineering. Even more so, many synthetic and natural polymers, hydrogel formulations, and composites, can be processed into three-dimensional matrices by this technology. It was observed that chondrocyte culture over nanoscale fibrous PCL scaffolds favored chondrocyte phenotype and ECM deposition (Li et al., 2003). The same group performed preliminary studies *in vivo* in a mini-pig model. PCL nanofibrous matrices seeded with chondrocytes and MSCs were implanted and well tolerated by animals. MSCs containing PCL matrices repair cartilage injuries *in vivo*, proving that they can promote cartilage regeneration (Li et al., 2009). Moreover, PCL-chitin nanofibrous mats showed a higher *in vitro* viability of human dermal fibroblasts (HDFs) for up to 7 days than pure PCL nanofibrous matrices, this increase being directly dependent on chitin concentration (Figure 8.2) (Kim et al., 2012). PCL nanofiber-coated PLA (poly(lactic acid)) microfiber scaffolds with 95% and 97% porosities were obtained, showing that scaffold porosity had great effects on cellular infiltration, with higher porosity resulting in increased infiltration (Thorvaldsson et al., 2008). This type of degradable polymer is a good material platform candidate for biomaterial-based cartilage repair, in particular when the fibers are of submicron diameters (Li et al., 2006a–c).

Schneider et al. studied the effect of fiber orientation on three different polymeric-based scaffolds (a synthetized copoly[ether ester urethane] [PDC], polyetherimide [PEI], and poly[p-dioxanone] [PPDO]). Better chondrocyte adhesion and proliferation were observed on the aligned matrices. Aligned scaffolds enhanced ECM production by seeded chondrocytes. Also, a more spindle-shaped

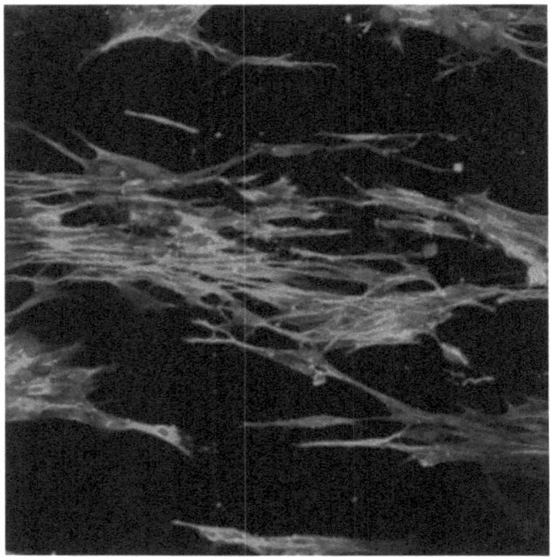

FIGURE 8.2

Human dermal fibroblast cultured on randomly oriented electrospun PCL fibers on day 7. Cell nuclei (blue) and actin filaments (green) were stained by DAPI and Alexa Fluor 488 phalloidin. Scale bar is 10 μm (Kim et al., 2012). (For interpretation of the references to color in this figure legend, the reader is referred to the web version of this book.)

morphology with better infiltration and rougher cell surfaces was produced over the aligned matrices. Among the three studied materials, the best results were obtained with PEI scaffolds independently of their topology (Schneider et al., 2012).

In another approach, scaffolds obtained from semisynthetic resorbable benzyl ester of hyaluronic acid (HYAFFt 11) allowed good viability and adhesivity of human nasoseptal chondrocytes with no need for any surface treatment. Furthermore, the cultured cells expressed cartilage-specific collagen type II, being able to retain a chondrocyte phenotype even after a long period of *in vitro* conditions (Aigner et al., 1998).

Garrigues et al. obtained PCL and PCL-CDM (cartilage-derived matrix) single scaffolds by continuous electrospinning or sequential collection of 60 layers from the surface of an aqueous grounded bath. Scaffold bioactivity was improved by multilayer assembly and slightly by CDM inclusion. The layered structure improved the homogeneous human adipose-derived stem cell (hASCs) seeding, whereas the inclusion of CDM enhanced chondrogenesis. However, the scaffold elastic modulus was inferior to human articular cartilage (Garrigues et al., 2014).

Despite the advances made in the last 20 years for cartilage tissue engineering, there is a long way to go in the area of clinical studies. Therefore, some important features of electrospun scaffolds have yet to be improved. Pore size enlargement to promote the formation of new vascularization, as well as cellular infiltration, is one of the principal challenges.

8.4.2 MUSCLE TISSUE ENGINEERING

Hierarchical tissues with highly organized morphology, like skeletal muscle, are hard to mimic with synthetic scaffolds (Riboldi et al., 2005; Huang et al., 2006). Muscle fibers work as a coordinated system, where each fiber is arranged parallel to the next one. It was observed that when myotubes grow on random surfaces this orientation and anisotropy is not achieved. This natural morphology is crucial for achieving a contracting skeletal muscle tissue. The use of oriented artificial scaffolds with guidance surfaces encourages a biomimetic myotube pattern (Dalby et al., 2003; Bashur et al., 2006).

Scaffolds produced by electrospinning are appealing for muscle tissue engineering since their topology and morphology can be tailor by controlling the process parameters (Courtney et al., 2006; Blackwood et al., 2008; Bian and Bursac, 2009; Wang et al., 2009). This technology has been employed to obtained matrices of biocompatible polyesters like PCL, PLA, poly(glycolic acid) (PGA), and their copolymer poly(D,L-lactide-*co*-glycolide) (PLGA) (Singh et al., 2004; Huang et al., 2005, 2006). Choi et al. developed a biodegradable, oriented, electrospun fibrous scaffold from a PCL/collagen blend. This study showed that highly oriented nanofibers significantly induced muscle cell alignment and myotube formation as compared to random nanofibers. The aligned nanofiber scaffolds seeded with skeletal muscle cells may provide implantable functional muscle for patients with large muscle defects (Choi et al., 2008).

McKeon-Fischer et al. developed coaxial electrospun scaffolds from PCL, multiwalled carbon nanotubes (MWCNT), and poly(acrylic acid)/poly(vinyl alcohol) (PAA/PVA) hydrogel, which respond to electrical stimulation mimicking the contraction and relaxation of natural skeletal muscle tissue. The scaffolds were tested for biocompatibility *in vivo* in Sprague–Dawley rat vastus lateralis muscle. Two different scaffolds were produced with good biocompatibility. Both of them presented an increase in myocytes with implantation time and evidence of neovascularization. However, one effect was more pronounced in each type of scaffold. Overall, the PCL–MWCNT–PAA/PVA scaffolds presented encouraging results for muscle tissue regeneration (McKeon-Fischer et al., 2014).

Riboldi et al. processed microfibrous matrices of biodegradable poly(ester urethane) block copolymer (DegraPol) by electrospinning. The scaffolds presented satisfactory mechanical properties for soft tissue engineering applications. Two cell lines (C2C12 and L6) and primary human satellite cells (HSCs) were culture *in vitro* and showed a promising response, with the presence of multinucleated myotubes on the membranes. These results confirmed the potentiality for skeletal muscle tissue engineering of electrospun DegraPol scaffolds (Riboldi et al., 2005).

The challenges on fibrous scaffolds for muscular tissue regeneration are not only related to fiber alignment. The use of composite materials to increase the conductivity of the scaffolds is also an important factor to consider in the achievement of muscular tissue regeneration.

8.4.3 CARDIOVASCULAR TISSUE ENGINEERING

Cardiovascular tissues possess an important mechanical function, generally anisotropic, non-linear, and viscoelastic. Therefore, not only is a biocompatible, non-cytotoxic scaffold required, but also one that can mimic the mechanical response under the pulsatile physiological regime. Cardiovascular tissue engineering is focused on the development of functional substitutes mainly for heart valves, arteries, and myocardium, these being tissues without a current long-term solution. Two strategies are being studied: the creation of tissue replacement *in vitro*, outside, or *in situ*, inside the human body. In some cases, like myocardial infarct, an off-the-shelf solution, with no *in vitro* long-term culture, is necessary. The electrospinning technique offers the ability to fine-tune mechanical properties, whilst also controlling the necessary biocompatibility, bioactivity, and structure of cardiovascular scaffolds.

8.4.3.1 Arteries

Most of the research in cardiovascular tissue engineering has been focused on vascular grafts. Among these, small-caliber arteries (<6 mm) are the target tissue, since no long-term synthetic replacement has been found to date. The success of a vascular graft lies, among other things, in manifesting values of internal diameter and mechanical properties, that comply, in particular, with native arteries. Electrospinning of polymeric solutions allows the production of biomimetic nanofibrous structures with ECM morphology concomitantly with the adjustment of the above-mentioned parameters. The electrospinning technique has been used, producing monolayer tubular scaffolds from pure polymers. Electrospun vascular grafts from PCL (Wu et al., 2010; Mugnai et al., 2013), biostable PU (Matsuda et al., 2005; Grasl et al., 2010; Miyazu et al., 2010; Bergmeister et al., 2013; Han et al., 2013a,b; He et al., 2013), and biodegradable PU (Han et al., 2011; Punnakitikashem et al., 2014) have presented encouraging properties. However, synthetic polymers do not display the same biological behavior as natural polymers. Among natural biopolymers, electrospun vascular grafts were made from silk fibroin (Marelli et al., 2010) and human recombinant tropoelastin (McKenna et al., 2012). These grafts presented poor mechanical properties and unstable dimensions caused by the premature dissolution and shrinkage in culture conditions (Sell et al., 2010).

In order to obtain scaffolds with improved mechanical and biological properties, small-diameter vascular grafts from polymer blends were produced. A few grafts were electrospun from synthetic polymer blends (Wang et al., 2012a, 2012b; Yu et al., 2012). However, most of the grafts produced from polymer blends were obtained from synthetic and natural polymers. Therefore, the graft takes advantage of the good mechanical properties and electrospinnability of synthetic polymers, and the biocompatibility, hydrophilicity, and cellular adhesion of natural polymers.

Atala and coworkers produced vascular grafts made from different synthetic polyesters, blended with collagen and elastin (Lee et al., 2008; Tillman et al., 2009). In a first approach, the mechanical properties and cytotoxicity of a PLGA, collagen, and elastin electrospun graft were analyzed (Stitzel et al., 2006). Good promising results were obtained, with compliance and burst pressure similar to those of natural arteries. Nevertheless, in a second *in vitro* study, the graft contraction and swelling were analyzed, as well as for blends with PCL, PLLA, poly (L-lactic acid-*co*-ε-caprolactone) (PLCL), and without a synthetic polymer (Lee et al., 2007). It was found that the grafts made from collagen and elastin alone collapsed on day 4 of culture *in vitro*. Furthermore, the blends with PLGA and PLCL suffered severe contractions after a month of culture, while PLLA and PCL blends kept their shape even after 2 months of culture. Later on, the group continued working with PCL and collagen blends, which resulted in high stability in a bioreactor culture and good mechanical properties (Lee et al., 2008). Even though the presented compliance value was in the natural arterial range, it was calculated at a more extended pressure range (0–120 mmHg). These scaffolds were studied *in vivo* and cultured in a bioreactor to study the growth of endothelium before implantation (Tillman et al., 2009). A good patency rate was observed after a month of implantation, and mechanical properties, although smaller, were kept within natural arterial values. However, the mechanical characterization was only studied in uniaxial traction, the dynamic pressure-diameter test being more representative of vascular graft mechanical response *in vivo*.

Vohra and coworkers developed a tubular scaffold from polyglecaprone (PGC, a copolymer of glycolide and ε-caprolactone), PCL, elastin, and gelatin (Zhang et al., 2011). The study was centered in a biological characterization, with emphasis on endothelium formation and platelet adhesion to the luminal surface. The formation of a confluent layer of endothelial cells was achieved in 24 h, which presents a possible time window for cardiovascular surgery. However, in this first study, the graft lacks a mechanical characterization which could show the viability against pulsatile physiological solicitations.

Yin et al. made vascular grafts from PLCL, collagen, and CS blends, and different polymer ratios were studied (Yin et al., 2013). The study was focused on the optimization of mechanical properties. Even though a good burst pressure value was obtained for almost all the studied ratios, the graft with the best general mechanical behavior presented a low compliance value.

Blended vascular grafts have improved both mechanical and biological responses, with respect to pure polymer grafts. However, the layered structure of natural arteries suggests that a better biomimeticity will be accomplished from bilayered or trilayered vascular grafts. Some groups have been centered in the development of multilayered grafts, in some cases hybrid grafts were produced, with an electrospun layer and another made from other technique to produce fibers or scaffolds (Soletti et al., 2010; Rapoport et al., 2012). Most researchers studied the electrospun multilayered grafts produced from different polymer blends, especially form natural and synthetic blends.

Matsuda et al. were the first to produce multilayered grafts using electrospinning. Their work was focused on the description of the sequential electrospinning technique, they produced a bilayered graft with a collagen inner layer and a biostable PU external layer (Kidoaki et al., 2005).

Vohra and coworkers have recently studied and optimized multilayered grafts (Thomas et al., 2007; Zhang et al., 2010a, 2010b). In a first approximation, bilayered and trilayered grafts with different porosity were produced from elastin, gelatin, and polyglyconate. Later, they continued their studies in monolayered blended grafts (Zhang et al., 2011), and produced bilayered grafts with an internal layer of PGC, PCL, elastin, and collagen, and an external layer of PGC, PCL, and elastin (Zhang et al., 2010a, 2010b). The mechanical properties were characterized in a more complete way, but no dynamic tests under physiological regimens were performed. The capacity of endothelium regeneration *in vitro* was also studied with good results.

Bowling and coworkers developed trilayered grafts made from PCL, elastin, and collagen or silk fibroin blends (McClure et al., 2010, 2012). The modification of the mechanical response by changing the internal and external layer blend ratios, as well as the effect of using collagen or silk fibroin, and two different crosslinking agents, was studied. The evaluation of mechanical properties after 4 weeks of hydrolytic degradation showed no significant variations. The study resulted in mechanical biomimetic vascular grafts, promising for small-diameter vessel replacement. However, cellular *in vitro* and *in vivo* studies must be done before clinical trials.

Our group also reported the development of bilayered PLLA and SPU blended tubular electrospun scaffolds for potential applications as small-diameter vascular grafts in cardiovascular tissue engineering (Montini Ballarin et al., 2014). Orientation of the nanofibers could be achieved by electric field modifications, using an auxiliary parallel plate collector. The blending of both polymers together resulted in lower crystallinity values with respect to their non-electrospun counterparts. The more amorphous polymers should favor a faster hydrolytic degradation. The hydrophilicity of PLLA was improved by blending it with SPU. Further studies regarding hydrolytic degradation, cytotoxicity tests, and complete mechanical characterization are being carried out.

Over the last few years, researchers have taken advantage of the nanofiber loading capacity, and multilayered vascular grafts with growth factors and anticoagulants agents were produced to improve cellular infiltration and avoid thrombus formation (Han et al., 2013a,b). The intentions are directed toward graft biofunctionalization in order to avoid an *in vitro* culture stage, and produce off-the-shelf vascular grafts ready for surgical implementation. There is still a need to obtain a successful small-diameter vascular graft, and electrospun constructs seem to be going in the right direction.

8.4.3.2 Myocardium

Cardiac tissue engineering recently gained great attention as it promises to revolutionize the treatment of patients with end-stage heart failure and provide new solutions to the serious problems of heart donor shortage. As vascular grafts, myocardial tissue is subjected to mechanical solicitations, and success lies in mimicking this behavior. Electrospun nanofibers have been considered great candidate scaffolds due to their tunable mechanical properties and orientation of fibers. Motivated by the development of cardiac-tissue-engineered scaffolds to restore cardiac function after myocardial infarction, Vacanti and coworkers studied the feasibility of PCL electrospun membranes as scaffolds for neonatal Lewis rat cardiomyocytes (Shin et al., 2004; Ishii et al., 2005). The cardiomyocytes attached well on the PCL meshes and expressed cardiac-specific proteins such as α-myosin heavy chain, connexin 43, and cardiac troponin I. The biological analysis converted this scaffold in a promising candidate; however, no mechanical characterization was made. Lelkes and coworkers (Li et al., 2006a–c) studied two different scaffolds. First, a blended scaffold of PLGA, and two natural proteins, gelatin and α-elastin, was made. The scaffold was cytocompatible, with good cellular attachment, proliferation, and infiltration. Nevertheless, its use as a myocardial substitute is questionable owing to its poor mechanical properties in the wet state. In a different approach, polyaniline (PANi) was blended with gelatin and electrospun to investigate its potential application as conductive scaffold for tissue engineering purposes. The authors demonstrated the biocompatibility of this scaffold by the attachment, migration, and proliferation of H9c2 rat cardiac myoblasts. These are preliminary results, and some specific tests on the effect of electrical stimulation on cell functionality and dynamic mechanical studies are necessary. Other groups also studied conducting intelligent substrates (Kai et al., 2011; Mooney et al., 2012). Mooney's approach was to prove a biomimetic electroactive cue through the manipulation of the mesenchymal stem cell differentiation pathway by harnessing the electrical properties of medium or scaffold containing carbon nanotubes. This study is promising for *in vitro* culture, nevertheless since the questionable biocompatibility of carbon nanotubes an *in vivo* application is not recommended.

In other works, the effect of substrate topography was analyzed (Zong et al., 2005; Orlova et al., 2011). These studies showed the influence of an aligned nanofibrous substrate on cellular orientation when cultured *in vitro*, with excellent cellular alignment in most of the cases. However, the setup to produce aligned nanofibers led in some cases (Orlova et al., 2011) to small surfaces, with 20 mm to a few cm widths, which are not big enough to cover an infarcted zone. Guan et al. developed an aligned scaffold that not only guided cell morphology but induced MSCs to differentiate into a cardiac lineage in the tissue constructs. The constructs were fabricated by concurrently electrospraying cells and electrospinning PU elastic fibers. The mechanical response of the grafts mimicked natural tissue anisotropy which also influenced cardiac cell differentiation. Therefore, this work shows how mechanical and topographical cues favor a cellular response.

These works in myocardial tissue engineering show the importance of topography and the election of biomaterials in mimicking the mechanical properties of natural myocardium. In spite of promising results, an electrical stimulation on cell functionality needs to be addressed in order to obtain a self-contractile regenerated tissue to compete with cell therapy and other developing treatments. The use of bioreactors with dynamic mechanical and electrical stimuli appears to be a promising form to achieve this.

8.4.3.3 Heart valves

Homografts, although limited in number, represent the most ideal choice among different options for heart valves due to their hemodynamic behavior. Besides, all currently available valve prostheses lack growth, remodeling, and adaptation capacity. Most of the tissue requirements (anisotropic mechanical behavior, highly porous structure, 3D structure, biocompatibility, among others) defined for heart valve tissue engineering can be accomplished by the electrospinning technique. Courtney et al. demonstrated that poly(ester urethane urea) (PEUU) electrospun scaffolds exhibited highly anisotropic mechanical properties closely resembling the native pulmonary heart valve leaflet (Courtney et al., 2006). Others have focused on the production of a biomimetic mechanical response with a two-dimensional structure (Masoumi et al., 2014). Only a few studies where a 3D construct was made have been carried out. By selecting and manufacturing the appropriate shape and dimensions of the mold used for electrospinning, native valve geometries were obtained (Del Gaudio et al., 2008; Simonet et al., 2011; Hinderer et al., 2014).

Van Lieshout et al. were the first to study the electrospinning process as a possible method to obtain valvular scaffolds with complex geometry with homogeneous thickness and sufficient mechanical integrity. They made a 3D nanofibrous structure from PCL and studied its mechanical and biological behavior. They proved that an electrospun valve with a complex geometry could be feasible, but also preferential deposition of the electrospun fibers due to an inhomogeneous electric field distribution on the mold valve was found. Therefore, the electrospinning method as presented is not suitable for valvular scaffold fabrication (Van Lieshout et al., 2006). Del Gaudio et al. also produced a PCL electrospun heart valve. Their results showed the technical feasibility to produce a functional heart valve with a uniform thickness and a correct functional response in a pulse duplicator. The valve did not undergo structural damage, nevertheless these studies were preliminary and the authors suggested the utilization of blends or copolymers to better resemble a biomimetic response (Del Gaudio et al., 2008).

Recently, Hinderer et al. developed a poly(ethylene glycol dimethacrylate)/PLA scaffold directly electrospun on a 3D collector with biomimetic structure and mechanical properties to native heart valve tissue (Hinderer et al., 2014). Good cell adherence, spreading and, viability for valvular interstitial cells (VICs) and valvular endothelial cells (VECs) were observed. To improve the scaffold bioactivity and obtain an off-the-shelf heart valve, different ECM proteins, responsible for human heart valve development, were adhered to the electrospun construct. As a consequence, a potentially bioactive heart valve scaffold was produced. However, in order to better mimic native tissue some features needs to be further improved.

A few studies were made with a 3D heart valve morphology and many of them were focused on the valve shape but not its material biomimeticity, or biological and mechanical properties. Future challenges in electrospun heart valve tissue engineering are to improve the mechanical and biological response, to obtain a truly off-the-shelf heart valve.

8.4.4 NERVE TISSUE ENGINEERING

Injuries occurring in the peripheral and central nervous systems are healed by slow or limited endogenous repair. In the cases of 20 mm or longer gaps, where neither repair nor suture of the nerve ends is possible, autografts or allografts are usually employed. However, due to the limited availability of these grafts, tissue engineering has become a possible solution. Significant effort has been placed on the development of efficient neural guidance conduits with the purpose of binding together damaged peripheral or central neurons gaps. The biomimetic ECM-like fibrous structure of nanofibers, as well as their ability to direct axon sprouting, converts electrospinning as an ideal technology for this application.

Nanofibers can be also loaded with neurotrophic factors to be released at the injury site.

Some studies were made with different random scaffolds obtained from synthetic and natural polymer blends, in which different neural cells improved their adherence by the incorporation of the natural component (Prabhakaran et al., 2008). Other studies were focused on the effect of topography in cellular morphology, adhesion, and axonal extension (Xie et al., 2009; He et al., 2010). These *in vitro* studies helped to understand the neural cellular behavior when in contact with nanofibers, and constituted a first stage toward the development of guidance conduits.

The first conduits with electrospun nanofiber guidance consisted of a film-based tubular construct with an internal electrospun coating or thin film (Kim et al., 2008; Clements et al., 2009). Panseri et al. developed a completely electrospun bilayered conduit made from PCL and a PCL/PLGA blend (Panseri et al., 2008). The conduit consisted of random oriented nanofibers, with micro- and nanometric sizes. The multiscaled electrospun nerve conduits were promising bioabsorbable scaffolds for stimulating and guiding peripheral nerve function regeneration. However, some modifications should be made to favor a functional and effective nervous regeneration, like polymer functionalization, incorporation of growth factors, and/or other biological cues. Koh et al. made a bilayered PLLA nanofibrous conduit with longitudinally aligned nanofibers in the lumen and randomly oriented ones on the outer surface. An intraluminal guidance channel made out of aligned PLGA nanofibrous yarns was incorporated inside the conduit. In addition, biomolecules such as laminin and nerve growth factor were incorporated (Koh et al., 2010). The nerve construct produced presented better sensory and motor functional recovery results than autografts, although axonal regeneration was observed to be greater in the autologous nerve grafts. Chew and coworkers developed two different electrospun nerve conduits (Chew et al., 2007; Liu et al., 2012; Jiang et al., 2014). Collagen and PCL spiral conduits were made with an emphasis on studying fiber orientation and size effect on neural recovery. These results could provide useful insights for future nerve guide designs. However, many improvements, such as tailoring the biocompatibility with blended materials, controlling the delivery of biomolecules, or improving the internal nerve guidance with channels, need to be done prior to a clinical trial.

Recently, Cirillo et al. produced random oriented electrospun tubular conduits from PCL and its blend with collagen (Cirillo et al., 2014). They studied the *in vitro* and *in vivo* conduit behavior, obtaining an opposite response. Even though collagen improved *in vitro* cellular adhesion and growth in respect to the PCL conduit, the latter displayed a better degradation behavior. These are preliminary results and several modifications were suggested in order to improve nerve regeneration. For example, the fabrication of a bilayered conduit by overlapping both studied conduits. Xie et al. also produced a PCL-based conduit, consisting of an axial aligned nanofibrous inner layer and a random outer layer (Xie et al., 2014). To improve neurite orientation over the scaffolds, Schwann cells were cultured in the conduit lumen. This resulted in good aligned neurites that copied the nanofibrous structure. Yu et al. made PCL/collagen blended conduits with MWCNT to enhance hydrophilicity, mechanical properties, and degradability (Yu et al., 2014). These electrospun conduits promoted nerve regeneration through a sciatic nerve defect in rats and prevented muscle atrophy. Even though promising results were obtained, the use of MWCNT in biodegradable matrices for *in vivo* applications is questionable. Dinis et al. studied the mechanical behavior and growth factor release of a silk/PEO electrospun conduit, with aligned and longitudinally oriented microchannels mimicking fascicles for peripheral nerve regeneration (Dinis et al., 2015). The construct incorporated a nerve growth factor and a ciliary neurotrophic factor. This conduit presented promising results with a sustained release and mechanical properties in the range of rat sciatic nerves. However, *in vivo* studies should be performed for better characterization.

A variety of nerve tissue-engineered conduits from natural and synthetic polymers, with different topographies, growth factors, and internal guidance characteristics were obtained. Although some of them presented very promising results, most of the studies were centered on the evaluation of their biological response. In order to fully characterize them, further studies should be carried out. Mechanical and degradation studies are needed before proceeding to a clinical stage.

8.4.5 SKIN TISSUE ENGINEERING

Skin tissue engineering is a mature field since it has been in clinical use for 25 years, having greatly developed in that time (Mac Neil, 2008; Geetha Priya et al., 2008). The current gold standard for skin regeneration is the use of autologous grafts for the permanent coverage of both acute and chronic wounds (Kumbar et al., 2008). Alternative treatments consist of the use of allogenic cadaver skin grafts or xenografts as temporary coverings to protect wounds. These therapies have several limitations regarding immunological rejection, the need for immunosuppressive treatments, and possible transmission of diseases, among others. Currently, there are many temporary or permanent commercially available skin equivalents, each one with its own limitations: high-cost grafts, limited shelf life, time-consuming manufacturing process, and reduced effectiveness (Shevchenko et al., 2010). Thus, many challenges still remain to be tackled.

The use of existing biomaterials presents several problems, which include: safety issues related to animal-derived materials, improving the take of cultured keratinocytes on wound beds, improving the rate of neovascularization of tissue-engineered constructs, and developing scaffolds that resist contraction and fibrosis.

Nowadays, there is much interest in producing scaffolds by electrospinning technology. Nanofiber scaffolds are good candidates for skin regeneration as they present tunable properties such as wettability, biodegradability, porosity, cell adhesive and antimicrobial properties, mechanical properties, and surgical handleability.

Novel modification techniques have been proposed to control and enlarge pore size in order to facilitate cell infiltration while retaining its ECM character (Zhu et al., 2008). In addition, other attempts explored the enhancement of cell penetration, including dynamic cell loading and dynamic culture conditions. The biological properties of electrospun scaffolds can be improved by changing the surface properties such as wettability, protein coatings, and peptide sequence. Moreover, fibers can be used as carriers for antibiotic, antimicrobial, gene, growth factor, and cell delivery systems. The development of nanofibrous scaffolds loaded with multiple growth factors (TGF-β, EGF, PDGF) may be the future direction of research on electrospun skin substitutes. The search for new functional scaffolds able to promote rapid wound healing, encourage better cell interactions, and angiogenesis without wound contraction and fibrosis (either in the short or long term) offers new insights into skin tissue engineering (Subramanian et al., 2011).

8.4.6 BLADDER TISSUE ENGINEERING

Disorders of the urinary bladder have no allograft solution. At the end-stage of bladder disease, the only existing treatment consists of the reconstruction of the bladder with vascularized segments of bowel. However, its highly developed ability to absorb water and salts, as opposite to the urothelium, results in the reabsorption of excreted products through the intestinal mucosa, which can cause salt and fluid imbalances. In addition, the intestinal mucosa can give rise to mucus and stone formations in the urinary bladder. An increased risk of developing malignancies has also been reported. Tissue engineering presents a possible solution to bladder disorders lacking treatments. The bladder wall is a trilayered tissue with high compliance, barrier function, and active bladder emptying. Extensive studies of electrospun matrices (e.g., the obtention of compliant tissues like cardiovascular) suggest that they could make a significant contribution to urinary tract reconstruction.

In the first approximation to electrospun bladder tissue engineering, studies were centered on the obtention of a scaffold and the evaluation of some basic aspects to analyze its potential as a urological tissue replacement. McManus et al. were the first to utilize an electrospun scaffold for urologic tissue engineering (McManus et al., 2007). They produced a fibrinogen-based scaffold that allowed human bladder smooth muscle cells to rapidly migrate into and remodel the scaffolds with deposition of native collagen fibrils. This response was enhanced by aprotinin-containing scaffolds. Stankus and coworkers produced an electrospun scaffold from urinary bladder ECM and PEUU. Although the obtained results were promising for its use in soft tissue engineering, more studies need to be carried out to determine its success as a bladder scaffold (Stankus et al., 2008). Baker and Southgate studied the effect of three-dimensional (3D) architecture on the differentiated phenotype of human smooth muscle cells derived from the stroma of the lower urinary tract (Baker and Southgate, 2008). Optimal differentiation conditions were achieved by coating electrospun polystyrene scaffolds with laminin, blocking serum protein adsorption, seeding cells in the absence of serum, and adding TGFb1 to the growth medium. This was mainly a proof-of-principle study, due to the use of a biostable polymer like polystyrene, which is not ideal for tissue engineering applications.

More recently, Kundu et al. developed a novel scaffold composed of PCL and PLLA generated by electrospinning directly onto spin-coated thin films (Kundu et al., 2011). Their results demonstrate that the addition of thin films onto electrospun scaffolds enhances urothelial cell proliferation, surface coverage, cell–cell interactions, and *in vitro* multilayering. Although mechanical characterization was not performed, the biological analysis suggests this hybrid scaffold could be a promising candidate for bladder tissue engineering. Horst et al. produced another hybrid scaffold from electrospun PLGA and bladder acellular matrix (Horst et al., 2013). This scaffold provided a natural barrier function and supported urothelial and smooth muscle regeneration. Moreover, it sustained normal bladder capacity after 8 weeks of implantation *in vivo*, which makes it a promising candidate for bladder tissue engineering. PLGA was also chosen by Ajalloueian et al. to make a hybrid construct with an electrospun layer, compressed collagen, and minced urothelium (Ajalloueian et al., 2014). A modified electrospinning approach favored the integration of PLGA nanofibers and a compressed collagen layer. The scaffold presented a mechanical response similar to human bladder tissue. The *in vitro* results showed a high rate of proliferation, reaching multilayer epithelium in 4 weeks. This scaffold is a good candidate for bladder tissue engineering, although *in vivo* studies are needed.

Even though some promising works with hybrid electrospun scaffolds for urological applications were made, to date a complete electrospinning scaffold has not been developed. This may be due to its highly porous structure which could complicate the barrier properties needed for bladder replacement. The combination of electrospinning technique with a barrier layer looks promising for finding a successful scaffold to treat bladder affections.

8.4.7 WOUND DRESSINGS

Wound dressings have undergone major changes over time. Initially, the wounds were merely covered with dressings from natural materials, but nowadays novel materials have been developed to exhibit many exceptional functions. Modern dressings and bandages made from electrospun natural and synthetic polymers could significantly enhance the healing of wounds compared to traditional fibrous bandages (such as gauze). Furthermore, therapeutic agents (antimicrobials, antibacterials, antifungals, and anti-inflammatories) could be incorporated into the fibrous bandages, to enhance wounds healing by means of their controlled release (Zahedi et al., 2010).

Electrospun fibrous matrices present excellent characteristics for use as wound dressing materials. Their fibrous structure and high porosity result are suitable for drainage of wound exudates and allow an appropriate permeation of atmospheric oxygen. Furthermore, non-woven fibrous structures could prevent possible infections generated by the attack of microbes, which could delay wound healing (Bhattarai et al., 2004). Electrospun fibrous bandages have significant properties as compared to conventional dressings. These advantages are mostly due to their high porosity, high surface-area-to-volume ratio, and small pore size. Some of these properties are: hemostasis, absorbability, semipermeability, conformability (due to the flexibility and resiliency of the dressings), functional ability (ease of incorporating therapeutic agents), and scar-free healing (Zhang et al., 2005).

Today, only a few polymers, such as PCL, PLLA, PVA, CS, and gelatin, have been studied by the electrospinning process for wound dressing applications (Venugopal and Ramakrishna, 2005). Duan et al. carried out cell proliferation tests on PCL nanofibers containing Ag-loaded zirconium phosphate nanoparticles. The results showed that the loaded PCL nanofibers have a higher rate of primary HDF proliferation than the pure PCL samples (Duan et al., 2007). Zhou et al. studied the adhesion and growth extent of mouse fibroblasts (L929) on the blend of crosslinked nanofibers of carboxyethyl chitosan (CECS) and PVA (CECS/PVA). It was observed that cell adhesion to the surface of nanofibers, reproduction, and growth along the nanofibers were very high, leading to epithelialization (Zhou et al., 2008). Chen et al. prepared nanofibrous membranes from collagen/CS and tested them as dressing materials. The rate of wound healing, that is, the rate of wound surface reduction in respect to time, was much higher for these membranes than gauze and commercial collagen sponge (Chen et al., 2008).

Khil et al. employed a histology test for the investigation of different phases of wound healing. Two different wound dressing materials were used: electrospun PU nanofibers and commercial Tegaderm™. Wounds performed on male adult guinea pigs were completely covered with the wound-dressing materials. Histology tests showed that the wounds presented granulation tissues along with cells rich from the inflammation phase and neovascularization. Some cells rich in collagen were also seen. After 15 days the epithelialization process was observed in both materials, but still some traces of inflammation phase cells for the Tegaderm™ group could be observed. For PU membranes, the rate of epithelialization process was higher and dermis was formed (Khil et al., 2003).

Kim et al. prepared blended nanofiber scaffolds using synthetic and natural polymers, PU, and gelatin, respectively. The obtained scaffolds had elasticity increased with higher PU content. Moreover, water uptake and cell proliferation increased with higher gelatin contents. Therefore, these gelatin/PU blended nanofiber scaffolds could have potential applications in wound dressings (Kim et al., 2009). An ultrafine gelatin fiber mat with antibacterial activity against some common bacteria found on burn wounds was prepared from a gelatin solution containing silver nanoparticles. The mat was further crosslinked with moist glutaraldehyde vapor to improve its stability in an aqueous medium. The antibacterial activity was highest against *Pseudomonas aeroginosa*, followed by *Staphylococcus aureus*, *Escherichia coli*, and methicillin-resistant *S. aureus* (Rujitanaroj et al., 2008).

The use of electrospinning technology to produce matrices for wound-dressing applications presents great proven advantages. The challenges in this area consist of the use of new natural–synthetic polymer blends, the incorporation of new therapeutic agents and the modulation of the agent delivery rate. For this purpose, some strategies related to multilayer electrospun matrices and coaxial fiber matrices are being investigated.

8.5 CONCLUDING REMARKS AND FUTURE DIRECTIONS

The design of scaffold microarchitecture to provide adequate spatial and temporal microenvironments is critical for inducing the desired cellular response, which is crucial for tissue engineering and organ regeneration. Electrospun nanofiber scaffolds offer many attractive advantages for the design of highly porous biomaterials widely used in tissue engineering and drug delivery systems. In the last few years, electrospinning has been widely explored as a powerful technique, and a huge number of publications have focused on material processing and properties, and new applications have appeared. Despite this, research on many aspects of electrospinning for biomedical applications, in particular in tissue engineering constructs, is needed, and many issues must be solved. The efforts are now addressed to control nanofiber scaffolds by modulating nanofiber morphology, two-dimensional structure of packing and alignment of nanofibers, as well as three-dimensional patterns and shapes. Thus, a controlled multilevel hierarchical structure of electrospun scaffolds still remains a challenge. Nanofibrous structures with large pore sizes and high porosities for cell infiltration and migration also need to be considered, including core-sheath nanofibers for encapsulating drug or growth factors for drug delivery systems or tissue engineering fields. Better understanding of the influence of nanofibers in cell behavior and tissue regeneration is still a challenge. In this sense, physiological and mechanotransductory signals need to be studied to optimize scaffold fabrication. The mechanical properties, integrity, and stability of scaffolds with high porosities are compromised. Thus, some recent advances to solve the cell infiltration problem were proposed. Direct electrospinning or coaxial electrospinning techniques allowed the incorporation of living cells simultaneously with nanofibers. Some results indicated that the viability of cells was not affected by the process, as a high fraction of cells remained viable after electrospinning. Many efforts also address the development of novel electrospun biomaterials, drug-loaded systems, electrospun nanocomposites, surface modifications, post-spinning processes, enhanced characterization tools and techniques, 3D functional structures, as well as novel applications of nanofibrous non-woven mats in the field of tissue engineering and regenerative medicine.

ACKNOWLEDGMENTS

This work is supported by the Argentinean National Agency of Scientific and Technological Promotion (Grant PICT 224), National Research Council CONICET (Grant PIP 089), and National University of Mar del Plata (Grant 15/G359). P.R.C.T. and F.M.B. thank CONICET for the fellowship awarded.

REFERENCES

Aigner, J., Tegeler, J., Hutzler, P., Campoccia, D., Pavesio, A., Hammer, C., et al., 1998. Cartilage tissue engineering with novel nonwoven structured biomaterial based on hyaluronic acid benzyl ester. J. Biomed. Mater. Res. 42, 172–181.

Ajalloueian, F., Zeiai, S., Fossum, M., Hilborn, J.G., 2014. Constructs of electrospun PLGA, compressed collagen and minced urothelium for minimally manipulated autologous bladder tissue expansion. Biomaterials 35, 5741–5748.

Araujo, J.V., Martins, A., Leonor, I.B., Pinho, E.D., Reis, R.L., Neves, N.M., 2008. Surface controlled biomimetic coating of polycaprolactone nanofiber meshes to be used as bone extracellular matrix analogues. J. Biomater. Sci. Polym. Ed. 19, 1261–1278.

Baker, S.C., Southgate, J., 2008. Towards control of smooth muscle cell differentiation in synthetic 3D scaffolds. Biomaterials 29, 3357–3366.

Bashur, C.A., Dahlgren, L.A., Goldstein, A.S., 2006. Effect of fiber diameter and orientation on fibroblast morphology and proliferation on electrospun poly(D,L-lactic-*co*-glycolic acid) meshes. Biomaterials 27, 5681–5688.

Beachley, V., Wen, X., 2010. Polymer nanofibrous structures: fabrication, biofunctionalization, and cell interactions. Progr. Polym. Sci. 35, 868–892.

Bergmeister, H., Schreiber, C., Grasl, C., Walter, I., Plasenzotti, R., Stoiber, M., et al., 2013. Healing characteristics of electrospun polyurethane grafts with various porosities. Acta Biomater. 9, 6032–6040.

Bhardwaj, N., Kundu, S.C., 2010. Electrospinning: a fascinating fiber fabrication technique. Biotechnol. Adv. 28, 325–347.

Bhattarai, S.R., Bhattarai, N., Yi, H.K., Hwang, P.H., Cha, D.I., Kim, H.Y., 2004. Novel biodegradable electrospun membrane: scaffold for tissue engineering. Biomaterials 25, 2595–2602.

Bian, W., Bursac, N., 2009. Engineered skeletal muscle tissue networks with controllable architecture. Biomaterials 30, 1401–1412.

Blackwood, K.A., McKean, R., Canton, I., Freeman, C.O., Franklin, K.L., Cole, D., et al., 2008. Development of biodegradable electrospun scaffolds for dermal replacement. Biomaterials 29, 3091–3104.

Burdick, J.A., Chung, C., Jia, X., Randolph, M.A., Langer, R., 2005. Controlled degradation and mechanical behavior of photopolymerized hyaluronic acid networks. Biomacromolecules 6, 386–391.

Buschmann, M.D., Gluzband, Y.A., Grodzinsky, A.J., Kimura, J.H., Hunziker, E.B., 1992. Chondrocytes in agarose culture synthesize a mechanically functional extracellular matrix. J. Orthop. Res. 10, 745–758.

Caracciolo, P.C., de Queiroz, A.A.A., Higa, O.Z., Buffa, F., Abraham, G.A., 2008. Segmented poly(esterurethane urea)s from novel urea–diol chain extenders: synthesis, characterization and *in vitro* biological properties. Acta Biomater. 4, 976–988.

Caracciolo, P.C., Buffa, F., Abraham, G.A., 2009a. Effect of the hard segment chemistry and structure on the thermal and mechanical properties of novel biomedical segmented poly(esterurethanes). J. Mater. Sci. Mater. Med. 20, 145–155.

Caracciolo, P.C., Thomas, V., Vohra, Y.K., Buffa, F., Abraham, G.A., 2009b. Electrospinning of novel biodegradable poly(ester urethane)s and poly(ester urethane urea)s for soft tissue-engineering applications. J. Mater. Sci. Mater. Med. 20, 2129–2137.

Caracciolo, P.C., Buffa, F., Thomas, V., Vohra, Y.K., Abraham, G.A., 2011. Biodegradable polyurethanes: comparative study of electrospun scaffolds and films. J. Appl. Polym. Sci. 121, 3292–3299.

Chang, S.C.N., Rowley, J.A., Tobias, G., Genes, N.G., Roy, A.K., Mooney, D.J., et al., 2001. Injection molding of chondrocyte/alginate constructs in the shape of facial implants. J. Biomed. Mater. Res. 55, 503–511.

Chen, J.P., Chang, G.Y., Chen, J.K., 2008. Electrospun collagen/chitosan nanofibrous membrane as wound dressing. Colloid Surf. A 313–314, 183–188.

Chew, S.Y., Mi, R., Hoke, A., Leong, K.W., 2007. Aligned protein-polymer composite fibers enhance nerve regeneration: a potential tissue-engineering platform. Adv. Funct. Mater. 17, 1288–1296.

Choi, J.S., Lee, S.J., Christ, G.J., Atala, A., Yoo, J.J., 2008. The influence of electrospun aligned poly(caprolactone)/collagen nanofiber meshes on the formation of self-aligned skeletal muscle myotubes. Biomaterials 29, 2899–2906.

Cirillo, V., Clements, B.A., Guarino, V., Bushman, J., Kohn, J., Ambrosio, L., 2014. A comparison of the performance of mono- and bi-component electrospun conduits in a rat sciatic model. Biomaterials 35, 8970–8982.

Clements, I.P., Kim, Y.-t, English, A.W., Lu, X., Chung, A., Bellamkonda, R.V., 2009. Thin-film enhanced nerve guidance channels for peripheral nerve repair. Biomaterials 30, 3834–3846.

Cortez Tornello, P.R., Feresin, G.E., Tapia, A., Veiga, I.G., Moraes, A.M., Abraham, G.A., et al., 2012. Dispersion and release of embelin from electrospun, biodegradable, polymeric membranes. Polym. J. 44, 1105–1111.

Courtney, T., Sacks, M.S., Stankus, J., Guan, J., Wagner, W.R., 2006. Design and analysis of tissue engineering scaffolds that mimic soft tissue mechanical anisotropy. Biomaterials 27, 3631–3638.

Dahlin, R.L., Kasper, F.K., Mikos, A.G., 2011. Polymeric nanofibers in tissue engineering. Tissue Eng. B Rev. 17, 349–364.

Dalby, M.J., Childs, S., Riechle, M.O., Johnstone, H.J.H., Affrossman, S., Curtis, A.S.G., 2003. Fibroblast reaction to island topography: changes in cytoskeleton and morphology with time. Biomaterials 24, 927–935.

Del Gaudio, C., Grigioni, M., Bianco, A., De Angelis, G., 2008. Electrospun bioresorbable heart valve scaffold for tissue engineering. Int. J. Artif. Organs 31, 68–75.

Díaz-Gómez, L., Montini Ballarin, F., Abraham, G.A., Concheiro, A., Alvarez-Lorenzo, C., 2014. Random and aligned PLLA:PRGF electrospun scaffolds for regenerative medicine. J. Appl. Polym. Sci. Available from: http://dx.doi.org/10.1002/app.41372.

Dinis, T.M., Elia, R., Vidal, G., Dermigny, Q., Denoeud, C., Kaplan, D.L., et al., 2015. 3D multi-channel bi-functionalized silk electrospun conduits for peripheral nerve regeneration. J. Mech. Behav. Biomed. 41, 43–55.

Duan, Y.Y., Jia, J., Wang, S.H., Yan, W., Jin, L., Wang, Z.Y., 2007. Preparation of antimicrobial poly(ϵ-caprolactone) electrospun nanofibers containing silver-loaded zirconium phosphate nanoparticles. J. Appl. Polym. Sci. 106, 1208–1214.

Duncan, R., 2011. Polymer therapeutics as nanomedicines: new perspectives. Curr. Opin. Biotechnol. 22, 492–501.

Elisseeff, J., McIntosh, W., Anseth, K., Riley, S., Ragan, P., Langer, R., 2000. Photoencapsulation of chondrocytes in poly(ethylene oxide)-based semi-interpenetrating networks. J. Biomed. Mater. Res. 51, 164–171.

Fang, J., Niu, H.-T., Lin, T., Wang, X.G., 2008. Applications of electrospun nanofibers. Chin. Sci. Bull. 53, 2265–2286.

Freed, L.E., Marquis, J.C., Nohria, A., Emmanual, J., Mikos, A.G., Langer, R., 1993. Neocartilage formation *in vitro* and *in vivo* using cells cultured on synthetic biodegradable polymers. J. Biomed. Mater. Res. 27, 11–23.

Freed, L.E., Hollander, A.P., Martin, I., Barry, J.R., Langer, R., Vunjak-Novakovic, G., 1998. Chondrogenesis in a cell-polymer-bioreactor system. Exp Cell Res. 240, 58–65.

Garrigues, N.W., Little, D., Sanchez-Adams, J., Ruch, D.S., Guilak, F., 2014. Electrospun cartilage-derived matrix scaffolds for cartilage tissue engineering. J. Biomed. Mater. Res. A 102, 3998–4008.

Geetha Priya, S., Junvid, H., Kumar, A., 2008. Skin tissue engineering for tissue repair and regeneration. Tissue Eng. B 14, 105–118.

Goldberg, M., Langer, R., Jia, X., 2007. Nanostructured materials for applications in drug delivery and tissue engineering. J. Biomater. Sci. Polym. Ed. 18, 241–268.

Grasl, C., Bergmeister, H., Stoiber, M., Schima, H., Weigel, G., 2010. Electrospun polyurethane vascular grafts: *in vitro* mechanical behavior and endothelial adhesión molecule expression. J. Biomed. Mater. Res 93A, 716–723.

Greiner, A., Wendorff, J.H., 2007. Electrospinning: a fascinating method for the preparation of ultrathin fibers. Angew. Chem. Int. Ed. 46, 5670–5703.

Han, F., Jia, X., Dai, D., Yang, X., Zhao, J., Zhao, Y., et al., 2013a. Performance of a multilayered small-diameter vascular scaffold dual-loaded with VEGF and PDGF. Biomaterials 34, 7302–7313.

Han, J., Cao, R.-W., Chen, B., Ye, L., Zhang, A.-Y., Zhang, J., et al., 2011. Electrospinning and biocompatibility evaluation of biodegradable polyurethanes based on L-lysine diisocyanate and L-lysine chain extender. J. Biomed. Mater. Res. 96A, 705–714.

Han, J., Farah, S., Domb, A.J., Lelkes, P.I., 2013b. Electrospun rapamycin-eluting polyurethane fibers for vascular grafts. Pharm. Res. 30, 1735–1748.

He, L., Liao, S., Quan, D., Ma, K., Chan, C., Ramakrishna, S., et al., 2010. Synergistic effects of electrospun PLLA fiber dimension and pattern on neonatal mouse cerebellum C17.2 stem cells. Acta Biomater. 6, 2960–2969.

He, W., Hu, Z., Xu, A., Liu, R., Yin, H., Wang, J., et al., 2013. The preparation and performance of a new polyurethane vascular prosthesis. Cell Biochem. Biophys. 66, 855–866.

Hinderer, S., Seifert, J., Votteler, M., Shen, N., Rheinlaender, J., Schäffer, T.E., et al., 2014. Engineering of a bio-functionalized hybrid off-the-shelf heart valve. Biomaterials 35, 2130–2139.

Horst, M., Madduri, S., Milleret, V., Sulser, T., Gobet, R., Eberli, D., 2013. A bilayered hybrid microfibrous PLGAeAcellular matrix scaffold for hollow organ tissue engineering. Biomaterials 34, 1537–1545.

Huang, N.F., Patel, S., Thakar, R.G., Wu, J., Hsiao, B.S., Chu, B., et al., 2006. Myotube assembly on nanofibrous and micropatterned polymers. Nano Lett. 6, 537–542.

Huang, Y.-C., Dennis, R.G., Larkin, L., Baar, K., 2005. Rapid formation of functional muscle *in vitro* using fibrin gels. J. Appl. Phys. 98, 706–713.

Ishii, O., Shin, M., Sueda, T., Vacanti, J., 2005. *In vitro* tissue engineering of a cardiac graft using a degradable scaffold with an extracellular matrix-like topography. J. Thorac. Cardiovasc. Surg. 130, 1358–1363.

Jiang, X., Mi, R., Hoke, A., Chew, S.Y., 2014. Nanofibrous nerve conduit-enhanced peripheral nerve regeneration. J. Tissue Eng. Regen. Med. 8, 377–385.

Johnstone, B., Alini, M., Cucchiarini, M., Dodge, G.R., Eglin, D., Guilak, F., et al., 2013. Tissue engineering for articular cartilage repair—the state of the art. Europ. Cells Mat. 25, 248–267.

Kai, D., Prabhakaran, M.P., Jin, G.R., Ramakrishna, S., 2011. Polypyrrole-contained electrospun conductive nanofibrous membranes for cardiac tissue engineering. J. Biomed. Mater. Res. A 99A, 376–385.

Khil, M.S., Cha, D.I., Kim, H.Y., Kim, I.S., Bhattarai, N., 2003. Electrospun nanofibrous polyurethane membrane as wound dressing. J. Biomed. Mater. Res. B 67, 675–679.

Kidoaki, S., Kwon, I.K., Matsuda, T., 2005. Mesoscopic spatial designs of nano- and microfiber meshes for tissue-engineering matrix and scaffold based on newly devised multilayering and mixing electrospinning techniques. Biomaterials 26, 37–46.

Kidoaki, S., Kwon, I.K., Matsuda, T., 2006. Structural features and mechanical properties of *in situ*-bonded meshes of segmented polyurethane electrospun from mixed solvents. J. Biomed. Mater. Res. B Appl. Biomater. 76B, 219–229.

Kim, M.S., Park, S.J., Gu, B.K., Kim, C.-H., 2012. Polycaprolactone-chitin nanofibrous mats as potential scaffolds for tissue engineering. J. Nanomater. 2012, 1–9.

Kim, S.E., Heo, D.N., Lee, J.B., Kim, J.R., Park, S.H., Jeon, S.H., et al., 2009. Electrospun gelatin/polyurethane blended nanofibers for wound healing. Biomed. Mater. 4, 1–11.

Kim, Y.-T., Haftel, V.K., Kumar, S., Bellamkonda, R.V., 2008. The role of aligned polymer fiber-based constructs in the bridging of long peripheral nerve gaps. Biomaterials 29, 3117–3127.

Koh, H.S., Yong, T., Teo, W.E., Chan, C.K., Puhaindran, M.E., Tan, T.C., et al., 2010. *In vivo* study of novel nanofibrous intra-luminal guidance channels to promote nerve regeneration. J. Neural Eng. 7, 046003 (14pp).

Kumari, A., Yadav, S.K., Yadav, S.C., 2010. Biodegradable polymeric nanoparticles based drug delivery systems. Colloids Surf. B Biointerfaces 75, 1–18.

Kumbar, S.G., Nukavarapu, S.P., James, R., Nair, L.S., Laurencin, C.T., 2008a. Electrospun poly(lactic acid-*co*-glycolic acid) scaffolds for skin tissue engineering. Biomaterials 29, 4100–4107.

Kumbar, S.G., Nukavarapu, S.P., James, R., Hogan, M.V., Laurencin, C.T., 2008b. Recent patents on electrospun biomedical nanostructures: an overview. Rec. Pat. Biomed. Eng. 1, 68–78.

Kundu, A.K., Gelman, J., Tyson, D.R., 2011. Composite thin film and electrospun biomaterials for urologic tissue reconstruction. Biotechnol. Bioeng. 108, 207–215.

Kuraishi, K., Iwata, H., Nakano, S., Kubota, S., Tonami, H., Toda, M., et al., 2009. Development of nanofiber-covered stents using electrospinning: *in vitro* and acute phase *in vivo* experiments. J. Biomed. Mater. Res. B Appl. Biomater. 88, 230–239.

Lannutti, J., Reneker, D., Ma, T., Tomasko, D., Farson, D., 2007. Electrospinning for tissue engineering scaffolds. Mater. Sci. Eng. C 27, 504–509.

Lee, S.J., Yoo, J.J., Lim, G.J., Atala, A., Stitzel, J., 2007. *In vitro* evaluation of electrospun nanofiber scaffolds for vascular graft application. J. Biomed. Mater. Res. 83A, 999–1008.

Lee, S.J., Liu, J., Oh, S.H., Soker, S., Atala, A., Yoo, J.J., 2008. Development of a composite vascular scaffolding system that withstands physiological vascular conditions. Biomaterials 29, 2891–2898.

Li, M., Guo, Y., Wei, Y., MacDiarmid, A.G., Lelkes, P.I., 2006a. Electrospinning polyaniline-contained gelatin nanofibers for tissue engineering applications. Biomaterials 27, 2705–2715.

Li, M., Mondrinos, M.J., Chen, X., Gandhi, M.R., Ko, F.K., Lelkes, P.I., 2006b. Co-electrospun poly(lactide-*co*-glycolide), gelatin, and elastin blends for tissue engineering scaffolds. J. Biomed. Mater. Res. A 79, 963–973.

Li, W.J., Danielson, K.G., Alexander, P.G., Tuan, R.S., 2003. Biological response of chondrocytes cultured in three-dimensional nanofibrous poly(epsilon-caprolactone) scaffolds. J. Biomed. Mater. Res. A 67, 1105–1114.

Li, W.J., Jiang, Y.J., Tuan, R.S., 2006c. Chondrocyte phenotype in engineered fibrous matrix is regulated by fiber size. Tissue Eng. 12, 1775–1785.

Li, W.J., Chiang, H., Kuo, T.F., Lee, H.S., Jiang, C.C., Tuan, R.S., 2009. Evaluation of articular cartilage repair using biodegradable nanofibrous scaffolds in a swine model: a pilot study. J. Tissue Eng. Regen. Med. 3, 1–10.

Liao, S., Li, B., Ma, Z., Wei, H., Chan, C., Ramakrishna, S., 2006. Biomimetic electrospun nanofibers for tissue regeneration. Biomed. Mater. 1, R45–R53.

Lim, S.H., Mao, H.-Q., 2009. Electrospun scaffolds for stem cell engineering. Adv. Drug Del. Rev. 61, 1084–1096.

Liu, T., Houle, J.D., Xu, J., Chan, B.P., Chew, S.Y., 2012. Nanofibrous collagen nerve conduits for spinal cord repair. Tissue Eng. A 18, 1057–1066.

Lutolf, M.P., Hubbell, J.A., 2005. Synthetic biomaterials as instructive extracellular microenvironments for morphogenesis in tissue engineering. Nat Biotechnol. 23, 47–55.

Lutolf, M.P., Lauer-Fields, J.L., Schmoekel, H.G., Metters, A.T., Weber, F.E., Fields, G. B., et al., 2003. Synthetic matrix metalloproteinase-sensitive hydrogels for the conduction of tissue regeneration: engineering cell-invasion characteristics. Proc. Natl. Acad. Sci. U.S.A. 100, 5413–5418.

Ma, P.X., 2008. Biomimetic materials for tissue engineering. Adv. Drug Del. Rev 60, 184–198.

Mac Neil, S., 2008. Biomaterials for tissue engineering of skin. Mater. Today 11, 26–35.

Marelli, B., Alessandrino, A., Farè, S., Freddi, G., Mantovani, D., Tanzi, M.C., 2010. Compliant electrospun silk fibroin tubes for small vessel bypass grafting. Acta Biomater. 6, 4019–4026.

Masoumi, N., Larson, B.L., Annabi, N., Kharaziha, M., Zamanian, B., Shapero, K.S., et al., 2014. Electrospun PGS:PCL microfibers align human valvular interstitial cells and provide tunable scaffold anisotropy. Adv. Healthcare Mater. 3, 929–939.

Matsuda, T., Ihara, M., Inoguchi, H., Kwon, I.K., Takamizawa, K., Kidoaki, S., 2005. Mechano-active scaffold design of small-diameter artificial graft made of electrospun segmented polyurethane fabrics. J. Biomed. Mater. Res. 73A, 125–131.

McClure, M.J., Sell, S.A., Simpson, D.G., Walpoth, B.H., Bowlin, G.L., 2010. A three-layered electrospun matrix to mimic native arterial architecture using polycaprolactone, elastin, and collagen: a preliminary study. Acta Biomater. 6, 2422–2433.

McClure, M.J., Simpson, D.G., Bowlin, G.L., 2012. Tri-layered vascular grafts composed of polycaprolactone, elastin, collagen, and silk: optimization of graft properties. J. Mech. Behav. Biomed. 10, 48–61.

McKenna, K.A., Hinds, M.T., Sarao, R.C., Wu, P.-C., Maslen, C.L., Glanville, R.W., et al., 2012. Mechanical property characterization of electrospun recombinant human tropoelastin for vascular graft biomaterials. Acta Biomater. 8, 225–233.

McKeon-Fischer, K.D., Rossmeisl, J.H., Whittington, A.R., Freeman, J.W., 2014. *In vivo* skeletal muscle biocompatibility of composite, coaxial electrospun, and microfibrous scaffolds. Tissue Eng. A, 1961–1970.

McManus, M., Boland, E., Sell, S., Bowen, W., Koo, H., Simpson, D., et al., 2007. Electrospun nanofibre fibrinogen for urinary tract tissue reconstruction. Biomed. Mater. 2, 257–262.

Miyazu, K., Kawahara, D., Ohtake, H., Watanabe, G., Matsuda, T., 2010. Luminal surface design of electrospun small-diameter graft aiming at *in situ* capture of endothelial progenitor cell. J. Biomed. Mater. Res. B Appl. Biomater. 94B, 53–63.

Montini Ballarin, F., Caracciolo, P.C., Blotta, E., Ballarin, V.L., Abraham, G.A., 2014. Optimization of poly(L-lactic acid)/segmented polyurethane electrospinning process for the production of bilayered small-diameter nanofibrous tubular structures. Mater. Sci. Eng. C 42, 489–499.

Mooney, E., Mackle, J.N., Blond, D.J.P., O'Cearbhaill, E., Shaw, G., Blau, W.J., et al., 2012. The electrical stimulation of carbon nanotubes to provide a cardiomimetic cue to MSCs. Biomaterials. 33, 6132–6139.

Moore, T., 2005. Design and synthesis of biodegradable thermoplastic polyurethanes for tissue engineering (PhD thesis). Swinburne University of Technology, Australia.

Mugnai, D., Tille, J.-C., Mrówczynski, W., de Valence, S., Montet, X., Möller, M., et al., 2013. Experimental noninferiority trial of synthetic small-caliber biodegradable versus stable vascular grafts. J. Thorac. Cardiovasc. Surg. 146, 400–407.

Nam, J., Huang, Y., Agarwal, S., Lannutti, J., 2007. Improved cellular infiltration in electrospun fiber via engineered porosity. Tissue Eng. 13, 2249–2257.

Orlova, Y., Magome, N., Liu, L., Chen, Y., Agladze, K., 2011. Electrospun nanofibers as a tool for architecture control in engineered cardiac tissue. Biomaterials 32, 5615–5624.

Panseri, S., Cunha, C., Lowery, J., Del Carro, U., Taraballi, F., Amadio, S., et al., 2008. Electrospun micro- and nanofiber tubes for functional nervous regeneration in sciatic nerve transections. BMC Biotechnology 8, 39.

Pham, Q.P., Sharma, U., Mikos, A.G., 2006. Electrospinning of polymeric nanofibers for tissue engineering applications: a review. Tissue Eng. 12, 1197–1211.

Prabhakaran, M.P., Venugopal, J.R., Chyan, T.T., Hai, L.B., Chan, C.K., Lim, A.Y., et al., 2008. Electrospun biocomposite nanofibrous scaffolds for neural tissue engineering. Tissue Eng. A 14, 1787–1797.

Punnakitikashem, P., Truong, D., Menon, J.U., Nguyen, K.T., Hong, Y., 2014. Electrospun biodegradable elastic polyurethane scaffolds with dipyridamole release for small diameter vascular grafts. Acta Biomater. 10, 4618–4628.

Ramakrishna, S., Fujihara, K., Teo, W.-E., Yong, T., Ma, Z., Ramaseshan, R., 2006. Electrospun nanofibers: solving global issues. Mater. Today 9, 40–50.

Ramalingam, M., Ramakrishna, S., 2006. Nano-featured scaffolds for tissue engineering: a review of spinning methodologies. Tissue Eng. 12, 435–447.

Ramalingam, M., Ramakrishna, S., 2007. Design strategies of tissue engineering scaffolds with controlled fiber orientation. Tissue Eng. 13, 1845–1866.

Rapoport, H.S., Fish, J., Basu, J., Campbell, J., Genheimer, C., Payne, R., et al., 2012. Construction of a tubular scaffold that mimics J-shaped stress/strain mechanics using an innovative electrospinning technique. Tissue Eng. C 18, 567–574.

Riboldi, S.A., Sampaolesi, M., Neuenschwander, P., Cossu, G., Mantero, S., 2005. Electrospun degradable polyesterurethane membranes: potential scaffolds for skeletal muscle tissue engineering. Biomaterials 26, 4606–4615.

Rujitanaroj, P.O., Pimpha, N., Supaphol, P., 2008. Wound-dressing materials with antibacterial activity from electrospun gelatin fiber mats containing silver nanoparticles. Polymer 49, 4723–4732.

Schneider, T., Kohl, B., Sauter, T., Kratz, K., Lendlein, A., Ertel, W., et al., 2012. Influence of fiber orientation in electrospun polymer scaffolds on viability, adhesion and differentiation of articular chondrocytes. Clin Hemorheol. Microcirc. 52, 325–336.

Sell, S., Barnes, C., Smith, M., McClure, M., Madurantakam, P., Grant, J., et al., 2007. Extracellular matrix regenerated: tissue engineering via electrospun biomimetic nanofibers. Polym. Int. 56, 1349–1360.

Sell, S.A., Wolfe, P.S., Garg, K., McCool, J.M., Rodriguez, I.A., Bowlin, G.L., 2010. The use of natural polymers in tissue engineering: a focus on electrospun extracellular matrix analogues. Polymers 2, 522–553.

Shevchenko, R.V., James, S.L., James, S.E., 2010. A review of tissue-engineered skin bioconstructs available for skin reconstruction. J. R. Soc. Interface 7, 229–258.

Shin, M., Ishii, O., Sueda, T., Vacanti, J.P., 2004. Contractile cardiac grafts using a novel nanofibrous mesh. Biomaterials 25, 3717–3723.

Sill, T.J., von Recum, H.A., 2008. Electrospinning: applications in drug delivery and tissue engineering. Biomaterials 29, 1989–2006.

Simonet, M., Driessen-Mol, A., Baaijens, F.P.T., Bouten, C.V.C., 2011. Heart valve tissue regeneration. In: Bosworth, L.A., Downes, S. (Eds.), Electrospinning for Tissue Regeneration. Woodhead Publishing, UK, pp. 202–224.

Singh, L., Kumar, V., Ratner, B.D., 2004. Generation of porous microcellular 85/15 poly (D,L-lactide-*co*-glycolide) foams for biomedical applications. Biomaterials 25, 2611–2617.

Soletti, L., Hong, Y., Guan, J., Stankus, J.J., El-Kurdi, M.S., Wagner, W.R., et al., 2010. A bilayered elastomeric scaffold for tissue engineering of small diameter vascular grafts. Acta Biomater. 6, 110–122.

Stankus, J.J., Freytes, D.O., Badylak, S.F., Wagner, W.R., 2008. Hybrid nanofibrous scaffolds from electrospinning of a synthetic biodegradable elastomer and urinary bladder matrix. J. Biomater. Sci. Polym. Ed. 19, 635–652.

Stitzel, J., Liu, J., Lee, S.J., Komura, M., Berry, J., Soker, S., et al., 2006. Controlled fabrication of a biological vascular substitute. Biomaterials. 27, 1088–1094.

Subramanian, A., Krishnan, U.M., Sethuraman, S., 2011. Skin tissue regeneration. In: Bosworth, L.A., Downes, S. (Eds.), Electrospinning for Tissue Regeneration. Woodhead Publishing, UK, pp. 298–316.

Thomas, V., Zhang, X., Catledge, S.A., Vohra, Y.K., 2007. Functionally graded electrospun scaffolds with tunable mechanical properties for vascular tissue regeneration. Biomed. Mater. 2, 224–232.

Thorvaldsson, A., Stenhamre, H., Gatenholm, P., Walkenstrom, P., 2008. Electrospinning of highly porous scaffolds for cartilage regeneration. Biomacromolecules 9, 1044–1049.

Tillman, B.W., Yazdani, S.K., Lee, S.J., Geary, R.L., Atala, A., Yoo, J.J., 2009. The *in vivo* stability of electrospun polycaprolactone-collagen scaffolds in vascular reconstruction. Biomaterials 30, 583–588.

Van Lieshout, M.I., Vaz, C.M., Rutten, M.C.M., Peters, G.W.M., Baaijens, F.P.T., 2006. Electrospinning versus knitting: two scaffolds for tissue engineering of the aortic valve. J. Biomater. Sci. Polym. Ed. 17, 77–89.

Venugopal, J., Ramakrishna, S., 2005. Applications of polymer nanofibers in biomedicine and biotechnology. Appl. Biochem. Biotechnol. 125, 147–158.

Venugopal, J., Low, S., Choon, A.T., Ramakrishna, S., 2008. Interaction of cells and nanofiber scaffolds in tissue engineering. J. Biomed. Mater. Res. B Appl. Biomater. 84B, 34–48.

Wan, L.-S., Xu, Z.-K., 2009. Polymer surfaces structured with random or aligned electrospun nanofibers to promote the adhesion of blood platelets. J. Biomed. Mat. Res. Part A 89A, 168–175.

Wang, H., Feng, Y., Fang, Z., Yuan, W., Khan, M., 2012a. Co-electrospun blends of PU and PEG as potential biocompatible scaffolds for small-diameter vascular tissue engineering. Mater. Sci. Eng. C 32, 2306–2315.

Wang, H., Feng, Y., An, B., Zhang, W., Sun, M., Fang, Z., et al., 2012b. Fabrication of PU/PEGMA crosslinked hybrid scaffolds by *in situ* UV photopolymerization favoring human endothelial cells growth for vascular tissue engineering. J. Mater. Sci. Mater. Med. 23, 1499–1510.

Wang, H.B., Mullins, M.E., Cregg, J.M., Hurtado, A., Oudega, M., Trombley, M.T., et al., 2009. Creation of highly aligned electrospun poly-L-lactic acid fibres for nerve regeneration applications. J. Nerual. Eng. 6, 1–15.

Williams, D.F., 2009. On the nature of biomaterials. Biomaterials 30, 5897–5909.

Wu, H., Fan, J., Chu, C.-C., Wu, J., 2010. Electrospinning of small diameter 3-D nanofibrous tubular scaffolds with controllable nanofiber orientations for vascular grafts. J. Mater. Sci. Mater. Med. 21, 3207–3215.

Xie, J., Li, X., Xia, Y., 2008. Putting electrospun nanofibers to work for biomedical research. Macromol. Rapid Commun. 29, 1775–1792.

Xie, J., Willerth, S.M., Li, X., Macewan, M.R., Rader, A., Sakiyama-Elbert, S.E., et al., 2009. The differentiation of embryonic stem cells seeded on electrospun nanofibers into neural lineages. Biomaterials 30, 354–362.

Xie, J., MacEwan, M.R., Liu, W., Jesuraj, N., Li, X., Hunter, D., et al., 2014. Nerve guidance conduits based on double-layered scaffolds of electrospun nanofibers for repairing the peripheral nervous system. Appl. Mater. Interfaces 6, 9472–9480.

Yarin, A.L., 2011. Coaxial electrospinning and emulsion electrospinning of core-shell fibers. Polym. Adv. Technol. 22, 310–317.

Yin, A., Zhang, K., McClure, M.J., Huang, C., Wu, J., Fang, J., et al., 2013. Electrospinning collagen/chitosan/poly(L-lactic acid-*co*-ε-caprolactone) to form a Cl and biological characterization. J. Biomed. Mater. Res. 101A, 1292–1301.

Yu, J., Wang, A., Tang, Z., Henry, J., Lee, B.L.-P., Zhu, Y., et al., 2012. The effect of stromal cell-derived factor-1a/heparin coating of biodegradable vascular grafts on the recruitment of both endothelial and smooth muscle progenitor cells for accelerated regeneration. Biomaterials 33, 8062–8074.

Yu, W., Jiang, X., Cai, M., Zhao, W., Ye, D., Zhou, Y., et al., 2014. A novel electrospun nerve conduit enhanced by carbon nanotubes for peripheral nerve regeneration. Nanotechnology 25, 165102 (13pp).

Zahedi, P., Rezaeian, I., Ranaei-Siadat, S.-O., Jafari, S.-H., Supaphol, P., 2010. A review on wound dressings with an emphasis on electrospun nanofibrous polymeric bandages. Polym. Adv. Technol. 21, 77–95.

Zhang, X., Thomas, V., Vohra, Y.K., 2010a. Two ply tubular scaffolds comprised of proteins/poliglecaprone/polycaprolactone fibers. J. Mater. Sci. Mater. Med. 21, 541–549.

Zhang, X., Thomas, V., Xu, Y., Bellis, S.L., Vohra, Y.K., 2010b. An *in vitro* regenerated functional human endothelium on a nanofibrous electrospun scaffold. Biomaterials 31, 4376–4381.

Zhang, X., Xu, Y., Thomas, V., Bellis, S.L., Vohra, Y.K., 2011. Engineering an antiplatelet adhesion layer on an electrospun scaffold using porcine endothelial progenitor cells. J. Biomed. Mater. Res. 97A, 145–151.

Zhang, Y., Lim, C.T., Ramakrishna, S., Huang, Z.M., 2005. Recent development of polymer nanofibers for biomedical and biotechnological applications. J. Mater. Sci. Mater. Med. 16, 933–946.

Zhang, Z., Hu, J., Ma, P.X., 2012. Nanofiber-based delivery of bioactive agents and stem cells to bone sites. Adv. Drug Del. Rev. 64, 1129–1141.

Zhou, Y., Yang, D., Chen, X., Xu, Q., Lu, F., Nie, J., 2008. Electrospun water-soluble carboxyethyl chitosan/poly(vinyl alcohol) nanofibrous membrane as potential wound dressing for skin regeneration. Biomacromolecules 9, 349–354.

Zhu, X., Cui, W., Li, X., Jun, Y., 2008. Electrospun fibrous mats with high porosity as potential scaffolds for skin tissue engineering. Biomacromolecules 9, 1795–1801.

Zong, X., Bien, H., Chung, C., Yin, L., Fang, D., Hsiao, B., et al., 2005. Electrospun fine-textured scaffolds for heart tissue constructs. Biomaterials 26, 5330–5338.

CHAPTER

9 Natural polymer-based hydrogels as scaffolds for tissue engineering

Manju Rawat Singh[1], Satish Patel[1] and Deependra Singh[1,2]

[1]University Institute of Pharmacy, Pt. Ravishankar Shukla University, Raipur, Chhattisgarh, India [2]NCNPR, School of Pharmacy, University of Mississippi, Oxford, MS, USA

9.1 INTRODUCTION

Research in the field of drug-delivery systems and tissue engineering has seen remarkable development in recent years due to their prospects of improving human health. Meanwhile, the developments of technology give diverse opportunities to characterize, control, and organize substances systematically. There has been a tremendous upsurge in the research and development of biomaterials for cell and tissue engineering due to advances in materials technology and cellular techniques. The roles of scaffolds in tissue engineering are very important and imperative.

Biomaterials, like nature-based polymers, have been used as controlled-release reservoirs and as artificial matrices for tissue engineering. Scaffolds can be primed with natural and controlled composition and morphology. Their properties can be influenced to increase biocompatibility, stability, solubility, immune compatibility, and cellular uptake. They can be used to deliver growth factors, stem cells, peptides, proteins, plasmid DNA, and synthetic nucleotides with natural tissue formation by intimately imitating the natural extracellular matrix (ECM).

Tissue engineering is also a part of drug-delivery system, where the objective is to achieve the controlled and sustained delivery of cells, proteins, peptides, etc. Controlled and organized release of therapeutic factors and actives would improve the efficacy of tissue engineering. From the point of view of materials, scaffolds for tissue engineering must be biocompatible and biodegradable with a suitable porosity and surface chemistry to permit addition, migration, proliferation, differentiation, and infiltration of the natural or engineered cells (Seidi and Ramalingam, 2012). It is the promising restorative approaches that merge cells, biomaterials, and other factors to provide a natural environment inducing different pathways and signals to promote tissue repair and functional restoration. The promising area in tissue engineering that has shown an increased surge of interest

Nanobiomaterials in Soft Tissue Engineering. DOI: http://dx.doi.org/10.1016/B978-0-323-42865-1.00009-X

includes engineered tissue material containing enzymes, drugs, growth factors, stem cells, nucleotides, proteins, etc., for better cell adherence, proliferation, and differentiation than noninformational polymers (Patricia, 2007).

Hydrogels have been extensively used as scaffolds in tissue engineering due to their excellent biocompatibility, soft tissue-like properties, and highly water-swollen networks that allow permeability for oxygen, nutrients, and water-soluble metabolites (Cushing and Anseth, 2007; Zhu and Marchant, 2011; Zhu, 2012). Biopolymer-derived hydrogels, such as those from collagen, fibrin, hyaluronic acid, alginate, and chitosan, usually also have some problem, such as weak mechanical strength, not absorbing exudates, allergic reaction, or contamination (Zhu and Marchant, 2011). Engineering of natural polymer-based hydrogels is a striking approach to develop scaffolds for tissue engineering, which gives information to recognize the interaction between cell or tissue with scaffold formation or regeneration of tissue or organ and their cellular responses.

9.2 TISSUE ENGINEERING

The area of tissue engineering has developed significantly since the beginning of the idea of combining cells or drug and scaffolds to generate artificial tissues. Tissue engineering researches have been directed toward the development of improved and better scaffolds as regenerative medicine and have become an important therapeutic strategy for present and future medicine. Over the last several years, the meaning of tissue engineering has transformed significantly from a material that acts as a neutral support for delivery and cell attachment, to serving as a more complex, dynamic environment for artificial tissue development. It is defined as an "Application of the principles and methods of engineering and the life sciences toward the fundamental understanding of structure–function relationships in normal and pathological mammalian tissues and the development of biological substitutes to restore, maintain, or improve functions" (Nerem 1991; Dang and Leong, 2006). This together with systematic discoveries in the field of drug-delivery systems, stem cells, and development of technology has provided the platform for future research that gives emphasis to the design and development of a biomimetic environment for artificial tissue development (Singh et al., 2013).

The main aim of tissue engineering is to restore, uphold, recover, or improve tissue functions that are faulty or have been lost by different pathological conditions, either by developing biological substitutes or by reconstructing tissues. Presently, the trend in tissue engineering is the delivery of growth factors, cells, proteins, peptides, and enzymes within the natural polymer or synthetic polymer-derived matrix as therapeutic strategy. Some limitations within such structures, such as cells, are arranged spatially in 3D with regard to one another but they still fix to a 2D surface and this arrangement does not display a phenotype that looks like the native tissue.

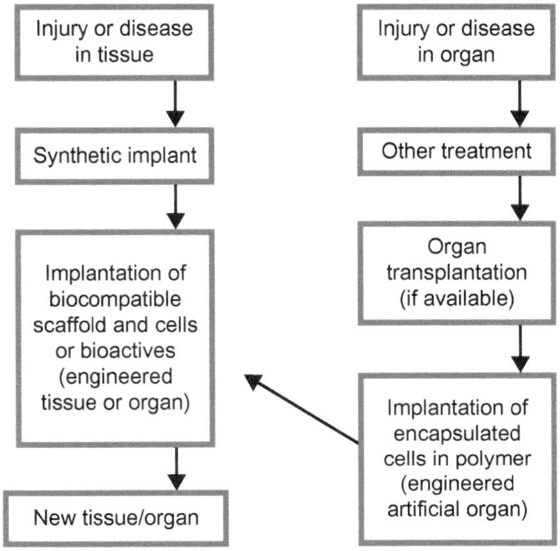

FIGURE 9.1

The evolution of tissue engineering for the repair and regeneration of injured tissue or organs.

Modified from Hoffman et al. (2002).

In tissue engineering, various strategies can be followed for the fabrication of new tissue, like isolated cells or cell substitutes, to provide the required action or tissue-inducing substances placed into target areas or cells sited on or within matrices which may be rooted and incorporated into the body or a combination of these (Figure 9.1; Langer and Vacanti, 1993).

9.3 NATURAL POLYMERS FOR HYDROGEL SCAFFOLDS IN TISSUE ENGINEERING

Polymers have been widely used as biomaterials for the production of medical devices and tissue engineering scaffolds. In biomedical applications, the criteria for selecting the materials as biomaterials are based on their material chemistry, molecular weight, solubility, shape and structure, hydrophilicity/hydrophobicity, lubricancy, surface energy, water absorption degradation, and erosion mechanism.

There are significant contributions of natural polymers in tissue engineering, particularly in the fabrication of scaffolds for delivery of therapeutic agents (Figure 9.2). Polymeric novel application, mainly due to its elite strength, has advanced tissue engineering. Novel and natural polymeric approaches are oriented toward improvement of various treatments. In natural polymeric approaches,

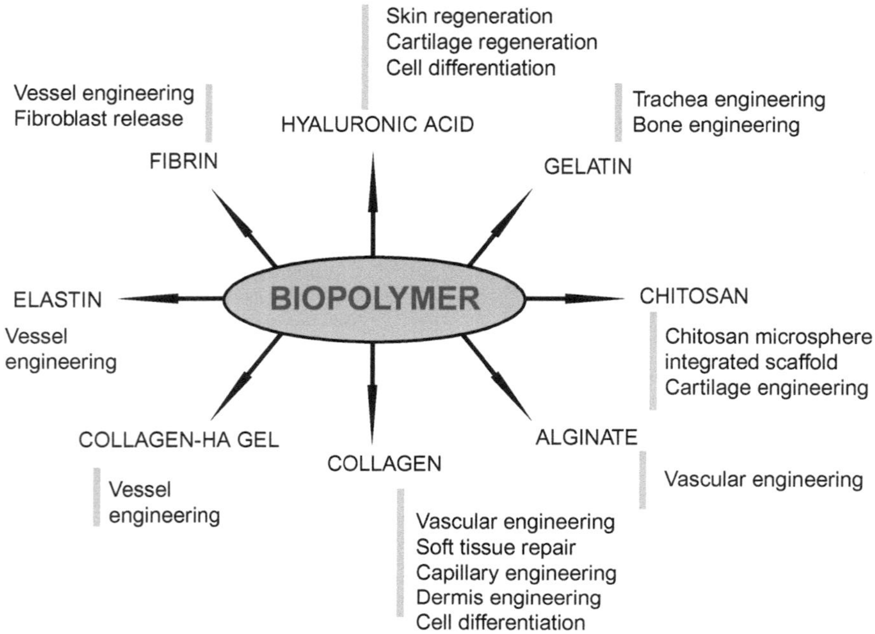

FIGURE 9.2

Various types of biopolymers used in tissue engineering.

accumulation of active cells and drugs in scaffolds and their target on specific sites is done in a controlled manner. The majority of natural polymers have reactive sites compliant for ligand conjugation, crosslinking, and other modifications that can provide a polymer tailored for a variety of clinical applications. Natural polymers also often possess good cytocompatibility and other advantages over synthetic polymers making them a popular option for tissue engineering scaffolding applications. Biopolymers, with their capacity to serve as carriers and tissue engineering scaffolds, have a significant role in the area of regenerative medicine (Dhandayuthapani et al., 2011). Scaffold materials may be natural or synthetic, degradable or nondegradable, depending on the intended use (Ramakrishna et al., 2001). The properties of polymers depend on the composition, structure, and arrangement of their constituent macromolecules. Natural polymers, owing to their bioactive properties, have better interactions with cells, which allows them to enhance tissue performance (Dhandayuthapani et al., 2011).

In recent years, there has been growing interest in the use of sustainable biopolymers. Natural and synthetic polymer-based novel approaches are used in tissue engineering and drug delivery. These polymers are excellent candidates for applications in tissue engineering growth because of their versatility, biocompatibility, and ability to degrade *in vivo* (Boudriot, 2012; Chereddy, 2014). One of the disadvantages of these biopolymers is their plausible group variation. This problem has been resolved using recombinant protein technologies by synthesizing monodisperse biopolymers with precisely defined properties, predictable site of crosslinking groups to bind moieties at specific sites along the polypeptide chain for drug delivery and tissue engineering (Rodriguez-Cabello et al., 2005).

The materials used for fabricating scaffolds in tissue engineering are capable of subsisting in the patient's body without affecting nearby cells or causing any significant or undesirable effects. Most biopolymer hydrogels are considered to be suitable for implantation due to the high water content and the minimal mechanical irritation inflicted on surrounding tissue, due to the soft, elastic properties of these hydrogels (Peppas, 2000). In contrast, synthetic hydrogels frequently display undesirable effects when implanted (Lee and Mooney, 2001).

Natural polymers have been used as scaffolds for tissue engineering due to their biocompatibility, inherent biodegradability, and critical biological functions. There are four major types of natural polymers, including (Zhu and Marchant, 2011):

- Proteins, including natural as well as genetically engineered proteins, such as collagen, gelatin, fibrin, silk, lysozyme, Matrigel™ (Ehrick et al., 2005; Glowacki and Mizuno, 2007; Kimelman-Bleich et al., 2009; Sakai et al., 2009; Sengupta and Heilshorn, 2010). Proteins mimick many features of ECM by directing the migration, growth, and organization of cells during tissue regeneration and wound healing and for stabilization of encapsulated and transplanted cells.
- Polysaccharides (Ramamurthi and Vesely, 2003; Denizli et al., 2004), such as hyaluronic acid, agarose, dextran, and chitosan.
- Protein/polysaccharide hybrid polymers (Stabenfeldt et al., 2006; Shikanov et al., 2009; Davidenko et al., 2010), such as collagen/HA, laminin/cellulose, gelatin/chitosan, and fibrin/alginate.
- DNA like X-, Y-, T-DNA, and linear plasmid DNA (Lee et al., 2008; Park et al., 2009; Xing et al., 2011).

Some natural polymers, like alginate, act as a reinforcing element for cell walls. At present, alginate fibers have become important materials in scaffolds because they have unique gel-forming characteristics (Augst, 2006). Alginate is prepared from polysaccharides obtained from various seaweeds and is a mixture of D-mannuronic acid and L-guluronic acid residues (Lee and Mooney, 2001). In compromised wounds and normal wounds, the gelled structure keeps the area between the dressing and the wound moist, and provides a natural moist environment for proper and complete healing. Such fibers are widely used for manufacturing modern dressing materials, and are suitable for use on medium to heavily oozing wounds and cavities. Scaffolds made from alginate fiber are bioabsorbable and nonadherent (Thomas, 1989). Alginate has a very restricted interaction with the bulk of cells due to its hydrophilic character, which promotes limited protein adsorption (Lee and Mooney, 2001). Commercially available products of alginate are Nu-Derm® (Johnson & Johnson, USA), Curasorb® (Kendall), and AlgiSite® (Smith & Nephew), which have been widely marketed as wound dressings.

Fibrin is another biocompatible polymer with high water content. Its mechanical properties resemble soft tissue. Fibrin derived from animals and humans is important in blood clotting (Janmey et al., 2009). It is used as a sealant, an adhesive in surgery, and for skin graft fixation (Lee and Mooney, 2001; Huang and Fu, 2010) useful in tissue engineering. Fibrin has the capability to be introduced in liquid form *in vivo* and transformed to a gel *in situ*. In cells, fibrin degrades rapidly due to the secretion of proteolytic enzymes and formulations have stability problems (Huang and Fu, 2010). Stability issues are resolved by use of inhibitors and fibrin stabilizers (Mol et al., 2005; Park et al., 2005). One of the advantages of fibrin is that it can be prepared from the patient blood so that no inflammatory or allergic responses would be expected. Also, no toxic degradation products form following degradation. The limited mechanical strength of fibrin gels has, however, limited use in clinical applications (Lee and Mooney, 2001).

Collagen is the most abundant form of protein in animals and humans, and is the main component of the ECM of skin, bone, cartilage, tendon, and ligament, and is mainly obtained from bovine skin. It is regarded as the best polymer for scaffold or matrix formation for tissue engineering as it is the chief protein component of the ECM that provides structural support to connective tissues such as skin, tendons, bones, cartilage, blood vessels, and ligaments (Lee et al., 2001a, 2001b; Foo and Kaplan, 2002). It has excellent biocompatibility, which makes it a popular component in tissue engineering and in delivery systems. Collagen can be pooled with other materials for tissue regeneration. Bioactives, growth factors, and stem cells have been included in collagen to augment healing of wounds. Collagen is also used as an absorbable suture material, used for sutures that are readily accepted by the body, a hemostat, an artificial skin, a bone-filling material, and as a wound dressing (Bret, 2008).

There are 27 different forms of collagen found in vertebrates with 42 distinct polypeptide chains have been identified, the most ubiquitous is type I collagen. Types I, II, III, V, XI, XXIV, XXVII collagen are fibril-forming collagens, containing triple-helical structures which are able to bundle into fibrils. Characteristic for collagen is the presence of hydroxyproline residues needed for stabilization of the collagen triple helix (Pachence, 1996). These fibril-forming collagen molecules utilized in tissue engineering applications consist of three polypeptide chains of glycine–X–Y (Gly–X–Y) amino acid repeats twined around one another to form triple helices (Berisio et al., 2002). The self-assembling tendencies of type I collagen have led to it be used as a hydrogel for use in tissue engineering. Collagen can be used to rebuild skin after wounding. Biocompatibility and low antigenicity make collagen a good natural polymer. Its weak feature is mechanical weakness (Brown, 2005). However, collagen can be chemically crosslinked using glutaraldehyde (Rault, 1996) or diphenylphosphoryl azide (Marinucci, 2003) to improve its physical strength. The hasty deprivation of collagen hydrogels in cells is also challenging. Researchers have tried to resolve these problems by using various crosslinkers including transglutimase, 1-ethyl-3-3-dimethylaminopropylcarbodiimide hydrochloride (Chau, 2005; Powell and Boyce, 2006) and by blending it with other polymers (i.e., poly[glycolic acid], poly[lactic-*co*-glycolic acid], chitosan, etc.). Various animal source collagen scaffolds have been successfully developed and marketed for tissue engineering. The first bioengineered skin to receive FDA approval in 1998 was Apligraf®, commercialized by Organogenesis. It consist of bilayered collagen gels incorporated with human fibroblasts in the lower part and human keratinocytes in the upper layer. Revitix™ (topical cosmetic product), VCTO1™ (bilayered bioengineered skin), or Forta-Derm™ Antimicrobial (antimicrobial wound dressing) and FUSE® Bone Graft (bone morphogenetic protein [BMP-2]) are other collagen-based products (Spiro and Polarek, 2004; Malafaya et al., 2007). Angiotech Pharmaceuticals, Inc., in Canada, commercialized Collagraft® which is a mixture of porous hydroxyapatite and tricalcium phosphate and animal-derived collagen I (Spiro and Polarek, 2004). Biomend® is a product of Integra LifeSciences Corp. in the United States and is used in the regeneration of periodontal tissue (Danielsson et al., 2006).

Another collagen-derived biodegradable and biocompatible polymer extensively used in the pharmaceutical industry is gelatin. Unlike collagen, gelatin is usually denatured and has relatively low antigenicity. Gelatin is a denatured protein obtained by acid and alkaline processing of collagen (Djagny et al., 2001). Hydrogel produced with the use of gelatin by chemical crosslinking, as it is insoluble in water, is tailored with water-soluble carbodiimides and glutaraldehyde. The gelatin-based hydrogels form polyion complexes with proteins which make it feasible for the release of proteins, which is controlled by matrix degradation (Young et al., 2005), and consequently the period for bioactive release can be controlled by modifying the extent of crosslinking thus regulating hydrogel degradation. The isoelectric point can be distorted to formulate gelatin appropriate for a wide range of uses with different pH. Bioactives, growth factors, human chondrocytes (Park et al., 2005), human preadipocytes (Kimura et al., 2003), and stem cells (Ponticiello et al., 2000) have been integrated with gelatine vehicles and used as controlled-release systems and scaffolds for tissues like skin in tissue regeneration. Gelatin can also be used as a vehicle for cells in skin regeneration (Huang and Fu, 2010). There are several commercially available gelatin-based carriers for drug delivery that are being applied in tissue engineering applications (Lindenhayn et al., 1999; Lee et al., 2002; Liao et al., 2005). The most commonly used ones are Gelfoam® commercialized now by Pfizer in the United States, Gelfilm® (absorbable gelatin film, Pfizer), Surgifoam® (absorbable gelatin disks, Ethicon, Inc.), and CultiSpher-G® (Percell Biolytica AB) (Malafaya et al., 2007).

Chitosan, derived from chitin, has been extensively used for many medical and pharmaceutical preparations due to its hemostatic properties, acceleration of bone formation and its regenerative effect on connective gum tissue. Various properties, like biocompatibility, nontoxicity, and solubility in weak acids, make it an excellent material for scaffold and in tissue engineering. It is positively charged, is a strong tissue adhesive, and forms gel easily. It has been proved to enhance the function of leukocytes, macrophages, and fibroblasts to enhance granulation and rebuilding of tissue (Huang and Fu, 2010). Commercially available products of chitosan include geniaBeads® (Genialab, Germany), HemCon® bandage (HemConMedical Technologies, Inc.), etc.

Hylauronic acid is commonly known as hyaluronan as it transforms *in vivo* into a poly-anion and not the protonated acid form. Hyaluronan and its allied networks have a lot of physiological functions that include tissue and matrix water regulation, structural, and space-filling properties, lubrication, and a number of other functions. It is a linear polysaccharide with alternate disaccharide units of α-1,4-D-glucuronic acid and β-1,3-*N*-acetyl-D-glucosamine, linked by β(1→3) bonds. Hyaluronan is a widely explored polymer in tissue engineering. Hyaluronan for tissue engineering has been focused on cartilage, bone, and osteochondral applications, most likely due to the fact that it is a major macromolecular component of the ECM (Liao et al., 2005; Malafaya et al., 2007). Commercially available products of hyaluronan are Hyalgan® and Hyalubrix® (Fidia, Italy), Artz® (Seikagaku Corporation, Japan), Bionect® (CSC Pharmaceutical, USA), Jossalind® (Hexal, Germany), Healon® (OVD, Advanced Medical Optics, USA), Opegan R® (Seikagaku, Japan), Opelead® (Shiseido, Japan), Orthovisc® (Anika, USA), and EmbryoGlue® (Vitrolife, USA) with widespread applications as support for the joints in osteoarthritis, surgery, and wound healing (Table 9.1).

9.4 HYDROGEL SCAFFOLDS

Hydrogels have exhibited tremendous research attention over recent decades for fundamental reasons as well as because of their potential for a wide range of applications. Hydrogels have been successfully used in biomedical fields due to their high water content and the consequent biocompatibility. Substances that absorb significant quantities of water are called gels or hydrogels. Naturally occurring materials with these properties play a very important role in all forms of life. Hydrogel is defined as a crosslinked three-dimensional polymeric network structure, which can absorb and retain considerable amounts of water (Rosiak and Yoshii, 1999). The water-holding capacity of hydrogels arises mainly due to the presence of hydrophilic groups, amino, carboxyl and hydroxyl groups, in the polymer chains.

Hydrogels are macromolecular networks that swell, but do not dissolve in water. The ability of hydrogels to absorb water arises from hydrophilic functional groups attached to the polymeric backbone, while their resistance to dissolution arises from crosslinks between network chains. Hydrogels have gained significant

Table 9.1 Classification of Natural Polymers with Their Specific Properties

S. No.	Polymer	Properties	Source	Gelation Method
1.	Cellulose and derivatives	Drug delivery	Plant sources	Physical, chemical crosslinking, or radical polymerization
2.	Carageenan	Drug delivery	Seaweed	Thermal and ionic crosslinking
3.	Alginates	Drug delivery and for cell entrapping	Seaweed	Thermal
4.	Gellan	Drug delivery	Bacteria	Thermal or ionotropic crosslinking
5.	Agarose	Low cell adhesivity and is nondegradable Drug delivery	Seaweed	Thermal
6.	Dextran	Drug delivery	Bacteria	Physical, chemical crosslinking, or radical polymerization
7.	Chitosan	Drug delivery, tissue regeneration	Crustaceans and fungi	Ionotrophic or covalent
8.	Hyaluronic acid	Drug delivery	Animal and human	Chemical crosslinking
9.	Poly (β-hydroxy butyrate) Poly (β-hydroxyvalerates)	Drug delivery	Bacteria	
10.	Collagen	Soft tissue, plastic surgery to fill up tissue defects and drug delivery	Animal and human	Neutralization
11.	Gelatin	Drug delivery	Animal and human	Thermal
12.	Fibrin	Different surgical applications to control bleeding and provide air and fluid tightness	Animal and human	Proteolytic cleavage

(*Continued*)

Table 9.1 Classification of Natural Polymers with Their Specific Properties *Continued*

S. No.	Polymer	Properties	Source	Gelation Method
13.	Poly(L-lactide)	Orthopedic surgery, oral and maxillofacial surgery	Synthetic	Physical, chemical crosslinking, or radical polymerization
14.	Poly(L-lactide-co-D, L-lactide) 70/30	Orthopedic surgery, oral and maxillofacial surgery	Synthetic	Physical, chemical crosslinking, or radical polymerization
15.	Polyanhydrides	Animal experiments	Synthetic	Physical, chemical crosslinking, or radical polymerization
16.	Polyorthoester	Drug delivery	Synthetic	Physical, chemical crosslinking, or radical polymerization
17.	Polycaprolacton	Drug delivery	Synthetic	Physical, chemical crosslinking, or radical polymerization

attention in last four or five decades, due to their wide range of applications. They also have a degree of flexibility very similar to natural tissues due to their large water content (Ahmed, 2015). They have advantages over other types of polymeric scaffolds, such as easy control of structural parameters, high water content, promising biocompatibility, and adjustable scaffold architecture. Generally hydrogels have biological character, such as high tissue-like water content and permeability for incursion of nutrients and excretion of metabolites. Cells entrapped in a 3D hydrogels milieu are surrounded by a gel matrix that does not promote attachment or potential phenotype differentiation, thus making hydrogels especially suitable for scaffolds in tissue engineering. These hydrophilic combination arrangements are being deliberated to imitate the transport and mechanical properties of natural soft tissue. Hydrogels can homogeneously incorporate and suspend cells as well as growth factors and other bioactive reagents while allowing rapid diffusion of hydrophilic nutrients and metabolites to the incorporated cells or surrounding tissue. One of the prerequisites for an effective tissue scaffold is that it degrades in a controlled manner so that when the bioreplacement is complete and functional *in vivo* none of the scaffolding materials remain (Ottenbrite et al., 2010).

Scaffolds for tissue engineering should fulfill the following requirements (Sokolsky-Papkov et al., 2007):

- It should have adequate mechanical properties corresponding to the tissue at which it implants satisfactorily to protect the cells from harmful or negative compressive or tensile forces without altering appropriate biomechanical indications.
- It possesses an acceptable biocompatibility and toxicity report.
- It should mimic the resident ECM, which acts as a signaling structure to aid in binding to tissues, cellular development, and morphogenesis.
- It should have adequate interstitial adherence so that cells or proteins can attach on the scaffold surface with improved cell–cell contact and cell migration.
- It should have an optimum degradation rate facilitating adsorption to the biological surface with a tendency to be replaced by growing tissue.

The natural polymer used to grow the initial living, tissue-engineered skin product was a collagen hydrogel. Even though the achievement of skin tissue engineering is cheering, efforts to fabricate other soft tissues have not shown comparable success. The progress in large measure is limited by inappropriate properties of the biomaterials currently available. The main features of hydrogels influencing their use in tissue engineering include (Kopeček, 2009):

- Chemical and biochemical stability;
- Shape stability and softness;
- Absence of extractable actives;

- High permeability for water-soluble nutrients and metabolites across the biomaterial–tissue interface;
- Suitable rheological properties;
- Good tissue compatibility;
- Convenience in handling;
- Ease of application;
- Excellent biocompatibility due to their high water content.

9.5 CLASSIFICATION OF HYDROGELS

The hydrogel products can be classified on different bases as:

A. Classification based on source
- Natural origin;
- Synthetic origin.

B. Classification based on polymeric composition
- Homopolymeric hydrogels: Polymer network derived from a single species of monomer;
- Copolymeric hydrogels: Comprised of two or more different monomer species with at least one hydrophilic component, arranged in a random, block, or alternating configuration along the chain of the polymer network;
- Multipolymer hydrogel: Made of two independent crosslinked synthetic and/or natural polymer components, contained in a network form.

C. Classification based on configuration/physical structure and chemical composition
- Amorphous;
- Semicrystalline;
- Crystalline.

D. Classification based on type of crosslinking
- Chemically crosslinked networks: Permanent junctions;
- Physical crosslinked networks: Transient junctions.

E. Classification based on physical appearance depending on the polymerization technique involved
- Matrix;
- Film;
- Microsphere.

F. Classification based on network electrical charge
- Nonionic (neutral);
- Ionic (including anionic or cationic);
- Amphoteric electrolyte (ampholytic);
- Zwitterionic (polybetaines).

9.6 METHOD OF FABRICATING HYDROGELS

Materials for the preparation of hydrogel scaffolds should be selected on the basis of their physical properties (mechanical strength and gel formation dynamics), the mass transport property (diffusion rations), and the biological interaction requirements (toxicity and allergic reaction) of each specific application. These properties are determined by the proposed scaffold application and surroundings into which the scaffold will be incorporated (Drury and Mooney, 2003). Hydrogels may be prepared in a variety of ways. These may include one-step procedures like polymerization or multiple-step procedures involving synthesis of polymer molecules having reactive groups and their subsequent crosslinking, possibly also by reacting polymers with suitable crosslinking agents (Ahmed, 2013).

A. Physical crosslinking
- **a.** Heating or cooling a polymer solution;
- **b.** Ionic interaction;
- **c.** Complex coacervation;
- **d.** Hydrogen bonding;
- **e.** Maturation or heat-induced aggregation;
- **f.** Freeze-thawing.

B. Chemical crosslinking
- **a.** Use of crosslinkers;
- **b.** Chemical grafting;
- **c.** Radiation grafting.

C. Radiation crosslinking
- **a.** Aqueous state radiation;
- **b.** Radiation in paste;
- **c.** Solid state radiation (crosslinking in solid state).

9.7 SCAFFOLD FABRICATION METHODS

- Dry–wet spinning;
- Emulsion templating extrusion;
- Solution casting and sphere leaching;
- Solvent-free solid-state foaming and ultrasound technique;
- Sodium chloride (NaCl) particulate leaching;
- Solvent-assisted room-temperature compression molding;
- Solvent casting;
- Spin casting;
- Modified slip-casting and supercritical-fluid processing;
- Thermal-induced phase separation (TIPS);
- Injection molding with rapid solvent evaporation;
- Paraffin-spheres-dissolution technique;

- Co-electrospinning;
- Controlled-rate freezing and lyophilization technique
- Sintering together composite chitosan/Poly(Lactide-co-Glycolide) (PLGA) microspheres;
- Melt-molding particulate-leaching method compression molding;
- Photocrosslinkable;
- Hydrogels: photopolymerization;
- Computer-controlled rapid prototyping selective laser sintering;
- Wet-spinning technique;
- Gas foaming technique;
- Freeze-drying method.

9.8 CURRENTLY APPLIED THREE-DIMENSIONAL SCAFFOLD FABRICATION TECHNOLOGIES

Following Technology use for three dimensional scaffold fabrication (Hutmacher, 2000).

- Solvent casting in combination with particular leaching;
- Membrane lamination;
- Fabrication of nonwoven;
- Melt molding;
- Extrusion in combination with particular leaching;
- Emulsion freeze-drying;
- TIPS;
- Supercritical-fluid technology;
- Supercritical-fluid technology in combination with particle leaching;
- 3D printing in and without combination of particle leaching;
- Fused deposition modeling.

9.9 CHARACTERIZATION OF HYDROGEL SCAFFOLD

A. Visual appearance

The hydrogels are visually inspected for clarity, color, and transparency, and further evaluated for the presence of any particles. Smears of gels are prepared on glass slides and observed under the microscope for the presence of any particle or grittiness.

B. pH of the hydrogel

The pH of gels is determined after diluting and dispersing it in distilled water (10%, w/v). One gram of hydrogel gel is mixed with 9 ml of water, and the pH of the resulting mixture is taken with a pH meter.

C. Clarity

The clarity of the hydrogel is determined by visual inspection under a black and white background.

D. Spreadability

To determine spreadability, a spreadability apparatus is used. It contains a wooden block having two glass plates. Initially, the hydrogel sample is placed between the two glass plates. Weight near 300 g is put on the top plate which expels the air to form a uniform gel layer. Afterwards, 100 g weight is used to drag the top plate by 10 cm using string attached to a hook. The time required to move the upper plate by 10 cm distance is noted, the less the time required for dragging the upper plate the better is the spreadability value. The spreadability value is determined with the help of the following formula:

$$S = \frac{M \times L}{T}$$

where, S is the spreadability value, L is the length of the glass slide, M is the weight tied to the upper plate, and T is the time taken to separate the glass slides.

E. Rheological study

Viscosities of cream are measured using viscometers, such as the Brookfield viscometer DV-E with spindle 3 at 3, 6, 12, 30, 60, 100 rpm under room temperature.

9.10 *IN VITRO* DRUG RELEASE

An *in vitro* release study is carried out in modified a Franz diffusion cell using treated semipermeable membrane in between the donor and receiver compartments. The normal surface of the Franz diffusion cells is 5.53 cm^2 and the receiver compartment has a capacity of approximately 100 ml. In drug release studies, semipermeable membranes are mounted in Franz diffusion cells and the membrane surface is dosed with drug-loaded hydrogel. Receptor fluid is added to the cell and the temperature is maintained at 37 ± 5 °C. The dissolution medium is stirred at 50–100 rpm using Teflon-coated magnetic beads. Aliquots, each of 5 ml volume, are withdrawn periodically at predetermined time intervals of 1–8 h, and replaced by an equal volume of the receptor medium. The aliquots are further subjected to analysis by various spectrophotometric methods.

9.11 APPLICATIONS OF HYDROGELS

The phenomenal properties of hydrogels continue to stimulate researchers and scientists to search for new ideas in the development of novel biomaterials and bioapplications. Hydrogels are smart polymers to use as scaffolds for tissue engineering (Peppas et al., 2006) and in a diverse range of applications, due to their structural similarities to body tissues (Drury and Mooney, 2003). Furthermore, they can be easily modified to alter their properties and can be directed to targeted delivery, increasing time, and a reduction in toxicity and side effects. Fibroblasts, osteoblasts, vascular smooth muscle cells, and chondrocytes successfully immobilize and attach to hydrogel scaffolds (Peppas et al., 2006). The combination of high water content, biocompatibility, excellent mechanical properties, and minimally invasive delivery capability makes hydrogels particularly attractive for tissue engineering applications (Drury and Mooney, 2003; Peppas et al., 2006). Hydrogels have been widely used as scaffolds for wound healing (Table 9.2), tissue engineering, and as immune-isolation barriers for microencapsulation technology in which allogeneic or xenogeneic cells are protected from the host's immune system through separation from the immune components via a semipermeable membrane. Successful examples of the application of hydrogel in the biomedical field includes soft contact lenses (Compan et al., 2002), wound dressings (Azad et al., 2004), super absorbents (Lionetto et al., 2003; Zohuriaan and Pourjavadi, 2003), and drug-delivery systems (Kim et al., 1992). The latest and stimulating applications of hydrogels are cell-based therapeutics (Jen et al., 1996; Lysaght, 1999) and soft tissue engineering (Lee et al., 2001a, 2001b). Hydrogel scaffolds are also being widely used in the area of nonload-bearing bone tissue engineering. In general, hydrogels do not possess the mechanical strength to be used in load-bearing applications, but can be placed into critical defects in a minimally invasive manner to promote regeneration, which would not otherwise occur. Both alginate and HA have been used in this application (Drury and Mooney, 2003).

Hydrogel scaffolds stabilize and deliver bioactive molecules and encapsulate secretory cells and stem cells. Currently, the majority of small- and large-molecule drugs are delivered into patients systemically without the use of a scaffold. The desired local effect requires large doses to avoid loss of drug by enzymatic degradation of the drug and nonspecific uptake by other tissues leading to other associated side effects. Hydrogel scaffolds are made up of three-dimensional networks of polymers providing a place for cells to adhere, proliferate, and differentiate. They also serve as signaling systems by lodging growth factors. Currently, hydrogel scaffolds are being used in an attempt to engineer a wide range of tissues, including cartilage, bone, muscle, fat, liver, and neurons. Various growth factors and stem cells are delivered by using a hydrogel scaffold (Table 9.3).

9.12 OTHER SCAFFOLDS

9.12.1 POROUS SCAFFOLD

Porous scaffolds are three-dimensional polymeric porous scaffolds with higher porosities and a homogeneous interconnected pore network are highly useful for tissue engineering. Sponge or foam porous scaffolds have been used in tissue engineering applications (Zhang, 1999; Dhandayuthapani et al., 2011).

Table 9.2 Natural Polymer Hydrogels as Scaffold for Wound Healing

S. No.	Types of Polymers	Characteristics for Wound Healing	Reference
1.	Collagen	Provides structural support and controls many cellular functions, including cell shape and differentiation, migration, and synthesis of a number of proteins essential in wound management	Shen et al. (2008)
2.	Hyaluronic acid and its derivatives	Interacts with protein proteoglycan growth factor and tissue components (biomolecule) which has vital importance in healing of various type of wound and acts with fibrin to support the influx of fibroblasts and endothelial cells into the wound site and the subsequent formation of granulation tissue	Park et al. (2003)
3.	Chitosan and its derivatives	Chitosan is the hemostatic agent which accelerates the formation of fibroblasts and increases early-phase reactions related to healing. It inhibits fibroplasia in wound healing and promotes tissue growth	Ueno et al. (1999)
4.	Fucoidan	Provides the moisture balance in wound/burn area, accelerates the migration of fibroblasts and provides re-epithelialization. It shows anticoagulant effect and heparin activity	Sezer et al. (2007)
5.	Poly-*N*-acetyl glucosamine	Wound and burn healing due to hemostatic property. It accelerates wound closure mainly by re-epithelialization and increased keratinocyte migration, granulation tissue formation, cell proliferation, and vascularization compared with control wounds	Pietramaggiori et al. (2008)
6.	Alginic acid and its salts	Alginate is the hemostatic agent which maintains a physiologically moist microenvironment that promotes healing and the formation of granulation tissue. Alginate dressings are very useful for moderate to heavily exudating wounds	Thomas et al. (1989)
7.	Microbial cellulose	Synthesized in abundance by *Acetobacter xylinum* shows vast potential as a novel wound-healing system	Czajaa et al. (2006)

(*Continued*)

Table 9.2 Natural Polymer Hydrogels as Scaffold for Wound Healing *Continued*

S. No.	Types of Polymers	Characteristics for Wound Healing	Reference
8.	Lysostaphin-functionalized cellulose fiber	Used as a antimicrobial matrix in wound-healing applications due to their good biocompatibility	Miao (2011)
9.	Sodium carboxymethyl cellulose	Partial-thickness wound healing	Ramli and Wong (2011)
10.	Dextran	Dextran-based hydrogels can serve as instructive scaffolds to promote neovascularization (critical determinant of wound-healing outcomes for deep burn injuries) and skin regeneration in third-degree burn wounds. It promotes dermal regeneration with complete skin appendages	
11.	Alginate + chitosan + polyglutamic acid	Used for full-thickness wound healing in diabetic rat model	Lee (2012)
12.	Gelatin	Used as a wound-healing material due to its excellent biocompatibility and controllable biodegradation	Yang and Xu et al. (2010)
13.	Fibronectin	Supports formation of proper substratum for migration and growth of cells with remodeling and resynthesis of the connective tissue matrix	George (1993)
14.	Hydroxyapatite and silk fibroin composites	Higher promotive effects on wound healing, re-epithelialization, and matrix formation	Okabayashi et al. (2009)

Table 9.3 Various Bioactives Delivered Using Hydrogel Scaffolds

Hydrogel System/Scaffold	Delivered	Outcome/Application	References
Gel	Platelet Derived Growth Factor (PDGF)	Increased angiogenesis, cell proliferation, and epithelialization	Li et al. (2008)
Collagen/gelatin sponge	Basic fibroblast growth factor	Improved wound healing	Morimoto et al. (2012)
Collagen gel	BMP-2 gene	Bone/cartilage tissue engineering application	Xu et al. (2005)
Collagen gel	PDGF-A and -B gene	Skin regeneration	Chandler et al. (2000)
Collagen/hydroxyapatite	Nerve growth factor	Bone tissue engineering application	Letic-Gavrilovic et al. (2003)
Glutaraldehyde crosslinked collagen sponges	Vascular Endothelial Growth Factor (VEGF)	Improved angiogenesis	Peters et al. (1998)
Heparin alginate gels	Basic fibroblast growth factor	Enhanced angiogenesis	Tabata et al. (2000)
Chitosan freeze-dried scaffolds	PDGF-BB	Enhanced bone formation	Lee et al. (2002)
Chitosan/collagen scaffolds	Human periodontal ligament cells	Periodontal tissue engineering	Zhang et al. (2006)
Fibrin gel in a fiber-based scaffold	Human venous myofibroblasts	Cardiovascular tissue engineering	Mol et al. (2005)
Photocrosslinkable chitosan hydrogel	Fibroblast growth factor-2	Stimulates wound healing	Obara et al. (2003)
Fibrin scaffold	Murine embryonic stem cells	Increased differentiation of stem cells	Willerth et al. (2006)
Gelatin (hydrogel)	Basic fibroblast growth factor	Increased protein release	Tabata and Ikada (1998)
Gelatin microspheres encapsulated in a hydrogel injectable matrix	TGF-β1 and IGF-I	Cartilage tissue engineering	Holland et al. (2005)
Transglutaminase crosslinked gelatin (hydrogel)	Vitronectin/fibronectin	–	Ito et al. (2003)

(*Continued*)

Table 9.3 Various Bioactives Delivered Using Hydrogel Scaffolds *Continued*

Hydrogel System/Scaffold	Delivered	Outcome/Application	References
Gelatin microspheres incorporated in collagen hydrogel	Fibroblast growth factor-2	Adipose tissue engineering	Vashi et al. (2006)
Fibrin–collagen gel	Embryonic chondrogenic cells	Increases joint cartilage repair	Perka et al. (2000)
Poly Lactide-Poly Ethylene Glycol (PLA-PEG) system	Bone morphogenic protein-2	Ectopic bone formation	Edelman et al. (1991)
Silk fibroin fiber scaffolds	Bone morphogenic protein-2	Bone tissue engineering	Li et al. (2006)
Freeze-dried chitosan scaffolds	Chondrocytes	Decreased collagen II deposition	Lee et al. (2001a, 2001b), Bryant and Anseth (2002)
Chitosan scaffolds	Insulin-like growth factor and TGF-β	Maintained chondrocytes in a proliferative state	Elisseeff et al. (2001)
Hyaluronic acid gel	Platelet	Enhance granulation tissue formation	Crovetti et al. (2004)
HA-containing alginate system	–	Increase both chondrocyte proliferation and protein secretion	Lindenhayn et al. (1999)
Hyaffs11 (commercially available HA) scaffold	Bone marrow stromal cells	Increase mineralization and healing	Facchini (2002)
Hydrogel	VEGF	Enhanced wound healing	Galiano et al. (2004)
Gel	Recombinant PDGF	Increases re-epithelialization	Cheng et al. (2007)
Chitosan crosslinked collagen sponge	Recombinant human acidic fibroblast growth factor	Decrease healing time	Wang et al. (2008)
Arginine and epidermal growth factor	Hyaluronic acid sponge	Decreased wound size by increasing the epithelialization	Matsumoto and Kuroyanagi (2010)
Collagen-gelatin sponge	Basic Fibroblast Growth Factor (bFGF)	Increased angiogenesis to promote wound healing	Kanda et al. (2014)
AL–CS–Polyglycolic Acid (PGA) hydrogel	–	Increase wound healing	Lee et al. (2012a, 2012b)

Carbopol hydrogel	Atorvastatin	Increased wound healing	Aly (2012)
5-Methyl pyrrolidinone chitosan dressing	Neurotensin	Reduced inflammatory status, improve wound healing, re-epithelialization	Moura et al. (2014a, 2014b)
Collagen dressings	Neurotensin	Reduced inflammatory cytokine, TNF-α, IL-1β, and Matrix Metalloproteinases (MMPs)	Moura et al. (2014a, 2014b)
PEG scaffolds	Adhesion proteins	Increase collagen production by smooth muscle cells	Kim et al. (2012)
Methylcellulose film	HoxD3 plasmid DNA	Significant acceleration of wound closure by increasing mRNA expression	Hansen et al. (2003)
Electrospun collagen scaffold	Mesenchymal stem cells	Enhancing wound healing	Nithya (2013)
Atelocollagen matrix	Adipose tissue-derived stromal cells	Accelerating wound healing	Nambu et al. (2009)
Poly Vinyl Alcohol (PVA)-gelatin hydrogel	Gentamicin and serratioeptidase co-delivery	Accelerated and complete wound healing	Singh and Rawat (2012)

9.12.2 FIBROUS SCAFFOLD

As indicated by the name, a fibrous scaffold consists of fibers and nanofibers. The development of nanofibers has improved the range of fabricating scaffolds that can potentially imitate the architecture of natural tissue at the lower scale. Nanofibers synthesized by self-assembly and phase separation have had comparatively restricted studies exploring their application as scaffolds for tissue engineering (Zhang, 1999; Dhandayuthapani et al., 2011).

9.12.3 MICROSPHERE SCAFFOLD

Microsphere-based tissue engineering scaffold designs have gathered significant attention in recent years. Microsphere scaffolds having spatial extension and temporal duration control, which provides the stiffness gradients for interfacial tissue engineering. Microsphere scaffolds are increasingly used as drug delivery systems and in advanced tissue engineering applications (Stephens et al., 2000; Singh et al., 2008, 2010; Dhandayuthapani et al., 2011).

9.12.4 ACELLULAR SCAFFOLD

Acellular tissue matrices can be primed by manufacturing artificial scaffolds or by removing cellular components from tissues by mechanical and chemical manipulation to produce collagen-rich matrices. These matrices slowly degrade on implantation and are generally replaced by the ECM proteins secreted by in-growing cells. Acellular tissue matrices have been proven to support cell in-growth and regeneration of genitourinary tissues, including urethra and bladder, with no evidence of immunogenic rejection (Dahms et al., 1998; Yoo, 1998; Dhandayuthapani et al., 2011).

9.13 FUTURE PERSPECTIVES

The field of tissue engineering has advanced dramatically in the last 10 years, offering the potential for regenerating almost every tissue and organ of the human body. Various types of natural and synthetic hydrogels are used for repairing and regenerating a wide variety of tissues and organs. Specifically, natural polymers have been critically evaluated as they provide the biophysical and biochemical environment for optimum expression of cellular behavior with effective tissue replacement and restoration. The skill to fabricate hydrogels has created new prospects in facing the challenges and obstacles in tissue engineering. Hydrogels are appealing materials for use as scaffolds in tissue engineering due to their large water content, which approximates the properties of soft tissue. Composition of hydrogels strongly mimics the combination of fibrous proteins and hydrophilic proteoglycans found *in vivo*. Fabricating of materials, proportions, and arrangement of the constituents of the scaffold allows for tuning with different cellular microenvironments. A variety of hydrogel scaffold systems has been prepared and studied for use in tissue engineering. Combinational and multiphase hydrogel systems have been established to improve troubles that arise throughout the duration of the scaffold *in vivo*. At the same time, the properties of materials used for fabricating scaffold are vastly dependent on fabricated and designed systems. Promising avenues of research include use of natural polymers for developing hydrogels, inclusion of stem cells and bioactives during scaffold fabrication. The use of hydrogel scaffolds has also allowed the ability to affect both systemic and topical or local properties. This chapter mainly focused on natural polymers used for fabricating hydrogel scaffolds, type, classification, property, and application of hydrogel as scaffolds in the treatment of wounds and other diseases, with the ultimate goal of clinical tissue regeneration. Scaffolds can also be promising models to examine cellular behavior, signaling pathways, and environmental interactions.

ACKNOWLEDGMENTS

The authors are thankful to Director, University Institute of Pharmacy, Pt. Ravishankar Shukla University, Raipur, Chhattisgarh, India for providing all necessary facilities for carrying out this work and University Grants Commission No. F. 7-341/2011 (BSR)/2014 and DST-FIST for financial assistance.

REFERENCES

Ahmed, E.M., 2013. Hydrogel: preparation, characterization, and application. J. Adv. Res. Available from: http://dx.doi.org/10.1016/j.jare.2013.07.006.

Ahmed, E.M., 2015. Hydrogel: preparation, characterization, and applications: a review. J. Adv. Res. 6 (2), 105–121.

Aly, U.F., 2012. Preparation and evaluation of novel topical gel preparations for wound healing in diabetics. Int. J. Pharm. Pharm. Sci. 4, 76–77.

Augst, A.D., Kong, H.J., Mooney, D.J., 2006. Alginate hydrogels as biomaterials. Macromol. Biosci. 6 (8), 623–633.

Azad, A.K., Sermsintham, N., Chandrkrachang, S., Stevens, W.F., 2004. Chitosan membrane as a wound-healing dressing: characterization and clinical application. J. Biomed. Mater. Res. 69, 216–222.

Berisio, R., Vitagliano, L., Mazzarella, L., Zagari, A., 2002. Recent progress on collagen triple helix structure, stability and assembly. Prot. Pept. Lett. 9, 107–116.

Boudriot, U., Dersch, R., Greiner, A., Wendorff, J.H., 2006. Electrospinning approaches toward scaffold engineering - a brief overview. Art. Organs 30, 785–792.

Brannon-Peppas, L., Harland, R.S., 1991. Absorbent polymer technology. J. Control. Release 173, 297–298.

Bret, D., 2008. A review of collagen and collagen-based wound dressings. Wounds 20, 12.

Brown, R.A., Bunting, S.C.J., Hall, S.M., Phillips, J.B., 2005. Tissue Eng. 11 (9–10), 1611–1617. Available from: http://dx.doi.org/10.1089/ten.2005.11.1611.

Bryant, S.J., Anseth, K.S., 2002. Hydrogel properties influence ECM production by chondrocytes photoencapsulated in poly(ethylene glycol) hydrogels. J. Biomed. Mater. Res. 59, 63–72.

Chandler, L.A., Gu, D.L., Ma, C.L., Gonzalez, A.M., Doukas, J., Nguyen, T., et al., 2000. Matrix-enabled gene transfer for cutaneous wound repair. Wound Repair Regen. 8, 473–479.

Chau, D.Y.S., Collighan, R.J., Verderio, E.A.M., Victoria, L., Addyc, V.L., Martin Griffinb, M., 2005. The cellular response to transglutaminase-cross-linked collagen. Biomaterials 26 (33), 6518–6529.

Cheng, B., Liu, H.W., Fu, X.B., Sun, T.Z., Sheng, Z.Y., 2007. Recombinant human platelet-derived growth factor enhanced dermal wound healing by a pathway involving ERK and c-fos in diabetic rats. J. Dermatol. Sci. 45, 193–201.

Chereddy, K.K., Her, C.H., Comune, M., Moia, C., Lopes, A., Porporato, P.E., et al., 2014. PLGA nanoparticles loaded with host defense peptide LL37 promote wound healing. J. Con. Rel. 194, 138–147.

Compan, V., Andrio, A., Lopez-Alemany, A., Riande, E., Refojo, M.F., 2002. Oxygen permeability of contact lenses with organo silicon moieties. Biomaterials 23, 2767–2772.

Crovetti, G., Martinelli, G., Issi, M., Barone, M., Guizzardi, M., Campanati, B., et al., 2004. Platelet gel for healing cutaneous chronic wounds. Transfus. Apher. Sci. 30, 145–151.

Cushing, M.C., Anseth, K.S., 2007. Hydrogel cell cultures. Science 316, 1133–1134.

Czajaa, W., Krystynowicza, A., Bieleckia, S., Brown Jr, R.M., 2006. Microbial cellulose—the natural power to heal wounds. Biomaterials 27, 145–151.

Dahms, S.E., Piechota, H., Dahiya, R., Lue, T.F., Tanagho, E.A., 1998. Composition and biomechanical properties of the bladder acellularmatrix graft: comparative analysis in rat, pig and human. Br. J. Urol. 82 (3), 411–419.

Dang, J.M., Leong, K.W., 2006. Natural polymers for gene delivery and tissue engineering. Adv. Drug Deliv. Rev. 58, 487–499.

Danielsson, C., Ruault, S., Basset-Dardare, A., Frey, P., 2006. Modified collagen fleece, a scaffold for transplantation of human bladder smooth muscle cells. Biomaterials 27, 1054–1060.

Davidenko, N., Campbell, J.J., Thian, E.S., Watson, C.J., Cameron, R.E., 2010. Collagen-hyaluronic acid scaffolds for adipose tissue engineering. Acta Biomater. 6 (10), 3957–3968.

Denizli, B.K., Can, H.K., Rzaev, Z.M.O., Guner, A., 2004. Preparation conditions and swelling equilibria of dextran hydrogels prepared by some crosslinked agents. Polymer 45 (19), 6431–6435.

Dhandayuthapani, B., Yoshida, Y., Maekawa, T., Kumar, D.S., 2011. Polymeric scaffolds in tissue engineering application: a review. Int. J. Poly. Sci.Article ID 290602,19. Available from: http://dx.doi.org/10.1155/2011/290602.

Djagny, K.B., Wang, Z., Xu, S., 2001. Gelatin: a valuable protein for food and pharmaceutical industries: review. Crit. Rev. Food Sci. Nutr. 41, 481–492.

Drury, J.L., Mooney, D.J., 2003. Hydrogels for tissue engineering: scaffold design variables and applications. Biomaterials 24, 4337–4351.

Edelman, E.R., Mathiowitz, E., Langer, R., Klagsbrun, M., 1991. Controlled and modulated release of basicfibroblast growth factor. Biomaterials 12, 619–626.

Ehrick, J.D., Deo, S.K., Browning, T.W., Bachas, L.G., Madou, M.J., Daunert, S., 2005. Genetically engineered protein in hydrogels tailors stimuli-responsive characteristic. Nat. Mater. 4, 298–302.

Elisseeff, J., McIntosh, W., Fu, K., Blunk, T., Langer, R., 2001. Controlled release of IGF-1 and TGF-b1 in a photopolymerizing hydrogel for cartilage tissue engineering. J. Orthop. Res. 19, 1098–1104.

Facchini, A., 2002. Osteogenesis of large segmental radius defects enhanced by basic fibroblast growth factor activated bone marrow stromal cells grown on non-woven hyaluronic acid-based polymer scaffold. Biomaterials 23, 1043–1051.

Foo, C.W.P., Kaplan, D.L., 2002. Genetic engineering of fibrous proteins: spider dragline silk and collagen. Adv. Drug Deliv. Rev. 54, 1131–1143.

Galiano, R.D., Tepper, O.M., Pelo, C.R., Bhatt, K.A., Callaghan, M., Bastidas, N., et al., 2004. Topical vascular endothelial growth factor accelerates diabetic wound healing through increased angiogenesis and by mobilizing and recruiting bone marrow-derived cells. Am. J. Pathol. 164, 1935–1947.

George, E.L., Labouesse, G., Patel-King, R.S., Rayburn, H., Hynes, R.O., 1993. Defects in mesoderm, neural tube and vascular development in mouse embryos lacking fibronectin. Development 119, 1079–1091.

Glowacki, J., Mizuno, S., 2007. Collagen scaffolds for tissue engineering. Biopolymers 89 (5), 338–344.

Hansen, S.L., Myers, C.A., Charboneau, A., Young, D.M., Boudreau, N., 2003. HoxD3 accelerates wound healing in diabetic mice. Am. J. Pathol. 163, 2421–2431.

Holland, T.A., Tabata, Y., Mikos, A.G., 2005. Dual growth factor delivery from degradable oligo(poly(ethylene glycol) fumarate) hydrogel scaffolds for cartilage tissue engineering. J. Control. Release 101, 111–125.

Huang, S., Fu, X., 2010. Naturally derived material-based cell and drug delivery systems in skin regeneration. J. Control. Release 142, 149–159.

Hutmacher, D.W., 2000. Scaffolds in tissue engineering bone and cartilage. Biomaterials 21, 2529–2543.

Ito, A., Mase, A., Takizawa, Y., Shinkai, M., Honda, H., Hata, K.I., et al., 2003. Transglutaminase-mediated gelatin matrices incorporating cell adhesion factors as a biomaterial for tissue engineering. J. Biosci. Bioeng. 95, 196–199.

Janmey, P.A., Winer, J.P., Weisel, J.W., 2009. Fibrin gels and their clinical and bioengineering applications. J. R. Soc. Interface 6 (30), 1–10. Available from: http://dx.doi.org/10.1098/rsif.2008.0327.

Jen, A.C., Wake, M.C., Mikos, A.G., 1996. Hydrogels for cell immobilization. Biotechnol. Bioeng. 50, 357–364.

Kanda, N., Morimoto, N., Ayvazyan, A.A., Takemoto, S., Kawai, K., Nakamura, Y., et al., 2014. Evaluation of a novel collagen-gelatin scaffold for achieving the sustained release of basic fibroblast growth factor in a diabetic mouse model. J. Tissue Eng. Regen. Med. 8, 29–40.

Kim, S.W., Bae, Y.H., Okano, T., 1992. Hydrogels: swelling, drug loading and release. Pharm. Res. 9, 283–290.

Kim, S.W., Zhang, H.Z., Guo, L., Kim, J.M., Kim, M.H., 2012. Amniotic mesenchymal stem cells enhance wound healing in diabetic NOD/SCID mice through high angiogenic and engraftment capabilities. PLoS One 7, e41105.

Kimelman-Bleich, N., Pelled, G., Sheyn, D., 2009. The use of a synthetic oxygen carrier-enriched hydrogel to enhance mesenchymal stem cell-based bone formation *in vivo*. Biomaterials 30 (27), 4639–4648.

Kimura, Y., Ozeki, M., Inamoto, T., Tabata, Y., 2003. Adipose tissue engineering based on human preadipocytes combined with gelatin microspheres containing basic fibroblast growth factor. Biomaterials 24, 2513–2521.

Kopeček, J.Y., 2009. Hydrogels from soft contact lenses and implants to self-assembled nanomaterials. J. Polym. Sci. A Polym. Chem. 47, 5929–5946.

Langer, R., Vacanti, J., 1993. Tissue engineering. Science 260, 920–926.

Lee, K.Y., Mooney, D.J., 2001. Hydrogel for tissue engineering. Chem. Rev. 101, 1869–1879.

Lee, Y.H., Chang, J.J., Yang, M.C., Chien, C.T., Lai, W.F., 2012. Acceleration of wound healing in diabetic rats by layered hydrogel dressing. Carbohydr. Polym. 88 (3), 809–819.

Lee, C.H., Singla, A., Lee, Y., 2001a. Biomedical applications of collagen. Int. J. Pharmacogn. 221, 1–22.

Lee, C.R., Grodzinsky, A.J., Spector, M., 2001b. The effects of cross-linking of collagen-glycosaminoglycan scaffolds on compressive stiffness, chondrocyte-mediated contraction, proliferation, and biosynthesis. Biomaterials 22, 3145–3154.

Lee, J.Y., Nam, S.H., Im, S.Y., Park, Y.J., Lee, Y.M., Seol, Y.J., et al., 2002. Enhanced bone formation by controlled growth factor delivery from chitosan-based biomaterials. J. Control. Release 78, 187–197.

Lee, C.K., Shin, S.R., Lee, S.H., Jeon, J.H., So, I., Kang, T.M., et al., 2008. DNA hydrogel fiber with self-entanglement prepared by using an ionic liquid. Angew. Chem. Int. Ed. 47 (13), 2470–2474.

Lee, Y., Chang, J.J., Yang, M.C., Chien, C.T., Lai, W.F., 2012a. Acceleration of wound healing in diabetic rats by layered hydrogel dressing. Carbohydr. Polym. 88, 809–819.

Lee, Y.H., Chang, J.J., Chien, C.T., Yang, M.C., 2012b. Antioxidant sol-gel improves cutaneous wound healing in streptozotocin-induced diabetic rats. Exp. Diabet. Res. 2012, 504693. Available from: http://dx.doi.org/10.1155/2012/504693.

Letic-Gavrilovic, A., Piattelli, A., Abe, K., 2003. Nerve growth factor beta delivery via a collagen/hydroxyapatite composite and its effects on new bone growth. J. Mater. Sci. Mater. Ed. 14, 95–102.

Li, C., Vepari, C., Jin, H.J., Kim, H.J., Kaplan, D.L., 2006. Electrospun silk-BMP-2 scaffolds for bone tissue engineering. Biomaterials 27, 3115–3124.

Li, H., Fu, X., Zhang, L., Huang, Q., Wu, Z., Sun, T., 2008. Research of PDGF-BB gel on the wound healing of diabetic rats and its pharmacodynamics. J. Surg. Res. 145, 41–48.

Liao, Y.H., Jones, S.A., Forbes, B., Martin, G.P., Brown, M.B., 2005. Hyaluronan: pharmaceutical characterization and drug delivery. Drug Deliv. 12, 327–342.

Lindenhayn, K., Perka, C., Spitzer, R.S., Heilmann, H.H., Pommerening, K., Mennicke, J., et al., 1999. Retention of hyaluronic acid in alginate beads: aspects for *in vitro* cartilage tissue engineering. J. Biomed. Mater. Res. 44, 149–155.

Lionetto, F., Sannino, A., Mensitieri, G., Maffezzoli, A., 2003. Evaluation of the degree of crosslinking of cellulose-based hydrogels: a comparison between different techniques. Macromol. Symp. 200, 199–207.

Lysaght, M.J., Reyes, J., 2001. The growth of tissue engineering. Tissue Eng. 7 (5), 485–493. Available from: http://dx.doi.org/10.1089/107632701753213110.

Malafaya, P.B., Silva, G.A., Reis, R.L., 2007. Natural−origin polymers as carriers and scaffolds for biomolecules and cell delivery in tissue engineering applications. Adv. Drug Del. Rev 59, 207−233.

Marinucci, L., Lilli, C., Guerra, M., Belcastro, S., Becchetti, E., Stabellini, G., et al., 2003. Biocompatibility of collagen membranes crosslinked with glutaraldehyde or diphenylphosphoryl azide: an in vitro study. J. Biomed. Mat. Res. A 67 (2), 504−509.

Matsumoto, Y., Kuroyanagi, Y., 2010. Development of a wound dressing composed of hyaluronic acid sponge containing arginine and epidermal growth factor. J. Biomater. Sci. Polym. Ed. 21, 715−726.

Miao, J., Pangule, R.C., Paskaleva, E.E., Hwang, E.E., Kane, R.S., Linhardt, R.J., et al., 2011. Lysostaphin-functionalized cellulose fibers with antistaphylococcal activity for wound healing applications. Biomaterials 32 (36), 9557−9567.

Mol, A., van Lieshout, M.I., Dam-de Veen, C.G., Neuenschwander, S., Hoerstrup, S.P., Baaijens, F.P.T., et al., 2005. Fibrin as a cell carrier in cardiovascular tissue engineering applications. Biomaterials 26, 3113−3121.

Morimoto, N., Yoshimura, K., Niimi, M., Ito, T., Tada, H., Teramukai, S., et al., 2012. An exploratory clinical trial for combination wound therapy with a novel medical matrix and fibroblast growth factor in patients with chronic skin ulcers: a study protocol. Am. J. Transl. Res. 4, 52−59.

Moura, L.I.F., Dias, A.M.A., Leal, E.C., Carvalho, L., De Sousa, H.C., Carvalho, E., 2014a. Chitosan-based dressings loaded with Neurotensin—an efficient strategy to improve early diabetic wound healing. Acta Biomater. 2, 843−857.

Moura, L.I.F., Dias, A.M.A., Suesca, E., Casadiegos, S., Leal, E.C., Fontanilla, M.R., et al., 2014b. Neurotensin-loaded collagen dressings reduce inflammation and improve wound healing in diabetic mice. Biochim. Biophys. Acta 1842, 32−43.

Nam, H.S., An, J., Chung, D.J., Kim, J.H., Chung, C.P., 2006. Controlled release behavior of bioactive molecules from photo-reactive hyaluronic acid-alginate scaffolds. Macromol. Res. 14, 530−538.

Nambu, M., Kishimoto, S., Nakamura, S., Mizuno, H., Yanagibayashi, S., Yamamoto, N., et al., 2009. Accelerated wound healing in healing-impaired db/db mice by autologous adipose tissue-derived stromal cells combined with atelocollagen matrix. Ann. Plast. Surg. 62, 317−321.

Nerem, R.M., 1991. Cellular engineering. Ann. Biomed. Eng. 19 (5), 529−545.

Nithya, T.G., 2013. Efficacy of mesenchymal stem cell incorporation in different composite electrospun collagen nanofibers for diabetic wound healing. Asian J. Pharm. Clin. Res. 6, 149−152.

Obara, K., Ishihara, M., Ishizuka, T., Fujita, M., Ozeki, Y., Maehara, T., et al., 2003. Photocrosslinkable chitosan hydrogel containing fibroblast growth factor-2 stimulates wound healing in healing-impaired db/db mice. Biomaterials 24, 3437−3444.

Okabayashi, R., Nakamura, M., Okabayashi, T., Tanaka, Y., Nagai, A., Yamashita, K., 2009. Efficacy of polarized hydroxyapatite and silk fibroin composite dressing gel on epidermal recovery from full-thickness skin wounds. J. Biomed. Mat. Res. B Appl Biomater. 90B (2), 641−646.

Ottenbrite, R.M., Park, K., Okano, T. (Eds.), 2010. Biomedical Applications of Hydrogels Handbook. Springer-Verlag, New York.

Pachence, J.M., 1996. Collagen-based devices for soft tissue repair. J. Biomed. Mat. Res. 33 (1), 35−40.

Park, Y.D., Tirelli, N., Hubbel, J.A., 2003. Photopolymerized hyaluronic acid-based hydrogels and interpenetrating networks. Biomaterials 24, 893–900.

Park, H., Temenoff, J.S., Holland, T.A., Tabata, Y., Mikos, A.G., 2005. Delivery of TGF-beta1 and chondrocytes via injectable, biodegradable hydrogels for cartilage tissue engineering applications. Biomaterials 26, 7095–7103.

Park, N., Kahn, J., Rice, E.J., Hartman, M.R., Funabashi, H., Xu, J., et al., 2009. High-yield cell-free protein production from P-gel. Nat. Protoc. 4 (12), 1759–1770.

Peppas, N.A., Hilt, J.Z., Khademhosseini, A., Langer, R., 2006. Hydrogels in biology and medicine: from molecular principles to bionanotechnology. Adv. Mater. 18, 1345–1360.

Peppasa, N.A., Buresa, P., Leobandunga, W., Ichikawab, H., 2000. Hydrogels in pharmaceutical formulations. Eur. J. Pharm. Biopharm. 50, 27–46.

Perka, C., Schultz, O., Lindenhayn, K., Spitzer, R.S., Muschik, M., Sittinger, M., et al., 2000. Joint cartilage repair with transplantation of embryonic chondrocytes embedded in collagen–fibrin matrices. Clin. Exp. Rheumatol. 18, 13–22.

Peters, M.C., Isenberg, B.C., Rowley, J.A., Mooney, D.J., 1998. Release from alginate enhances the biological activity of vascular endothelial growth factor. J. Biomater. Sci. Polym. Ed. 12, 1267–1278.

Pietramaggiori, G., Yang, H.J., Scherer, S.S., Kaipainen, A., Chan, R.K., Alperovich, M., et al., 2008. Effects of poly-N-acetyl glucosamine (pGlcNAc) patch on wound healing in db/db mouse. J. Trauma 64, 803–808.

Ponticiello, M.S., Schinagl, R.M., Kadiyala, S., Barry, F.P., 2000. Gelatin-based resorbable sponge as a carrier matrix for human mesenchymal stem cells in cartilage regeneration therapy. J. Biomed. Mater. Res. 52, 246–255.

Powella, H.M., Boycea, S.T., 2006. EDC cross-linking improves skin substitute strength and stability. Biomaterials 27 (34), 5821–5827.

Ramakrishna, S., Mayer, J., Wintermantel, E., Leong, K.W., 2001. Biomedical applications of polymer-composite materials: a review. Comp. Sci. Technol. 61 (9), 1189–1224.

Ramamurthi, A., Vesely, I., 2003. Ultraviolet light-induced modification of crosslinked hyaluronan gels. J. Biomed. Mater. Res. A 66 (2), 317–329.

Ramli, N.A., Wong, T.W., 2011. Sodium carboxymethylcellulose scaffolds and their physicochemical effects on partial thickness wound healing. Int. J. Pharm. 403 (1–2), 73–82.

Rault, I., Frei, V., Herbage, D., Abdul-Malak, N., Huc, A., 1996. Evaluation of different chemical methods for cros-linking collagen gel, films and sponges. J. Mat. Sci. Mater. Med. 7 (4), 215–221.

Rodriguez-Cabello, J.C., Reguera, J., Girotti, A.M., Testera, A.M., 2005. Developing functionality in elastin-like polymers by increasing their molecular complexity: the power of the genetic engineering approach. Prog. Polym. Sci. 30, 1119–1145.

Rosiak, J.M., Yoshii, F., 1999. Hydrogels and their medical applications. Nucl. Inst. Meth. Phy. Res. B Beam Inter. Mat. Atoms 151 (1), 56–64.

Sakai, S., Hirose, K., Taguchi, K., Ogushi, Y., Kawakami, K., 2009. An injectable, *in situ* enzymatically gellable, gelatin derivative for drug delivery and tissue engineering. Biomaterials 30 (20), 3371–3377.

Seidi, A., Ramalingam, M., 2012. Protocols for biomaterial scaffold fabrication. In: Ramalingam, M., Haidar, Z., Ramakrishna, S., Kobayashi, H., Haikel, Y. (Eds.), Integrated Biomaterials in Tissue Engineering. Scrivener Publishing LLC, Salem, MA, pp. 1–24.

Sengupta, D., Heilshorn, S., 2010. Protein-engineered biomaterials: highly tunable tissue engineering scaffolds. Tissue Eng. B 16 (3), 285–293.

Sezer, A.D., Hatipoglu, F., Cevher, E., Oğurtan, Z.A.L., Akbuğa, J., 2007. Chitosan film containing fucoidan as a wound dressing for dermal burn healing: preparation and *in vitro/in vivo* evaluation. AAPS Pharm. Sci. Technol. 8 (2), E94–E101.

Shen, Z.L., Dodge, M.R., Kahn, H., Ballarini, R., Eppell, S.J., 2008. Stress-strain experiments on individual collagen fibrils. Biophys. J. 95, 3956–3963.

Shikanov, A., Xu, M., Woodruff, T.K., Shea, L.D., 2009. Interpenetrating fibrin-alginate matrices for *in vitro* ovarian follicle development. Biomaterials 30 (29), 5476–5485.

Singh, D., Rawat, M.R., 2012. Development of antibiotic and debriding enzyme loaded PLGA microspheres entrapped in PVA-Gelatin hydrogel for complete wound management. Artif. Cells Blood Substit. Biotechnol.: Int. J. 40 (5), 345–353.

Singh, M., Morris, C.P., Ellis, R.J., Detamore, M.S., Berkland, C., 2008. Microsphere-based seamless scaffolds containing macroscopic gradients of encapsulated factors for tissue engineering. Tissue Eng. C 14 (4), 299–309.

Singh, M., Sandhu, B., Scurto, A., Berkland, C., Detamore, M.S., 2010. Microsphere-based scaffolds for cartilage tissue engineering: using subcritical CO2 as a sintering agent. Acta Biomater. 6 (1), 137–143.

Singh, M.R., Saraf, S., Vyas, A., Jain, V., Singh, D., 2013. Innovative approaches in wound healing: trajectory and advances. Artif. Cells Blood Substit. Biotechnol.: Int. J.epub. Informa Healthcare.

Sokolsky-Papkov, M., Agashi, K., Olaye, A., Shakesheff, K., Domb, A.J., 2007. Polymer carriers for drug delivery in tissue engineering. Adv. Drug Deliv. Rev. 59, 187–206.

Spiro, R., Polarek, J.W., 2004. The application of recombinant human collagen in tissue engineering. Bio. Drugs 18, 103–119.

Stabenfeldt, S.E., Garcia, A.J., LaPlaca, M.C., 2006. Thermoreversible laminin-functionalized hydrogel for neural tissue engineering. J. Biomed. Mater. Res. A 77 (4), 718–725.

Stephens, D., Li, L., Robinson, D., Chen, S., Chang, H., Liu, R.M., et al., 2000. Investigation of the *in vitro* release of gentamicin from a polyanhydride matrix. J. Control. Release 63 (3), 305–317.

Tabata, Y., Ikada, Y., 1998. Protein release from gelatin matrices. Adv. Drug Deliv. Rev. 31, 287–301.

Tabata, Y., Miyao, M., Ozeki, M., Ikada, Y., 2000. Controlled release of vascular endothelial growth factor by use of collagen hydrogels. J. Biomater. Sci. Polym. Ed. 11, 915–930.

Thomas, S., 1989. Pain and wound management. Comm. Outlook., 11–15.

Thomas, V., Donahoe, T., Nyairo, E., Dean, D.R., Vohra, Y.K., 2011. Electrospinning of biosyn (R)-based tubular conduits: structural, morphological, and mechanical characterizations. Acta. Biomater. 7, 2070–2079.

Ueno, H., Yamada, H., Tanaka, I., Kaba, N., Matsuura, M., Okumura, M., et al., 1999. Accelerating effects of chitosan for healing at early phase of experimental open wound in dogs. Biomaterials 20 (15), 1407–1414.

Vashi, A.V., Abberton, K.M., Thomas, G.P., Morrison, W.A., O'Connor, A.J., Cooper-White, J.J., et al., 2006. Adipose tissue engineering based on the controlled release of fibroblast growth factor-2 in a collagen matrix. Tissue Eng. 12, 3035–3043.

Wang, W., Lin, S., Xiao, Y., Huang, Y., Tan, Y., Cai, L., et al., 2008. Acceleration of diabetic wound healing with chitosan crosslinked collagen sponge containing recombinant human acidic fibroblast growth factor in healing-impaired STZ diabetic rats. Life Sci. 82, 190–204.

Willerth, S.M., Arendas, K.J., Gottlieb, D.I., Sakiyama-Elbert, S.E., 2006. Optimization of fibrin scaffolds for differentiation of murine embryonic stem cells into neural lineage cells. Biomaterials 27, 5990–6003.

Xing, Y., Cheng, E., Yang, Y., Chen, P., Zhang, T., Sun, Y., et al., 2011. Self-assembled DNA hydrogels with designable thermal and enzymatic responsiveness. Adv. Mater. 23 (9), 1117–1121.

Xu, X.L., Lou, J., Tang, T.T., Ng, K.W., Zhang, J.H., Yu, C.F., et al., 2005. Evaluation of different scaffolds for BMP-2 genetic orthopedic tissue engineering. J. Biomed. Mater. Res. B Appl. Biomater. 75B, 289–303.

Yang, C., Xu, L., Zhou, Y., Zhang, X., Huang, X., Wang, M., et al., 2010. A green fabrication approach of gelatin/CM-chitosan hybrid hydrogel for wound healing. Carbohydr. Polym. 82 (4), 1297–1305.

Young, S., Wong, M., Tabata, Y., Mikos, A.G., 2005. Gelatin as a delivery vehicle for the controlled release of bioactive molecules. J. Control. Release 109, 256–274.

Zhang, R., Ma, P.X., 1999. Synthetic nano-scale fibrous extracellular matrix. J. Biomed. Mat. Res. 46 (1), 60–72.

Zhang, Y., Cheng, X., Wang, J., Wang, Y., Shi, B., Huang, C., et al., 2006. Novel chitosan/collagen scaffold containing transforming growth factor-beta1 DNA for periodontal tissue engineering. Biochem. Biophys. Res. Commun. 344, 362–369.

Zhu, J., 2012. Biomimetic hydrogels as scaffolds for tissue engineering. J. Biochips Tissue Chips 2, e119. Available from: http://dx.doi.org/10.4172/2153-0777.1000e119.

Zhu, J., Marchant, R.E., 2011. Design properties of hydrogel tissue-engineering scaffolds. Expert. Rev. Med. Devices 8, 607–626.

Zohuriaan, M.J., Pourjavadi, A., 2003. Superabsorbent hydrogels from starch-g-PAN: effect of some reaction variables on swelling behavior. J. Polym. Mater. 20, 113–120.

CHAPTER

Bioactive nanomaterials for cartilage and muscle regeneration

10

Alina Maria Holban[1,2,3], Ecaterina Andronescu[1], Carmen Curutiu[2,3], Lia-Mara Ditu[2,3], Mariana Carmen Chifiriuc[2,3] and Veronica Lazar[2,3]

[1]Department of Science and Engineering of Oxide Materials and Nanomaterials, Faculty of Applied Chemistry and Materials Science, University Politehnica of Bucharest, Bucharest, Romania [2]Microbiology Immunology Department, Faculty of Biology, University of Bucharest, Bucharest, Romania [3]Research Institute of the University of Bucharest, Bucharest, Romania

10.1 CARTILAGE TISSUE

Cartilage is a flexible connective tissue found in many areas of the human body, including joints, ribs, nose, ear, trachea, and intervertebral discs (Oseni et al., 2011). Human cartilage could be organized into three types, differing by structure, elasticity, and strength, i.e., *hyaline/articular cartilage* (covering joint surfaces), *fibrocartilage* (found in the knee meniscus and vertebral discs, ligaments, and tendons), and *elastic cartilage* (found in the outer ear, nose) (Hauser, 2015). Thereby, the cartilage provides support for adjacent tissues, acting as structural scaffold and maintaining the shape or absorbing shocks during physical exercises (Oseni et al., 2011).

Cartilage is a specialized structure with a relatively hard, resistant outer surface of collagen fibers covering a flexible, porous collagen structure. The extracellular matrix (ECM) of cartilage consists of a network of macromolecules including collagen, elastin, glycoproteins, and proteoglycans, each of which is present in varying amounts, depending on the type and function of cartilage (Oseni et al., 2011).

Articular cartilage is produced by a single cell type represented by chondrocytes, derived from the mesenchymal stem cells (MSCs) and can be organized into four major zonal compartments: superficial (10–20%), middle (40–60%), lower (30%), and calcified (5%) (Campos et al., 2012; Mow and Ratcliffe, 1997).

Human adult articular cartilage is a complex tissue of matrix proteins that varies from superficial to deep layers, composed of the ECM containing

Nanobiomaterials in Soft Tissue Engineering. DOI: http://dx.doi.org/10.1016/B978-0-323-42865-1.00010-6

collagen, proteoglycans, and water. The chondrocytes produce various types of collagen (type II and small amounts of types V, VI, IX, X, and XI) interconnected by proteoglycans and hyaluronan (known as *hyaluronic acid*, HA), and the ECM is more abundant close to the calcified zone. Chondrocyte aerobic metabolism depends on different local factors: matrix composition, growth factors (GFs), electrical fields, hydrostatic pressures, and mechanical loads (Campos et al., 2012).

Articular cartilage damage is the most commonly encountered type and, once injured, it has very limited self-repairing capacity, having no direct blood supply (Steinert et al., 2008). The usual tissue response to injury is the occurrence of inflammation, which depends on the intrinsic vascularization of the tissue (Lipowitz, 2015). Cartilage regeneration and remodeling are thus dependent upon articular chondrocytes and their metabolism, including synthesis of ECM molecules (Campos et al., 2012). The reparative processes are not coordinated by the chondrocyte progenitor cells present in blood and marrow because they cannot access the damaged region. Moreover, resident articular chondrocytes do not migrate to the lesion, and therefore, the production of a reparative matrix by these cells cannot occur (Steinert et al., 2008). The resulting fibrocartilaginous repair tissue is of inferior quality, rather classified as scar tissue, a fact which is associated with an increased risk for gradual development of secondary osteoarthritis (Van Osch et al., 2009).

Fibrocartilage is a tough form of cartilage that consists of chondrocytes scattered among clearly visible dense bundles of collagen fibers within the matrix. Fibrocartilage does not have perichondrium. Fibrocartilage merges with the dense fibrous connective tissue in tendons and ligaments. Tendons serve primarily to transfer the tension of muscles to bone and ligaments. Both are characterized by their great tensile strength and are dominated by collagen fibers (In and Ralphs, 1998; Thomopoulos et al., 2011). Fibrocartilage is also found in the pubic symphysis and the annulus fibrosus of intervertebral discs.

The development of functionally equivalent fibrocartilage remains elusive despite efforts to engineer tissues such as the knee menisci, intervertebral disc, considering that fibrocartilage lacks an innate ability to self-repair following disease or injury (MacBarb et al., 2013).

Elastic cartilage is histologically similar to hyaline cartilage but contains many elastic fibers lying in a solid matrix and chondrocytes and does not normally ossify or calcify (Kim et al., 2011). Collagen fibers give great flexibility, so that elastic cartilage is able to withstand repeated bending, and perichondrium is present. Perichondrocytes are differentiated into mature chondrocytes and form an elastic cartilage rich in proteoglycans and elastic fibers (Kobayashi et al., 2011). In the human body, elastic cartilage tissue forms auditory (Eustachian) tubes, external ear (auricle), and epiglottis, provides support to surrounding structures, and helps to define and maintain the shape of the area in which it is present.

10.1.1 CARTILAGE TISSUE PATHOLOGY

Musculoskeletal pathologies are a diverse group of diseases anatomically linked and by their association with pain and impaired physical function (Figure 10.1).

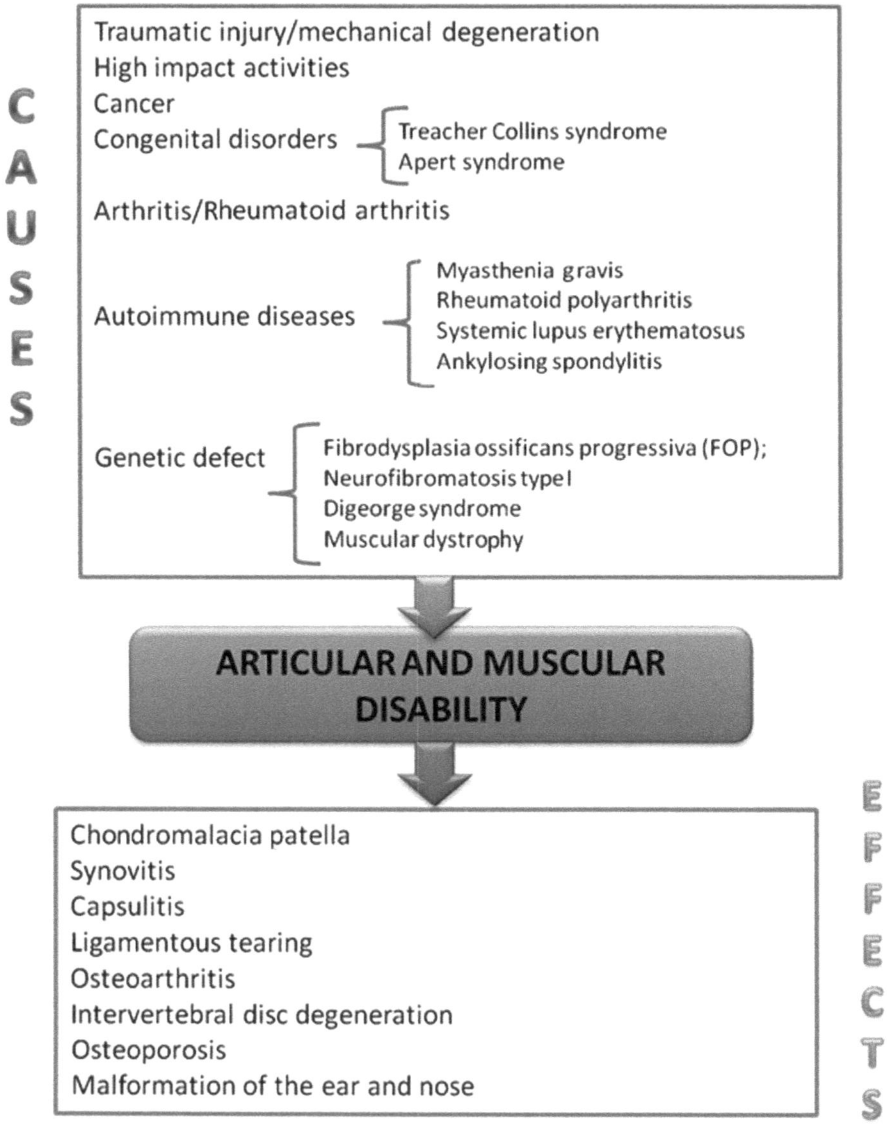

FIGURE 10.1

The most common causes and complications of articular and muscular disabilities.

They are the most common cause of severe long-term pain and physical disability (Woolf and Pfleger, 2003).

10.1.1.1 Osteoarthritis

Osteoarthritis (OA) affects the whole joint structure with progressive changes in cartilage, menisci, ligaments, and subchondral bone, and synovial inflammation (Lotz el al., 2013), being the most common chronic health conditions and a leading cause of pain and disability among adults (Johnson and Hunter, 2014). As in other disease processes in the body, the etiology and/or progression of OA is multifactorial: age (senescence) associated with other risk factors (obesity and metabolic syndrome, nutritional and vitamin factors, bone density and bone mass, smoking), traumatic joint injury (the major risk factor for osteoarthritis, particularly at the knee), joint shape, muscle strength and mass, leg length inequality, occupation, and physical activity (Allen and Yvonne, 2015). Recent studies discovered the implication of a genetic and epigenetic predisposition represented by the presence of over 80 gene mutations involved in the pathogenesis of OA, among which the most relevant is a single nucleotide polymorphism responsible for the development, maintenance, and repair of synovial joints.

The best candidates for biomarkers in osteoarthritis are structural molecules or fragments measured in the synovial fluid, blood, or urine, linked to cartilage, bone, or synovium which may indicate tissue degradation or tissue synthesis (Lotz el al., 2013). Many are associated with the metabolism of collagen (type II) and aggrecan in cartilage or subchondral bone (type I collagen). Type II collagen fragments (C-terminal telopeptide of collagen type II, type II collagen α-chain collagenase neoepitope, type II collagen propeptides, type II collagen cleavage product, collagen type-II-specific neoepitope, pyridinoline, and Glc-Gal-PYD, etc.) (Kraus et al., 2011; Rousseau and Garnero, 2012; Williams and Spector, 2008; Mobasheri, 2012) and aggrecan (chondroitin sulfate epitope 846 and monoclonal antibody 3B3, keratane sulfate) (Karsdal et al., 2008, 2013), the most abundant proteins in the cartilage matrix, are promising targets for diagnostics. Also, there are biomarkers related to a range of noncollagenous proteins that have a role in other metabolic pathways in the joint, including glycoproteins, proteoglycans, metalloproteinases, and advanced glycation endproducts, as well as HA, which is a constituent of both cartilage and synovium (Karsdal et al., 2011). Finally, there are a number of biomarkers associated with other processes, such as inflammation or fibrosis (uric acid, hs-CRP, IL-1β, IL-6, factors indicating fibrosis, and complement) (van Spil et al., 2010). The ability to detect biomarkers of cartilage degradation in body fluids may enable clinicians to diagnose subclinical OA, as well as determining the course of disease progression (Mobasheri, 2011).

Clinically, the condition is characterized by joint pain, tenderness, limitation of movement, crepitus, occasional effusion, and variable degrees of local inflammation. It can occur in any joint but is most common in the hip, knee, and the joints of the hand, foot, and spine (Lotz el al., 2013). The impairment of the chondrocytes and the ECM lead to a decreased capacity of the joint to adapt to different stress conditions, both chemical and mechanical, the chondrocytes having a limited number of divisions (approximately 30–40), known as the "Hayflick limit" (Musumeci et al., 2015). The senescence of chondrocytes is the main factor responsible for the development and progression of OA, the senescent cells losing their ability to maintain and repair the ECM of cartilage (Mobasheri, 2011). Under normal physiological conditions, chondrocytes maintain a balance between the synthesis and degradation of ECM components, regulating the structural and functional integrity of cartilage. Chondrocyte apoptosis is associated with matrix degradation and calcification that suggest an important role of cell death/survival mechanisms in OA pathogenesis (Musumeci et al., 2015).

The OA-associated molecules, including IL-1β, TNF-α, RAGE, leptin, insulin-like growth factor (IGF)-1, transforming growth factor (TGF)-β1, iNOS, MMP13, laminin, fibronectin, integrin, and collagen, are involved in chondrocyte activation. These molecules contribute to the pathogenesis of OA by destroying the cartilage in the joints or serving as the substrates for ECM destruction (i.e., laminin, fibronectin, and collagen type II).

10.1.1.2 Rheumatoid arthritis

Rheumatoid arthritis (RA) is a chronic, systemic, destructive arthritis, in which the inflammatory process widely involves the synovial joint. It is the most common form of chronic polyarthritis and it predominantly affects the peripheral joints. Because persistent synovitis leads to joint destruction, the RA results in long-term morbidity and increased mortality (Woolf and Pfleger, 2003). Based on the presence of autoantibodies (rheumatoid factor (RF) and anticitrullinated protein antibody (ACPA)) detected in the previous stage of clinical phase of RA (Aletaha et al., 2010), RA is considered an autoimmune disease. Autoimmunity and the overall systemic and articular inflammatory load drive the destructive progression of the disease.

However, RA is a multifactorial disease sustained by environmental and genetic factors, including dietary factors (alcohol, inhaled particulate air pollution), occupational exposures (such as mineral oils, silica dust), reproductive and hormonal factors (steroid hormones, especially in women), infections, and smoking, as well as epigenetic factors (Korczowska, 2014; Karlson and Deane, 2012). The genetic factors are responsible for susceptibility to the disease and the phenotype, having a contribution to the disease of 30–60% (Deane et al., 2010). Several genes have been implicated so far in the pathogenesis of RA, the most important encoding the human leukocyte antigen (HLA) molecules contributing to approximately half of the genetic susceptibility of RA. These seem to be necessary, but not sufficient in the disease development, nonetheless they can be responsible for different clinical pictures and responses to therapy, and they can represent potential therapeutic targets (Perricone et al., 2011).

The clinical evaluation of RA should include quantitative assessment of serum CRP concentration, which is the most clinically useful biomarker (Smolen et al.,

2008), ACPA (formerly, anticyclic citrullinated peptide antibody) serologic test, which has high specificity ($>$90%) and moderate sensitivity ($\sim$60%) for RA. RF may also be used as a serologic marker of the disease, although it has considerably lower specificity ($<$70%) (Davis and Matteson, 2012).

There are four identified phases of RA development, characterized by differing pathogenesis and physical changes. Transition between phases may be caused by interactions between genetic and environmental factors, and/or changes in immune reactivity, the biological mechanisms involved in these transitions being a real challenge for the field (Korczowska, 2014). The initial phase is characterized by the presence of the genetic risk for RA, during which no biomarkers of active autoimmunity and inflammation or symptoms are present. *Phase 1* may last for years, and is followed by environmental and additional genetic influences that lead to *Phase 2* of disease development—asymptomatic autoimmunity—characterized by the presence of RA-related autoantibodies and other immunologic factors such as T- and B-cell autoreactivity, and sometimes, elevated inflammatory markers. *Phase 2* may be of variable length, probably being influenced by genetic, environmental or endogenous factors such as age or gender. *Phases 1 and 2* are asymptomatic, so, they may be termed "preclinical" RA. Finally, there is a transition from asymptomatic autoimmunity to *Phase 3*, or clinically apparent disease. During the final *Phase 4*, patients will have symptoms and signs of active RA, and numerous autoimmune and inflammatory biomarkers present as well as clear evidence of end-organ damage (Deane et al., 2010).

10.1.1.3 Osteoporosis

Osteoporosis (*porous bone*) is a silent disease characterized by reduced bone mass and microarchitectural deterioration of bone tissue. This leads to an increased risk of bone fragility and fractures (hip fractures, vertebral fractures, forearm fractures and pelvis, rib, humerus, tibia, fibula, clavicle, scapula, sternum, and other femoral fractures), which represent the main clinical consequence of the disease (Svedbom et al., 2013). It is a major public health problem, affecting hundreds of millions of people worldwide, predominantly postmenopausal women (Cosman et al., 2014).

In 1994, the World Health Organization defined the diagnostic criteria for osteoporosis on the basis of measurement of bone mineral density and relating it to the mean bone mineral density of young adult women (*T*-score). Thus, when bone mineral density is more than 2.5 standard deviations below the mean bone mineral density of young adult women (bone mineral density *T*-score <-2.5), it is called osteoporosis. When bone mineral density value is between 1 and 2.5 standard deviations below the mean bone mineral density of young adult women ($-2.5<$ bone mineral density *T*-score <-1), it is called osteopenia (low bone mass) (Woolf and Pfleger, 2003).

The risk factors associated with development of osteoporosis can be classified in unmodifiable factors, such as age, genetic factors, calcium-deficient diet, family history of osteoporosis, low body weight, use of medication, and modifiable factors, such as estrogen-deficient state, excessive alcohol intake, and smoking.

Basic mechanisms responsible for development of osteoporosis are poor bone mass acquisition during growth and development and accelerated bone loss in the period after peak bone mass is achieved. Both processes are modulated by environmental and genetic factors. A healthy skeleton is maintained throughout life by the constant process of bone remodeling that is regulated by the balanced activities of bone-resorbing osteoclasts and bone-forming osteoblasts to maintain normal physiological structure and mineral content. Osteoporosis is caused by an uncoupling of bone resorption from bone formation such that the activities of osteoclasts far outweigh those of osteoblasts. Peak bone mass is achieved in early adulthood and, following this point, both women and men lose bone with increasing age. However, this process is accelerated in postmenopausal women whereby the loss of estrogen is associated with an increase in osteoclast activity (Das and Crockett, 2013). It has been demonstrated that long-term hormone replacement therapy with estrogen plus progestin prevents bone loss and fractures (Cervellati et al., 2014).

10.1.2 MEDICAL IMPACT OF CARTILAGE TISSUE-ASSOCIATED DISEASES

Musculoskeletal joint conditions are among the most prevalent disease processes and common causes of pain and disability, resulting in significant healthcare costs. These disease processes are secondary only to heart disease in causing significant disability that affects work status (Deryk, 2009). The cost of musculoskeletal injury or disease is greater than breast cancer, stroke, and cardiovascular disease combined and results in greater disability. Annual total costs for bone and joint health in the United States alone are estimated at $849 billion and one in two adults age 18 and older report suffering from a musculoskeletal condition that lasted more than 3 months (Bonewald et al., 2013, Mitchell et al., 2012). The Centers for Disease Control and Prevention predicted that by 2020 arthritis will gain more new patients than any other disease form in America (Deryk, 2009).

Osteoarthritis is the most common joint disease and a major cause of disability, characterized by joint pain and dysfunction and, in advanced stages, joint contractures, muscle atrophy, and limb deformity (Heijink et al., 2012). According to the *National Institutes of Health guidelines*, 20% of men and 25% of women are categorized as obese and the number has increased by 50% over the past 10–15 years. Studies have demonstrated that obese individuals can reduce their risk of developing osteoarthritis and decrease the severity of clinical symptoms through weight loss (Deryk, 2009).

RA is a chronic, systemic inflammatory disease of unknown etiology that affects 0.5–1.0% of the general population. The prevalence of RA increases considerably with age, affecting approximately 6% of the white population older than 65 years. In the United States, the lifetime risk of developing RA is 3.6% in women and 1.7% in men. There is some indication that the risk of developing RA has increased somewhat in recent years, at least in women (Davis and Matteson, 2012). Generally, the lifetime risk of inflammatory autoimmune rheumatic disease development is substantial, being 1:12 for women and 1:20 for men (Crowson et al., 2011). Although heterogeneous, RA is primarily characterized by symmetric, erosive synovitis, which, if uncontrolled, can lead to joint and cartilage damage, multiple comorbidities, significant disability, and a reduction in quality of life (Mitchell et al., 2012).

Osteoporosis is the most common bone disease in humans, representing a major public health problem. A relatively recent "Osteoporosis in the European Union: Medical Management, Epidemiology and Economic Burden" report claims that, in 2010, 22 million women and 5.5 million men were estimated to have osteoporosis in the EU; and 3.5 million new fragility fractures were sustained (620,000 hip fractures, 520,000 vertebral fractures, 560,000 forearm fractures, and 1,800,000 other fractures). The economic burden of incident and prior fragility fractures was estimated at €37 billion and the costs are expected to increase by 25% in 2025 (Svedbom et al., 2013). Osteoporotic fractures have serious consequences on the individual and the societal levels. Fracture patients often have a decreased functional mobility and health-related quality of life, and face an increased mortality (Bleibler et al., 2014).

10.1.3 CARTILAGE REPARATIVE STRATEGIES

Hyaline cartilage is avascular and low metabolic, leading the currently available therapies largely ineffective at producing a robust and healthy repair tissue.

Many researches and clinical studies have been made to restore the integrity of cartilage. There are several different techniques available, some of which have the same principles. The choice of the most appropriate technique for each patient is very important and represents a major responsibility of the surgeon in order to obtain a full recovery of the cartilage function for active lifestyle of the patient.

In treating articular cartilage lesions, several factors must be considered to make a decision: surface, depth, location, history, associated injuries, knee stability, meniscal injuries, limb mechanical axis, the patient's age, and not least patient's requests related to functionality. Cartilage repair procedures may be divided into primary, simple procedures that can be performed arthroscopically as first-line treatment, and secondary, which are more complex, aimed at restoring lasting cartilage surface.

The methods presently used are: (i) arthroscopic lavage and debridement, as palliative procedures; (ii) bone marrow stimulation (abrasion arthroplasty, drilling, microfractures) as cartilage reparative strategies, determining a fibrocartilage healing response; and (iii) osteochondral allograft or/and autograft transplantation and autologous chondrocyte implantation (ACI) or matrix-induced autologous chondrocyte implantation (MACI) as cartilage restorative techniques which suppose a replacement of the injured cartilage (Rodrıguez-Merchan and de la Corte-Garcıa, 2012). Not all the methods are clearly delimitated, some of them interfering by using different type of cells, bioactive molecules (GFs, platelet-rich plasma (PRP)), and scaffolds.

Arthroscopic lavage and debridement are used for patients with low mechanical stress of the joint with unique and relatively small lesions and which do not wish to undergo a lasting treatment for recovery. In this method the chondral tissue debris is removed and inflammatory molecules are released by synovial membrane, with good results in terms of alleviating pain, for patients with acute or degenerative chondral lesions. However, either lavage or debridment are not a definitive treatment, as the lesions are not repaired. Moreover, some studies have recently argued that the positive effect felt by patient could be only a placebo effect after surgery. These procedures are accepted only for a short time, and only for patients with early osteoarthritis (Özmeriç et al., 2014).

Arthroscopic procedures used for cartilage repair are abrasion arthroplasty, drilling, and microfractures.

In *abrasion arthroplasty*, with an automated burr, 1–3 mm of subchondral bone is removed to access the vasculature. The technique is accompanied by debridement, the boundary of the articular cartilage injured is debrided, and a uniform edge of new collagen appears, making possible the adherence of a fibrin clot formed by perfusion of blood into the lesion. Abrasion arthroplasty is recommended especially in the case of some sclerotic degenerative arthritic lesions (Craig et al., 2003). The results of this technique vary in different studies, in recent years it has become no longer used due to some disadvantages, such as excessive trauma of the bone and thermal necrosis (Falah et al., 2010).

Drilling stimulates bleeding by drilling the subchondral bone with multiple drill holes through trabecular bone. Similar to abrasion arthroplasty, fibrin clot will be formed by perfusion of blood into the lesion, this will start the injury repair, by formation of a mixed cartilage: hyaline and fibrocartilage (Pridie, 1959; Craig et al., 2003). It seems that compared with microfracture, the drill holes create more generous channels for cell migration, but also have the disadvantage of thermal necrosis (Chen et al., 2009).

The *microfracture* technique developed by Steadman et al. involves the debridement of damaged cartilage down to the subchondral bone using small awls to realize multiple drill holes, approximately 2–3 mm apart. The consequences are bleeding, formation of a blood clot, and fibrous tissue repair development. The technique is similar to drilling, but it eliminates the thermal effects of a drill, because the holes are made with an arthroscopic awl (Steadman et al., 1997).

Microfracture is recommended in focal chondral defects smaller than 2.5 cm^2, and in patients younger than 40 years old (Özmeriç et al., 2014). However, in time the newly formed hyaline-like cartilage becomes a fibrous-type cartilage with lower biomechanical and viscoelastic properties, and the symptoms will reappear. In order to eliminate this drawback, a combination between scaffold and this technique was developed (Matsiko et al., 2013).

Associated with cartilage restorative techniques, new structures such as *scaffolds* (implants) were developed, allowing the *acellular matrix-induced microfracture* approaches. These structures improved morrow function, and represent good support for stability of mesenchymal cells and tissue differentiation. Host tissue will cover the scaffold that in time will be resorbed and replaced with new tissue. The advantages of this technique are represented by the fact that the implants are introduced in one step, and the procedure is less expensive and time-consuming, compared with other techniques in which two surgical operations and also an intermediary phase for *in vitro* cell cultivation are necessary.

Bioscaffolds are represented by biological materials, either natural (collagens, HA, fibrin glue, etc.) or synthetic (polycaprolactone (PCL), poly L-lactic acid (PLA), and polyglycolic acid (PGA), etc.), used as templates for cellular propagation (Craig et al., 2003). These scaffolds should be stable in terms of structure and mechanical properties, biocompatible, and capable of interacting with other bioactive molecules and to promote cellular differentiation. The most well-known natural scaffolds are matrices with HA and collagen, these components being normally found in the structure of the articular cartilage. Examples of such commercial scaffolds are Chondrotissue®, Hyalofast®, AMIC®, CAIS®, Alginate Beads®, Trufit®, and Maiorege n® (Filardo et al., 2013). Good results were reported in a recent study with 27 patients, 87% of them presenting significant clinical healing after a period of 37 months (Gille et al., 2013). It was recommended that osteochondral scaffolds be used in the case of lesions where the subchondral layer is also implicated (Özmeriç et al., 2014).

Hyalograft CTM, a HA-based scaffold was already used for treatment of cartilage defects. On this scaffold, autologous chondrocytes were implanted directly into the defect area, without a periosteal flap, and it appeared that 96.7% of patients developed hyaline-like cartilage.

Another example is the use, with good results, of some synthetic alginate-based *scaffolds*, containing human mature chondrocytes, for the treatment of knee cartilage defects (Almqvist et al., 2009).

Osteochondral autograft transplantations (AOTs) consist of transplantation of the human articular cartilage tissue collected from nonload-bearing regions of the articular cartilage into injured areas, in a single or multiple smaller grafts (multiple grafts = mosaicplasty). The advantage is represented by the fact that this is a single operation for the patient, the tissue is taken from one site and immediately transplanted to the lesion site. Mosaicplasty is recommended in cases of $1-5\ cm^2$ focal chondral defects and for patients under 50 years old and with desire for an active life (Hangody et al., 2004). By comparing microfracture and AOT, Gudas et al. (2012) observed that patients treated with microfracture presented good results immediately, but not over time, compared with AOT, many of the patients (sportsmen) being capable of resuming their activities. A disadvantage of this procedure is the dislodgement of the transplanted tissue in rare cases.

Osteochondral allograft transplantation, introduced by Yamashita et al. (1985) and universalized by Hangody et al. (1997), represents the transplantation of a composite cadaveric graft from subchondral bone and overlying hyaline cartilage in the patient's defect area. Allografts should be taken from young, healthy people with good bones and cartilage.

Transplanted tissue is used for many sites: the femoral condyle, the patella, trochlea, and the medial and lateral tibial plateau. This technique is used with better results in the case of moderate articular lesions (up to 8 cm^2) in relatively active patients. In a recent study, Chahal et al. (2013) observed that osteochondral allograft transplantation for focal and diffuse chondral defects were practiced with good results. Allografts should be fresh, increasing the risk of potential disease transmission. Other drawbacks are represented by the cost and size mismatch.

Cell transplantation-based repair. Chondrocytes are the only cell type present in the articular cartilage surrounded by a rich ECM. Their ability to synthesize *in vitro* cartilage-like matrix demonstrates the regeneration capacity of these cells. Therefore, chondrocytes gain the attention of clinicians that choose to use these cells for repairing chondral lesions in ACI. ACI was described for the first time by Mats Brittberg et al. in Sweden for the treatment of full-thickness chondral lesions (Brittberg et al., 1994). In ACI, cells are extracted initially by arthroscopy from nonweight-bearing regions of the articular cartilage, e.g., from lateral trochlear ridge (Frisbie et al., 2008). The isolated cells are digested enzymatically and then expanded *in vitro* for 6 weeks in a GMP laboratory. The next step is the arthrotomy, the expanded cells being injected at the lesion and covered with a sutured periosteal flap. ACI is indicated for active 20- to 50-year-old patients with an isolated traumatic femoral chondral lesion. The resulting tissue is more durable and has biomechanical properties similar to the native hyaline-like cartilage tissue (Brittberg et al., 1994; Minas, 1998; Peterson et al., 2010). Different studies revealed good results for patients regarding pain and joint function, even a long period of time after the procedure: 72% of patients monitored for 24 months in a study realized by Minas (1998), or 84% of the patients 3 years after the intervention from another study (Micheli et al., 2001). A clinical study that investigated patients aged 2–9 years also demonstrated good results in 80% of them (Peterson et al., 2000).

On the other hand, ACI involves a two-step procedure, with a long period of time necessary for chondrocytes to expand sufficiently *in vitro*, a low dedifferentiation of cells following implantation, long operation time, large incision size, sometimes difficulty in accessing certain areas for suturing, and long rehabilitation time. Other negative aspects that could occur are periosteal hypertrophy or loss of implanted cells from the lesion (Zaslav et al., 2009; Niemeyer et al., 2008).

To eliminate some disadvantages related to the periosteal flap, the use of a collagen membrane to cover and close the cartilage lesion is practiced under the name of collagen-covered autologous chondrocyte implantation (CACI) or autologous matrix-induced chondrogenesis (AMIC).

AMIC is used for cartilage repair using the patient's stem cells. Good results were obtained mostly in larger lesions and in early osteoarthritis (Steinwachs, 2008).

Steinwachs and Kreuz (2007) reported the results on 63 patients treated by ACI, but expanded cells within the defect were covered with a type I/III collagen membrane. They observed that no patient presented the symptoms of graft hypertrophy, so the use of collagen membrane rather than a periosteal flap eliminates the risk of graft hypertrophy.

D'Anchise et al. (2005) described a second-generation *MACI* procedure, in which the collagen membrane (type I/III) is inoculated on autologous chondrocytes. On one side of the chondrocytes attachment and neomatrix synthesizing occurs, the other smooth side allows sliding of the chondral surface. The novelty of the procedure lies in the use of fibrin glue, more exactly a combination between fibrinogen and thrombin. This glue sticks together the collagen membrane and the chondral surface. The benefits of this technique are the absence of a suture, the absence of periosteal harvesting, and the less invasive procedure and rapid patient mobilization (Bentley, 2008). Disadvantages are represented by price and the long rehabilitation (Falah et al., 2010).

Another type of cell used for cartilage lesion repair instead of chondrocytes is adult *MSCs* derived from different sources: bone-marrow-derived stem cells, adipose-derived stem cells (ADSCs), infrapatellar fat-pad-derived stem cells (IPFSCs), or synovium-derived stem cells. The use of MSCs is due to their great capacity to differentiate, self-regenerate, and secrete some important cellular factors, such as cytokines or GFs. The bone marrow is one of the most important sources for progenitor cells. It contains multipotent MSCs, mostly in infancy (Caplan, 2007). *In vitro* and *in vivo* studies proved the capacity of bone-marrow-derived MSCs to differentiate down a chondrocytic lineage (Farrell et al., 2006). MSCs isolated from lipoaspirates, so-called ADSCs demonstrated *in vitro* their ability to differentiate into cartilage-like cells (Awad et al., 2004; Guilak et al., 2004) and *in vivo* to produce some cartilage matrix molecules (Erickson et al., 2002). The same capacity to produce cartilage-like matrix was observed in the case of IPFSCs, which are in fact MSCs isolated from the fat pads of joints, and also in the case of synovial membrane-derived stem cells (SMSCs), MSCs isolated from synovial tissue (Matsiko et al., 2013).

PRP is based on the use of a natural concentrate of autologous blood GFs. It was observed that therapy with PRP injections reduced patient pain and improved the quality of life for a short time. The procedure is simple, almost noninvasive, and low cost. PRP was used in many medical fields, for articular cartilage lesions its role was explored by Kon et al. (2010). The initial results are good in terms of reducing pain in young patients with small articular defects.

GFs promote cell migration and proliferation. For cartilage defects, most interest is given to TGF-β, and bone morphogenetic protein (BMP), due to the chondrogenic and osteogenic properties (Ueda et al., 2002; Farnworth, 2000). The drawbacks of TGF-β use are the relatively high cost and also the appearance of some mineral deposition due to chondrocyte hypertrophy as a response to the high amounts of this GF. A combination of TGF-β with other GFs could eliminate this disadvantage and also lead to a greater chondrogenic response (Fukumota et al., 2003; Yaeger et al., 1997). Some studies indicated that OP-1 (BMP-7, Osteo Progenitor-1) was capable of inducing articular cartilage and joint surface restoration. The use of GFs in this kind of therapy presents the risk of ectopic tissue formation *in vivo*. An example is represented by BMP-2 that elicits ectopic bone formation, after it was approved by the FDA for use in tissue engineering. Fibroblast growth factor (FGF) proved to also have chondrogenic capacity in some studies (Buckley and Kelly, 2012), but it cannot act alone as a secondary factor is necessary for complete tissue regeneration. Parathyroid hormone-related peptide and platelet-derived growth factor are two other GFs that stimulate cartilage matrix production (Guo et al., 2006; Kieswetter et al., 1997). Some commercial products based on GFs are already available and approved for use in the clinical field: Stryker's OP-1® and Medtronic's INFUSE® for bone tissue applications (Matsiko et al., 2013). A disadvantage of all GFs in this kind of application is their short-range diffusion, it being necessary for carrier molecules to ensure correct delivery at the target area and control of the right dosage. A new approach in this regard could be the use of *gene therapy*, that uses the manipulation of cells (progenitor cells or chondrocytes) to express genes encoding GFs involved in osteochondral repair (Pecina et al., 2002, 2006). A new technique based on gene therapy, *gene-activated matrices* (GAMs), in which scaffolds are used as carrier structures for plasmid DNA has been developed (Bonadio et al., 1999). GAMs are scaffolds carrying vectors with genes encoding for the desired gene expression and elicit a chondrogenic effect on seeded cells (Bolliet et al., 2008; Im et al., 2011) (Figure 10.2).

Cells (cultures, tissue fragments, MSCs, etc.), bioscaffolds (natural/synthetic), as well as GFs, could be useful for good regeneration of cartilage, and all of these should be accompanied by the treatment of misalignment, patella femoral problems, meniscus tears, and/or ligament instabilities. The "gold standard methods" for the treatment of cartilage defects are not a suitable for all situations. Many approaches are used, depending on many factors regarding the type of cartilage defect, the needs and lifestyles of patients, but also the surgeon experience and medical center possibilities.

10.1.4 BIOACTIVE SCAFFOLDS FOR CARTILAGE REPAIR

Tissue engineering is focusing on investigating several types of cells, different biodegradable and biocompatible scaffolds, and multiple GFs to offer new insights into the repair of articular cartilage.

Scaffolds represent an important parameter for successful cartilage repair, since they are three-dimensional (3D) structures that can favor or inhibit the

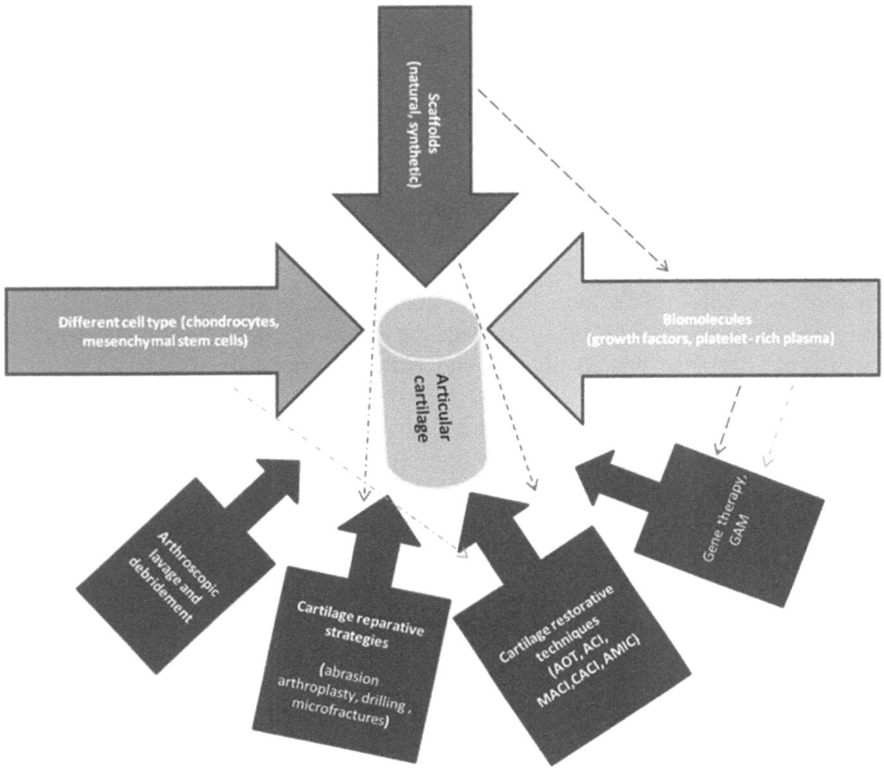

FIGURE 10.2

Graphic representation of factors and methods involved in cartilage regeneration and relationship between them. AOT, osteochondral allograft or/and autograft transplantation; ACI, autologous chondrocyte implantation; MACI, matrix-induced autologous chondrocyte implantation; CACI, covered autologous chondrocyte implantation; AMIC, autologous matrix-induced chondrogenesis; GAMs, gene-activated matrices.

adhesion and proliferation of cartilage cells and also mediate cell-to-cell signaling and interaction. Therefore, the physicochemical properties, the biocompatibility, and the architectural type of the scaffolding material represent key factors in the success of cartilage regeneration and repair. An adequate scaffolding material used for cartilage repair should fulfill the following basic requirements: good biocompatibility, biodegradability, be easily obtained in a highly porous structure, suitable for cell attachment, proliferation and differentiation, osteoconductive, noncytotoxic, flexible and elastic, and nonantigenic.

The current research in an applicative field regarding regenerative medicine divides biomaterials into (i) biological materials and (ii) synthetic polymers (Kuo et al., 2006).

10.1.4.1 Biological materials

Collagen is a native biological material, representing more than 90% of ECM (Cen et al., 2008). In articular cartilages, type II collagen is the most common component, representing approximately 60% of the dry weight of the tissue.

Collagen has excellent tissue compatibility, little toxicity, and facile biodegradation. Moreover, the resulting products after collagen degradation are easily absorbed without the occurrence of inflammation (Badylak et al., 2009). Native collagen has been extensively investigated as a scaffold for tissue engineering. Because of the different chemical and physical treatments that apply for collagen extraction (usually made from collagen-rich native natural tissues), the native organization of its microstructure is usually destroyed. This is leading to a less-resistant collagen-based support; therefore recent scientific progress is focusing on investigating different approaches to increase the mechanical properties of collagen (Rajan et al., 2008).

Proteoglycan scaffolds have also been investigated as native biological-derived scaffolds suitable for soft tissue engineering. HA also represents an important component of the ECM of cartilage and is extensively used in tissue engineering and scaffolding due to its biocompatibility, and structural and signaling roles in a variety of tissues. Its scaffolding properties are related to the fact that the carboxylate group of glucuronic acid allows for facile crosslinking and chemical modification of HA to form hydrogels or sponges. This natural material has interesting physical and biochemical properties, when used in solution or as a hydrogel, which make it very useful for cartilage repair (Allison and Grande-Allen, 2006). HA-based scaffolds can bind to proteins and cells through different cell surface receptors, being involved in the wound-healing process and tissue regeneration and repair.

HA presents different bioactivities; this trait is highly dependent on the molecular weight of the polymer and its associations with other proteins and ECM components (Unterman et al., 2012).

HA scaffolds are often utilized as hydrogels due to water retention and chondrogenic induction. Recently, Unterman and coworkers designed an HA-interacting hydrogel scaffold that noncovalently binds HA, in order to achieve a more natural presentation of HA. The authors conjugated a phage-derived HA-binding peptide to a synthetic hydrogel scaffold based on poly(ethylene glycol) (PEG) diacrylate and observed that this scaffold can interact with HA in the local ECM environment, including cell-secreted HA and exogenously supplied HA. The results showed that the HA-interacting hydrogel improves chondrogenesis of bone-marrow-derived MSCs in an *in vitro* culture system model. The developed model also proved its efficiency *in vivo*, using a rat osteochondral defect model, demonstrating that it might be used in cartilage repair (Unterman et al., 2012).

Recent studies have reported the preparation of hybrid scaffolds composed of HA and collagen to be tested for cartilage regeneration. The hybrid scaffolds presented a 3D structure with interconnected pores (with different amounts of collagen, i.e., 0.1, 0.3, 0.5 wt.%) and revealed an increase in the tensile strength with increasing collagen concentration. The *in vitro* results demonstrated that the degradation period of the hybrid scaffolds increased with increasing collagen concentration and that the cell growth in the hybrid scaffolds increased with increasing collagen concentration. This effect was observed for 2 weeks of cell culture. The *in vivo* tests demonstrated that after the hybrid scaffolds with different collagen concentrations were implanted into cartilage defects of rabbit ears for 6 months, cartilage tissue was easily formed in the collagen-containing scaffolds, the effect being dependent on the collagen concentration. These results demonstrated that collagen-containing porous scaffolds can be effectively used for cartilage regeneration (Kim et al., 2012).

Polysaccharides, such as agarose, alginate, and chitosan, were also recently investigated for developing cartilage repair scaffolds. All these biological materials have some properties which recommend them for medical use, such as great biocompatibility and ability to form hydrogels making them suitable for injectable implantation. Agarose and alginate proved an enhanced ability to induce cartilage growth but they also promote an immunogenic response and inflammation. For this reason there are not many available *in vivo* long-term test results. On the other hand, chitosan proved to be more appropriate for long-term approaches. The hydrogels formed by crosslinking with chondroitin sulfate are thermosensitive and may be injected at room temperature, while producing gels at 37°C.

Because of their different properties, recent studies have proposed the fabrication of mixed scaffolds containing two or more polysaccharides. Gupta et al. (2014a,b), investigated the potential of a chitosan–agarose–gelatin cryogel scaffold for the repair of subchondral cartilage defects. The authors surgically implanted the cryogel scaffold in the knee joint of female New Zealand White rabbits, with surgically created subchondral defects. Macroscopic evaluation revealed the successful integration of the scaffold with the surrounding tissue, while SEM analysis and histological staining of the remnants of implanted cryogel scaffold showed infiltration of the host cells. Their data showed significant cartilage regeneration 4 weeks after implantation. Moreover, the regenerated tissue was confirmed by immunohistochemical approaches as being hyaline cartilage and no hypertrophy markers were observed. This study also highlighted that the mixed polymeric scaffold did not show any adverse immunological rejection or inflammatory reaction (Gupta et al., 2014a,b).

Silk-based scaffolds represent an efficient alternative to other biodegradable biopolymers for soft and hard tissue engineering. These scaffolds are usually composed of natural silk protein, fibroin, and sericin protein. Fibroin 3D scaffolds have been extensively investigated for cartilage repair. Silk scaffolds have many advantages, the most important being the excellent mechanical properties offered to the material, also supporting bone formation.

In order to promote cartilage regeneration a study combined adult human chondrocytes with aqueous-derived porous silk fibroin scaffolds. This study demonstrated that the deposition of cartilage-specific ECM was significantly enhanced by this combinatorial treatment, the inserted cellular density being important for the final results. These data suggest that engineered 3D silk fibroin scaffolds may be successfully used for autologous cell-based tissue engineering, especially to generate engineered cartilage-like tissues (Wanga et al., 2006).

Fibrin originates from blood and has no immunogenicity. This biological material is widely applied in many clinical treatments. Besides its excellent biocompatibility, fibrin can effectively promote the adhesion of different cell types. However, the main disadvantage of fibrin is its weak mechanical properties and unstable degradation rate which limit its application in tissue engineering. Despite these disadvantages, an increasing number of studies utilize this blood component, responsible for hemostasis, as a biopolymer scaffold in tissue engineering. Fibrin can be obtained by various methods, usually from autologous plasma, and is widely available as glue or as engineered microbeads. Moreover, commercially available fibrinogen and thrombin may be combined to form a fibrin hydrogel. In this hydrogel structure it may be incorporated with several bioactive peptides and GFs through a heparin-binding delivery system to improve the functionality of fibrin as a specific scaffold. The novel technological progress facilitated the control of the fibrin structure and geometry into appropriate and predictable forms. Fibrin can be used for the development of different biological scaffolds for the regeneration of different soft tissues, such as adipose tissue, cartilage, tendons, ligaments, liver, nervous tissue, cardiac tissue, ocular tissue, and also skin. Recent studies reported fibrin as a versatile biopolymer, with great potential in tissue regeneration and wound healing (Ahmed et al., 2008).

10.1.4.2 Synthetic polymeric materials

Synthetic polymers aimed at cartilage repair should be molded easily in order to have tunable mechanical properties and a suitable degradation kinetics. Most polymers display increased mechanical properties, making them desirable for many scaffolding applications, including cartilage tissue engineering. However, synthetic materials are more expensive than natural materials and usually they have weaker cell-adhesive abilities.

Recent studies focus on the development and use of injectable polymeric scaffolding materials for *in vivo* cartilage tissue regeneration, since this approach allows cell implantation through minimally invasive surgical procedures.

Poly(lactic-co-glycolic acid) (PLGA) is a biocompatible polymer, successfully used for cartilage repair. This polymer is suitable for biomedical applications, including tissue engineering due to multiple properties: (i) biocompatibility; (ii) tailored biodegradation rate; (iii) approval for clinical use in humans by the Food and Drug Administration (FDA); (iv) potential to modify its surface properties to provide better interaction with biological materials; and (v) suitability for export to countries and cultures where implantation of animal-derived products is inappropriate (Gentile et al., 2014).

PLGA in the form of microspheres was used as an injectable scaffold to engineer cartilage tissue in the subcutaneous space of athymic mice. Recent studies also reported that injectable scaffolding nonporous PLGA microspheres can also be used to regenerate hyaline cartilage in the osteochondral defects of rabbit knees (Kang et al., 2006). The same research group further demonstrated that open macroporous PLGA microspheres utilized as injectable scaffolds provide a larger surface area for cell adhesion and a larger void space for cartilage tissue regeneration. Using this type of polymeric scaffold, the cartilage regeneration is faster and of a higher quality than in the case of nonporous PLGA microspheres (Kang et al., 2009).

Poly(lactic acid) (PLA) is widely used in tissue engineering of cartilage. Porous D,D-L,L-polylactic acid was utilized as a carrier for delivering repair cells obtained from rib perichondrium into full-thickness articular cartilage defects of adult New Zealand White rabbits. The results demonstrated that these scaffolds support the growth of cartilaginous repair tissue and are compatible with *in vitro* and *in vivo* survival of chondrogenic cells (Chu et al., 1995).

Hydrogels based on PEG are also used for soft tissue engineering. Their properties, such as water content, elasticity, biocompatibility, and ability to permit diffusion of nutrients and bioactive molecules, make these polymers suitable candidates for cartilage engineering (Sharma et al., 2007).

PCL can maintain the phenotype and promote the proliferation of chondrocytes. The most significant advantages of PCL are its slow degradation rate and high drug permeability, traits that make this polymer suitable for cartilage engineering (Baker et al., 2012).

Even though significant progress was observed when utilizing these polymers separately, novel approaches developed combinations of natural and synthetic materials for enhancing their cartilage tissue repair property.

A novel tool for articular cartilage repair, consisting of a triple composite of an interconnected porous hydroxyapatite (IP-CHA), recombinant human bone morphogenetic protein-2 (rhBMP-2), and a synthetic biodegradable polymer (PLA-PEG) as a carrier for rhBMP-2 was reported recently. This triple composite was proven to induce the regeneration of articular cartilage, only 1 week after implantation. Results demonstrated rapid and enhanced repair in the subchondral defect, revealing agglomerations of mesenchymal cells which had migrated from the surrounding bone marrow either directly, or indirectly, via the interconnecting pores of the IP-CHA scaffold. The study demonstrated that the initial defects are completely repaired 6 weeks post-implantation. Moreover, the regenerated cartilage manifested a hyaline-like appearance, with a mature matrix and a columnar organization of chondrocytes, demonstrating that a tested triple composite of rhBMP-2, PLA-PEG, and IP-CHA promotes the repair of full-thickness articular cartilage defects. The authors stated that this novel cell-free implant biotechnology could mark a new development in the field of articular cartilage repair (Tamai et al., 2005).

A recent comparative study revealed that PLGA scaffolds are better for inducing cartilage tissue formation as compared to the PLA scaffolds. Histological and immunohistochemical results demonstrated that chondrocytes seeded into PLGA retained their morphological phenotype to a greater extent than those seeded into PLA scaffolds (Lee et al., 2009).

10.1.4.3 Nanomaterials and nanotechnology

The science of nanomaterials and the recent progress of nanotechnology have developed new methods for improving the quality of scaffold intended for cartilage repair. The most utilized nanomaterials include nanoparticles, nanoclusters, nanocrystals, nanotubes, nanofibers, nanowires, nanorods, and nanofilms.

Novel techniques, such as electrospinning and 3D fiber deposition, were applied in the engineering at the nanoscale level of scaffolds. In order to add nanoscale features to a matrix structure, recent methods incorporate different nanoparticles into a polymeric material, offering high specificity of the final product. Scaffolds obtained by these methods are more similar to the extracellular matrix environment found in native cartilage tissue. The implication of nanomaterials in scaffold engineering leads to an increased cellular interaction with the scaffold and improved the quality of the produced constructs (Oseni et al., 2011). Nanomaterials aimed for regenerative medicine can be made of metals, ceramics, polymers, organic materials, and composites.

The main advantage of nanomaterials is their ability to grow in an organized and controlled manner and self-assembly into nanotubes or nanofibers which can accurately simulate the dimensions of natural entities, such as collagen, HA, fibrin, and alginate fibers. Also, the fact that after decreasing the material size into the nanoscale range, the surface area is dramatically increased, leading to better control of the roughness and surface-area-to-volume ratios, creating materials with superior physiochemical properties. Along with their dimensional similarity to cartilage tissue, nanomaterials also exhibit unique surface properties (such as surface topography, surface chemistry, surface wettability, and surface energy) as compared to conventional scaffolding materials.

Recent studies reported a functional nanostructured self-assembled hydrogel scaffold, containing the peptide (KLD-12, Lys-Leu-Asp), intended for biomedical use in cartilage repair. By using this nanostructured self-assembly, researchers created a biologically inspired 3D scaffold with self-assembled biomimetic features, suitable for reconstructing 3D cartilage tissue. A derived chondrocyte encapsulated scaffold, tested for cartilage regeneration, supported chondrocyte differentiation and promoted the synthesis of a cartilage-like ECM (Kisiday et al., 2002; Zhang and Webster, 2009).

Synthetic and natural polymers, such as PGA, PLGA, gelatin, collagen, and chitosan, are excellent candidates for the fabrication of nanoporous or nanofibrous polymer matrices intended for cartilage regeneration. Various nanostructured materials can be fabricated by several typical methods such as electrospinning, phase separation, particulate leaching, chemical etching, and 3D printing (Li et al., 2008).

Another technique of particular interest for cartilage engineering relies on the incorporation of chondrocytes or progenitor cells into a 3D polymer or nanostructured composite scaffold. Recent studies demonstrated that, depending on their structure, nanostructured scaffolds may be used to trigger a particular effect regarding cartilage and bone regeneration (Zhang and Webster, 2009).

10.2 MUSCLE TISSUE

Muscle is a highly complex and heterogeneous tissue serving a multitude of functions in the organism. The process of generating muscle—myogenesis—can be divided into several distinct phases (Tajbakhsh, 2009). With the exception of head muscles, all skeletal muscles are derived from mesodermal precursor cells, which originate from the somites (Karalaki et al., 2009). Somites are formed sequentially as segments of the paraxial mesoderm on each side of the neural tube, from anterior to posterior, at regular time intervals (Tee and Peppelenbosch, 2010). During embryonic myogenesis, mesoderm-derived structures generate the first muscle fibers of the body proper, and in subsequent waves additional fibers are generated along these template fibers (Sambasivan and Tajbakhsh, 2007). In the perinatal phase, muscle-resident myogenic progenitors initially proliferate extensively but later decrease as the number of myonuclei reaches a steady state and myofibrillar protein synthesis peaks. Once the muscle has matured, these progenitors will enter quiescence and henceforth reside within in it as satellite cells (SCs) that have the potential to differentiate into new fibers (Davis and Fiorotto, 2009). It is now generally accepted that SCs are closely related to progenitors of somitic origin (Bentzinger et al., 2012). Adult skeletal muscle, like all renewing organs, relies on a mechanism that compensates for the turnover of terminally differentiated cells to maintain tissue homeostasis (Pellettieri and Alvarado, 2007).

Somites represent transient structures able to differentiate into different types of tissue structures such as sclerotome (precursor of bones, cartilage, and tendons), myotome (precursor of muscle), and dermatome (precursor of the dermis). At a certain point, some myoblasts may irreversibly exit the cell cycle, align with each other, and fuse, forming multinucleated myotubes. Soon after primary myogenesis, secondary myoblasts in the dermomyotome use the primary myotome as a scaffold to attach to and fuse with each other, forming secondary myotubes (Bryson-Richardson and Currie, 2008). A similar myogenesis molecular process occurs after birth and this process aims to recruit adult muscle precursors for producing new myofibers during skeletal muscle damage (Tee and Peppelenbosch, 2010).

Tissue and organ regeneration proceed in a coordinated manner to restore proper function after trauma. Vertebrate skeletal muscle has a remarkable ability to regenerate after repeated and complete destruction of the tissue, yet limited information is available on how muscle stem and progenitor cells, and other non-muscle cells, reestablish homeostasis after the regenerative process (Tajbakhsh, 2009).

10.2.1 MUSCLE TISSUE PATHOLOGY

Muscle diseases (MDs) are a group of conditions that can be acquired or genetic, and which result in progressive shrinking and weakness of the skeletal muscle such as to cause varying degrees of disability (Sadjadi et al., 2011). MDs lead to muscle fiber degeneration, impairment of mobility, and in some cases premature death. Many of these muscular diseases are largely idiopathic (Gupta et al., 2014a,b). It has already been mentioned that many factors can influence muscle structure: genetic abnormalities, toxins, inflammation, infection, and hormonal and electrolyte imbalances (Bentzinger et al., 2012).

Myopathies may be divided into two main categories: inherited and acquired, including a very large number of muscular diseases (Table 10.1). The two types of myopathies are distinguished by the temporal course, the pattern of muscle weakness, and the absence or presence of a family history (Muthusamy, 2010). The underlying disease can involve muscles at both structural and functional levels including metabolism as well as muscle ion channel.

Diagnosis of these disorders is contingent on a targeted history and examination, biochemical and neurophysiological assessment, muscle biopsy, and genetic testing (Cardamone et al., 2008).

Myopathies are characterized by motor symptoms in the absence of any sensory involvement. Most myopathies manifest with weakness involving the proximal muscles. Some myopathies are associated with atypical distributions of weakness, such as inclusion body myositis, an inflammatory myopathy seen typically in older men that manifests with weakness in the finger flexors and quadriceps.

10.2.2 MEDICAL IMPACT

Muscular diseases affect millions of individuals each year, causing muscle atrophy, weakness, and/or pain, and often lead to muscle fiber degeneration, impairment of mobility, and even premature death. The individual MDs differ in their age of onset, their rate of progression, and their pattern of weakness, which in turn dictates the nature and extent of the disability that they cause. The disability caused by MD impacts upon quality of life (Sadjadi et al., 2011).

Table 10.1 The More Commonly Seen Inherited and Acquired Myopathies

	Acquired Myopathies		Inherited Myopathies
Inflammatory myopathy	Polymyositis	Muscular dystrophy	Dystrophinopathy (Duchenne muscular dystrophy, Becker muscular dystrophy)
	Dermatomyositis		Myotonic dystrophy 1 and 2
	Inclusion body myositis		Facioscapulohumeral muscular dystrophy
Infection	Viral infections (HIV, influenza virus, Epstein–Barr virus)		Oculopharyngeal muscular dystrophy
	Bacterial pyomyositis (*Staphylococcus aureus* and streptococci are common organisms)		Limb girdle muscular dystrophy
	Spirochete (Lyme disease)	Congenital myopathy	Nemaline myopathy
	Parasitic infections such as trichinosis		Central core myopathy
Toxic myopathy	Medications:	Metabolic myopathy	Acid maltase or acid alpha-1,4-glucosidase deficiency (Pompe disease)
	• Steroids		
	• Cholesterol-lowering medications: statins, fibrates, niacin, and ezetimibe		
	• Propofol		
	• Amiodarone		
	• Colchicine		
	• Chloroquine		
	• Antivirals and protease inhibitors		
	• Omeprazole		
	• Tryptophan		
	Toxins:		Glycogen storage disorders 3–11
	• Alcohol		
	• Toluene		

Myopathy associated with systemic diseases	Endocrine disorders: • Thyroid • Parathyroid • Pituitary or adrenal dysfunction Systemic inflammatory diseases: • Systemic lupus erythematosus • Rheumatoid arthritis • Scleroderma • Mixed connective disease • Sarcoidosis Electrolyte imbalance • Potassium or magnesium abnormalities • Hypophosphatemia Critical illness myopathy: • Non-depolarizing neuromuscular blocking agents • Steroids Critical illness myopathy • Non-depolarizing neuromuscular blocking agents • Steroids Amyloid myopathy: • Primary amyloidosis • Familial amyloidosis (TTR mutation)		Carnitine deficiency Fatty acid oxidation defects Carnitine palmitoyl transferase deficiency.
		Mitochondrial myopathy	Myoclonic epilepsy and ragged red fibers (MERRF) Mitochondrial myopathy, lactic acidosis, and strokes (MELAS) Mitochondrial neurogastrointestinal encephalomyopathy (MNGIE) Progressive external ophthalmoplegia (PEO)

Adapted from Muthusamy (2010).

10.2.3 MUSCLE REGENERATION

Muscle tissue damaged (skeletal, smooth, or cardiac muscle) either by injury or due to some degenerative diseases is able to regenerate new muscle fiber. The regeneration process depends on the magnitude of the initial lesion, the status of the host, and some other environmental factors (including ECM). In mammals, skeletal muscle has a great regeneration capacity, but this is much reduced for cardiac muscle.

The key cells involved in regeneration of muscle tissue are represented by a population of cells localized at periphery of adult myofiber named, for this reason, SCs; besides these, other cells have been proven to have myogenic capacity *in vitro*, or after transplantation: pericytes, endothelial cells, and interstitial cells (Tedesco et al., 2010). Other factors also contribute to muscle regeneration such as hepatocyte growth factor, FGFs, TGF-β, IGFs, and TNF-α.

Other cells with myogenic activity originally from tissues other than skeletal muscle are cells from ectoderm, such as neural stem cells, hematopoietic cells, cells derived from mesoderm (other than hematopoietic cells), pluripotent stem cells, such as embryonic stem cells (Thomson et al., 1998) or induced pluripotent stem cells (Yamanaka, 2009).

For the regeneration of damaged muscle tissue, similar steps to those from embryogenesis are followed. Initially, necrosis of the myofiber of the damaged tissue and inflammation, repair, and remodeling occur. Ultimately, SCs also known as this stage as myoblasts or myogenic precursor cells are activated and begin proliferation (Price et al., 2007) and differentiate under the control of myogenic regulatory factor 5, myogenic differentiation 1 (MyoD), and transcription factor paired box 7 (Pax7). Large numbers of new myofibers are generated in a few days (Whalen et al., 1990) after some asymmetric division and other SCs return to quiescence in order to maintain a pool of progenitors.

10.2.3.1 Therapeutic ultrasound

Therapeutic ultrasound is recommended and used in the treatment of muscle injuries. The treatment works as pain relief, and also enhances the initial stage of muscle regeneration, however the scientific proofs obtained till now using animal studies are not so promising.

10.2.3.2 Hyperbaric oxygen therapy

Hyperbaric oxygen therapy was another therapeutic option for the regeneration of the injured skeletal muscle, but the results are still controversial (Järvinen et al., 2013).

10.2.3.3 Cell therapy/tissue engineering

Because of their powerful myogenic activity, SCs were the first candidates used in cell therapy for muscular diseases. Some initial studies using intramuscular injections of myoblasts were realized on mice with lack of dystrophin. Although the results seemed promising, clinical trials that followed were unsuccessful due to low survival and migration of cells, or due to their rejection as a result of the immune response of the patient (Cossu and Sampaolesi, 2004). Also, these cells did not have the capacity to cross endothelial membrane for systemic transmission.

Rossi et al. (2011) designed and developed the delivery of SCs embedded in a hyaluronan-based hydrogel, hyaluronic acid–photoinitiator (HA-PI) complex for solving this problem and observed that SCs embedded in HA-PI promote regeneration of the tissue.

To this day, SCs are use in clinical trials in pathologies such as muscular dystrophy, stress urinary incontinence, or heart diseases (Tedesco et al., 2010).

In the case of skeletal muscle defects involving the loss of volume of the tissue, known as volumetric muscle loss (VML), regeneration is more difficult. The remaining functional myofibers are incapable of covering the gap formed, so an implant will be necessary also allowing the development of new functional myofibers, blood vessels, and nerves. In this case, *autologous tissue* from another area of the patient's body is transferred to the damaged zone, however, there remains the risk of donor-site morbidity, and the technique is not applicable for large defects in load-bearing muscles. A solution could be the use of a scaffold seeded with progenitor cells for regeneration of the tissue. A good choice for a scaffold could even be the ECM remaining after skeletal muscle tissue is decellularized.

Some defects repaired with ECM scaffold seeded with myocardial cells improve myocardial function in some studies (Kochupura et al., 2005). However, *in vivo*, the growth of new myofibers was limited and the functional recovery was not fully satisfactory (Kin et al., 2007). Researchers found solutions, and the use of MSCs could be a real option in this case, because MSCs are multipotent cells derived from bone morrow capable of differentiating into different tissues, including muscle, vascular tissue, and nerves. These cells participate in skeletal muscle regeneration physiologically. Therefore, the next step was the addition of MSCs to acellular ECM implants in the myocardium, and it was then observed that new myofibers were formed and attached to the ventricular surface (Chang et al., 2007; Wei et al., 2006), proving the potential of this technique in cardiac and skeletal muscle regeneration (Merritt et al., 2010).

A recent study (Ward et al., 2015) suggests the use of autologous *minced muscle grafts* instead of whole-muscle grafts for VML. The muscle, minced into small pieces, was used with success in a rodent VML model and in improving urinary incontinence in humans. A possible advantage of this technique is represented by the potential of expansion of this minced tissue in a conductive biomaterial, permitting regeneration of large muscle cells starting from a small amount of donor tissue (Ward et al., 2015).

Muscle regeneration is a complex process involving the use of different cells or scaffolds. Continuous research regarding development of new biomaterials and methods for treating various muscular diseases is of great interest and highly appreciated.

10.2.4 BIOACTIVE SCAFFOLDS AND NANOMATERIALS FOR MUSCLE REPAIR

Even though muscle (especially skeletal muscle) has an impressive capacity to regenerate after injury and damage, severe traumatic injuries result in a significant loss of muscle mass, the natural repairing processes being unable to bridge the gap between the remaining tissue. Even though tissue engineering using progenitor cells offers significant clinical progress, the success of this approach is significantly increased when the cells are used in combination with 3D scaffolds to faster repair, replace, and restore the essential functions of lost or damaged muscle tissue (Chaturvedi et al., 2011).

Recent approaches developed cell-free scaffolds made of different functional biomaterials to allow the endogenous myogenic cells to migrate, proliferate, and differentiate using the bioscaffold as a template to produce new muscle. Particular attention should be paid to the type of biomaterial used for the regenerative scaffold, to create an artificial niche, which allows the natural processes of stem cell activation, proliferation, differentiation, and self-renewal to occur.

An appropriate skeletal scaffold intended for muscle engineering should be biocompatible, biodegradable, have appropriate porosity, have the correct balance of stability and elasticity, and also mimic the ECM of the muscle tissue. These properties facilitate the success of the therapy and increase the probability that surrounding cells will be stimulated to proliferate, migrate, and differentiate to produce new, functional muscle tissue (Koning et al., 2009).

Recent studies reported that for functional skeletal muscle restoration it can be used a functional bioscaffold able to simultaneously act as an inductive microenvironment and as a cell- or drug-delivery vehicle to encourage muscle growth. Four types of material may be successfully used for muscle engineering: (i) biologically active, naturally derived materials (such as collagen, fibronectin, elastin, fibrin, hyaluronin and laminin), (ii) engineered synthetic silicones, (iii) polymers (such as PLA, PGA, PCL), and (iv) their copolymers (e.g., PLGA) (Wolf et al., 2015). Recent approaches at the development of hybrid scaffolds, comprising both naturally derived and synthetic materials, would combine the advantageous properties of these components to create an optimal platform for cell and drug delivery, and facilitate the engineering of muscle tissues.

10.2.4.1 Natural materials

Studies have reported a variety of naturally occurring scaffolds composed of ECM able to support the engineering and regeneration of skeletal muscle. These natural materials can be configured as two-dimensional sheets, simple tubular or hollow constructs, 3D whole-organ shapes, and also as hydrogels for expanded clinical applications (Wolf et al., 2015). Although individual ECM components have been isolated from native tissues to investigate the specific effects of these molecules on cell behavior and scaffolding properties, the complex constitution of the matrix is important for fast and efficient muscle regeneration. Collagen, gelatin, chitosan, silk fibroin, alginate, and agarose may be prepared as hydrogels and molded into shapes conducive for myogenesis. Moreover, more complex patterns can be introduced in such hydrogels to create myotube networks that yield improved viability and differentiation of muscle cells (Badylak et al., 2011).

In the available literature many *in vitro* and *in vivo* studies regarding the clinical and preclinical impact of naturally derived scaffolding materials on muscle engineering can be found. It is estimated that over 4 million patients have been implanted with a biocompatible scaffold containing naturally derived materials. The most common reasons for such a scaffold implantation are: extremity musculotendinous reinforcement, ventral hernia repair, and esophageal reconstruction. Recent studies reported a scaffolding implant, derived from ECM components, which revealed *de novo* formation of skeletal muscle cells, increased force production of the affected muscle group, and improved daily activities of the patients (Sicari et al., 2014).

10.2.4.2 Synthetic scaffolding materials

The most investigated materials for muscle tissue engineering are polypropylene, polyesters and their copolymers, and also various polyurethanes. Among these, the copolymer *PLGA* is one of the most extensively investigated and used synthetic biomaterials in skeletal muscle tissue engineering. Studies demonstrated that biodegradable porous PLGA promotes cell adherence, proliferation, formation of new 3D tissues, and also host-mediated vascularization and cell infiltration *in vivo*. PLGA was used in combination with another synthetic polymer, *poly (ε-caprolactone)* (PCL) (which is FDA approved for the fabrication of scaffolds for skeletal muscle engineering). PCL–PGA copolymer fibers were successfully used to obtain efficient scaffolds for different biomedical applications, including tissue engineering (Bellon et al., 2007).

Polyurethanes represent a diverse class of polymers that are able to incorporate numerous other chemical moieties to efficiently control the properties of the scaffolding material, such as *in vivo* degradation rate, mechanics, and hydrophobicity. Polyurethanes proved their usefulness in skeletal engineering by specifically influencing cellular phenotype and enabling physiologic muscle function.

Since musculoskeletal tissues are composed of highly organized nanostructured materials, with self-healing capability, nanomaterials have attracted much attention to create novel tissue engineering scaffolds for muscle repair in severe injury.

Because most nanostructured materials can be synthesized with controlled composition, size, geometry, and morphology they present enhanced biocompatibility and cell adhesion, being suitable for different applications in the development of musculoskeletal tissue scaffolds (Peng et al., 2014).

10.3 CONCLUSIONS

Since articular and muscle damage represent a major cause of disability, affecting an increasing percentage of the population, a wide range of therapeutic approaches are currently available to treat these disorders.

Many traditional therapeutic approaches are still the first-line choices because of their efficiency and low cost. However, for difficult-to-treat or untreatable cartilage and MDs, recent biomedical and technological progress has led to the development of novel therapeutic and preventive methods, which may successfully be applied in clinics.

Tissue and organ engineering is now possible, due to the identification and synthesis of natural and artificial materials, at micro- and nanometric scales, which could help the regeneration and repair or even structural and/or functional replacement of human body tissues. Engineered scaffolds were developed for the treatment of the most severe cartilage and muscle disorders and their applicative potential and impact are huge. However, despite the recent technological and clinical success there are several queries regarding the wide utilization of such therapeutic approaches, mainly related to the poor clinical knowledge regarding the long- and mid-term impact of such nanostructured biomaterials within the human body.

ACKNOWLEDGMENTS

This work was supported by a grant of the Romanian National Authority for Scientific Research and Innovation, CNCS – UEFISCDI, project number "PN-II-RU-TE-2014-4-2269".

REFERENCES

Ahmed, T.A., Dare, E.V., Hincke, M., 2008. Fibrin: a versatile scaffold for tissue engineering applications. Tissue Eng. Part B Rev. 14 (2), 199–215.

Aletaha, D., Neogi, T., Silman, A.J., Funovits, J., Felson, D.T., Bingham III, C.O., et al., 2010. Rheumatoid arthritis classification criteria: an American College of Rheumatology/European League Against Rheumatism collaborative initiative. Arthritis Rheum. 62 (9), 2569–2581.

Allen, K.D., Yvonne, M.G., 2015. Epidemiology of osteoarthritis: state of the evidence. Curr. Opin. Rheumatol. 27 (3), 276–283.

Allison, D.D., Grande-Allen, K.J., 2006. Review. Hyaluronan: a powerful tissue engineering tool. Tissue Eng. 12 (8), 2131–2140.

Almqvist, K.F., Dhollander, A.A., Verdonk, P.C., Forsyth, R., Verdonk, R., Verbruggen, G., 2009. Treatment of cartilage defects in the knee using alginate beads containing human mature allogenic chondrocytes. Am. J. Sports Med. 37 (10), 1920–1929.

Awad, H.A., Quinn Wickham, M., Leddy, H.A., Gimble, J.M., Guilak, F., 2004. Chondrogenic differentiation of adipose-derived adult stem cells in agarose, alginate, and gelatin scaffolds. Biomaterials 25, 3211–3222.

Badylak, S.F., Freytes, D.O., Gilbert, T.W., 2009. Extracellular matrix as a biological scaffold material: structure and function. Acta Biomater. 5, 1–13.

Badylak, S.F., Hoppo, T., Nieponice, A., Gilbert, T.W., Davison, J.M., Jobe, B.A., 2011. Esophageal preservation in five male patients after endoscopic inner-layer circumferential resection in the setting of superficial cancer: a regenerative medicine approach with a biologic scaffold. Tissue Eng. Part A 17 (11–12), 1643–1650.

Baker, M.I., Walsh, S.P., Schwartz, Z., Boyan, B.D., 2012. A review of polyvinyl alcohol and its uses in cartilage and orthopedic applications. J. Biomed. Mater. Res. B Appl. Biomater. 100 (5), 1451–1457.

Bellon, J.M., Rodriguez, M., Garcia-Honduvilla, N., Pascual, G., Bujan, J., 2007. Partially absorbable meshes for hernia repair offer advantages over nonabsorbable meshes. Am. J. Surg. 194, 68–74.

Bentley, G., 2008. Advances in cartilage cell transplantation. In: Symposium on Cartilage Repair. 8th EFFORT Congress, Nice, France.

Bentzinger, C.F., Wang, Y.X., Rudnicki, M.A., 2012. Building muscle: molecular regulation of myogenesis. Cold Spring Harb. Perspect. Biol. 4 (2), a008342.

Bleibler, F., Rapp, K., Jaensch, A., Becker, C., König, H.-H., 2014. Expected lifetime numbers and costs of fractures in postmenopausal women with and without osteoporosis in Germany: a discrete event simulation model. BMC Health Serv. Res. 14, 284.

Bolliet, C., Bohn, M.C., Spector, M., 2008. Non-viral delivery of the gene for glial cell line-derived neurotrophic factor to mesenchymal stem cells *in vitro* via a collagen scaffold. Tissue Eng. C Methods 14, 207–219.

Bonadio, J., Smiley, E., Patil, P., Goldstein, S., 1999. Localized, direct plasmid gene delivery *in vivo*: prolonged therapy results in reproducible tissue regeneration. Nat. Med. 5, 753–759.

Bonewald, L.F., Kiel, D., Clemens, T., Esser, K., Orwoll, E., O'Keefe, R., et al., 2013. Forum on bone and skeletal muscle interactions: summary of the proceedings of an ASBMR workshop. J. Bone Miner. Res. 28 (9), 1857–1865.

Brittberg, M., Lindahl, A., Nilsson, A., Ohlsson, C., Isaksson, O., Peterson, L., 1994. Treatment of deep cartilage defects in the knee with autologous chondrocyte transplantation. New Engl. J. Med. 331, 889–895.

Bryson-Richardson, R.J., Currie, P.D., 2008. The genetics of vertebrate myogenesis. Nat. Rev. Genet. 9, 632–646.

Buckley, C.T., Kelly, D.J., 2012. Expansion in the presence of FGF-2 enhances the functional development of cartilaginous tissues engineered using infrapatellar fat pad derived MSCs. J. Mech. Behav. Biomed. Mater. 11, 102–111.

Campos, D.F.D., Drescher, W., Rath, B., Tingart, M., Fischer, H., 2012. Supporting biomaterials for articular cartilage repair. Cartilage 3 (3), 205–221.

Caplan, A.I., 2007. Adult mesenchymal stem cells for tissue engineering versus regenerative medicine. J. Cell. Physiol. 213, 341–347.

Cardamone, M., Darras, B.T., Ryan, M.M., 2008. Inherited myopathies and muscular dystrophies. Semin. Neurol. 28 (2), 250–259.

Cen, L., Liu, W., Cui, L., Zhang, W., Cao, Y., 2008. Collagen tissue engineering: development of novel biomaterials and applications. Pediatr. Res. 63, 492–496.

Cervellati, C., Bonaccorsi, G., Cremonini, E., Romani, A., Fila, E., Castaldini, M.C., et al., 2014. Oxidative stress and bone resorption interplay as a possible trigger for postmenopausal osteoporosis. Biomed. Res. Int. 2014, 569563.

Chahal, J., Gross, A.E., Gross, C., Mall, N., Dwyer, T., Chahal, A., et al., 2013. Outcomes of osteochondral allograft transplantation in the knee. Arthroscopy 29, 575–588.

Chang, Y., Lai, P.H., Wei, H.J., Lin, W.W., Chen, C.H., Hwang, S.M., et al., 2007. Tissue regeneration observed in a basic fibroblast growth factor-loaded porous acellular bovine pericardium populated with mesenchymal stem cells. J. Thorac. Cardiovasc. Surg. 134, 65, 73. e1.

Chaturvedi, V., Dye, D., Coombe, D., Grounds, M., 2011. Bioactive scaffolds in skeletal muscle regeneration and tissue engineering. Aust. Biochem. 42 (3).

Chen, H., Sun, J., Hoemann, C.D., Lascau-Coman, V., Ouyang, W., McKee, M.D., et al., 2009. Drilling and microfracture lead to different bone structure and necrosis during bone-marrow stimulation for cartilage repair. J. Orthop. Res. 27, 1432–1438.

Chu, C.R., Coutts, R.D., Yoshioka, M., Harwood, F.L., Monosov, A.Z., Amiel, D., 1995. Articular cartilage repair using allogeneic perichondrocyte-seeded biodegradable porous polylactic acid (PLA): a tissue-engineering study. J. Biomed. Mater. Res. 29 (9), 1147–1154.

Cosman, F., de Beur, S.J., LeBoff, M.S., Lewiecki, E.M., Tanner, B., Randall, S., et al., 2014. Clinician's guide to prevention and treatment of osteoporosis. Osteoporos. Int. 25 (10), 2359–2381.

Cossu, G., Sampaolesi, M., 2004. New therapies for muscular dystrophy: cautious optimism. Trends. Mol. Med. 10 (10), 516–520.

Craig, W., David, J.W., Ming, H.Z., 2003. A current review on the biology and treatment of the articular cartilage defects (part I & part II). J. Musculoskelet. Res. 7 (3&4), 157–181.

Crowson, C.S., Matteson, E.L., Myasoedova, E., Michet, C.J., Ernste, F.C., Warrington III, K.J., et al., 2011. The lifetime risk of adult-onset rheumatoid arthritis and other inflammatory autoimmune rheumatic diseases. Arthritis. Rheum. 63 (3), 633–639.

D'Anchise, R., Manta, N., Prospero, E., Bevilacqua, C., Gigante, A., 2005. Autologous implantation of chondrocytes on a solid collagen scaffold: clinical and histological outcomes after two years of followup. J. Orthop. Traumatol. 6, 36–43.

Das, S., Crockett, J.C., 2013. Osteoporosis—a current view of pharmacological prevention and treatment. Drug Des. Dev. Ther. 7, 435–448.

Davis III, J.M., Matteson, E.L., 2012. My treatment approach to rheumatoid arthritis. Mayo. Clin. Proc. 87 (7), 659–673.

Davis, T.A., Fiorotto, M.L., 2009. Regulation of muscle growth in neonates. Curr. Opin. Clin. Nutr. Metab. Care. 12, 78–85.

Deane, K.D., Norris, J.M., Holers, V.M., 2010. Pre-clinical rheumatoid arthritis: identification, evaluation and future directions for investigation. Rheum. Dis. Clin. North. Am. 36 (2), 213–241.

Deryk, G.J.M.D., 2009. Articular cartilage degeneration: etiologic association with obesity. Ochsner J. 9 (3), 137–139.

Erickson, G.R., Gimble, J.M., Franklin, D.M., Rice, H.E., Awad, H., Guilak, F., 2002. Chondrogenic potential of adipose tissue-derived stromal cells *in vitro* and *in vivo*. Biochem. Biophys. Res. Commun. 290, 763–769.

Falah, M., Nierenberg, G., Soudry, M., Hayden, M., Volpin, G., 2010. Treatment of articular cartilage lesions of the knee. Int. Orthop. (SICOT) 34, 621–630.

Farnworth, L., 2000. Osteochondral defects of the knee. Orthopaedics 23 (2), 146–157.

Farrell, E., O'Brien, F.J., Doyle, P., Fischer, J., Yannas, I., Harley, B.A., et al., 2006. A collagen-glycosaminoglycan scaffold supports adult rat mesenchymal stem cell differentiation along osteogenic and chondrogenic routes. Tissue Eng. 12, 459–468.

Filardo, G., Kon, E., Roffi, A., Di Martino, A., Marcacci, M., 2013. Scaffold-based repair for cartilage healing: a systematic review and technical note. Arthroscopy 29, 174–186.

Frisbie, D.D., Bowman, S.M., Colhoun, H.A., DiCarlo, E.F., Kawcak, C.E., McIlwraith, C. W., 2008. Evaluation of autologous chondrocyte transplantation via a collagen membrane in equine articular defects—results at 12 and 18 months. Osteoarthr. Cartil. 16, 667–679.

Gentile, P., Chiono, V., Carmagnola, I., Hatton, P.V., 2014. An overview of poly(lactic-*co*-glycolic) acid (PLGA)-based biomaterials for bone tissue engineering. Int. J. Mol. Sci. 15, 3640–3659.

Gille, J., Behrens, P., Volpi, P., de Girolamo, L., Reiss, E., Zoch, W., et al., 2013. Outcome of autologous matrix induced chondrogenesis (AMIC) in cartilage knee surgery: data of the AMIC registry. Arch. Orthop. Trauma Surg. 133, 87–93.

Gudas, R., Gudaite, A., Pocius, A., Gudiene, A., Cekanauskas, E., Monastyreckiene, E., et al., 2012. Ten-year follow-up of a prospective, randomized clinical study of mosaic osteochondral autologous transplantation versus microfracture for the treatment of osteochondral defects in the knee joint of athletes. Am. J. Sports. Med. 40, 2499–2508.

Guilak, F., Awad, H.A., Fermor, B., Leddy, H.A., Gimble, J.M., 2004. Adipose-derived adult stem cells for cartilage tissue engineering. Biorheology 41, 389–399.

Guo, J., Chung, U.-I., Yang, D., Karsenty, G., Bringhurst, F.R., Kronenberg, H.M., 2006. PTH/PTHrP receptor delays chondrocyte hypertrophy via both Runx2-dependent and -independent pathways. Dev. Biol. 292, 116–128.

Gupta, A., Bhat, S., Jagdale, P.R., Chaudhari, B.P., Lidgren, L., Gupta, K.C., et al., 2014a. Evaluation of three-dimensional chitosan-agarose-gelatin cryogel scaffold for the repair of subchondral cartilage defects: an *in vivo* study in a rabbit model. Tissue. Eng. Part A 20 (23–24), 3101–3111.

Gupta, S., Kim, S.-M., Wang, Y., Dinasarapu, A.R., Subramaniam, S., 2014b. Statistical insights into major human muscular diseases. Hum. Mol. Genet. 23 (14), 3772–3778.

Hangody, L., Kish, G., Kárpáti, Z., Szerb, I., Udvarhelyi, I., 1997. Arthroscopic autogenous osteochondral mosaicplasty for the treatment of femoral condylar articular defects. A preliminary report. Knee Surg. Sports Traumatol. Arthrosc. 5, 262–267.

Hangody, L., Ráthonyi, G.K., Duska, Z., Vásárhelyi, G., Füles, P., Módis, L., 2004. Autologous osteochondral mosaicplasty. Surgical technique. J. Bone Joint. Surg. Am. 86-A (Suppl. 1)), 65–72.

Hauser, R., 2015. Treatment of degenerative joint disease. http://www.caringmedical.com/treatment/degenerative-joint-disease/.

Heijink, A., Gomoll, A.H., Madry, H., Drobnič, M., Filardo, G., Espregueira-Mendes, J., et al., 2012. Biomechanical considerations in the pathogenesis of osteoarthritis of the knee. Knee Surg. Sports Traumatol. Arthrosc. 20 (3), 423–435.

Im, G.I., Kim, H.J., Lee, J.H., 2011. Chondrogenesis of adipose stem cells in a porous PLGA scaffold impregnated with plasmid DNA containing SOX trio (SOX-5,-6 and -9) genes. Biomaterials 32, 4385–4392.

In, B.M., Ralphs, J.R.J., 1998. Fibrocartilage in tendons and ligaments—an adaptation to compressive load. Anatomie 193, 481–494.

Järvinen Tero, A.H., Järvinen, M., Kalimo, H., 2013. Regeneration of injured skeletal muscle after the injury. Muscles Ligaments Tendons J 3 (4), 337–345.

Johnson, V.L., Hunter, D.J., 2014. The epidemiology of osteoarthritis. Best. Pract. Res. Clin. Rheumatol. 28, 5–15.

Kang, S.W., Yoon, J.R., Lee, J.S., Kim, H.J., Lim, H.W., Lim, H.C., et al., 2006. The use of poly(lactic-*co*-glycolic acid) microspheres as injectable cell carriers for cartilage regeneration in rabbit knees. J. Biomater. Sci. Polym. Ed. 17 (8), 925–939.

Kang, S.W., La, W.G., Kim, B.S., 2009. Open macroporous poly(lactic-*co*-glycolic acid) microspheres as an injectable scaffold for cartilage tissue engineering. J. Biomater. Sci. Polym. Ed. 20 (3), 399–409.

Karalaki, M., Fili, S., Philippou, A., Koutsilieris, M., 2009. Muscle regeneration: cellular and molecular events. In Vivo 23, 779–796.

Karlson, E.W., Deane, K., 2012. Environmental and gene-environment interactions and risk of rheumatoid arthritis. Rheum. Dis. Clin. North. Am. 38 (2), 405–426.

Karsdal, M.A., Madsen, S.H., Christiansen, C., Henriksen, K., Fosang, A.J., Sondergaard, B.C., 2008. Cartilage degradation is fully reversible in the presence of aggrecanase but not matrix metalloproteinase activity. Arthritis Res. Ther. 10, R63.

Karsdal, M.A., Woodworth, T., Henriksen, K., Maksymowych, W.P., Genant, H., Vergnaud, P., et al., 2011. Biochemical markers of ongoing joint damage in rheumatoid arthritis—current and future applications, limitations and opportunities. Arthritis Res. Ther. 13 (2), 215.

Karsdal, M.A., Nielsen, M.J., Sand, J.M., Henriksen, K., Genovese, F., Bay-Jensen, A.C., et al., 2013. Extracellular matrix remodeling: the common denominator in connective tissue diseases possibilities for evaluation and current understanding of the matrix as more than a passive architecture, but a key player in tissue failure. Assay. Drug Dev. Technol. 11, 70–92.

Kieswetter, K., Schwartz, Z., Alderete, M., Dean, D.D., Boyan, B.D., 1997. Platelet derived growth factor stimulates chondrocyte proliferation but prevents endochondral maturation. Endocrine 6, 257–264.

Kim, H.J., Kim, K.K., Park, I.K., Choi, B.S., Kim, J.H., Kim, M.S., 2012. Hybrid scaffolds composed of hyaluronic acid and collagen for cartilage regeneration. Tissue Eng. Regen. Med. 9 (2), 57–62.

Kim, S.Y., Hong, D.K., Im, M., Lee, Y., Lee, J.H., Seo, Y.J., 2011. A case of auricular ossification. Ann. Dermatol. 23 (Suppl. 2), S261–S263.

Kin, S., Hagiwara, A., Nakase, Y., Kuriu, Y., Nakashima, S., Yoshikawa, T., et al., 2007. Regeneration of skeletal muscle using in situ tissue engineering on an acellular collagen sponge scaffold in a rabbit model. ASAIO. J. 53, 506–513.

Kisiday, J., Jin, M., Kurz, B., Hung, H., Semino, C., Zhang, S., et al., 2002. Self-assembling peptide hydrogel fosters chondrocyte extracellular matrix production and cell division: implications for cartilage tissue repair. Proc. Natl. Acad. Sci. U.S.A. 99, 9996.

Kobayashi, S., Takebe, T., Inui, M., Iwai, S., Kan, H., Zheng, Y.-W., et al., 2011. Reconstruction of human elastic cartilage by a $CD44^+$ $CD90^+$ stem cell in the ear perichondrium. Proc. Natl. Acad. Sci. U.S.A. 108 (35), 14479–14484.

Kochupura, P.V., Azeloglu, E.U., Kelly, D.J., Doronin, S.V., Badylak, S.F., Krukenkamp, I.B., et al., 2005. Tissue-engineered myocardial patch derived from extracellular matrix provides regional mechanical function. Circulation 112 (Suppl. 9), I144.

Kon, E., Buda, R., Filardo, G., Di Martino, A., Timoncini, A., Cenacchi, A., et al., 2010. Platelet-rich plasma: intra-articular knee injections produced favorable results on degenerative cartilage lesions. Knee Surg. Sports Traumatol. Arthrosc. 18, 472–479.

Koning, M., Harmsen, M.C., van Luyn, M.J., Werker, P.M., 2009. Current opportunities and challenges in skeletal muscle tissue engineering. J. Tissue Eng. Regen. Med. 3, 407–415.

Korczowska, I., 2014. Rheumatoid arthritis susceptibility genes: an overview. World J. Orthop. 5 (4), 544–549.

Kraus, V.B., Burnett, B., Coindreau, J., Cottrell, S., Eyre, D., Gendreau, M., Osteoarthritis Biomarkers Working Group, et al., 2011. Application of biomarkers in the development of drugs intended for the treatment of osteoarthritis. Osteoarthr. Cartil. 19 (5), 515–542.

Kuo, C.K., Li, W.J., Mauck, R.L., Tuan, R.S., 2006. Cartilage tissue engineering: its potential and uses. Curr. Opin. Rheumatol. 18 (1), 64–73.

Lee, N.K., Oh, H.J., Hong, C.M., Suh, H., Hong, S.H., 2009. Comparison of the synthetic biodegradable polymers, polylactide (PLA), and polylactic-*co*-glycolic acid (PLGA) as scaffolds for artificial cartilage. Biotechnol. Bioprocess Eng. 14 (2), 180–186.

Li, W.J., Jiang, Y.J., Tuan, R.S., 2008. Cell-nanofiber-based cartilage tissue engineering using improved cell seeding, growth factor, and bioreactor technologies. Tissue Eng. Part A 14, 639.

Lipowitz, A.J., 2015. Degenerative joint disease and traumatic arthritis (Chapter 87), Charles D. Newton. http://cal.vet.upenn.edu/projects/saortho/chapter_87/87mast.htm/.

Lotz, M., Martel-Pelletier, J., Christiansen, C., Brandi, M.-L., Bruyère, O., Chapurlat, R., et al., 2013. Value of biomarkers in osteoarthritis: current status and perspectives. Ann. Rheum. Dis. 72 (11), 1756–1763.

MacBarb, R.F., Makris, E.A., Hu, J.C., Athanasiou, K.A., 2013. A chondroitinase-ABC and TGF-β1 treatment regimen for enhancing the mechanical properties of tissue engineered fibrocartilage. Acta Biomater. 9 (1), 4626–4634.

Matsiko, A., Levingstone, T.J., O'Brien, F.J., 2013. Advanced strategies for articular cartilage defect repair. Materials 6, 637–668.

Merritt, E.K., Cannon, M.V., Hammers, D.W., Le Long, N., Gokhale, R., Sarathy, A., et al., 2010. Repair of traumatic skeletal muscle injury with bone-marrow-derived mesenchymal stem cells seeded on extracellular matrix. Tissue Eng. Part A 16 (9), 2871–2881.

Micheli, L.J., Browne, J.E., Erggelet, C., Fu, F., Mandelbaum, B., Moseley, J.B., et al., 2001. Autologous chondrocyte implantation of the knee: multicenter experience and minimum 3-year follow-up. Clin. J. Sport. Med. 11, 223–228.

Minas, T., 1998. Nonarthroplasty management of knee arthritis in the young individual. Curr. Opin. Orthop. 9, 46–52.

Mitchell, W.K., Williams, J., Atherton, P., Larvin, M., Lund, J., Narici, M., 2012. Sarcopenia, dynapenia, and the impact of advancing age on human skeletal muscle size and strength; a quantitative review. Front. Physiol. 3, 260.

Mobasheri, A., 2011. Applications of proteomics to osteoarthritis, a musculoskeletal disease characterized by aging. Front. Physiol. 2.

Mobasheri, A., 2012. Osteoarthritis year 2012 in review: biomarkers. Osteoarth. Cartil. 20, 1451–1464.

Mow, V.C., Ratcliffe, A., 1997. Structure and Function of Articular Cartilage and Meniscus, second ed. Lippincott Raven, Philadelphia, PA.

Muthusamy, P., 2010. Myopathy. Center for continuing education, Cliveland clinic. http://www.clevelandclinicmeded.com/.

Niemeyer, P., Pestka, J.M., Kreuz, P.C., Erggelet, C., Schmal, H., Suedkamp, N.P., et al., 2008. Characteristic complications after autologous chondrocyte implantation for cartilage defects of the knee joint. Am. J. Sports. Med. 36, 2091–2099.

Oseni, A.O., Crowley, C., Boland, M.Z., Butler, P.E., Seifalian, A.M., 2011. Cartilage tissue engineering: the application of nanomaterials and stem cell technology. In: Eberli, E. (Ed.), Tissue Engineering and Regenerative Medicine "Tissue Engineering for Tissue and Organ Regeneration", InTech, Berlin. ISBN 978-953-307-688-1.

Özmeriç, A., Bahadır, A.K., Hürriyet, A.N., 2014. Treatment for cartilage injuries of the knee with a new treatment algorithm. World J. Orthop. 5 (5), 677–684.

Pecina, M., Jelic, M., Martinovic, S., Haspl, M., Vukicevic, S., 2002. Articular cartilage repair: the role of bone morphogenetic proteins. Int. Orthop. 26 (3), 131–136.

Pecina, M., Jelic, M., Ivkovic, A., Hudetz, D., 2006. Gene therapy applications in orthopaedics. Int. Orthop. 30 (3), 215–216.

Pellettieri, J., Alvarado, S.A., 2007. Cell turnover and adult tissue homeostasis: from humans to planarians. Annu. Rev. Genet. 41, 83–105.

Peng, H., Liu, X., Wang, R., Jia, F., Dongd, L., Wang, Q., 2014. Emerging nanostructured materials for musculoskeletal tissue engineering. J. Mater. Chem. B 2, 6435–6461.

Perricone, C., Ceccarelli, F., Valesini, G., 2011. An overview on the genetic of rheumatoid arthritis: a never-ending story. Autoimmun. Rev. 10, 599–608.

Peterson, L., Minas, T., Brittberg, M., Nilsson, A., Sjogren Jansson, E., Lindahl, A., 2000. Two- to 9-year outcome after autologous chondrocyte transplantation of the knee. Clin. Orthop. 374, 212–234.

Peterson, L., Vasiliadis, H.S., Brittberg, M., Lindahl, A., 2010. Autologous chondrocyte implantation. Am. J. Sports. Med. 38, 1117–1124.

Price, F.D., Kuroda, K., Rudnicki, M.A., 2007. Stem cell based therapies to treat muscular dystrophy. Biochim. Biophys. Acta 1772 (2), 272–283.

Pridie, A.H., 1959. The method of resurfacing osteoarthritic knee. J. Bone Joint. Surg. [Br] 41, 618–623.

Rajan, N., Lagueux, J., Couet, F., Pennock, W., Mantovani, D., Sionkowska, A., 2008. Low doses of ultraviolet radiation stimulate cell activity in collagen-based scaffolds. Biotechnol. Prog. 24 (4), 884–889.

Rodnguez-Merchan, E.C., De la Corte-Garcıa, H., 2012. Regeneration of articular cartilage of the knee: basic concepts. In: Rodríguez-Merchán, E.C. (Ed.), Articular Cartilage Defects of the Knee. Springer-Verlag, Italia.

Rossi, C.A., Flaibani, M., Blaauw, B., Pozzobon, M., Figallo, E., Reggiani, C., et al., 2011. *In vivo* tissue engineering of functional skeletal muscle by freshly isolated satellite cells embedded in a photopolymerizable hydrogeli. FEBS J. 25, 2296–2304.

Rousseau, J.C., Garnero, P., 2012. Biological markers in osteoarthritis. Bone 51, 265–277.

Sadjadi, R., Vincent, K.A., Carr, A.J., Walburn, J., Brooks, V.L., Pandya, S., Muscle Study Group, et al., 2011. Validation of the individualised neuromuscular quality of life for the USA with comparison of the impact of muscle disease on those living in USA versus UK. Health Qual. Life Outcomes 9, 114.

Sambasivan, R., Tajbakhsh, S., 2007. Skeletal muscle stem cell birth and properties. Semin. Cell. Dev. Biol. 18, 870–882.

Sharma, B., Williams, C.G., Khan, M., Manson, P., Elisseeff, J.H., 2007. *In vivo* chondrogenesis of mesenchymal stem cells in a photopolymerized hydrogel. Plast. Reconstr. Surg. 119, 112–120.

Sicari, B.M., Dearth, C.L., Badylak, S.F., 2014. Tissue engineering and regenerative medicine approaches to enhance the functional response to skeletal muscle injury. Anat. Rec. 297, 51–64.

Smolen, J.S., Aletaha, D., Grisar, J., Redlich, K., Steiner, G., Wagner, O., 2008. The need for prognosticators in rheumatoid arthritis: biological and clinical markers: where are we now? Arthritis Res. Ther. 10 (3), 208.

Steadman, J.R., Rodkey, W.G., Singleton, S.B., Briggs, K.K., 1997. Microfracture technique for full-thickness chondral defects: technique and clinical results. Operat. Tech. Orthop. 7, 300–307.

Steinert, A.F., Nöth, U., Tuan, R.S., 2008. Concepts in gene therapy for cartilage repair. Injury 39 (Suppl. 1), S97–113.

Steinwachs, M., 2008. Cell based articular cartilage repair strategies. In: Symposium on Cartilage Repair. 8th EFFORT Congress, Nice, France.

Steinwachs, M., Kreuz, P.C., 2007. Autologous chondrocyte implantation in chondral defects of the knee with a type I/III collagen membrane: a prospective study with a 3-year follow-up. Arthroscopy 23 (4), 381–387.

Svedbom, A., Hernlund, E., Ivergård, M., Compston, J., Cooper, C., Stenmark, J., et al., 2013. Osteoporosis in the European Union: a compendium of country-specific reports. Arch. Osteoporos. 8 (1–2), 137.

Tajbakhsh, S., 2009. Skeletal muscle stem cells in developmental versus regenerative myogenesis. J. Intern. Med. 266 (4), 372–389.

Tamai, N., Myoui, A., Hirao, M., Kaito, T., Ochi, T., Tanaka, J., et al., 2005. A new biotechnology for articular cartilage repair: subchondral implantation of a composite of interconnected porous hydroxyapatite, synthetic polymer (PLA-PEG), and bone morphogenetic protein-2 (rhBMP-2). Osteoarth. Cartil. 13 (5), 405–417.

Tedesco, F.S., Dellavalle, A., Jordi, D.-M., Graziella, M., 2010. Repairing skeletal muscle: regenerative potential of skeletal muscle stem cells. J. Clin Invest. 120 (1), 11–19.

Tee, J.-M., Peppelenbosch, M.P., 2010. Anchoring skeletal muscle development and disease: the role of ankyrin repeat domain containing proteins in muscle physiology. Crit. Rev. Biochem. Mol. Biol. 45 (4), 318–330.

Thomson, J.A., Itskovitz-Eldor, J., Shapiro, S.S., Waknitz, M.A., Swiergiel, J.J., Marshall, V.S., et al., 1998. Embryonic stem cell lines derived from human blastocysts. Science 282 (5391), 1145–1147.

Ueda, H., Hong, L., Yamamoto, M., Shigeno, K., Inoue, M., Toba, T., et al., 2002. Use of collagen sponge incorporating transforming growth factor-beta1 to promote bone repair in skull defects in rabbits. Biomaterials 23 (4), 1003–1010.

Unterman, S.A., Gibson, M., Lee, J.H., Crist, J., Chansakul, T., Yang, E.C., et al., 2012. Hyaluronic acid-binding scaffold for articular cartilage repair. Tissue Eng. Part A 18 (23–24), 2497–2506.

Van Osch, G.J., Brittberg, M., Dennis, J.E., Bastiaansen-Jenniskens, Y.M., Erben, R.G., Konttinen, Y.T., et al., 2009. Cartilage repair: past and future—lessons for regenerative medicine. J. Cell. Mol. Med. 13 (5), 792–810.

van Spil, W.E., Degroot, J., Lems, W.F., Oostveen, J.C., Lafeber, F.P., 2010. Serum and urinary biochemical markers for knee and hip-osteoarthritis: a systematic review applying the consensus BIPED criteria. Osteoarth. Cartil. 18, 605–612.

Wanga, Y., Dominick, J.B., Kimb, H.-J., Kimc, H.S., Kaplan, D.L., 2006. Cartilage tissue engineering with silk scaffolds and human articular chondrocytes. Biomaterials 27 (25), 4434–4442.

Ward, C.L., Ji, L., Corona, B.T., 2015. An autologous muscle tissue expansion approach for the treatment of volumetric muscle loss. BioRes. Open Access 4, 198–208. Available from: http://dx.doi.org/10.1089/biores.2015.0009/.

Wei, H.J., Chen, S.C., Chang, Y., Hwang, S.M., Lin, W.W., Lai, P.H., et al., 2006. Porous acellular bovine pericardia seeded with mesenchymal stem cells as a patch to repair a myocardial defect in a syngeneic rat model. Biomaterials 27, 5409–5419.

Whalen, R.G., Harris, J.B., Butler-Browne, G.S., Sesodia, S., 1990. Expression of myosin isoforms during notexininduced regeneration of rat soleus muscles. Dev. Biol. 141 (1), 24–40.

Williams, F.M., Spector, T.D., 2008. Biomarkers in osteoarthritis. Arthritis Res. Ther. 10, 101.

Wolf, M.T., Dearth, C.L., Sonnenberg, S.B., Loboa, E.G., Badylak, S.F., 2015. Naturally derived and synthetic scaffolds for skeletal muscle reconstruction. Adv. Drug. Deliv. Rev. 84, 208–221.

Woolf, A.D., Pfleger, B., 2003. Burden of major musculoskeletal conditions. Bull. World. Health. Organ. 81 (9), 646–656.

Yaeger, P.C., Masi, T.S.L., de Ortiz, J.L.B., Binette, F.O., Tubo, R., McPherson, J.M., 1997. Synergistic action of transforming growth factor-[beta] and insulin-like growth factor-I induces expression of type II collagen and aggrecan genes in adult human articular chondrocytes. Exp. Cell. Res. 237, 318–325.

Yamanaka, S., 2009. A fresh look at iPS cells. Cell. 137 (1), 13–17.

Yamashita, F., Sakakida, K., Suzu, F., Takai, S., 1985. The transplantation of an autogeneic osteochondral fragment for osteochondritis dissecans of the knee. Clin. Orthop. Relat. Res. 201, 43–50.

Zaslav, K., Cole, B., Brewster, R., DeBerardino, T., Farr, J., Fowler, P., et al., 2009. A prospective study of autologous chondrocyte implantation in patients with failed prior treatment for articular cartilage defect of the knee: results of the study of the treatment of articular repair (STAR) clinical trial. Am. J. Sports. Med. 37, 42–55.

Zhang, L., Webster, T.J., 2009. Nanotechnology and nanomaterials: promises for improved tissue regeneration. Nano Today 4, 66–80.

CHAPTER

Fabrication of complex biomaterial scaffolds for soft tissue engineering by electrospinning

11

Aaron S. Goldstein[1,2] and Patrick S. Thayer[2]

[1]Department of Chemical Engineering, Virginia Tech, Blacksburg, VA, USA [2]School of Biomedical Engineering and Sciences, Virginia Tech, Blacksburg, VA, USA

11.1 INTRODUCTION

Mammalian cells are dynamic, continuously probing their microenvironment and changing their morphology and phenotype in response to local stimuli. Consequently, critical to the achievement of functional engineered tissues is the fabrication of biomaterial scaffolds that incorporate the appropriate topographical, mechanical, and biochemical stimuli to guide cell proliferation, differentiation, and assembly into tissue-like structures. This is easier said than done. Although a plethora of approaches to generate functional scaffolds have been described, many fall short of achieving this goal. Techniques such as particle sintering (Duan et al., 2010), fused deposition modeling (Leong et al., 2003), or porogen leaching (Gao et al., 2006; Yang et al., 2001; Laurencin et al., 1999) of hydrophobic synthetic polymers (e.g., polycaprolactone (PCL), polyglycolide (PGA), polylactide (PLA)) result in mechanically robust scaffolds with high surface areas and extensive networks of large (~100–500 μm) and interconnected pores. However, *in vitro* cell adhesion is limited to the pore surfaces and the extracellular matrix (ECM) is relatively disorganized (Gao et al., 2006; Zeltinger et al., 2001; Huang et al., 2004). Furthermore, these polymeric scaffolds often degrade slowly, are difficult for cells to remodel, and can obstruct nutrient transport and organization of tissue-like structures. Alternatively, techniques built around hydrogel materials (e.g., fibrin, collagen, various polysaccharides, and degradable polyethylene glycol (PEG) networks) can allow unrestricted cell migration and nutrient transport (Ahmed et al., 2008; Cross et al., 2010; Miller et al., 2010). However, these materials are frequently very soft, making them difficult to handle and primarily suited as injectable cell carriers, void-fillers, and bulking agents (Young et al., 2011; Bryan et al., 2009). In addition, neither of these two families of techniques

Nanobiomaterials in Soft Tissue Engineering. DOI: http://dx.doi.org/10.1016/B978-0-323-42865-1.00011-8

is ideal for guiding cell alignment: a property central to the development of oriented soft tissues and organs (e.g., muscle, tendons and ligaments, blood vessels, tubular organs).

In contrast, anisotropic fibrous scaffolds—which are strong in tension and compliant in bending and compression—have been developed for the replacement of vascular structures (Takahashi et al., 2009) and the repair of abdominal hernias (Boukerrou et al., 2007) and torn ligaments and tendons (Freeman et al., 2007). These large scaffolds are formed by braiding, knitting, or compressing (Wang et al., 2011) fibers prepared from silk fibroin (Altman et al., 2002), PLA (Freeman et al., 2007), and various polyurethanes (Liljensten et al., 2002). However, the individual fibers—typically prepared by wet- and melt-spinning processes—have diameters of 25–200 μm, which are too large to guide cell alignment.

On the other hand, scaffolds that incorporate microfibers (defined here as fibers with diameters of 0.1–10 μm) can both introduce mechanical anisotropy and provide topographic features to guide cell alignment. Importantly, these materials may be able to organize cells into oriented tissue-like structures. In this chapter, we discuss the fabrication of such microfiber "meshes" through solution electrospinning (Section 11.2), and how changing fiber diameter and degree of alignment can influence cell behavior through contact guidance and mechanical effects (Section 11.3). Next, we describe various techniques for chemically modifying the fibers to present biochemical cues (Section 11.4). This is followed by a discussion of methods to form complex fibrous meshes that incorporate multiple material types and phases, and when arranged in a graded or laminated manner may be utilized for the generation of complex tissue structures (Section 11.5). Finally, we close this chapter with a brief outlook on the future and the challenges with incorporating electrospinning into an effective strategy for regenerating damaged tissues and organs (Section 11.6).

11.2 ELECTROSPINNING OF FIBROUS SCAFFOLDS

Solution electrospinning is a simple and inexpensive polymer-processing technique for the fabrication of dense, nonwoven fibrous meshes, which can guide cell alignment (Manwaring et al., 2004) and modulate development of an organized ECM (Lee et al., 2005). To fabricate an electrospun mesh, the polymer of choice is dissolved in a moderately volatile solvent (e.g., hexafluoroisopropanol, trifluoroethanol, dichloromethane, chloroform (Jarusuwannapoom et al., 2005)), delivered to a spinneret, and exposed to a voltage potential (between the spinneret and a collecting surface) (Doshi and Reneker, 1995; Figure 11.1a). At a sufficient voltage differential, the electrostatic force acting on the polymer solution overcomes the surface tension and generates a Taylor cone at the tip of the spinneret, from which a polymer jet is drawn. Under the right solution conditions

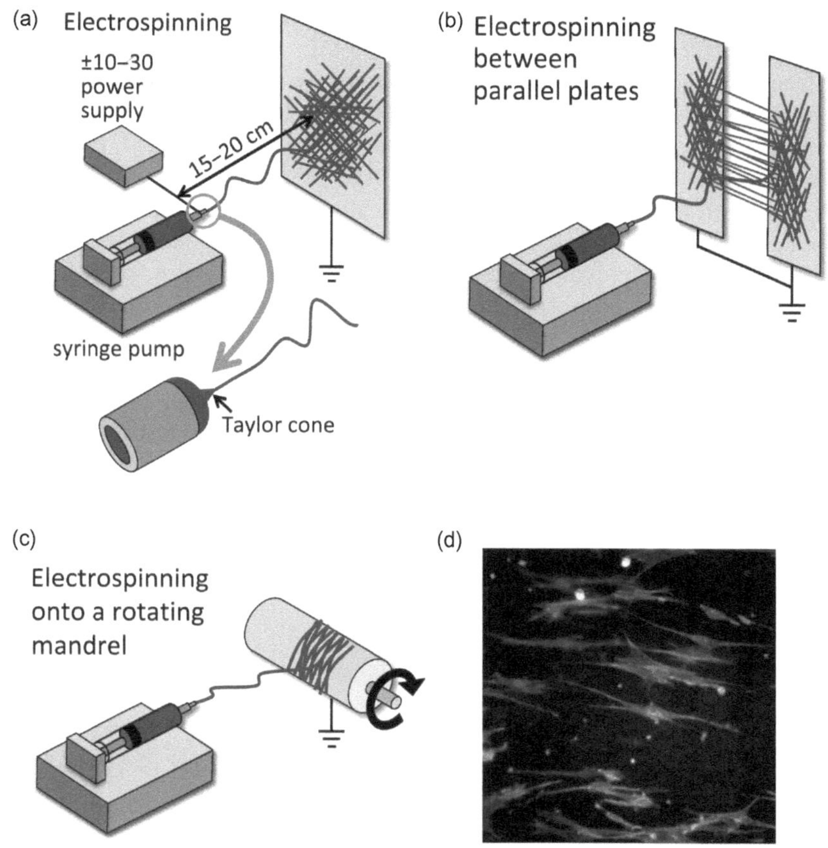

FIGURE 11.1

(a) Diagram of a typical electrospinning system with a syringe pump to deliver a polymer solution (red) to a charged needle. A polymer jet is ejected from the needle tip by an electric potential of ±10–25 kV, and is collected on a grounded collector situated 15–20 cm away. Aligned fibers can be collected by (b) electrospinning between two grounded collectors or (c) onto a grounded rotating mandrel. (d) Image of mesenchymal stem cells elongated on horizontally aligned PCL fibers.

(e.g., viscosity, polymer molecular weight), polymer chain entanglements prevent the jet from breaking into droplets (i.e., electrospraying) (Shenoy et al., 2005), while rapid evaporation of the solvent consolidates the jet into a fiber. Electrostatic repulsion and bending instability cause chaotic whipping of the fiber, leading to fiber drawing and deposition on the target with a random orientation (Reneker et al., 2000). Residual solvent in the fibers facilitates interfiber bonding that confers mechanical integrity to the resultant mesh. However, the deposition process is relatively slow; meshes of 25–150 μm can be prepared in under an hour, but 1-mm-thick meshes can require several hours of electrospinning (Baker and Mauck, 2007).

Electrospinning is most typically performed with unbranched polymers of intermediate molecular weights (i.e., 50–500 kDa) that either have a small pendant groups (e.g., polystyrene, PLA) or no pendant group (e.g., PEO, PGA, PCL). Electrospinning of structural proteins has been described (e.g., silk (Li et al., 2006), collagen (Rho et al., 2006)), but typically involves denaturing the protein to disrupt secondary, tertiary, and quaternary structures and blending the protein with synthetic linear polymers (Zeugolis et al., 2008). Likewise, polysaccharide materials have been electrospun (e.g., alginate (Bonino et al., 2011), chitosan (Bhattarai et al., 2005)), but typically as blends with linear polymers.

Nevertheless, electrospinning is a versatile platform from which a wide of range of mesh architectures (e.g., fiber diameters and orientations), mechanical properties, and compositions (e.g., surface chemistry, bioactivity) can be generated through careful variation of electrospinning conditions. Furthermore, complex materials can be achieved using more elaborate approaches, such as coaxial electrospinning, electrospinning from multiple spinnerets, electrospinning onto specialized collectors or by integrating electrospinning with other scaffold fabrication techniques. These strategies are described in detail in the subsequent sections.

11.3 INFLUENCE OF ARCHITECTURE OF MICROFIBER MESHES ON CELL BEHAVIOR

The architecture of electrospun meshes can be easily tuned by variation of both the electrospinning conditions and the properties of the target on which the fibers are collected. Specifically, fiber diameter can be increased from ~100 nm to ~10 μm by increasing the polymer concentration, increasing the solution viscosity, or decreasing the throw distance (Tan et al., 2005). At the same time, highly aligned fiber meshes (angular standard deviations below 20°) can be formed by collecting fibers in a gap between parallel grounded targets (Jha et al., 2011) (Figure 11.1b), while differing degrees of alignment (angular standard deviations of 20–40°) can be achieved by varying the rotational speed of a grounded mandrel (Bashur et al., 2006; Figure 11.1c).

The architecture of electrospun fiber meshes (i.e., fiber diameter, fiber orientation) can have a pronounced effect on cell adhesion, morphology, proliferation, and differentiation (Sutherland et al., 2005). Biomaterial surfaces with topographical features (e.g., grooves, ridges) 70 nm (Teixeira et al., 2003) to 5 μm (Nikkhah et al., 2012) in size have been shown to spatially regulate cell adhesion, spreading and migration by a phenomenon known as contact guidance. Specifically, anchorage-dependent mammalian cells establish adhesive contacts to biomaterials via integrin adhesion receptors, which subsequently cluster into focal adhesions.

Focal adhesions, in turn, contain various plaque proteins involved in cell signaling (e.g., vinculin, paxillin, focal adhesion kinase (Cukierman et al., 2001)), serve as anchor points for the actin cytoskeleton (Alenghat and Ingber, 2002), and allow cells to exert contractile forces on their microenvironments. Consequently, topographic features on the biomaterial surface can guide the size, density, and spatial distribution of these focal adhesions. In turn, this impacts cytoskeletal organization (e.g., Figure 11.1d) and cell behavior (Feinberg et al., 2008; Geiger et al., 2009). Specifically, through modulation of the actin cytoskeleton (Dalby, 2005), the topographic features can influence signaling pathways involved in cell proliferation (Provenzano et al., 2008), differentiation, and the deposition and organization of ECM proteins (Manwaring et al., 2004).

11.3.1 EFFECT OF FIBER DIAMETER AND ORIENTATION ON CELL PROLIFERATION

One of the easiest topographical features to control is fiber diameter (Tan et al., 2005), and several studies have demonstrated that attachment and proliferation rates differ between cells on small (<0.5 μm), intermediate (0.5–1.2 μm), and large (>1.2 μm) diameter fiber meshes. For example, Chen and Su, (2011) reported that NIH 3T3 cells attached more rapidly on small-diameter fiber PCL meshes (<0.50 μm) as compared to intermediate- and large-diameter fiber PCL meshes (>0.50 μm), while cell proliferation was slower on intermediate-diameter fiber meshes relative to meshes comprised of small (<0.50 μm) or large (>1.5 μm) diameter fibers. Badami et al. (2006), who also explored the effect of fiber diameter, reported higher MC3T3-E1 osteoprogenitor cell densities on large-diameter fiber meshes (2.1 μm) relative to cells on small-diameter meshes (0.14 μm). In contrast, Erisken et al. (2013), who cultured human tendon fibroblasts on electrospun fiber meshes for 28 days, reported that DNA content was greater on the smallest-diameter fiber (0.32 μm) meshes compared to intermediate- (0.68 μm) and large-diameter (1.8 μm) fiber meshes. Together, these results indicate that fiber diameter affects cell proliferation rate, but differences between the three studies suggest other factors (e.g., cell type, mesh chemistry, mesh compliance) may also be important.

11.3.2 EFFECT OF FIBER DIAMETER AND ORIENTATION ON CELL PHENOTYPE

A second topographical feature of electrospun meshes that is both easy to control and that can influence the development of aligned tissues is fiber alignment. In conjunction with fiber diameter, fiber alignment has been shown to affect the expression of phenotypic markers of connective (e.g., tendon, ligament), nervous, vascular, and muscle (e.g., skeletal, smooth, and cardiac) tissues.

11.3.2.1 Tendon and ligament

With regard to the tendon and ligament phenotypes, a number of research groups have examined the effect of fiber diameter within aligned and randomly oriented fiber meshes. Erisken et al., who examined aligned fiber meshes, reported increased expression of collagen types I, III, and V and tenomodulin for human tendon fibroblasts grown for 14 days on large-diameter (1.80 μm) aligned fiber meshes, and increased deposition of glycosaminoglycans by cells grown on small-diameter (0.32 μm) aligned fiber meshes relative to intermediate-diameter (0.68 μm) aligned fiber meshes (Erisken et al., 2013). Similarly, Cardwell et al. reported that on large-diameter (2.1 μm) aligned fibers C2H10T1/2 mesenchymal progenitor cells expressed more collagen I and scleraxis mRNA than cells grown on small-diameter (0.50 μm) aligned fiber meshes (Cardwell et al., 2014). In contrast, when fibers were randomly oriented, Bashur et al. reported that the expression of collagen 1α1 and decorin by mesenchymal stem cells was elevated in small-diameter (0.28 μm) fiber meshes relative to large-diameter (2.3 μm) fiber meshes (Bashur et al., 2009). Together, these studies suggest that fiber diameter and orientation act together to affect development of the tendon/ligament phenotype.

11.3.2.2 Nervous tissue

Likewise, development of nervous tissue is modulated by both diameter and alignment of electrospun fibers. However, unlike cells within tendon and ligament tissues—which are primarily fibroblastic—nervous tissue consists of neurons and a variety of supporting cell types (e.g., microglia, astrocytes, oligodendrocytes in the central nervous system, Schwann cells in the peripheral nervous system). Consequently, electrospun fibers intended to guide formation of nervous tissue must present surface topographies that support the development of a balance of cell phenotypes. Christopherson et al., who probed the effect of fiber diameter on randomly oriented meshes, reported that neural stem cells exhibited a glial cell morphology and differentiated toward the oligodendrocytic lineage on small-diameter (0.28 μm) meshes (Christopherson et al., 2009). In contrast, on intermediate- (0.75 μm) and large-diameter (1.45 μm) fiber meshes neural stem cells elongated and differentiated toward a neuronal lineage. Separately, Chew et al. explored how alignment of electrospun PCL fiber meshes influences the maturation of human Schwann cells (Chew et al., 2008). They showed that both random and aligned fibers supported induction of myelin-associated glycoprotein (an early myelin marker) and suppressed expression of neural cell-adhesive molecule-1 (an immature Schwann cell marker) compared to smooth surfaces. In addition, they reported that the myelin-specific gene, *P0*, was upregulated by cells on the aligned meshes as compared to cells on randomly oriented fiber meshes and smooth surfaces. Furthermore, Schwann cells were highly elongated on aligned 1.0-μm-diameter fibers, but remained unoriented on randomly oriented 2.3-μm-diameter fibers. These data show that topographical features (e.g., fiber diameter and alignment) can play an important role in development of the different cell types found within nervous tissue.

11.3.2.3 Vascular tissue

Vascular tissue—like nervous tissue in the previous example—is composed of multiple cell types. In arteries and veins these cells are spatially arranged in three layers (the *tunica intima*, the *tunica media*, and the *tunica adventitia*), each with a different ECM composition and organization. The *tunica intima*, the inner-most layer, consists of a dense polysaccharide matrix and a monolayer of endothelial cells, which are in direct contact with the blood, and acts as a nonthrombogenic barrier. Interested in engineering a *tunica intima*, Kwon et al. fabricated poly (caprolactone-*co*-lactide) (PLCL) meshes with different fiber diameters (Kwon et al., 2005). On small- (0.3 μm) and intermediate-diameter (1.2 μm) fibers human endothelial cells formed adhesive contacts to multiple fibers and proliferated well. In contrast, on large-diameter (7 μm) fibers endothelial cells adhered to single fibers, assumed a more rounded morphology, and proliferated more slowly. The *tunica media*, the middle layer, is comprised of circumferentially oriented smooth muscle cells within an oriented collagen- and elastin-rich ECM. Toward developing an engineered *tunica media*, Zhu et al. examined the effect of alignment of large-diameter ($\sim$10 μm) PCL fiber meshes on human smooth muscle cell morphology and phenotype (Zhu et al., 2010). Culture for 7 days on aligned fiber meshes resulted in the generation of a highly organized, oriented cell monolayer which exhibited a more contractile phenotype as shown by the presence of α-smooth muscle actin. In contrast, cells seeded on randomly oriented meshes exhibited no preferred orientation and α-smooth muscle actin remained relatively unorganized. Together, these data suggest that a multilayer deposition strategy for preparing electrospun meshes with distinct properties for the *tunica intima* and *tunica media* may be advantageous for vascular applications. (This strategy is discussed in Section 11.5.1.)

11.3.2.4 Muscle tissue

Development of functional muscle tissue is a complex problem, requiring a biomaterial scaffold that supports formation of organized muscle fibers consisting of enervated and multinucleated myotubes, a supporting capillary network, and a dense ECM. Focusing on the potential role of aligned electrospun fibers in myotube formation, Choi et al. fabricated 0.30-μm PCL/collagen meshes with varying degrees of fiber orientation (Choi et al., 2008a). Human skeletal muscle cells—seeded onto fiber meshes—developed longer and more highly aligned myotubes when the fibers were aligned, as compared to fibers that were randomly oriented. Likewise, Aviss et al. reported that C2C12 skeletal muscle cells elongated and oriented their actin cytoskeletons more rapidly on aligned poly(lactic-*co*-glycolic acid) (PLGA) microfibers than on randomly oriented fibers (Aviss et al., 2010). Additionally, a greater percentage of cells fused into multinucleated myotubes with highly aligned sarcomeric myosin structures on aligned fibers. Similarly,

Ricotti et al. analyzed the behavior of both skeletal (C2C12) and cardiac (H9c2) muscle cell lines on random and aligned 0.20–0.40-μm poly(hydroxybutyrate) (PHB) fiber meshes (Ricotti et al., 2012). While cell proliferation was similar on both randomly oriented and aligned fibers, aligned fibers resulted in the formation of significantly more multinucleated myotubes. Furthermore, in both C2C12 and H9c2 cells, the expression of relevant genes such as *MLP*, *Acta1*, *MYH1*, *-2*, and *-4* was significantly increased on aligned fiber meshes as compared to randomly oriented fiber meshes. Together, these studies demonstrate that formation of aligned myotubes is facilitated by an aligned microfiber architecture. While we posit that aligned fibers create a topography that is conducive to myoblast alignment, we cannot discount the role of mechanical properties in cell alignment and maturation. Indeed Ricotti et al. reported that the modulus of their aligned PHB fiber meshes was 50% higher than that of their random fiber meshes (Ricotti et al., 2012). Therefore, the role of mechanical properties is the focus of the next section.

11.3.3 MECHANICAL CONSIDERATIONS OF CELL RESPONSE TO FIBER DIAMETER AND ORIENTATION

In the preceding sections, we showed a variety of examples that highlight how cell adhesion, proliferation, morphology, and phenotype are sensitive to the diameter and orientation of electrospun fibrous meshes. However, care must be taken in interpreting these data as such trends may reflect differences in the mechanical properties of the electrospun meshes. It has been well-established that biomaterial compliance can affect stem cell behavior (Engler et al., 2006). In general, soft materials have been shown to guide differentiation toward soft tissues such as fat (Rowlands et al., 2008) and neuronal tissue (Leipzig and Shoichet, 2009), while stiffer materials have been shown to facilitate development of stiff tissues such as bone (Kelly and Jacobs, 2010). Efforts to tune electrospun fiber diameter and alignment can impact the mechanical properties of the resultant meshes. For example, Kwon et al., who prepared 50/50 PLCL meshes with fiber diameters of 0.3, 1.2, and 7.0 μm (by varying the electrospinning conditions), found that the smaller-diameter fiber meshes were stiffer than the larger (Young's moduli of 2.2, 1.8, and 0.8 MPa, respectively) (Kwon et al., 2005). Similarly, Stylianopoulos et al. demonstrated that when polyurethane was electrospun onto a rotating collector, systematic increases in mandrel speed (0, 2.0, or 4.4 m/s) resulted in decreases in fiber diameter (0.90 μm, 0.63 μm, and 0.57 μm) and angular standard deviation (54.6°, 41.2°, and 29.9°, respectively), and an increase in the tensile modulus (0.89, 1.41, and 3.04 MPa) (Stylianopoulos et al., 2008). One factor contributing to this trend could be polymer morphology. Wong et al. used X-ray diffraction and single-fiber tensile testing to show that stiffer smaller-diameter PCL fibers had higher degrees of crystallinity and molecular orientation compared to softer large-diameter fibers (Wong et al., 2008), possibly through a process of strain crystallization.

To isolate the effect of mechanical properties, Nam et al. leveraged coaxial electrospinning (Figure 11.2a) to fabricate chemically and architecturally similar meshes with different elastic moduli (Nam et al., 2011). Specifically, two meshes were fabricated: one composed of PCL (modulus of 7.1 MPa) and one consisting of a poly(ether sulfone) core phase and a PCL shell (modulus of 30.6 MPa). Mouse C3H10T1/2 mesenchymal progenitor cells were seeded on both materials and cultured under either chondrogenic or osteogenic conditions. Under chondrogenic conditions, cells on the softer fibers had a greater deposition of glycosaminoglycans and expression of sox9, collagen type II, and aggrecan as compared to cells on the stiffer fibers. Conversely, under osteogenic conditions, cells on stiffer

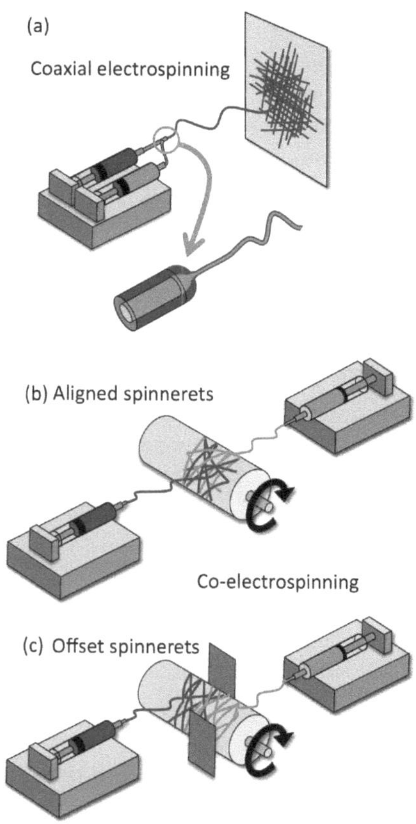

FIGURE 11.2

Diagrams of more complex electrospinning approaches. (a) Coaxial electrospinning where two needles (one inside the other) deliver the core (light gray) and shell (dark gray) phases simultaneously. (b and c) Co-electrospinning to create a mesh consisting of two different types of fibers. Spatial arrangement of the spinnerets can be used to create (b) depthwise and (c) lateral gradients of material properties.

fibers had greater alkaline phosphatase activity and expressed more Runx2, alkaline phosphatase, and osteocalcin mRNA compared to cells on the softer fibers. Further, cells on stiff fibers were more spread out and actin stress fibers were more pronounced, while on soft fibers cells appeared more rounded.

11.3.4 EFFECT OF FIBER DIAMETER ON MACROPHAGE RESPONSE

Up to this point, we have only considered examples of how electrospun fiber diameter, alignment, and mechanical properties affect the behavior of cells associated with soft tissues and organs. However, components of the immune system play critical roles in normal tissue remodeling as well as foreign body responses to implanted materials, and therefore require some discussion.

An emerging theme in tissue engineering is the role of a competent immune system. To guide tissue regeneration, biomaterial scaffolds must elicit an inflammatory response, recruit macrophages, and direct them toward a proregenerative phenotype. Consequently, an understanding of how scaffolds interact with the major components of the immune system is of keen interest. Saino et al. investigated macrophage response to intermediate- ($\sim$0.6 μm) and large-diameter ($\sim$1.6 μm) PLLA fibers with either random or aligned orientations (Saino et al., 2011). Murine macrophage-like RAW 264.7 cells cultured for 7 days on meshes exhibited lower levels of cytokine release on intermediate-diameter fibers (compared to macrophages on large fibers) regardless of mesh orientation. Garg et al. extended this study, and analyzed the polarization of naïve mouse bone-marrow-derived macrophages (M0) toward inflammatory (M1) and regenerative (M2) phenotypes on randomly oriented polydioxanone meshes with fiber diameters of 0.96, 2.2, and 2.8 μm (Garg et al., 2013). On the largest-diameter meshes macrophages exhibited a more pronounced M2 phenotype, as indicated by increased expression of transforming growth factor (TGF)-β1, vascular endothelial growth factor (VEGF), and fibroblast growth factor (FGF)-2. Furthermore, the authors showed that conditioned media collected from naïve macrophage culture on the largest-diameter fibers were angiogenic and stimulated sprouting of capillary-like structures from endothelial cell-coated beads.

11.3.5 CONCLUDING REMARKS ON FIBER ARCHITECTURE

In this section, we presented examples of how variation in the architecture, topography, and mechanical properties of biocompatible materials affect cell behavior, and can be designed to elicit tissue-specific responses. The key point is that most “biocompatible” materials are not bio-inert; cells are able to establish adhesive contacts to them and probe their properties. In the next section, we consider approaches to modify the biomaterial surface to facilitate specific cell/surface contacts.

11.4 SURFACE MODIFICATION

Surface chemistry of electrospun fibers can guide cell fate in a manner that is both significant and complementary to biomaterial architecture, topography, and compliance. However, conventional biocompatible polymers (e.g., PLGA, PCL, PEG) are not intrinsically bioactive. In contrast, the ECM—consisting of structural proteins (e.g., collagens, laminin), glycosaminoglycans (e.g., hyaluronic acid, heparans, dermatans), and growth factors and morphogens—consists of a rich milieu of bioactive factors that can interact with cells through receptor-mediated binding, and can control cell phenotype and fate through the modulation of biochemical signaling pathways. Therefore, the decoration of conventional biocompatible polymers with peptides or proteins—through physisorption or covalent grafting—could be a powerful means to stimulate cell function. In addition, a variety of simple nonspecific modification techniques are available to improve material hydrophilicity and cell adhesion.

11.4.1 NONSPECIFIC MODIFICATION

Nonspecific surface modification involves chemical changes to the fiber surfaces that improve overall biocompatibility without introducing molecular species that target specific cell receptors. A broad array of chemical treatments have been described in the literature to nonspecifically modify biomaterial surfaces, and include exposure of fibers to oxygen (Chen and Su, 2011), argon (Baker et al., 2006), or ammonia plasma (Cheng et al., 2014), and immersion in poly-lysine- or serum-containing solutions. Plasma treatments can introduce oxygen and nitrogen groups that can improve the wettability of otherwise hydrophobic fiber meshes. Further, positive charges conferred by ammonia plasma treatment or poly-lysine adsorption can interact with negative polysaccharides displayed on cell membranes to facilitate cell adhesion. In contrast, immersion of electrospun meshes in serum-containing culture media permits adsorption of various proteins (e.g., fibronectin, vitronectin) that are recognized by integrin adhesion receptors (Figure 11.3a). One can consider this nonspecific modification as it produces a heterogeneous and poorly characterized surface that is analogous to the protein absorption that occurs *in vivo* due to contact with blood and other body fluids (Horbett, 1993). This approach is beneficial if simple adhesion is desired; however, nonspecific protein absorption can lead to unintended consequences, including surface fouling, nondesired differentiation, and host immune responses (Anderson et al., 2008; Gristina, 1994).

11.4.2 SPECIFIC MODIFICATION

Specific modification includes the physisorption of large proteins or covalent grafting of small proteins and biomolecules to biomaterial surfaces such that they

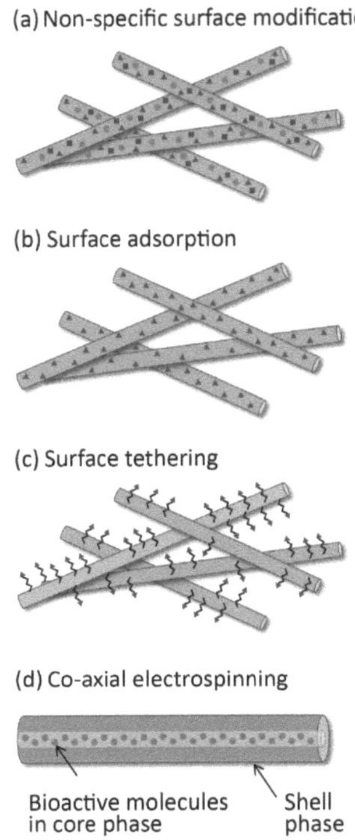

FIGURE 11.3

Methods for incorporating bioactive molecules onto fibers. (a) Adsorption of serum results in a poorly characterized mixture of different proteins. (b) Adsorption and (c) covalent tethering of a single protein. (d) Incorporation of a single protein into the core phase of coaxial fibers.

may interact with specific cell receptors (Figure 11.3b and c). The former group includes structural ECM proteins laminin, fibronectin, and collagen, which are known to interact with specific members of the integrin adhesion receptor family (Frith et al., 2012). Due to their large sizes (>100 kDa), these proteins typically become irreversibly adsorbed to biomaterials surface, permitting long-term stable functionalization. In contrast, physisorption of smaller proteins (e.g., growth factors, morphogens) can be transient, as these biomolecules may be displaced by larger proteins (e.g., from blood plasma or serum-containing culture media). This displacement—known as the Vroman effect—can be prevented by covalently linking the biomolecules to biomaterial surfaces. This, in turn, often requires modification of the biomaterial to incorporate chemistries amenable to surface grafting. Both the blending of the biomaterial with graftable macromolecules prior to electrospinning (Yu et al., 2014, Kim and Park, 2006) and various chemical treatments (e.g., plasma (Cheng et al., 2014; Chen and Su, 2011), aminolysis (Horne et al., 2009; Zhang and Hollister, 2009), and acid or alkali etching (Hayami et al., 2010) have been reported. In the two following sections, we review efforts to modify electrospun fibers with cell-adhesive, mitogenic and morphogenic biomolecules.

11.4.3 ADHESIVE BIOMOLECULES

While entire proteins such as collagens, fibronectin, and fibrin can be physisorbed from solution onto electrospun fibers, a number of smaller peptide sequences—derived from these larger proteins—have been identified that can mediate adhesion via specific integrin adhesion receptors. The tripeptide sequence Arg-Gly-Asp (RGD)—that is found in fibronectin and vitronectin—is recognized by many integrin heterodimers (and among many cell types) (Shekaran and Garcia, 2011), making it one of the most commonly grafted adhesive sequences (Ruoslahti and Pierschbacher, 1987). Similarly, the laminin-derived Tyr-Ile-Gly-Ser-Arg (YIGSR) sequence (Malinda and Kleinman, 1996) has also been used to promote cell adhesion. However, in contrast to fibronectin, which is ubiquitous throughout the ECM, laminin is primarily localized to the basement membranes of tissues, and can be utilized to target ECM-specific cell integrin receptors such as those found in epithelial and neuronal cells. Beyond these two peptide sequences, a wide variety of other ECM and tissue-specific peptide fragments have been described (Shekaran and Garcia, 2011) that can also be grafted to impart adhesion to electrospun fibers.

11.4.4 GROWTH FACTORS AND MORPHOGENS

Similar to adhesive proteins and peptides, growth factors and morphogens can directly influence cellular differentiation through their interaction with specific cell receptors. Because of their relatively low molecular weight, growth factors and morphogens can be displaced from the biomaterial surface by the Vroman effect, necessitating either surface grafting or incorporation of these macromolecules within the bulk of the fiber. Incorporation of growth factors and morphogens (e.g., insulin like growth factor-1, hepatocyte growth factor, FGF-2) into electrospinning solutions has been described previously in the literature (Nelson et al., 2011; Sahoo et al., 2010), but concern exists that the solvents and electric fields—used in the electrospinning process—can denature proteins (Zeugolis et al., 2008). Alternatively, proteins in aqueous solutions have been incorporated into the core phase of coaxially electrospun fibers (Figure 11.3d) (Sahoo et al., 2010). However, this can make the rate of delivery dependent on the rate of degradation of the shell phase.

Surface conjugation can ensure immediate availability of growth factors and morphogens to adherent cells. A variety of factors, including epidermal growth factor (EGF) (Choi et al., 2008b), nerve growth factor (NGF) (Cho et al., 2010), and brain-derived neurotrophic factor (BDNF) (Horne et al., 2009), have been covalently tethered to electrospun fibers. Alternatively, because a large number of growth factors and morphogens possess heparin-binding domains (e.g., members of the FGF and TGF-β families), covalent grafting of heparin to fibers followed by ionic tethering of growth factors or morphogens to the heparin may be a tractable alternative to present such bioactive molecules. Indeed, Lee et al. used this approach to conjugate platelet-derived growth factor (PDGF)-BB to PCL/gelatin fibers (Lee et al., 2012).

11.4.5 SPECIFIC MODIFICATION OF FIBER SURFACE FOR TISSUE ENGINEERING APPLICATIONS

In the following subsections we summarize recent efforts to modify electrospun fiber surfaces to facilitate the development of connective, vascular, nervous, and dermal tissues.

11.4.5.1 Connective tissue applications

For potential application in engineering of connective tissues (e.g., tendon, ligament), Kim et al. grafted RGD to electrospun PLGA fibers (Kim and Park, 2006). Specifically, an amine-terminated PLGA-PEG diblock copolymer was blended with PLGA and electrospun to form fiber meshes displaying primary amine groups. These surface amine groups were subsequently used to tether the RGD-containing pentapeptide Gly-Arg-Gly-Asp-Tyr. The authors then demonstrated more rapid adhesion and proliferation of NIH 3T3 fibroblasts on the RGD-functionalized fibers as compared to the unmodified fibers. Further, the authors reported a more defined actin cytoskeleton after 2 and 12 h postseeding, compared to rounder and less spread out cells on the unmodified fibers.

11.4.5.2 Vascular applications

For application in engineering a *tunica intima*, Choi et al. tethered an RGD-containing peptide to electrospun fibers to improve cell adhesion. Briefly, the researchers first surface-modified polyurethane meshes with amine-terminated PEG groups (where the PEG block served as a spacing arm) and then tethered the pentapeptide Gly-Arg-Gly-Asp-Ser (GRGDS) to the primary amines (Choi et al., 2008c). Human umbilical vein endothelial cells seeded on these functionalized meshes showed greater viability as compared to cells on unmodified meshes. Separately, Lee et al. sought to improve the bioactivity of PCL/gelatin electrospun fibers for application as an engineered *tunica media* by adsorption of PDGF-BB. To this end, Lee et al. formed randomly oriented fiber meshes (1.0 and 3.0 μm), tethered heparin to primary amines on the fibers, and adsorbed PDGF-BB to the fiber surfaces (Lee et al., 2012). Comparison of the release of PDGF-BB from heparin-conjugated and plain PCL/gelatin fibers showed a more sustained release without a burst when heparin was included. Subsequently, cell culture experiments indicated increased human smooth muscle cell proliferation rate and infiltration depth on the large-diameter (3.0 μm) heparin-conjugated PCL/gelatin fibers containing PDGF-BB.

11.4.5.3 Neural applications

As described in Section 11.3, aligned meshes lead to the orientation of seeded cells along the fibers, inducing the development of aligned tissues. Consequently, aligned nanofiber meshes have been extensively applied toward neural tissue targets due to the need for oriented axonal extension to restore functional tissues such as peripheral nerves. Concurrently, additional factors, such as adhesive peptides and neuronal growth factors, can be conjugated to these aligned fibers to provide synergistic cues to promote the differentiation and development of mature neuronal tissues. For example, Bockelmann et al. grafted GRGDS onto electrospun blends of PCL and isocyanate-terminated PEG star polymers (Bockelmann et al., 2010). When dorsal root ganglia (DRGs) were plated onto RGD-modified fiber meshes, Schwann cells migrated out of DRGs and divided more rapidly than on unmodified fiber meshes. In addition, axonal growth by sensory neurons in DRGs was faster on RGD-modified fiber meshes. Separately, Smith Callahan et al. grafted the cell-adhesive peptide fragment YIGSR, found within laminin, to both aligned and randomly oriented fiber meshes that were electrospun from 4-dibenzyocyclooctynol (DIBO) terminated PLLA (Smith Callahan et al., 2013). Mouse embryonic stem cells cultured on YIGSR-functionalized aligned fibers expressed higher levels of neuron-specific class III β-tubulin and microtubule-associated protein 2 compared to the nonfunctionalized equivalents. Interestingly, this effect was not observed on the YIGSR-functionalized randomly oriented fiber meshes, indicating that topographical characteristics are important to neuronal differentiation of embryonic stem cells.

In another set of studies, Cho et al. compared grafting and physisorption of NGF to aligned and randomly oriented electrospun blends of PCL and amine-terminated PCL-PEG (Cho et al., 2010). Release profiles revealed desorption of ~80% of physisorbed NGF within 1 day, compared to a negligible release from NGF-immobilized fibers. NGF-immobilized fibers induced greater expression of neuronal markers, such as nestin, tubulin βIII, and map2 by bone-marrow-derived stem cells, as compared to NGF-absorbed fibers. Further, this effect was enhanced on aligned fibers. These results indicate that cell differentiation can be enhanced when physical and biochemical cues are combined. Separately, Horne et al. examined the effect of BDNF on neural stem cells on PCL fiber meshes. In comparison to glass slide controls, neural stem cell proliferation was enhanced on both randomly oriented and aligned fiber surfaces in the presence of BDNF (whether conjugated to the fibers or added to the media) (Horne et al., 2009), though the effect was greater on the conjugated fibers. Furthermore, immunostaining revealed elevated numbers of neurons and oligodendrocytes on the fibers in the presence of BDNF, with greater numbers on the conjugated fibers regardless of fiber alignment.

11.4.5.4 Dermal and epithelial tissues

In dermal and epithelial tissues, local delivery of growth factors and morphogens can facilitate wound contraction and healing. For potential treatment of diabetic skin ulcers, Choi et al. explored the bioconjugation of EGF to the surface of electrospun PCL/amine-terminated PCL-PEG fibers (Choi et al., 2008b). Using a full-thickness dermal wound in a diabetic mouse model, the authors reported greater percentages of wound closure with EGF-tethered fiber meshes as compared to treatments with either EGF physisorbed to the fiber meshes or with plain fiber meshes (no EGF) after 7 and 14 days.

11.4.6 CONCLUDING REMARKS ON SURFACE MODIFICATION

In the preceding examples we highlighted strategies to utilize electrospun fibers to locally deliver adhesive molecules, growth factors, and morphogens to guide tissue formation. Despite the conceptual simplicity of these approaches, presentation and delivery of such molecules is intrinsically challenging and factors such as protein denaturation and release can play prominent roles in their efficacy. In addition, other types of bioactive agents (e.g., hormones, cytokines, antibiotics, polysaccharides) can be incorporated into electrospun fiber and stimulate cell differentiation, modulate foreign body responses, and mitigate infection. For the sake of brevity, we did not delve into these topics.

11.5 COMPLEX SCAFFOLDS

In the previous sections we considered the design of homogeneous scaffolds for the development of simple tissue structures. However, most tissues and organs are complex and heterogeneous, containing a variety of cell types and ECM structures that are arranged in a lamellar or spatially graded manner. This spatial organization not only regulates the different cell phenotypes within complex tissues but also maintains the function of the particular tissue or organ. Techniques to fabricate electrospun fiber meshes with spatial gradients include multilayer deposition processes (to create depthwise gradients, Figure 11.4a and b) (Soliman et al., 2010) and co-electrospinning from two or more off-set spinnerets (to create lateral gradients, Figure 11.4c) (Samavedi et al., 2011). In addition, because most tissues are larger than the typical thickness of electrospun meshes (100–300 μm), techniques are required to increase mesh thickness by either combining multiple meshes together or integrating electrospinning with other scaffold fabrication techniques. For example, composite scaffolds can be fabricated by combining several electrospun meshes together via layering (Li et al., 2004) or rolling (Ekaputra et al., 2009) and then subsequently bonding them together with another component such as a hydrogel. Ultimately, we envision that—to achieve tissue scaffolds composed

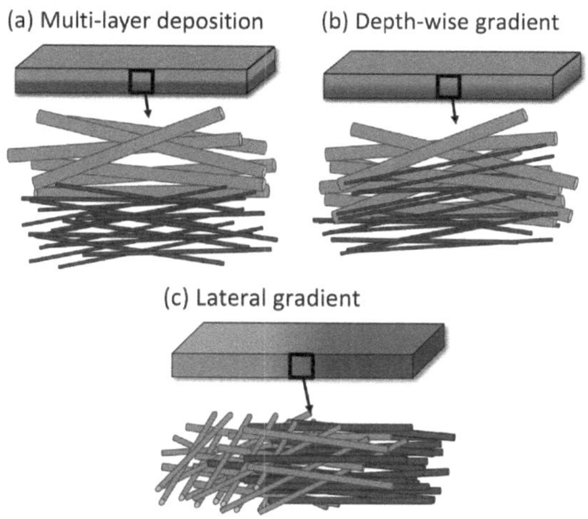

FIGURE 11.4

Complex scaffolds formed by electrospinning from two or more spinnerets. (a) Deposition of one layer (small fibers) followed by a second layer (large fibers). (b) Deposition of depthwise gradient by increasing the deposition rate of one polymer (small fibers) while decreasing the rate of the other (large fibers). (c) Deposition of a lateral gradient by co-electrospinning two polymers from off-set spinnerets (left: smaller randomly oriented fibers; right: larger aligned fibers).

of multiple phenotypes with hierarchical organization in several dimensions—strategies to construct spatial gradients will need to be combined with approaches to form thick composite scaffolds.

11.5.1 ARCHITECTURE GRADIENTS

In Sections 11.3.1 and 11.3.2, we described examples of how mesh architecture (e.g., fiber diameter, alignment) modulates cell behavior (i.e., adhesion, proliferation, morphology, phenotype). In those cases, we considered only spatially homogeneous architectures. Now, we describe examples of depthwise and lateral gradations in architecture (by multilayer and co-electrospinning methods) to elicit different cell responses as a function of position. This section is not comprehensive, but it highlights current efforts and approaches.

11.5.1.1 Depthwise spatial heterogeneity

Multilayering of electrospun fibers is an attractive means to form the different layers found within vascular and dermal tissues. Vaz et al. applied this approach to prepare tubular meshes—for vascular tissue engineering—that consisted of randomly oriented PCL fibers (for the *tunica intima*) and circumferentially oriented PLA fibers (for the *tunica media*) (Vaz et al., 2005). While this technique resulted in a stiff but pliable tubular scaffold, cell infiltration was limited due to the high fiber density. Similarly, Yang at al. utilized a layer-by-layer fabrication technique for dermal tissue engineering (Yang et al., 2008). Specifically, randomly oriented PCL/collagen fibers were deposited into a tissue culture plate followed by the seeding of a monolayer of cells. A second fiber layer was then deposited on top of the first and more cells were seeded. This process was repeated until 18 layers of dermal fibroblasts and two layers of human keratinocytes were deposited. Histological examination after 14 days of culture indicated significant cell proliferation and glycosaminoglycan deposition, clearly defined epidermal and dermal layers, and evidence of construct contraction.

In a variation of multilayering, Grey et al. utilized a unique two-chambered electrospinning syringe to deliver both high (200 mg/ml) and low (100 mg/ml) concentration PCL solutions to the electrospinning needle (Grey et al., 2013). By independently controlling delivery of the two solutions, the research team was able to generate a continuous depthwise gradient in electrospun fiber diameter from 0.29 to 0.89 μm without having to halt the electrospinning process. In another variation of the multilayering approach, He et al. fabricated an incomplete layer of randomly oriented fibers atop a complete layer of oriented fibers (He et al., 2014). Specifically, after collection of aligned fibers on a rapidly rotating mandrel, the authors deposited randomly oriented fibers on a limited region (by rotating the mandrel through a small angle). The resultant mesh surface displayed a lateral gradient where fiber orientation changed from random to aligned over a length of 7 cm.

11.5.1.2 Lateral heterogeneity

Lateral gradients can be readily formed by co-electrospinning from off-set spinnerets (Figures 11.2c and 11.4c). For example, Samavedi et al. demonstrated that a topography gradient could be formed by electrospinning large (1.9 μm diameter) polyurethane fibers from one spinneret and small (0.47 μm diameter) nano-hydroxyapatite/PCL fibers from an off-set spinneret (Samavedi et al., 2011). Over a gradient region of roughly 7 cm, the authors showed a transition from large fibers, to a mixture of large and small fibers, to small fibers. Subsequently, Samavedi et al. showed that lateral gradients in both fiber alignment and diameter can be achieved with off-set spinnerets (Samavedi et al., 2014). Specifically, one spinneret delivered a PCL solution into a 2.5-cm gap between a pair of slowly rotating drums (Figure 11.5a). This caused the PCL fibers to be collected in an aligned manner across the gap, while a separate spinneret dispensed PLGA onto each of the two drums (and was collected as a network of randomly oriented fibers). In this way, the resultant mesh contained an aligned PCL fiber region (white), flanked by two randomly oriented PLGA fiber regions (pink, Figure 11.5b). The authors then went on to show that the aligned and random regions had different mechanical properties.

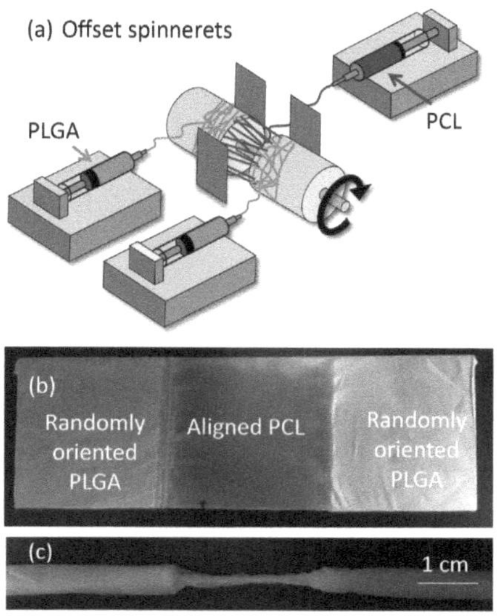

FIGURE 11.5

Co-electrospinning from off-set spinnerets onto a dual-drum collector. (a) Diagram of the apparatus. (b) Resultant mesh (on a glass slide) where the lateral regions are PLGA and the central region is PCL. (c) Rolled mesh bonded with a PEG hydrogel.

11.5.2 MECHANICAL GRADIENTS

Gradients of mechanical properties are a key characteristic of many tissue types. For example, tendons and ligaments possess mechanical gradients where they attach to muscles and bones. Therefore, scaffolds designed to guide regeneration of such tissues should possess the appropriate gradients to ensure robust integration. Toward this end, Ladd et al. sought to construct an elastic modulus gradient—for repair of the muscle–tendon junction—by co-electrospinning PCL/collagen and PLLA/collagen from off-set spinnerets (Ladd et al., 2011). The deposited fibers resulted in a mesh with three distinct regions: a stiff PLLA/collagen region, an overlap region with intermediate properties, and a soft PCL/collagen region. Elastic moduli were 27.6, 20.1, and 4.49 MPa, while strain-at-failures were 35%, 42%, and 130% for the three regions, respectively. Similarly, Samavedi et al. used electrospinning from off-set spinnerets to create a spatial gradient of mechanical properties for ligament tissue engineering (Samavedi et al., 2012, 2011). Dispensing of polyurethane from one spinneret resulted in a modulus of 0.22 MPa, while PCL (embedded with nano-hydroxyapatite particles) produced a modulus of 0.64 MPa. The overlap region had a modulus of 0.58 MPa. In addition, the authors showed that immersing the different regions in simulated body fluid selectively deposited hydroxyapatite mineral on the PCL region and increased its modulus to 2.4 MPa without affecting the moduli of the other regions.

In the previous example the authors went on to show that the different regions of their laterally graded meshes exhibited different osteogenic potentials. However, it is not known whether this effect is related to spatial differences in mechanical properties or surface chemistries (or both). Therefore, we turn now to efforts to create spatial gradients of bioactivity.

11.5.3 BIOACTIVITY

Biochemical gradients *in vivo* play central roles in a broad range of biological processes including development, angiogenesis, wound healing, and tissue remodeling. Consequently, gradients of bioactivity can be employed to induce cell alignment, migration, and differentiation into a spatial gradient of phenotypes. In the following paragraphs we describe the extension of techniques to incorporate bioactivity (described in Section 11.4) into the formation of meshes with gradients of bioactivity. Specifically, we consider depthwise gradients of bioactivity for vascular applications and lateral gradients for nerve applications. While this is far from comprehensive, it includes examples of protein absorption, growth factor encapsulation, and covalent tethering of adhesive peptides.

For vascular applications, Zhang et al. created tubular meshes by multilayer electrospinning (Zhang et al., 2013). Specifically, an intimal layer was prepared by coaxial electrospinning a chitosan hydrogel core phase containing VEGF along with a poly(ethylene glycol)-*b*-poly(L-lactide-*co*-caprolactone) (PEG-PLCL) shell phase. Next, a medial layer was prepared by coaxial electrospinning an emulsion of PEG-PLGA and PDGF-BB as the core phase and PEG-PLCL as the shell phase. *In vitro*, VEGF release from the inner layer was rapid, with 60% released after 3 days and 80% released after 9 days. In contrast, PDGF release from the outer layer was slower with only 30% and 50% released after 3 and 9 days, respectively. These dual-growth factor meshes were then used to replace the carotid arteries of rats. Immunohistochemical staining indicated endothelialization of the lumen by 2 weeks, and accumulation of smooth muscle cells by 4 weeks. Minimal host response to the graft was exhibited. Additionally, a lack of cell infiltration into the bulk of the mesh was observed, perhaps due to insufficient pore size.

A potential limitation with the approach of Zhang et al. (2013) is that the uniform concentrations of bioactive molecules within individual layers (e.g., *tunica intima, tunica media*) may not provide a sufficient chemotactic gradient to drive cell infiltration. In contrast, Bonani et al. developed a double-electrospinning system (using two independent spinnerets in tandem, Figure 11.2b) to create multilayered gradient meshes (Bonani et al., 2011). The authors then used their system to create multilayered tubular meshes with depthwise gradients of fluorescein- and rhodamine-conjugated albumin (Figure 11.4b; Bonani et al., 2012). Fluorescence imaging confirmed the different layers as well as gradients of the model protein albumin within the individual layers. Separately, Sundararaghavan et al. developed a system in which a single spinneret is fed by two programmable syringe pumps (Sundararaghavan and Burdick, 2011). By simultaneously ramping one flow rate up and the other down, the authors were able to create crosslinked methacrylated hyaluronic acid fibers that displayed a depthwise gradient of the cell-adhesive peptide RGD. Cell culture confirmed differences in cell spreading with RGD content. In addition, the authors reported better infiltration of cells into meshes with a low-to-high RGD gradient as compared to meshes with a high-to-low gradient or a uniform RGD concentration.

Perhaps more challenging than a depthwise gradient is the development of a lateral gradient. Nevertheless, Shi et al. constructed a simple lateral gradient of physisorbed fibronectin by slowly (0.17 mm/min) immersing an electrospun mesh into a 1 mg/ml solution of fluorescein-conjugated fibronectin (Shi et al., 2010). Fluorescence imaging confirmed a spatial gradient in protein concentration that correlated with incubation time. Cell density on meshes also varied spatially with protein concentration. Separately, Dinis et al. fabricated aligned electrospun silk fiber meshes with gradients of NGF as a potential means to guide nerve regeneration (Dinis et al., 2014). Specifically, NGF gradients were formed through a process of fiber deposition and subsequent cropping of aligned silk/NGF fibers. First, aligned fibers containing a high concentration of NGF were deposited onto a strip of nonconductive tape (between two collectors) and the resultant mesh trimmed to 4 mm (in the direction of fiber alignment). Next, aligned fibers containing an intermediate NGF concentration were deposited atop the first layer and trimmed to 7 mm (in the direction of fiber alignment). Then, aligned fibers containing a low NGF concentration were deposited and trimmed to 10 mm. Finally, aligned fibers containing no NGF were deposited. Rat primary sensory neuron cells cultured on these NGF gradients averaged two neurite extensions compared to up to four extensions on meshes with uniform NGF concentrations. Furthermore, extensions on gradient meshes were longer and oriented in the direction of the gradient compared to the shorter and more random extensions on uniform meshes.

11.5.4 FIBER–HYDROGEL COMPOSITES

In the preceding examples, cells seeded onto electrospun meshes were guided by the topographical, mechanical, and biochemical properties of the fibers to assume various target morphologies and phenotypes. However, in nearly all cases explored, the efficacy of the electrospun meshes was diminished by two intrinsic limitations of electrospun materials: poor cell infiltration (due to pore sizes on the order of fiber diameters) and low mesh thickness (due to the slow and electrically driven deposition process). The fabrication of electrospun fiber–hydrogel composites has been proposed as a solution to both of these limitations due to the ability for hydrogels to increase interfiber spacing of electrospun meshes and to bond together multiple electrospun mesh layers. Several techniques exist for incorporating hydrogels into electrospun meshes during or after mesh fabrication. One of the simplest is concurrent electrospraying of a hydrogel component (with or without cells) during the electrospinning process. Alternatively, addition of the hydrogel phase postfabrication permits the creation of multilayered composites where several electrospun layers are bonded together via hydrogels which are polymerized around or grafted to the fibers.

Concurrent electrospraying of a hydrogel phase during the electrospinning of fibers has been explored by several research groups, including Ekaputra et al. and Stankus et al. Ekaputra et al. fabricated fiber–hydrogel composite meshes by electrospraying either gelatin, PEO, or Heprasil concurrently with the deposition of PCL/collagen fibers onto a slowly rotating mandrel (Ekaputra et al., 2009). The hydrogel component of the resultant composites was either leached away (in the case of gelatin and PEO) or retained by gelation (in the case of Heprasil). While leaching of gelatin and PEO did not improve human fetal osteoblast infiltration, inclusion of the Heprasil gel greatly enhanced cellularization of the composite meshes. This suggests that leaching of the hydrogel may cause consolidation of the fiber meshes, preventing cell infiltration. In a follow-up study by the same group, the electrosprayed Heprasil was utilized as a carrier for the growth factors VEGF and PDGF-BB. Human umbilical vein endothelial cells and lung fibroblasts were seeded onto the PCL/collagen fiber–Heprasil hydrogel composites and cultured for 14 days. The release of the growth factors from the Heprasil phase promoted cell proliferation and formation of a microvascular network as compared to composites without growth factors (Ekaputra et al., 2011). A similar approach was used by Stankus et al. to rapidly cellularize polyurethane electrospun meshes (Stankus et al., 2006). Concurrent electrospraying of rat vascular smooth muscle cells in a gelatin solution resulted in complete cellularization of the electrospun meshes. In addition, cell viability was maintained using perfusion culture. Importantly, this technique has potential in vascular tissue engineering applications as the tubular composites possessed good suture retention strength, and exhibited static and dynamic compliances and burst strengths similar to native tissues (Stankus et al., 2007).

As an alternative to concurrent deposition of fiber and hydrogel phases, a number of research groups have used hydrogels to bond together successive electrospun fiber layers. For example, McMahon et al. fabricated tubular composites for vascular applications by rolling a cell-seeded aligned polyurethane fiber mesh around a cylindrical mandrel and filling the pores with a PEG-fibrin gel (McMahon et al., 2011). The resultant composites exhibited circumferential stress–strain curves with similar toe-in and linear regions to native coronary artery. The authors then applied pulsatile perfusion culture of cell-seeded composites under physiological conditions for 12 days, and reported that this conditioning period facilitated ECM deposition and some cell infiltration into the layers. Similarly, Thayer et al. fabricated composite polyurethane-PEG scaffolds for ligament tissue applications (Thayer et al., 2013). Cellularized polyurethane meshes were prepared by concurrent electrospinning of fibers and electrospraying of cells. Resultant meshes were then rolled, filled with PEG diacrylate, and

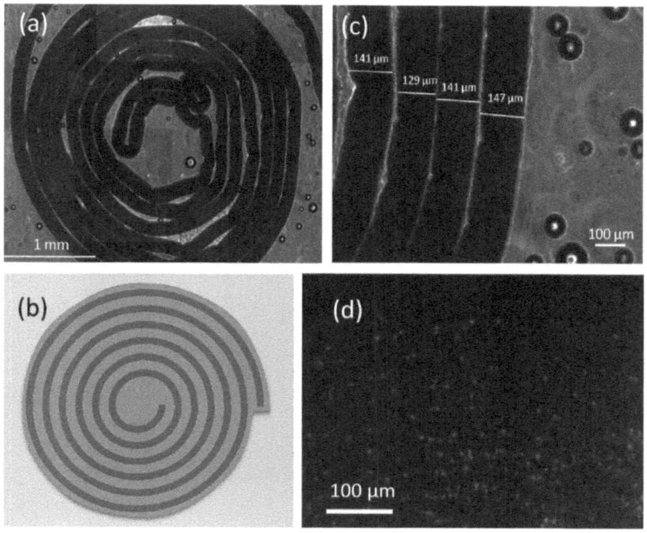

FIGURE 11.6

Fiber–hydrogel composites. (a) Histological section and (b) diagram of a rolled fiber–hydrogel composite. (c) Separate layers are tightly packed together, and (d) cells nuclei appear as bright dots can be distributed throughout the composite by co-electrospraying.

photocross linked (Figure 11.6). Incorporation of a small amount of PEG diacrylate into the polyurethane electrospinning solution reduced the mechanical properties of the fibers but improved integration of the gel and fiber phases. However, cell proliferation was not observed in this system, and this was likely due to the high fiber density and the nondegradable hydrogel phase. In contrast, Deepthi et al. used a chitosan–hyaluronic acid gel to bond successive electrospun fiber meshes (Deepthi et al., 2015). The authors showed that this gel increased rabbit fibroblast proliferation compared to uncoated controls and proposed the gel could function as a reservoir for growth factors to induce cell infiltration and differentiation.

11.5.5 SPARSE FIBER–HYDROGEL COMPOSITES

As a final example of composites, we consider two cases where a low density of electrospun fibers was dispersed within a hydrogel phase. Under this condition, the fibers do not contribute significantly to the overall mechanical properties of the gel, but can provide clues to guide cell alignment (Figure 11.7). Kriebel et al. fabricated low-density fiber–gel composites for topographical guidance of neuronal cells within a larger gel medium (Kriebel et al., 2014). Collagen gels containing DRGs were cast around low-density highly aligned three-dimensional fiber arrays. Schwann cells in contact with the fibers exhibited spindle-shaped

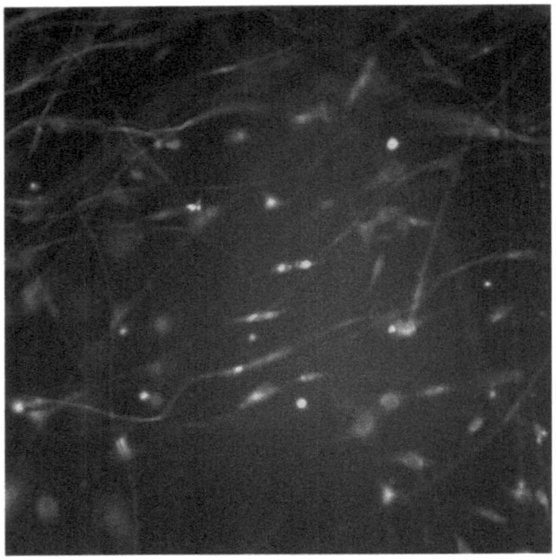

FIGURE 11.7

Mesenchymal stem cells within a sparse PCL fiber–collagen hydrogel composite.

morphologies and sensory neurons extended axons along the fibers. In contrast, cells within pure collagen gels exhibited no preferential orientation, with axonal extensions in random directions. Subsequently, these fiber–collagen composites were placed within nerve conduits and demonstrated similar behaviors. In an analogous approach, Laco et al. generated sparse fiber–hydrogel composites that could guide capillary formation for microvascular applications (Laco et al., 2013). Randomly oriented and aligned electrospun meshes were fabricated, onto which collagen gels containing human lymphatic microvascular endothelial cells were cast. Cells within the collagen gels migrated to the fibers and aligned with the orientation of the fiber. Interestingly, alignment was also observed among neighboring cells that were not in direct contact with the fibers.

11.5.6 CONCLUDING REMARKS

In this section we discussed strategies to create electrospun meshes that exhibit lateral and depthwise gradients in architecture, mechanical properties, and bioactivity, as well as methods to incorporate a hydrogel phase within the fibers and create thick fiber–hydrogel composites. Importantly, these strategies can be readily integrated. Architectural, topographic, and mechanical properties are intrinsically coupled, allowing one to create gradients in all three properties by judicious selection of materials. Further, a hydrogel phase can be readily integrated during or after the electrospinning process. Thus, the most difficult component to incorporate is gradients of bioactivity, although coaxial (e.g., Zhang et al., 2013) and co-electrospinning (e.g., Bonani et al., 2011) may be promising approaches (Figure 11.2).

11.6 LIMITATIONS WITH ELECTROSPINNING AND FUTURE OPPORTUNITIES

In this chapter, we have described a broad variety of methods to adapt the electrospinning process for the engineering of specific soft tissues, including muscle, nerve, tendon, ligament, skin, and vascular applications. However, clinical efficacy of these materials is presently impeded by a pair of intrinsic limitations with electrospinning. The first is that traditional electrospinning methods are slow and not amenable to the fabrication of thick scaffolds. While it may be tractable to use electrospun materials for the repair of thin tissues such as skin and small blood vessels, fabrication of scaffolds with dimensions necessary for repairing tendons, ligaments, muscle, and even large hollow organs may not be feasible without integrating electrospinning with other techniques. In Section 11.5.5, we described efforts to combine electrospun fibers with hydrogels. Perhaps integrating electrospun fibers with other scaffold manufacturing processes (e.g., organ printing, fused deposition modeling) could be a solution. Under the proper fabrication conditions, the micron-scale electrospun fibers may be able to confer anisotropic properties to the scaffold and guide cells to align and organize into oriented tissue-like structures.

The second limitation is the poor ability of cells to infiltrate into and populate electrospun meshes. This may stem from two separate issues: small pore dimensions and slow migration of cells into meshes. Efforts to address the first have had mixed results. The introduction of porogens (e.g., co-electrospun PEO (Baker et al., 2008), electrosprayed gelatin (Ekaputra et al., 2009)) can lead to subsequent mesh consolidation, but the introduction of a hydrogel phase (e.g., Hepracil (Ekaputra et al., 2009), fibrin (McMahon et al., 2011), PEG (Thayer et al., 2013)) may delay this consolidation. The second issue is cell infiltration and tissue formation within meshes. The introduction of porogens and hydrogels can enlarge interfiber spacing (Baker et al., 2008), but this alone does not ensure subsequent cell infiltration. Co-electrospraying of cells is one approach to achieve high initial cellularity (Stankus et al., 2006). Alternatively, the construction of a depthwise gradient of adhesive peptides (e.g., RGD (Sundararaghavan and Burdick, 2011)) or a bioactive factor gradient may guide cell infiltration into meshes.

Ultimately, these limitations will likely be resolved over the next several years. Then, electrospun materials—with anisotropic and graded properties, contact guidance features, and bioactive molecules—will begin to be used to regenerate soft tissues such a ligament, tendon, muscle, and blood vessels as well as various tubular and hollow organs.

REFERENCES

Ahmed, T.A., Dare, E.V., Hincke, M., 2008. Fibrin: a versatile scaffold for tissue engineering applications. Tissue Eng. B Rev. 14, 199–215.

Alenghat, F.J., Ingber, D.E., 2002. Mechanotransduction: all signals point to cytoskeleton, matrix, and integrins. Sci. STKE 119.

Altman, G.H., Horan, R.L., Lu, H.H., Moreau, J., Martin, I., Richmond, J.C., et al., 2002. Silk matrix for tissue engineered anterior cruciate ligaments. Biomaterials 23, 4131–4141.

Anderson, J.M., Rodriguez, A., Chang, D.T., 2008. Foreign body reaction to biomaterials. Sem. Immunol. 20, 86–100.

Aviss, K., Gough, J., Downes, S., 2010. Aligned electrospun polymer fibres for skeletal muscle regeneration. Eur. Cell Mater. 19, 193–204.

Badami, A.S., Kreke, M.R., Thompson, M.S., Riffle, J.S., Goldstein, A.S., 2006. Effect of fiber diameter on spreading, proliferation, and differentiation of osteoblastic cells on electrospun poly(lactic acid) substrates. Biomaterials 27, 596–606.

Baker, B.M., Mauck, R.L., 2007. The effect of nanofiber alignment on the maturation of engineered meniscus constructs. Biomaterials 28, 1967–1977.

Baker, B.M., Gee, A.O., Metter, R.B., Nathan, A.S., Marklein, R.A., Burdick, J.A., et al., 2008. The potential to improve cell infiltration in composite fiber-aligned electrospun scaffolds by the selective removal of sacrificial fibers. Biomaterials 29, 2348–2358.

Baker, S.C., Atkin, N., Gunning, P.A., Granville, N., Wilson, K., Wilson, D., et al., 2006. Characterisation of electrospun polystyrene scaffolds for three-dimensional *in vitro* biological studies. Biomaterials 27, 3136–3146.

Bashur, C.A., Dahlgren, L.A., Goldstein, A.S., 2006. Effect of fiber diameter and orientation on fibroblast morphology and proliferation on electrospun poly (D, L-lactic-*co*-glycolic acid) meshes. Biomaterials 27, 5681–5688.

Bashur, C.A., Shaffer, R.D., Dahlgren, L.A., Guelcher, S.A., Goldstein, A.S., 2009. Effect of fiber diameter and alignment of electrospun polyurethane meshes on mesenchymal progenitor cells. Tissue Eng. A 15, 2435–2445.

Bhattarai, N., Edmondson, D., Veiseh, O., Matsen, F.A., Zhang, M., 2005. Electrospun chitosan-based nanofibers and their cellular compatibility. Biomaterials 26, 6176–6184.

Bockelmann, J., Klinkhammer, K., von Holst, A., Seiler, N., Faissner, A., Brook, G.A., et al., 2010. Functionalization of electrospun poly (ε-caprolactone) fibers with the extracellular matrix-derived peptide GRGDS improves guidance of schwann cell migration and axonal growth. Tissue Eng. A 17, 475–486.

Bonani, W., Maniglio, D., Motta, A., Tan, W., Migliaresi, C., 2011. Biohybrid nanofiber constructs with anisotropic biomechanical properties. J. Biomed. Mater. Res. B Appl. Biomater. 96, 276–286.

Bonani, W., Motta, A., Migliaresi, C., Tan, W., 2012. Biomolecule gradient in micropatterned nanofibrous scaffold for spatiotemporal release. Langmuir 28, 13675–13687.

Bonino, C.A., Krebs, M.D., Saquing, C.D., Jeong, S.I., Shearer, K.L., Alsberg, E., et al., 2011. Electrospinning alginate-based nanofibers: from blends to crosslinked low molecular weight alginate-only systems. Carbohydr. Polym. 85, 111–119.

Boukerrou, M., Boulanger, L., Rubod, C., Lambaudie, E., Dubois, P., Cosson, M., 2007. Study of the biomechanical properties of synthetic mesh implanted *in vivo*. Eur. J. Obstet. Gynecol. Reprod. Biol. 134, 262–267.

Bryan, N., Rhodes, N.P., Hunt, J.A., 2009. Derivation and performance of an entirely autologous injectable hydrogel delivery system for cell-based therapies. Biomaterials 30, 180–188.

Cardwell, R.D., Dahlgren, L.A., Goldstein, A.S., 2014. Electrospun fibre diameter, not alignment, affects mesenchymal stem cell differentiation into the tendon/ligament lineage. J. Tissue Eng. Regen. Med. 8, 937–945.

Chen, J.P., Su, C.H., 2011. Surface modification of electrospun PLLA nanofibers by plasma treatment and cationized gelatin immobilization for cartilage tissue engineering. Acta Biomater. 7, 234–243.

Cheng, Q., Komvopoulos, K., Li, S., 2014. Plasma-assisted heparin conjugation on electrospun poly(L-lactide) fibrous scaffolds. J. Biomed. Mater. Res. A 102, 1408–1414.

Chew, S.Y., Mi, R., Hoke, A., Leong, K.W., 2008. The effect of the alignment of electrospun fibrous scaffolds on Schwann cell maturation. Biomaterials 29, 653–661.

Cho, Y.I., Choi, J.S., Jeong, S.Y., Yoo, H.S., 2010. Nerve growth factor (NGF)-conjugated electrospun nanostructures with topographical cues for neuronal differentiation of mesenchymal stem cells. Acta Biomater. 6, 4725–4733.

Choi, J.S., Lee, S.J., Christ, G.J., Atala, A., Yoo, J.J., 2008a. The influence of electrospun aligned poly(ε-caprolactone)/collagen nanofiber meshes on the formation of self-aligned skeletal muscle myotubes. Biomaterials 29, 2899–2906.

Choi, J.S., Leong, K.W., Yoo, H.S., 2008b. *In vivo* wound healing of diabetic ulcers using electrospun nanofibers immobilized with human epidermal growth factor (EGF). Biomaterials 29, 587–596.

Choi, W.S., Bae, J.W., Lim, H.R., Joung, Y.K., Park, J.-C., Kwon, I.K., et al., 2008c. RGD peptide-immobilized electrospun matrix of polyurethane for enhanced endothelial cell affinity. Biomed. Mater. 3, 044104.

Christopherson, G.T., Song, H., Mao, H.-Q., 2009. The influence of fiber diameter of electrospun substrates on neural stem cell differentiation and proliferation. Biomaterials 30, 556–564.

Cross, V.L., Zheng, Y., Won Choi, N., Verbridge, S.S., Sutermaster, B.A., Bonassar, L.J., et al., 2010. Dense type I collagen matrices that support cellular remodeling and microfabrication for studies of tumor angiogenesis and vasculogenesis *in vitro*. Biomaterials 31, 8596–8607.

Cukierman, E., Pankov, R., Stevens, D.R., Yamada, K.M., 2001. Taking cell-matrix adhesions to the third dimension. Sci. Signal 294, 1708.

Dalby, M.J., 2005. Topographically induced direct cell mechanotransduction. Med. Eng. Phys. 27, 730–742.

Deepthi, S., Jeevitha, K., Nivedhitha Sundaram, M., Chennazhi, K.P., Jayakumar, R., 2015. Chitosan–hyaluronic acid hydrogel coated poly(caprolactone) multiscale bilayer scaffold for ligament regeneration. Chem. Eng. J. 260, 478–485.

Dinis, T.M., Elia, R., Vidal, G., Auffret, A., Kaplan, D.L., Egles, C., 2014. Method to form a fiber/growth factor dual-gradient along electrospun silk for nerve regeneration. ACS Appl. Mater. Interfaces 6, 16817–16826.

Doshi, J., Reneker, D.H., 1995. Electrospinning process and applications of electrospun fibers. J. Electrostatics 35, 151–160.

Duan, B., Wang, M., Zhou, W.Y., Cheung, W.L., Li, Z.Y., Lu, W.W., 2010. Three-dimensional nanocomposite scaffolds fabricated via selective laser sintering for bone tissue engineering. Acta Biomater. 6, 4495–4505.

Ekaputra, A.K., Zhou, Y., Cool, S.M., Hutmacher, D.W., 2009. Composite electrospun scaffolds for engineering tubular bone grafts. Tissue Eng. A 15, 3779–3788.

Ekaputra, A.K., Prestwich, G.D., Cool, S.M., Hutmacher, D.W., 2011. The three-dimensional vascularization of growth factor-releasing hybrid scaffold of poly (ε-caprolactone)/collagen fibers and hyaluronic acid hydrogel. Biomaterials 32, 8108–8117.

Engler, A.J., Sen, S., Sweeney, H.L., Discher, D.E., 2006. Matrix elasticity directs stem cell lineage specification. Cell 126, 677–689.

Erisken, C., Zhang, X., Moffat, K.L., Levine, W.N., Lu, H.H., 2013. Scaffold fiber diameter regulates human tendon fibroblast growth and differentiation. Tissue Eng. A 19, 519–528.

Feinberg, A.W., Wilkerson, W.R., Seegert, C.A., Gibson, A.L., Hoipkemeier-Wilson, L., Brennan, A.B., 2008. Systematic variation of microtopography, surface chemistry and elastic modulus and the state dependent effect on endothelial cell alignment. J. Biomed. Mater. Res. A 86A, 522–534.

Freeman, J.W., Woods, M.D., Laurencin, C.T., 2007. Tissue engineering of the anterior cruciate ligament using a braid–twist scaffold design. J. Biomech. 40, 2029–2036.

Frith, J.E., Mills, R.J., Hudson, J.E., Cooper-White, J.J., 2012. Tailored integrin–extracellular matrix interactions to direct human mesenchymal stem cell differentiation. Stem Cells Dev. 21, 2442–2456.

Gao, J., Crapo, P.M., Wang, Y., 2006. Macroporous elastomeric scaffolds with extensive micropores for soft tissue engineering. Tissue Eng. 12, 917–925.

Garg, K., Pullen, N.A., Oskeritzian, C.A., Ryan, J.J., Bowlin, G.L., 2013. Macrophage functional polarization (M1/M2) in response to varying fiber and pore dimensions of electrospun scaffolds. Biomaterials 34, 4439–4451.

Geiger, B., Spatz, J.P., Bershadsky, A.D., 2009. Environmental sensing through focal adhesions. Nat. Rev. Mol. Cell Biol. 10, 21–33.

Grey, C.P., Newton, S.T., Bowlin, G.L., Haas, T.W., Simpson, D.G., 2013. Gradient fiber electrospinning of layered scaffolds using controlled transitions in fiber diameter. Biomaterials 34, 4993–5006.

Gristina, A.G., 1994. Implant failure and the immuno-incompetent fibro-inflammatory zone. Clin. Orthop. Rel. Res. 298, 106–118.

Hayami, J.W.S., Surrao, D.C., Waldman, S.D., Amsden, B.G., 2010. Design and characterization of a biodegradable composite scaffold for ligament tissue engineering. J. Biomed. Mater. Res. A 92A, 1407–1420.

He, J., Qin, T., Liu, Y., Li, X., Li, D., Jin, Z., 2014. Electrospinning of nanofibrous scaffolds with continuous structure and material gradients. Mater. Lett. 137, 393–397.

Horbett, T.A., 1993. Principles underlying the role of adsorbed plasma proteins in blood interactions with foreign materials. Cardiovasc. Pathol. 2, 137–148 (Chapter 13).

Horne, M.K., Nisbet, D.R., Forsythe, J.S., Parish, C.L., 2009. Three-dimensional nanofibrous scaffolds incorporating immobilized BDNF promote proliferation and differentiation of cortical neural stem cells. Stem Cells Dev. 19, 843–852.

Huang, W., Carlsen, B., Wulur, I., Rudkin, G., Ishida, K., Wu, B., et al., 2004. BMP-2 exerts differential effects on differentiation of rabbit bone marrow stromal cells grown in two-dimensional and three-dimensional systems and is required for *in vitro* bone formation in a PLGA scaffold. Exp. Cell Res. 299, 325–334.

Jarusuwannapoom, T., Hongrojjanawiwat, W., Jitjaicham, S., Wannatong, L., Nithitanakul, M., Pattamaprom, C., et al., 2005. Effect of solvents on electro-spinnability of polystyrene solutions and morphological appearance of resulting electrospun polystyrene fibers. Eur. Polym. J. 41, 409–421.

Jha, B.S., Colello, R.J., Bowman, J.R., Sell, S.A., Lee, K.D., Bigbee, J.W., et al., 2011. Two pole air gap electrospinning: fabrication of highly aligned, three-dimensional scaffolds for nerve reconstruction. Acta Biomater. 7, 203–215.

Kelly, D.J., Jacobs, C.R., 2010. The role of mechanical signals in regulating chondrogenesis and osteogenesis of mesenchymal stem cells. Birth Defects Res. C Rev. 90, 75–85.

Kim, T.G., Park, T.G., 2006. Biomimicking extracellular matrix: cell adhesive RGD peptide modified electrospun poly (D, L-lactic-*co*-glycolic acid) nanofiber mesh. Tissue Eng. 12, 221–233.

Kriebel, A., Rumman, M., Scheld, M., Hodde, D., Brook, G., Mey, J., 2014. Three-dimensional configuration of orientated fibers as guidance structures for cell migration and axonal growth. J. Biomed. Mater. Res. B Appl. Biomater. 102, 356–365.

Kwon, I.K., Kidoaki, S., Matsuda, T., 2005. Electrospun nano- to microfiber fabrics made of biodegradable copolyesters: structural characteristics, mechanical properties and cell adhesion potential. Biomaterials 26, 3929–3939.

Laco, F., Grant, M.H., Black, R.A., 2013. Collagen–nanofiber hydrogel composites promote contact guidance of human lymphatic microvascular endothelial cells and directed capillary tube formation. J. Biomed. Mater. Res. A 101, 1787–1799.

Ladd, M.R., Lee, S.J., Stitzel, J.D., Atala, A., Yoo, J.J., 2011. Co-electrospun dual scaffolding system with potential for muscle–tendon junction tissue engineering. Biomaterials 32, 1549–1559.

Laurencin, C.T., Ambrosio, A., Borden, M., Cooper Jr., J., 1999. Tissue engineering: orthopedic applications. Ann. Rev. Biomed. Eng. 1, 19–46.

Lee, C.H., Shin, H.J., Cho, I.H., Kang, Y.-M., Kim, I., Park, K.-D., et al., 2005. Nanofiber alignment and direction of mechanical strain affect the ECM production of human ACL fibroblast. Biomaterials 26, 1261–1270.

Lee, J., Yoo, J.J., Atala, A., Lee, S.J., 2012. The effect of controlled release of PDGF-BB from heparin-conjugated electrospun PCL/gelatin scaffolds on cellular bioactivity and infiltration. Biomaterials 33, 6709–6720.

Leipzig, N.D., Shoichet, M.S., 2009. The effect of substrate stiffness on adult neural stem cell behavior. Biomaterials 30, 6867–6878.

Leong, K.F., Cheah, C.M., Chua, C.K., 2003. Solid freeform fabrication of three-dimensional scaffolds for engineering replacement tissues and organs. Biomaterials 24, 2363–2378.

Li, C., Vepari, C., Jin, H.-J., Kim, H.J., Kaplan, D.L., 2006. Electrospun silk-BMP-2 scaffolds for bone tissue engineering. Biomaterials 27, 3115–3124.

Li, D., Wang, Y., Xia, Y., 2004. Electrospinning nanofibers as uniaxially aligned arrays and layer-by-layer stacked films. Adv. Mater. 16, 361–366.

Liljensten, E., Gisselfalt, K., Edberg, B., Bertilsson, H., Flodin, P., Nilsson, A., et al., 2002. Studies of polyurethane urea bands for ACL reconstruction. J. Mater. Sci. Mater. Med. 13, 351–359.

Malinda, K.M., Kleinman, H.K., 1996. The laminins. Int. J. Biochem. Cell Biol. 28, 957–959.

Manwaring, M.E., Walsh, J.F., Tresco, P.A., 2004. Contact guidance induced organization of extracellular matrix. Biomaterials 25, 3631–3638.

McMahon, R.E., Qu, X., Jimenez-Vergara, A.C., Bashur, C.A., Guelcher, S.A., Goldstein, A.S., et al., 2011. Hydrogel–electrospun mesh composites for coronary artery bypass grafts. Tissue Eng. C Methods 17, 451–461.

Miller, J.S., Shen, C.J., Legant, W.R., Baranski, J.D., Blakely, B.L., Chen, C.S., 2010. Bioactive hydrogels made from step-growth derived PEG–peptide macromers. Biomaterials 31, 3736–3743.

Nam, J., Johnson, J., Lannutti, J.J., Agarwal, S., 2011. Modulation of embryonic mesenchymal progenitor cell differentiation via control over pure mechanical modulus in electrospun nanofibers. Acta Biomater. 7, 1516–1524.

Nelson, D.M., Baraniak, P.R., Ma, Z., Guan, J., Mason, N.S., Wagner, W.R., 2011. Controlled release of IGF-1 and HGF from a biodegradable polyurethane scaffold. Pharm. Res. 28, 1282–1293.

Nikkhah, M., Edalat, F., Manoucheri, S., Khademhosseini, A., 2012. Engineering microscale topographies to control the cell–substrate interface. Biomaterials 33, 5230–5246.

Provenzano, P.P., Inman, D.R., Eliceiri, K.W., Trier, S.M., Keely, P.J., 2008. Contact guidance mediated three-dimensional cell migration is regulated by Rho/ROCK-dependent matrix reorganization. Biophys. J. 95, 5374–5384.

Reneker, D.H., Yarin, A.L., Fong, H., Koombhongse, S., 2000. Bending instability of electrically charged liquid jets of polymer solutions in electrospinning. J. Appl. Phys. 87, 4531.

Rho, K.S., Jeong, L., Lee, G., Seo, B.-M., Park, Y.J., Hong, S.-D., et al., 2006. Electrospinning of collagen nanofibers: effects on the behavior of normal human keratinocytes and early-stage wound healing. Biomaterials 27, 1452–1461.

Ricotti, L., Polini, A., Genchi, G.G., Ciofani, G., Iandolo, D., Vazão, H., et al., 2012. Proliferation and skeletal myotube formation capability of C2C12 and H9c2 cells on isotropic and anisotropic electrospun nanofibrous PHB scaffolds. Biomed. Mater. 7, 035010.

Rowlands, A.S., George, P.A., Cooper-White, J.J., 2008. Directing osteogenic and myogenic differentiation of MSCs: interplay of stiffness and adhesive ligand presentation. Am. J. Physiol. Cell Physiol. 295, C1037–C1044.

Ruoslahti, E., Pierschbacher, M., 1987. New perspectives in cell adhesion: RGD and integrins. Science 238, 491–497.

Sahoo, S., Ang, L.T., Goh, J.C., Toh, S.L., 2010. Growth factor delivery through electrospun nanofibers in scaffolds for tissue engineering applications. J. Biomed. Mater. Res. A 93, 1539–1550.

Saino, E., Focarete, M.L., Gualandi, C., Emanuele, E., Cornaglia, A.I., Imbriani, M., et al., 2011. Effect of electrospun fiber diameter and alignment on macrophage activation and secretion of proinflammatory cytokines and chemokines. Biomacromolecules 12, 1900–1911.

Samavedi, S., Olsen Horton, C., Guelcher, S.A., Goldstein, A.S., Whittington, A.R., 2011. Fabrication of a model continuously graded co-electrospun mesh for regeneration of the ligament–bone interface. Acta Biomater. 7, 4131–4138.

Samavedi, S., Guelcher, S.A., Goldstein, A.S., Whittington, A.R., 2012. Response of bone marrow stromal cells to graded co-electrospun scaffolds and its implications for engineering the ligament-bone interface. Biomaterials 33, 7727–7735.

Samavedi, S., Vaidya, P., Gaddam, P., Whittington, A.R., Goldstein, A.S., 2014. Electrospun meshes possessing region-wise differences in fiber orientation, diameter, chemistry and mechanical properties for engineering bone-ligament-bone tissues. Biotechnol. Bioeng. 111, 2549–2559.

Shekaran, A., Garcia, A.J., 2011. Extracellular matrix-mimetic adhesive biomaterials for bone repair. J. Biomed. Mater. Res. A 96, 261–272.

Shenoy, S.L., Bates, W.D., Frisch, H.L., Wnek, G.E., 2005. Role of chain entanglements on fiber formation during electrospinning of polymer solutions: good solvent, non-specific polymer–polymer interaction limit. Polymer 46, 3372–3384.

Shi, J., Wang, L., Zhang, F., Li, H., Lei, L., Liu, L., et al., 2010. Incorporating protein gradient into electrospun nanofibers as scaffolds for tissue engineering. ACS Appl. Mater. Interfaces 2, 1025–1030.

Smith Callahan, L.A., Xie, S., Barker, I.A., Zheng, J., Reneker, D.H., Dove, A.P., et al., 2013. Directed differentiation and neurite extension of mouse embryonic stem cell on aligned poly(lactide) nanofibers functionalized with YIGSR peptide. Biomaterials 34, 9089–9095.

Soliman, S., Pagliari, S., Rinaldi, A., Forte, G., Fiaccavento, R., Pagliari, F., et al., 2010. Multiscale three-dimensional scaffolds for soft tissue engineering via multimodal electrospinning. Acta Biomater. 6, 1227–1237.

Stankus, J.J., Guan, J., Fujimoto, K., Wagner, W.R., 2006. Microintegrating smooth muscle cells into a biodegradable, elastomeric fiber matrix. Biomaterials 27, 735–744.

Stankus, J.J., Soletti, L., Fujimoto, K., Hong, Y., Vorp, D.A., Wagner, W.R., 2007. Fabrication of cell microintegrated blood vessel constructs through electrohydrodynamic atomization. Biomaterials 28, 2738–2746.

Stylianopoulos, T., Bashur, C.A., Goldstein, A.S., Guelcher, S.A., Barocas, V.H., 2008. Computational predictions of the tensile properties of electrospun fibre meshes: effect of fibre diameter and fibre orientation. J. Mech. Behav. Biomed. Mater. 1, 326–335.

Sundararaghavan, H.G., Burdick, J.A., 2011. Gradients with depth in electrospun fibrous scaffolds for directed cell behavior. Biomacromolecules 12, 2344–2350.

Sutherland, J., Denyer, M., Britland, S., 2005. Contact guidance in human dermal fibroblasts is modulated by population pressure. J. Anat. 206, 581–587.

Takahashi, H., Yokota, T., Uchimura, E., Miyagawa, S., Ota, T., Torikai, K., et al., 2009. Newly developed tissue-engineered material for reconstruction of vascular wall without cell seeding. Ann. Thor. Surg. 88, 1269–1276.

Tan, S.H., Inai, R., Kotaki, M., Ramakrishna, S., 2005. Systematic parameter study for ultra-fine fiber fabrication via electrospinning process. Polymer 46, 6128–6134.

Teixeira, A.I., Abrams, G.A., Bertics, P.J., Murphy, C.J., Nealey, P.F., 2003. Epithelial contact guidance on well-defined micro- and nanostructured substrates. J. Cell Sci. 116, 1881–1892.

Thayer, P.S., Dimling, A.F., Plessl, D.S., Hahn, M.R., Guelcher, S.A., Dahlgren, L.A., et al., 2013. Cellularized cylindrical fiber/hydrogel composites for ligament tissue engineering. Biomacromolecules 15, 75–83.

Vaz, C., Van Tuijl, S., Bouten, C., Baaijens, F., 2005. Design of scaffolds for blood vessel tissue engineering using a multi-layering electrospinning technique. Acta Biomater. 1, 575–582.

Wang, X., Han, C., Hu, X., Sun, H., You, C., Gao, C., et al., 2011. Applications of knitted mesh fabrication techniques to scaffolds for tissue engineering and regenerative medicine. J. Mech. Behav. Biomed. Mater. 4, 922–932.

Wong, S.-C., Baji, A., Leng, S., 2008. Effect of fiber diameter on tensile properties of electrospun poly(ε-caprolactone). Polymer 49, 4713–4722.

Yang, S., Leong, K.-F., Du, Z., Chua, C.-K., 2001. The design of scaffolds for use in tissue engineering. Part I. Traditional factors. Tissue Eng. 7, 679–689.

Yang, X., Shah, J.D., Wang, H., 2008. Nanofiber enabled layer-by-layer approach toward three-dimensional tissue formation. Tissue Eng. A 15, 945–956.

Young, D.A., Ibrahim, D.O., Hu, D., Christman, K.L., 2011. Injectable hydrogel scaffold from decellularized human lipoaspirate. Acta Biomater. 7, 1040–1049.

Yu, J., Lee, A.R., Lin, W.H., Lin, C.W., Wu, Y.K., Tsai, W.B., 2014. Electrospun PLGA fibers incorporated with functionalized biomolecules for cardiac tissue engineering. Tissue Eng. A 20, 1896–1907.

Zeltinger, J., Sherwood, J.K., Graham, D.A., Müeller, R., Griffith, L.G., 2001. Effect of pore size and void fraction on cellular adhesion, proliferation, and matrix deposition. Tissue Eng. 7, 557–572.

Zeugolis, D.I., Khew, S.T., Yew, E.S.Y., Ekaputra, A.K., Tong, Y.W., Yung, L.-Y.L., et al., 2008. Electro-spinning of pure collagen nano-fibres—just an expensive way to make gelatin? Biomaterials 29, 2293–2305.

Zhang, H., Hollister, S., 2009. Comparison of bone marrow stromal cell behaviors on poly (caprolactone) with or without surface modification: studies on cell adhesion, survival and proliferation. J. Biomater. Sci. Polym. Ed. 20, 1975–1993.

Zhang, H., Jia, X., Han, F., Zhao, J., Zhao, Y., Fan, Y., et al., 2013. Dual-delivery of VEGF and PDGF by double-layered electrospun membranes for blood vessel regeneration. Biomaterials 34, 2202–2212.

Zhu, Y., Cao, Y., Pan, J., Liu, Y., 2010. Macro-alignment of electrospun fibers for vascular tissue engineering. J. Biomed. Mater. Res. B Appl. Biomater. 92, 508–516.

CHAPTER

12 Oxygen-generating nanobiomaterials for the treatment of diabetes: a tissue engineering approach

Mazaher Gholipourmalekabadi[1], Vahid Jajarmi[1,2], Zahra Rezvani[3], Maryam Ghaffari[4], Keshav Deo Verma[5], Haji Shirinzadeh[6] and Masoud Mozafari[3]

[1]Biotechnology Department, School of Advanced Technologies in Medicine, Shahid Beheshti University of Medical Sciences, Tehran, Iran [2]Cellular and Molecular Biology Research Center, Shahid Beheshti University of Medical Sciences, Tehran, Iran [3]Bioengineering Research Group, Nanotechnology and Advanced Materials Department, Materials and Energy Research Center (MERC), Tehran, Iran [4]Biomaterials Group, Faculty of Biomedical Engineering (Center of Excellence), Amirkabir University of Technology, Tehran, Iran [5]Department of Physics, S.V. (P.G.) College, Aligarh, Uttar Pradesh, India [6]Device Fabrication Group, Semiconductors Department, Materials and Energy Research Center (MERC), Tehran, Iran

LIST OF ABBREVIATIONS

Acronym	Definition
UV	Ultraviolet
ES cells	Embryonic stem cells
3D	Three dimensional
2D	Two dimensional
ECM	Extracellular matrices
IDDM	Insulin dependent diabetes mellitus
NIDDM	Non-insulin-dependent diabetes mellitus
T1DM	Type 1 diabetes mellitus
T2DM	Type 2 diabetes mellitus
CSII	Continuous subcutaneous insulin infusion
MDI	Multiple daily injection
WOP	Whole-organ pancreatic
IT	Islet transplantation
PEG	Poly (ethylene glycol)
PLGA	Poly(lactic-co-glycolic acid)

Nanobiomaterials in Soft Tissue Engineering. DOI: http://dx.doi.org/10.1016/B978-0-323-42865-1.00012-X

PVP	Poly(vinyl pyrrolidone)
PFCs	Perfluorocarbons
VEGF	Vascular endothelial growth factors
PDMS	Polydimethylsiloxane

12.1 INTRODUCTION

One of the promising fields that have a considerable effect on human health is nanotechnology. In fact, nanotechnology is a science with the aim of construction, design, characterization, and application of constructions, systems, and devices through a controlled method of size and form at a nanometer-length scale (10^{-9} m) to enhance the quality and properties of materials. In recent decades, progress in the technology of nanobiomaterials has improved tremendously. Nanobiomaterials are substances with fundamental structural units, particles, fibers, or other basic components of smaller size than 100 nm in at least one dimension (Siegel and Fougere, 1995; Gao and Xu, 2009; Zhang and Webster, 2009) that have attracted a great deal of attention in developing disease prohibition, diagnosis, and cure (Zhang and Webster, 2009), also, the number of nanotechnology researchers in the field of tissue engineering and drug delivery is increasing rapidly. The applications of nanotechnology in medical sciences are described as "nanomedicine" or "nano-biomedicine." Nanobiomaterials can be constructed by two methods: "top-down" and "bottom-up." In the top-down method, materials are broken down into more fundamental building blocks and commonly utilizes thermal and chemical techniques (Sahoo and Labhasetwar, 2003; Peppas, 2004). On the other hand, in the bottom-up method, compound structures are built by combining simple atomic-level constituents techniques (Ferrari, 2005).

Several of the significant bottom-up and top-down nanoconstruction methods are phase separation, electrospinning, chemical etching, thin film deposition, chemical vapor deposition, self-assembly processes, photolithography, nano-imprinting, and electron beam or nanospherelithographies (Zhang and Webster, 2009) which have been developed to fabricate nanobiomaterials with random or ordered nano-topographies (Chen and Ma, 2004; Zhang and Webster, 2009; Nezafati et al., 2012). By decreasing material size into the nanoscale, the aspect ratio of surface to volume is considerably increased, which accordingly can lead to enhancement of some properties such as multifunctionality, solubility, and greater physiochemistry (i.e., electrical, mechanical, catalytic, optical, magnetic properties, etc.) (Medintz et al., 2005; Dankers and Meijer, 2007; El-Sadik et al., 2010).

Whereas nanobiomaterials can mimic natural tissues and cooperate with biological methods at a molecular level (Bogunia-Kubik and Sugisaka, 2002), nanobiomaterials play a key role in motivating cell growth and function while guiding tissue restoration, and utilization of these materials may solve the above-described difficulties (Liu and Webster, 2007; Ye and Mahato, 2008; Zhang and Webster, 2009). Also, by using several methods including ultraviolet (UV), ethylene oxide, filtration with 0.22-μm filters, and plasma, nanobiomaterials can be sterilized simply. By modifying the surface of nanobiomaterials with recently advanced nano-methods, the cell–biomaterial interaction can be improved (Hoshino et al., 2004; Wang et al., 2009).

Nanotechnology has been used in a variety of fields, such as information storage capacity (Juang and Bogy, 2005), electronics (Peng and Cho, 2000; Bohr, 2002), food and agriculture (Morrissey, 2006), chemistry (as catalysts), drug delivery (Farokhzad and Langer, 2009), pharmaceutics (Uchegbu, 2006), DNA sequencing (using nanopores; Clarke et al., 2009), DNA delivery into cells (Stupp et al., 1997; Stupp and Ciegler, 2004), cell tracking and separation, diagnosis and cure of disease (Jain, 2003; Wang et al., 2008), and tissue engineering (Shin et al., 2003; Juang and Bogy, 2005; Dankers and Meijer, 2007; Liao et al., 2008; Mozafari et al., 2015).

12.2 TISSUE ENGINEERING

Recently, there have been several attempts to fabricate the structures that mimic natural tissues, including the physicochemical properties (Lanza et al., 2007; Baghbani et al., 2012; Mobini et al., 2013; Gholipourmalekabadi et al., 2015b). The aim of tissue engineering as a field of research is to increase biological replacements to repair injured tissues and reform their functionality by a triplet of biomaterial scaffolds and growth factors in conjunction with cells (i.e., stem cells) (Mooney et al., 1996; Shin et al., 2003; Ma, 2004, 2008; Juang and Bogy, 2005; Rice et al., 2005). Utilizing stem and progenitor cells has opened an innovative border in regenerative medicine. Stem cells are undifferentiated cells endowed with the capacity to self-regenerate, as well as clonogenic and multiline age separation (Weissman, 2000; Samadikuchaksaraei, 2006). These cells can be separated to at least two different cell lines and have a many applications in tissue engineering (Pera et al., 2000; Samadikuchaksaraei, 2006). Embryonic stem cells are pluripotent stem cells that are obtained from the internal cell mass of a blastocyst of an early-stage embryo. Adult stem cells, such as hematopoietic, mesenchymal stem cells are also multipotent stem cells that exist in bone marrow, marginal blood, and other tissues. Stem cells' behavior is regulated by the components lied in their extracellular microenvironment. It is recognized that stem cells can react to genetic signals such as those communicated by nucleic acids, to develop lineage-specific differentiation. However, before they reach therapeutic relevance, accurate techniques need to be developed to control stem cell differentiation (Donovan and Gearhart, 2001; Thomson, 2001; Samadikuchaksaraei, 2006). Some of the most significant objects for using these cells in tissue engineering are preservation of stem cells in the undifferentiated stage, directing stem cells to differentiate into a particular cell line, in other words preventing undesired differentiation, and delivery of cells into an exact tissue (Bianco and Robey, 2001; Sato et al., 2003).

Langer and Vacanti (1993) described tissue engineering as "an interdisciplinary field that utilizes the principles of engineering and life sciences toward the improvement of biological replacements that repair, maintain, or enhance tissue function or a whole organ" (Lanza et al., 2007).

Every year, the world's population increases rapidly. Therefore, it is anticipated that the number of patients requiring organ substitute treatment will increase in the near future as well. The two conventional tissue replacements are autografts and allografts. In autografts, replacement tissue or organ transfer is into a new part of the body of the same person but in allograft substitutes, transplant of an tissue or organ is from one person to another of the same kind but with a different genotype. These methods have a range of problems, such as deficiency of donor organs and transplant rejection (Strain and Neuberger, 2002; Dankers and Meijer, 2007), which do not meet high standards required for today's patients (Bohr, 2002; Lanza et al., 2007). In addition, two-dimensional (2D) cell culture systems, a glass flask, and Petri dish cannot fully mimic the natural tissue microenvironment. For example, substrate rigidity limits cell spreading and cytoskeleton assembly, as well as directional movement. There are numerous advantages to tissue engineering over conventional methods (autografts and allografts), as a typical example this technique would reduce the need for multiple surgeries associated with the removal of metallic implants (Lanza et al., 2007). One of the methods to overcome these problems is using three-dimensional (3D) tissue scaffolds as a template for restoration of tissue engineering. Generally, 3D scaffolds provide surroundings designed to advance self-assembly of natural components to tissue microenvironments. In this method, environmental mechanical forces acting upon cells can be operated by engineering the scaffold mechanical characteristics. Scaffolds also prepare a microenvironment for cells and adjust cell proliferation and separation, while allowing for a uniform cell population completely that is necessary for the tissue renovation process (Shin et al., 2003; Liu and Ma, 2004; Gelain et al., 2006; Ma, 2008; Mobini et al., 2013; Gholipourmalekabadi et al., 2014a). In the body, natural tissues or organs are in a nanoscale and cells directly interact with nanostructured extracellular matrices (ECM). Therefore, it is essential for the engineered implants to interrelate biologically with cells and the ECM (Zhang and Webster, 2009; Gholipourmalekabadi et al., 2015a).

In the tissue engineering field, a principal biomaterial has to perform favorable and optimal mechanical and biomaterial attributes for a given application. Also, it has to possess tunable biocompatibility and biodegradability. In principle, nanobiomaterials should mimic the natural environment or natural ECM where the materials are to be delivered or implanted (Hench and Polak, 2002; Dankers and Meijer, 2007; Zhang and Webster, 2009) and it should assist cell differentiation, adhesion, proliferation, and neo-tissue production (Shin et al., 2003; Oh et al., 2009a). To achieve this goal, many methods have been adopted to modify scaffolds to reclaim biodegradability, biocompatibility, and their mechanical properties (Ma and Langer, 1995; Ma et al., 2000; Skarja and Woodhouse, 2001; Chen and Ma, 2006). To date, bioengineers have utilized various biomaterials in scaffold construction. However, these materials are not optimal for fabrication of an appropriate scaffold (Zhang and Webster, 2009).

Tissue or organs with a collective level of complexity targeted for repair would require an increase in the complexity of the tissue engineering approach. Solid organs like the liver and pancreas have the utmost level of tissue complexity (Mikos et al., 2006). Tissue engineering in solid organs must recreate the extracellular microenvironment with adequate functionality to restore damaged tissue. Therefore, several approaches have been studied to overcome these complexities (see Figure 12.1; Dvir et al., 2011). Among the complexities, oxygenation of cell

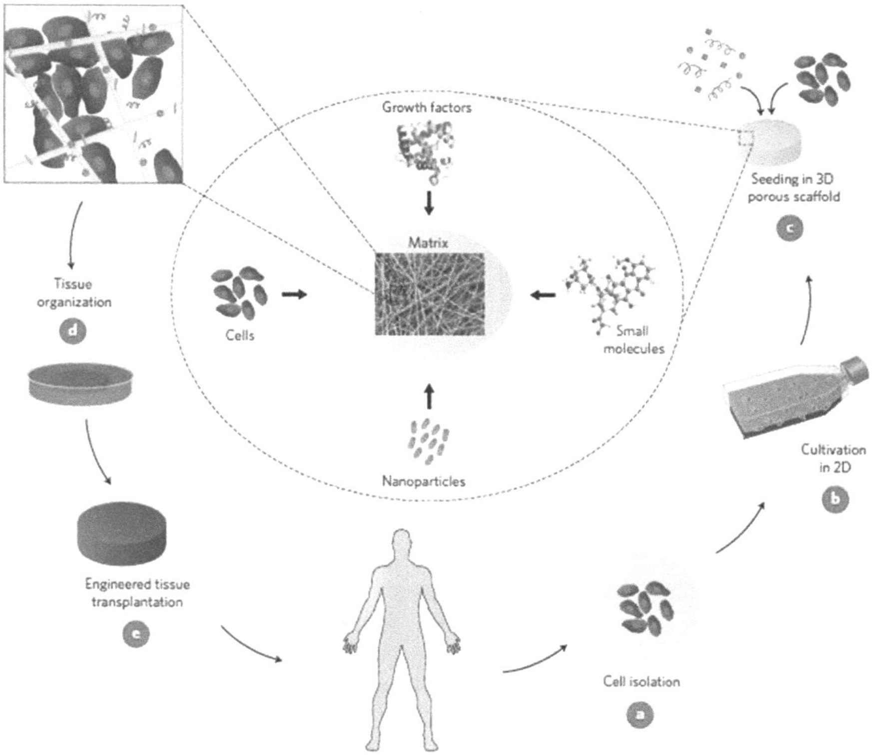

FIGURE 12.1

An example of a tissue engineering concept that involves seeding cells within porous nanobiomaterial scaffolds. (a) Cells are isolated from the patient and may be cultivated (b) *in vitro* on 2D surfaces for efficient expansion. (c) Next, the cells are seeded in porous scaffolds together with growth factors, small molecules, and micro- and/or nanoparticles. The scaffolds serve as a mechanical support and a shape-determining material, and their porous nature provides high mass transfer and waste removal. (d) The cell constructs are further cultivated in bioreactors to provide optimal conditions for organization into a functioning tissue. (e) Once a functioning tissue has been successfully engineered, the construct is transplanted onto the defect to restore function.

With permission from Nature Publishing Group (Dvir et al., 2011).

seeding is a new subject in the tissue engineering field. The next generation of materials would be dynamic nanobiomaterial that has a potential to revolutionize the healing process in solid organ tissue engineering, especially in tissues with high metabolic activity like beta cells in the pancreas (Amer et al., 2014; Huang et al., 2015). One class of these materials is oxygen-generating nanobiomaterials. Since oxygen diffusion limitation is one of the key factors in the failure of tissue engineering, oxygen-producing nanobiomaterials are capable of reducing hypoxia in the scaffold microenvironment. In fact, as a result of the long-term presence of oxygen in the microenvironment, cell apoptosis and necrosis are decreased. In addition, oxygen-releasing vectors are able to potentially improve angiogenesis and neovascularization (Colton, 2014). Oxygen carriers can be classified into natural and synthetic nanobiomaterials. Natural oxygen-generating biomaterial designs are based on a photosynthesis process, like the process that takes place in algae (Hopfner et al., 2014). The object of this chapter is synthetic oxygen-generating biomaterials which have the potential to be used in diabetes tissue engineering treatment. The importance of these materials is clear when we know that despite decades of research, oxygenation of cells in *in vitro* tissue engineering still remains as a major concern.

12.3 DIABETES

The increasing occurrence of diabetes mellitus all over the world has led to the labeling of diabetes as an epidemic of the twenty-first century (Montanya, 2004). Diabetic patients suffer from increased cardiovascular mortality and are afflicted by destructive microvascular complexities such as neuropathy, nephropathy, or retinopathy (Butler et al., 2003; Efrat, 2004; Montanya, 2004).

Diabetes mellitus, a metabolic disorder, is characterized by impaired cellular uptake of glucose. It is becoming one of the main threads to human health with a prevalence of 382 million people by 2013 and this is forecast to be reach 592 people by 2035 (Guariguata et al., 2014). Mechanistically, it is a complex disease caused by a combination of multiple gene alterations and environmental factors triggering a sequence of events conducted to elevate blood glucose concentration (hyperglycemia).

It is categorized into three main types including type 1 or insulin-dependent diabetes mellitus, type 2 or noninsulin-dependent diabetes mellitus, and finally, diabetes caused by defective metabolism or function of beta cells followed by various mutations in regulatory genes (Bell et al., 1996; Froguel and Velho, 1999; WHO Consultation Group, 1999; Association, 2008). Type 1 diabetes mellitus (T1DM) is T-lymphocyte-mediated pancreatic beta cell destruction. It contributes to chronic inflammation of the pancreas that may last for years (ranging from several months to over 20 years) (Bell et al., 1996; Herold et al., 2011) leading to more beta cell death. This results in reduction of blood insulin; in most cases, developing to complete loss (Bell et al., 1996). The destruction of islet cells is progressive and at the time when the beta cell mass is reduced by 80–90% clinical symptoms of diabetes are initiated. Several autoantibodies relevant to T1DM have been identified. It is found that the number of distinguished autoantibodies in a family may help to predict the risk of developing the disease over the following years (Bell et al., 1996; Verge et al., 1996; Turner et al., 1997; Froguel and Velho, 1999). Only less than 10% of genetically susceptible individuals may present subsequently with T1DM. This validates the noticeable role of environmental factors like viruses (Bell et al., 1996; Froguel and Velho, 1999), bacteria (Herold et al., 2011), diet (Hu, 2011; Katz, 2014), and weight gain (Colditz et al., 1995; Norris et al., 2012) in the onset and progression of the disease.

Type 2 diabetes mellitus (T2DM) which takes into account about 90–95% of all diabetics, is relatively different from T1DM in terms of etiology and the time of onset of the clinical phenotype, where T1DM appears mostly in infants and juveniles while T2DM generally occurs among middle-aged and older adults. However, in recent decades, because of changing lifestyles, more overweight and obese children have acquired T2DM. Peripheral insulin resistance and impaired function of beta cells are the reasons for hyperglycemia which may develop to hyperlipidemia. These two events cooperatively and progressively worsen the prognosis.

In both types of diabetes, chronically elevated levels of glucose are toxic for beta cells and prolonged exposure to glucose has deleterious effects on pancreatic beta cell function, leading to insulin insufficiency (Robertson et al., 2003, 2004). This loss of function is reversible at first but it becomes irreversible after a certain time point. Additionally, it should be noted that steady hyperglycemia may also induce apoptosis leading to reduced beta cell mass (Bell et al., 1996; Froguel and Velho, 1999; Jung et al., 2008).

12.4 THERAPEUTIC APPROACHES

12.4.1 COMMON APPROACHES

12.4.1.1 Oral medication

Ideally, oral diabetes drugs should improve macrovascular and microvascular results and decrease mortality. Treatment of T2DM varies depending on the severity of the disease. Several studies of the treatment of T2DM indicate that enhanced glycemic control decreases microvascular risks (Bolen et al., 2007). On the contrary, the effects of therapy on macrovascular risk are more controversial (Vijan et al., 1997; Pitale et al., 2000; Bolen et al., 2007), and to compare the effects of oral diabetes agents on clinical consequences is still less certain. Therefore, in general there are two approaches to treatment. Common oral medications like thiazolidinediones, sulfonylureas, and metformin are considered as the first line and as the disease develops, patients will require insulin regimen (Nathan et al., 2009). As recent oral drugs, such as thiazolidinediones and meglitinides, are progressively marketed more commonly, clinicians and patients must decide whether they prefer these usually more costly medications over older drugs, such as sulfonylureas and metformin (Vijan et al., 1997; Pitale et al., 2000). However, compared with newer medications, metformin and second-generation sulfonylureas share three extra advantages: longer use in practice, lower cost, and more intensive examination in long-term experiments with clinically related endpoints. Optimal glycemic control often needs multidrug therapy (Derosa et al., 2003; Papa et al., 2006).

12.4.1.2 Exogenous insulin

A prolonged increase in blood glucose is associated with chronic and consecutive complications including nephropathy, neuropathy, retinopathy, and hyperlipidemia leading to cardiovascular disease. Therapeutic strategies usually take into account different approaches to enhance the efficiency of the treatment. The administration of exogenous insulin as the treatment of choice, in combination with physical exercise and management of diet, is used for T1DM and severe cases of T2DM (Bell et al., 1996; Cooke and Plotnick, 2008; Inzucchi et al., 2012). New formulations of insulin (e.g., lispro and glargine analogs), continuous glucose-sensing devices, or continuous subcutaneous insulin infusion (CSII) have improved the control of the disease (Bell et al., 1996).

Evidence indicates that methods such as CSII have offered advantages over the traditional method of multiple daily injection (Bell et al., 1996; Froguel and Velho, 1999; Willi et al., 2003; Weinzimer et al., 2004); these strategies are capable of temporarily reducing of symptoms. In addition, prolonged insulin injections or uncontrolled concentrations of insulin are associated with hypoglycemia which causes other complications. Therefore, the development of new approaches for sustained production of insulin is becoming a new field of research aiming to control blood glucose in a physiological manner.

12.4.2 RECENT DEVELOPING APPROACHES

12.4.2.1 Gene-based therapies

Primary attempts were conducted on insulin production in nonbeta cells using insulin genes under the control of a promoter. Constitutively activated promoters were first used for this purpose. However, the main concern is the necessity to design a strategy in which release of insulin becomes controllable. Although regulatory promoters involved in glucose metabolism and responsive to elevated levels of glucose were promising *in vitro*, they failed tight control, robust, and prompt release of insulin in response to increased levels of blood glucose. However, construction of chimeric promoters may have potential for better regulation of insulin production *in vivo* (Chen et al., 2001; Alam and Sollinger, 2002; Olson et al., 2003; Kozlowski et al., 2007; Won et al., 2009; Han et al., 2012; Jajarmi et al., 2013).

12.4.2.2 Tissue engineering

Tissue engineering has opened a new window for treatment of diabetes. This area of science has had many successes in the development of substitutes for repair of damaged tissues and restoration of their functionality (Mooney et al., 1996; Shin et al., 2003; Ma, 2004; Rice et al., 2005; Nezafati et al., 2012; Mobini et al., 2013; Gholipourmalekabadi et al., 2014a, 2014b). Islet transplantation (IT) to bring back the beta cell mass in T1DM or to compensate for the reduced number of beta cells in T2DM may improve the insulin production impairment. However, organ shortages and the requirement for immunosuppressive agents for transplantation clearly are the main obstacles for clinical use of this approach (Bell et al., 1996; Shapiro et al., 2000). The generation of beta cells from stem cells with an embryonic or hematopoietic source would be an ideal approach to prepare adequate quantities of beta cell mass. On the other hand, organ transplantation is becoming a viable alternative to insulin therapy, which relies on providing adequate beta cell mass to restore normoglycemia. Whole-organ pancreatic (WOP) transplantation and IT as two parallel curative strategies have been performed to alleviate T1DM. Encouraging reports of successful WOP transplantation have been made during recent decades and it has been shown that simultaneous transplantation of pancreas and kidney may improve the results (Bell et al., 1996; Shapiro et al., 2000; Frank et al., 2004; Hakim, 2006). It was shown that the chance of graft survival during the first year of transplantation of simultaneous kidney and pancreas, pancreas after kidney transplantation, and pancreas alone was 89%, 86%, and 82%, respectively, while it was decreased to 71%, 65%, and 58%, respectively, within 5 years after transplantation (Gruessner and Gruessner, 2011). Therefore, many organ recipients need to be re-transplanted a few years later. Xenotransplantation was introduced as a solution to overcome the organ shortage; however, it is associated with an increased risk of graft rejection and viral transmission.

It is well established that solid organ transplantation may be associated with various complications. As an example, transplant recipients may develop diabetes which itself is considered a source of a variety of consequences leading to loss of the graft (Hasse et al., 1998; Hopt and Drognitz, 2000). High susceptibility to fungal, bacterial, and viral infections is another important concern in this strategy (Paya, 1993; Couchoud, 1998; Snydman, 1999; Kotton et al., 2010). The same phenomenon can affect islet cell transplantation which may complicate the success of engraftments.

Several regulator agents and mechanisms have been reported to be involved in β cell ingrowth both *in vitro* and *in vivo*. The transplanted cells were seeded on a 3D scaffold that acted like a barrier against the immune system besides providing adequate transportation of nutrients, oxygen, and waste products. In an artificial pancreas concept, there must be adequate access to oxygen and glucose and removal of metabolic waste products (Aoki et al., 2005; see Figure 12.2). In fact, tissue engineering has been explored to define the related agents and utilize them

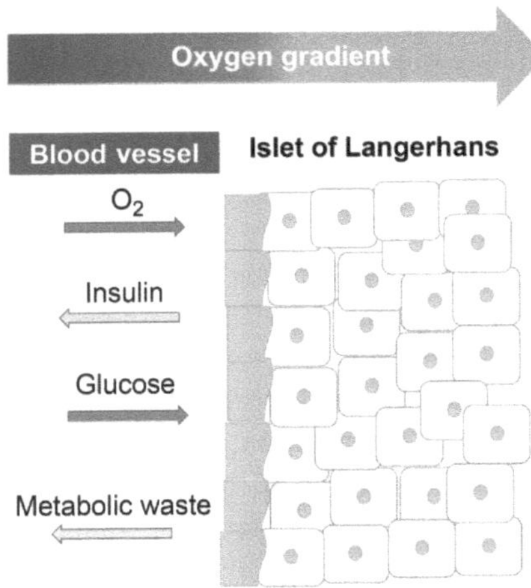

FIGURE 12.2

Essential elements of an implanted device illustrated in a conceptual biohybrid artificial pancreas.

within the 3D microenvironment with the aim of supporting islet cell viability and functionality (Alismail and Jin, 2014). For instance, it has been evidenced that the cell–cell adherent junction has a critical role in functionality and viability of insulin-secreting cells (Kelly et al., 2010; Bernard et al., 2012). Several studies have reported that poly(ethylene glycol) (PEG) hydrogel scaffolds could provide and mimic the cell–cell adherent junction in the microenvironment of insulin-secreting β cells (Weber et al., 2007a, 2007b; Lin and Anseth, 2011). Bernard et al. (2012) designed a cell culture system made from a PEG hydrogel-based microwell. They observed that β cells form aggregates within the hydrogels. The aggregated cells showed more cell viability and functionality (secretion of insulin) than single-cell cultures. Kelly et al. (2010) developed a PEG–ECM to mimic the islet–microenvironment interaction. For this purpose, a hydrogel containing PEG, collagen type I, collagen type IV, fibrinogen, fibronectin, laminin, and vitronectin was fabricated. The insulin-secreting cells were then encapsulated within the PEG–ECM hydrogel. A significant increase in cell viability and level of insulin secretion was reported by this group. The main complication associated with aggregation of islet cells is hypoxia conditions occurring in the site due to an insufficient level of oxygen, leading to necrosis and cell death.

12.4.3 OXYGEN-GENERATING NANOBIOMATERIALS

Islet cells are one of most oxygen-demanding cells due to their high metabolic activity. In the pancreas, islets consist of two types of endocrine hormone-producing cells (α- and ß-cells). ß-Cells are responsible for the secretion of insulin. An insufficient oxygen supply can profoundly affect the functionality of these cells and result in diabetes. Additionally, free radicals are produced during the hypoxia conditions that cause cell cycle arrest through damaging DNA (Wang and Semenza, 1993; Reynolds et al., 1996). Therefore, supplying adequate nutrition distribution, especially oxygen, is critical for success in diabetes therapy. Many attempts have been made to overcome such concerns (Wu et al., 1999; Bloch et al., 2006a; Pedraza et al., 2012; Colton, 2014). For the first time, Bloch et al. (2006b) introduced a novel technique in natural photosynthesis to generate oxygen for encapsulated pancreatic islets. In a similar study, the islet cells were encapsulated in agar, alginate, and chitosan to selectively receive oxygen and remove waste products (Colton, 2014). However, inaccessibility to a sufficient level of oxygen has still remained problematic. Recently, researchers have adopted some novel nanobiomaterials with the capability of producing oxygen to explore a way for overcoming delivery of oxygen. Oxygen-generating nanobiomaterials decompose to oxygen when they are exposed to water. The most common oxygen-generating nanobiomaterials, as well as their oxygenation mechanisms, are described below.

12.4.3.1 Solid inorganic peroxides

During the last decade, solid inorganic peroxides such as sodium percarbonate (Na_2CO_3) (Harrison et al., 2007), calcium peroxide (CaO_2) (Oh et al., 2009b), and magnesium peroxide (MgO_2) (Waite et al., 1999; Harrison et al., 2007) have been widely used in tissue engineering applications. These materials are decomposed to hydrogen peroxide (H_2O_2) when react with water. The related reactions are shown in Eqns (12.1)–(12.3):

$$CaO_2(s) + 2H_2O \rightarrow Ca(OH)_2(s) + H_2O_2 \tag{12.1}$$

$$MgO_2(s) + 2H_2O \rightarrow Mg(OH)_2(s) + H_2O_2 \tag{12.2}$$

$$(Na_2CO_3)_2 + 3H_2O_2 \rightarrow 4Na + 2CO_3^{-2} + 3H_2O_2 \tag{12.3}$$

CaO_2, due to its high purity (70% purity) and commercial availability, has become one of the most interesting oxygen-generating nanobiomaterials (White et al., 1998). On the other hand, MgO_2 has the slowest reaction rate due to its low solubility (Waite et al., 1999).

The production of metal hydroxides and hydrogen peroxide during the decomposition of oxygen-generating nanobiomaterials is one of the most important concerns associated with using these materials in tissue engineering (Pedraza et al., 2012). The production of such byproducts influences the pH level of the microenvironment through which they affect oxygenation. The pH could be stabilized by the use of some buffers (Waite et al., 1999).

Furthermore, accumulation of H_2O_2 profoundly stimulates formation of free radicals and affects cell viability. Catalase, as an antioxidant agent, has been utilized to warrant the decomposition of H_2O_2 to oxygen (Sinensky et al., 1995; Abdi et al., 2011). Therefore, concerns arising from the toxicity of H_2O_2 have been resolved by adding catalase to cell culture medium or scaffolds (Sinensky et al., 1995; Abdi et al., 2011). The mechanisms by which catalase decomposes the H_2O_2 are shown in Eqns (12.4) and (12.5):

$$H_2O_2(aq) + 2Fe^{3+}(aq) \rightarrow O_2(g) + 2Fe^{2+}(aq) + 2H^+(aq) \tag{12.4}$$

$$H_2O_2(aq) + 2Fe^{2+}(aq) + 2H^+(aq) \rightarrow 2H_2O(l) + 2Fe^{3+}(aq) \tag{12.5}$$

In their study, Harrison et al. (2007) engineered a construct made from sodium percarbonate-incorporated poly(lactic-co-glycolic acid) (PLGA). They reported that the complete release of oxygen occurred over 3 days. To slow down the oxygenation, the same research group carried out another study (Oh et al., 2009b). In this case, they encapsulated the CaO_2 in PLGA and showed its consistent oxygen release up to 10 days *in vitro*. They also evaluated the effect of different molar ratios of CaO_2 (ranging from 0% to 10%) in CaO_2–PLGA construct in efficiency of oxygenation. According to their results, 5 w/v%-CaO_2 was shown to be more effective compared with other concentrations when exposed to cells.

12.4.3.2 Hydrogen peroxide (H_2O_2)

The rate of spontaneous hydrogen peroxide decomposition to oxygen is very low. On the other hand, accumulation of H_2O_2 in tissue threatens the fate of cells through mediation of free radical formation. To overcome such obstacles, the catalase enzyme is added in medium (for *in vitro* applications) or tissue engineering scaffolds (for *in vivo* applications). Catalase, as an antioxidant enzyme, converts oxygen species' hydrogen peroxide to water and oxygen and thereby minimizes its cytoxicity. Microencapsulation of H_2O_2 in some nanobiomaterials is an efficient strategy for safe, consistent, and localized delivery of oxygen (Abdi et al., 2011; Li et al., 2012). A prolonged oxygenation was achieved by synthesis of PVP/H_2O_2/PLGA/catalase/hydrogel (Li et al., 2012). For this purpose, H_2O_2 was attached to poly(vinyl pyrrolidone) (PVP) and the resulting PVP/H_2O_2 complex was encapsulated in PLGA to form a core-shell microsphere. The microsphere was then incorporated in catalase-containing hydrogel. The authors showed that the release of oxygen in this construct was sustained for up to 14 days.

Abdi et al. (2011) successfully sustained oxygenation by microencapsulating the H_2O_2 particles in a two-layered construct. They placed the hydrogen peroxide in an intrinsic layer of PLGA that was surrounded by a secondary layer composed of alginate. They showed that H_2O_2 particles are released from PLGA to the secondary layer and decomposed to oxygen by catalase enzyme bounded to alginate.

12.4.3.3 *Fluorinated materials*

Perfluorocarbons (PFCs), as a promising oxygen-generating nanobiomaterial, have attracted the attention of researchers due to their ability to produce a large amount of oxygen. PFCs decompose to oxygen and carbon dioxide upon being exposed to water. Encapsulating the PFC within alginate was found to be an efficient strategy to sustain and localize delivery of oxygen, increasing oxygenation up to 1 week (Khattak et al., 2007). The authors suggested the potential applications of such a strategy in encapsulating the cells, especially islet cells.

In addition to biocompatibility, the oxygen release rate of oxygen-generating nanobiomaterials is another important factor which could directly influence tissue maturation. With the aim of delivering a satisfactory amount of oxygen, the rate of oxygenation requires to be adjusted to avoid bursts or very prolonged release of oxygen. There are some factors such as temperature, pH, amount of peroxide, and type of medium that could profoundly affect the amount and consistency of oxygenation from the oxygen-generating nanobiomaterials (Soleymani et al., 2011). For instance, the rate of oxygenation reduces with a decrease in the environmental temperature. On the other hand, as mentioned earlier in this chapter, incorporation of peroxide particles in some polymers is a way to adjust the rate and durability of oxygen release. For example, in contrast to hydrophobic compounds, hydrophilic materials increase the release of oxygen due to the fast diffusion of oxygen within them (Harrison et al., 2007; Fraker et al., 2011). Seifu et al. (2011) have recently introduced fluorinated zeolite particles as novel oxygen-generating nanobiomaterials in tissue engineering. They indicated that the fluoriated zeolite particles uniformly embedded in polyurethane scaffolds and oxygen concentration increased significantly. Based on cell culture results and cell viability measurements this kind of scaffold could safely provide oxygen delivery to cells.

12.4.4 OXYGEN-GENERATING NANOBIOMATERIALS IN DIABETES THERAPY

The delivery of ß-cells as insulin-producing cells to the pancreas is one of the most efficient strategies for diabetes therapy. Nevertheless, there are some challenges associated with such a strategy, including body immune response, inability to provide sufficient oxygen supply, and removal of waste byproducts that need to be addressed. After each implantation, especially in large engraftments, early neovascularization requires enough time to be achieved (around a couple of weeks). Therefore, the release of oxygen should be sustained to provide enough time for neovascularization and maturation of the engineered tissues (Pedraza et al., 2012). Elimination of the hypoxia period between transplantation and neovascularization formation could dramatically reduce hypoxia-induced cell death and necrosis. Several strategies were developed for sufficient delivery of oxygen to cells (Zisch et al., 2003; Ehrbar et al., 2004; Bloch et al., 2006b; Pileggi et al., 2006; Ludwig et al., 2010; Pedraza et al., 2012), for example, stimulation of preneovascularization in implantation site (Pileggi et al., 2006), promotion of early neovascularization using angiogenic factors such as endothelial cells and vascular endothelial growth factors (Nomi et al., 2002; Coppi et al., 2005; Kaigler et al., 2006), utilization of oxygen carriers within nanobiomaterials (Adlercreutz and Mattiasson, 1982), and *in situ* generation of oxygen by oxygen-generating nanobiomaterials (Harrison et al., 2007; Oh et al., 2009b). Among the above-mentioned strategies, *in situ* oxygenation is considered the most desirable strategy due to its ability to provide sufficient oxygen upon implantation without the need for additional surgeries. Various biomaterials have been investigated for their oxygenation ability. Despite the great success, quick release of oxygen by oxygen-generating nanobiomaterials still remains challenging (Pedraza et al., 2012). It needs to be emphasized that the chemical components of oxygen-generating nanobiomaterials could profoundly affect the release rate of oxygen (Harrison et al., 2007). It has also been found that incorporation of oxygen-generating nanobiomaterials into the hydrophobic polymers (Oh et al., 2009b) could slow down the oxygenation. Recently, researchers have focused on development of an appropriate strategy to incorporate the oxygen-generating nanobiomaterials into tissue engineering constructs (Harrison et al., 2007; Ward et al., 2013). In fact, oxygen-generating scaffolds can be classified as a new generation of scaffolds in tissue engineering, especially in large tissue masses which need more blood supply to enhance survival of cells. Thus, oxygen-releasing systems provide oxygen for stem cells sustainably, which overcomes oxygen diffusion limitations in bioengineering tissues (Khademhosseini et al., 2006). In this way, oxygen-generating nanobiomaterials are combined with the scaffolds. Harrison's group at Wake Forest University has frequently combined oxygen-generating nanobiomaterials with tissue engineering scaffolds (Harrison et al., 2007; Oh et al., 2009b). In a recent study, they used calcium-peroxide-based oxygen-generating particles in a 3D PLGA scaffold. The results showed enhanced cell survival besides neovascularization after implantation. These features would be helpful in tissue engineering of large tissues (Harrison et al., 2007; Oh et al., 2009b). For this purpose, various forms of scaffolds, such as films (Harrison et al., 2007), electrospun nanofibers (Wang et al., 2010), and hydrogels (Li et al., 2012), were achieved by incorporating the oxygen-generating nanobiomaterials into the tissue engineering constructs.

Pedraza et al. (2012) have developed a novel composite made of polydimethylsiloxane (PDMS)-encapsulated solid calcium peroxide (PDMS-CaO_2). They aimed to increase oxygen availability during the early engraftment period while an inevitable delay in angiogenesis occurs. For this purpose, the effect of synthesized construct on cell viability of β-cell line and pancreatic rat islets

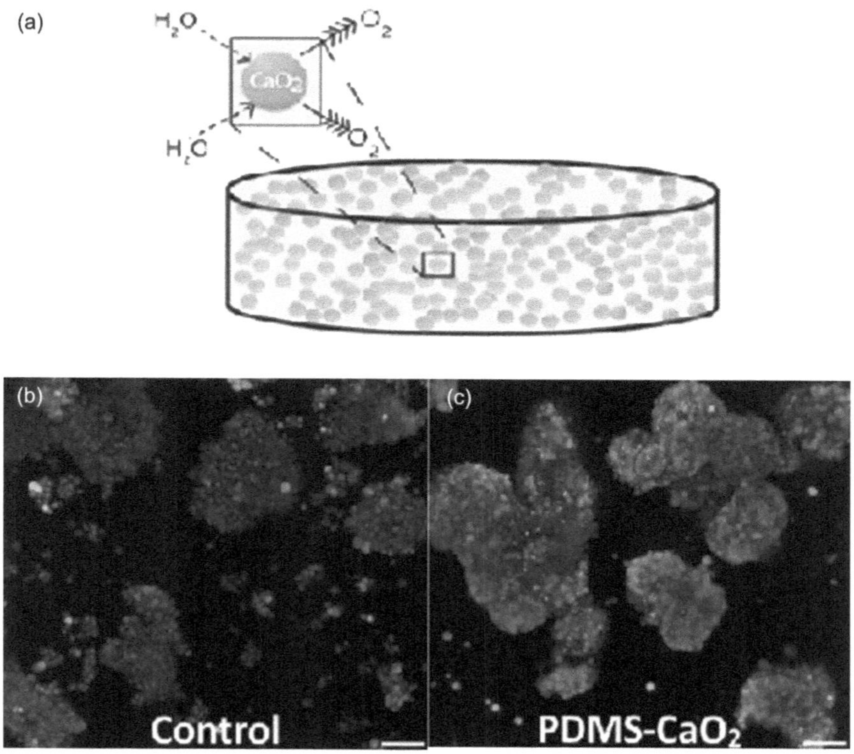

FIGURE 12.3

Schematic of an oxygen-generating biomaterial, fabricated using PDMS-CaO_2. Water diffusion is hindered by the hydrophobicity of the PDMS, whereas oxygen, generated via a hydrolytic reaction with calcium peroxide, quickly diffuses out of the PDMS material. (b, c) Representative confocal z-stacked images of islets, stained for live/dead (live, green; dead, red), after 6 h of culture at 0.05 mM oxygen without (control) or with a PDMS-CaO_2 disk. (Scale bar 100 μm.) (For interpretation of the references to colour in this figure legend, the reader is referred to the web version of this book.)

was determined. They showed that PMDS, as a highly hydrophobic and stable biopolymer, prolonged the release of oxygen from PDMS-CaO_2 through a decrease in water uptake, so that each sample released 0.026 mM oxygen per day, for up to 42 days. According to their results, the PDMS-CaO_2 significantly minimized the negative effects of hypoxia conditions on MIN6 ß-cell line and rat pancreatic islets for up to 14 days when compared with CPO-free PDMS (see Figure 12.3). The authors strongly suggested the potential application of such a construct in sustained generation and delivery of oxygen within the implants. However, further investigations need to be carried out to ensure the *in vivo* applications of these materials.

12.5 CONCLUSIONS

One of the concerns in tissue engineering is the angiogenic response, which is crucial for the survival of cells. Since oxygenation and nutrition of cells in the constructs are limited by diffusion, it is necessary to provide oxygen to enhance cell survival until tissue neovascularization. The chemical decomposition of oxygen-generating nanobiomaterials produces oxygen over a period of time. This sustained oxygen release is capable of enhancing cell survivability and subsequently providing a tissue engineering approach for diabetes therapy. This strategy may provide a new perspective in the treatment of diabetes. Despite reasonable success in this field, there are still challenges in the use of oxygen-generating nanobiomaterials. On the one hand, the rate of oxygen released from the particles is not fully determined, in which the excessive oxygen release would be cytotoxic. On the other hand, oxygen-generating nanobiomaterial incorporation should not affect the biomechanical properties of the prepared constructs.

REFERENCES

Abdi, S.I.H., Ng, S.M., Lim, J.O., 2011. An enzyme-modulated oxygen-producing micro-system for regenerative therapeutics. Int. J. Pharm. 409, 203–205.

Adlercreutz, P., Mattiasson, B., 1982. Oxygen supply to immobilized cells. Eur. J. Appl. Microbiol. Biotechnol. 16, 165–170.

Alam, T., Sollinger, H.W., 2002. Glucose-regulated insulin production in hepatocytes. Transplantation 74, 1781–1787.

Alismail, H., Jin, S., 2014. Microenvironmental stimuli for proliferation of functional islet β-cells. Cell Biosci. 4, 12.

Amer, L.D., Mahoney, M.J., Bryant, S.J., 2014. Tissue engineering approaches to cell-based type 1 diabetes therapy. Tissue Eng. Part B Rev. 20, 455–467.

Aoki, T., Hui, H., Umehara, Y., Licalzi, S., Demetriou, A.A., Rozga, J., et al., 2005. Intrasplenic transplantation of encapsulated genetically engineered mouse insulinoma cells reverses streptozotocin-induced diabetes in rats. Cell Transplant. 14, 411–421.

Association, A.D., 2008. Diagnosis and classification of diabetes mellitus. Diabetes Care 31, S55–S60.

Baghbani, F., Moztarzadeh, F., Nazari, A.G., Kamran, A.R., Tondnevis, F., Nezafati, N., et al., 2012. Biological response of biphasic hydroxyapatite/tricalcium phosphate scaffolds intended for low load-bearing orthopaedic applications. Adv. Compost. Lett. 21, 16–24.

Bell, G.I., Pilkis, S., Weber, I.T., Polonsky, K.S., 1996. Glucokinase mutations, insulin secretion, and diabetes mellitus. Annu. Rev. Physiol. 58, 171–186.

Bernard, A.B., Lin, C.-C., Anseth, K.S., 2012. A microwell cell culture platform for the aggregation of pancreatic β-Cells. Tissue Eng. Part C Methods 18, 583–592.

Bianco, P., Robey, P.G., 2001. Stem cells in tissue engineering. Nature 414, 118–121.

Bloch, K., Papismedov, E., Yavriyants, K., Vorobeychik, M., Beer, S., Vardi, P., 2006a. Immobilized microalgal cells as an oxygen supply system for encapsulated pancreatic islets: a feasibility study. Artif. Organs 30, 715–718.

Bloch, K., Papismedov, E., Yavriyants, K., Vorobeychik, M., Beer, S., Vardi, P., 2006b. Photosynthetic oxygen generator for bioartificial pancreas. Tissue Eng. 12, 337–344.

Bogunia-Kubik, K., Sugisaka, M., 2002. From molecular biology to nanotechnology and nanomedicine. Biosystems 65, 123–138.

Bohr, M.T., 2002. Nanotechnology goals and challenges for electronic applications. IEEE Trans. Nanotechnol. 1, 56–62.

Bolen, S., Feldman, L., Vassy, J., Wilson, L., Yeh, H.-C., Marinopoulos, S., et al., 2007. Systematic review: comparative effectiveness and safety of oral medications for type 2 diabetes mellitus. Ann. Intern. Med. 147, 386–399.

Butler, A.E., Janson, J., Soeller, W.C., Butler, P.C., 2003. Increased β-cell apoptosis prevents adaptive increase in β-cell mass in mouse model of type 2 diabetes evidence for role of islet amyloid formation rather than direct action of amyloid. Diabetes 52, 2304–2314.

Chen, V.J., Ma, P.X., 2004. Nano-fibrous poly (L-lactic acid) scaffolds with interconnected spherical macropores. Biomaterials 25, 2065.

Chen, V.J., Ma, P.X., 2006. The effect of surface area on the degradation rate of nano-fibrous poly (L-lactic acid) foams. Biomaterials 27, 3708–3715.

Chen, R., Meseck, M.L., Woo, S.L., 2001. Auto-regulated hepatic insulin gene expression in type 1 diabetic rats. Mol. Ther. 3, 584–590.

Clarke, J., Wu, H.C., Jayasinghe, L., Patel, A., Reid, S., Bayley, H., 2009. Continuous base identification for single-molecule nanopore DNA sequencing. Nat. Nanotechnol. 4, 265–270.

Colditz, G.A., Willett, W.C., Rotnitzky, A., Manson, J.E., 1995. Weight gain as a risk factor for clinical diabetes mellitus in women. Ann. Intern. Med. 122, 481–486.

Colton, C.K., 2014. Oxygen supply to encapsulated therapeutic cells. Adv. Drug Deliv. Rev. 67, 93–110.

WHO Consultation Group, 1999. Definition, diagnosis and classification of diabetes mellitus and its complications, Part 1: Diagnosis and classification of diabetes mellitus WHO/NCD/NCS/99. World Health Organization, Geneva.

Cooke, D.W., Plotnick, L., 2008. Type 1 diabetes mellitus in pediatrics. Pediatr. Rev. 29, 374–385.

Coppi, P.D., Delo, D., Farrugia, L., Udompanyanan, K., Yoo, J.J., Nomi, M., et al., 2005. Angiogenic gene-modified muscle cells for enhancement of tissue formation. Tissue Eng. 11, 1034–1044.

Couchoud, C. 1998. Cytomegalovirus prophylaxis with antiviral agents for solid organ transplantation. The Cochrane Library (published online).

Dankers, P.Y.W., Meijer, E., 2007. Supramolecular biomaterials. a modular approach towards tissue engineering. Bull. Chem. Soc. Jpn 80, 2047–2073.

Derosa, G., Mugellini, A., Ciccarelli, L., Crescenzi, G., Fogari, R., 2003. Comparison between repaglinide and glimepiride in patients with type 2 diabetes mellitus: a one-year, randomized, double-blind assessment of metabolic parameters and cardiovascular risk factors. Clin. Ther. 25, 472–484.

Donovan, P.J., Gearhart, J., 2001. The end of the beginning for pluripotent stem cells. Nature 414, 92–97.

Dvir, T., Timko, B.P., Kohane, D.S., Langer, R., 2011. Nanotechnological strategies for engineering complex tissues. Nat. Nanotechnol. 6, 13–22.

Efrat, S., 2004. Regulation of insulin secretion: insights from engineered β-cell lines. Ann. N. Y. Acad. Sci. 1014, 88–96.

Ehrbar, M., Djonov, V.G., Schnell, C., Tschanz, S.A., Martiny-Baron, G., Schenk, U., et al., 2004. Cell-demanded liberation of VEGF121 from fibrin implants induces local and controlled blood vessel growth. Circ. Res. 94, 1124–1132.

El-Sadik, A.O., El-Ansary, A., Sabry, S.M., 2010. Nanoparticle-labeled stem cells: a novel therapeutic vehicle. Clin. Pharmacol. 2, 9.

Farokhzad, O.C., Langer, R., 2009. Impact of nanotechnology on drug delivery. ACS Nano 3, 16–20.

Ferrari, M., 2005. Cancer nanotechnology: opportunities and challenges. Nat. Rev. Cancer 5, 161–171.

Fraker, C.A., Mendez, A.J., Stabler, C.L., 2011. Complementary methods for the determination of dissolved oxygen content in perfluorocarbon emulsions and other solutions. J. Phys. Chem. B. 115, 10547–10552.

Frank, A., Deng, S., Huang, X., Velidedeoglu, E., Bae, Y.-S., Liu, C., et al., 2004. Transplantation for type I diabetes: comparison of vascularized whole-organ pancreas with isolated pancreatic islets. Ann. Surg. 240, 631.

Froguel, P., Velho, G., 1999. Molecular genetics of maturity-onset diabetes of the young. Trends Endocrinol. Metab. 10, 142–146.

Gao, J., Xu, B., 2009. Applications of nanomaterials inside cells. Nano Today 4, 37–51.

Gelain, F., Bottai, D., Vescovi, A., Zhang, S., 2006. Designer self-assembling peptide nanofiber scaffolds for adult mouse neural stem cell 3-dimensional cultures. PLoS One 1, e119.

Gholipourmalekabadi, M., Mozafari, M., Bandehpour, M., Salehi, M., Sameni, M., Caicedo, H.H., et al., 2014a. Optimization of nanofibrous silk fibroin scaffolds as a delivery system for bone marrow adherent cells. Biotechnol. Appl. Biochem.

Gholipourmalekabadi, M., Mozafari, M., Bojnordi, M.N., Hashemi-soteh, M., Salimi, M., Rezaei, N., et al., 2014b. *In vitro* and *in vivo* evaluations of three-dimensional hydroxyapatite/silk fibroin nanocomposites scaffolds. Biotechnol. Appl. Biochem. 62, 441–450.

Gholipourmalekabadi, M., Mozafari, M., Salehi, M., Seifalian, A., Bandehpour, M., Ghanbarian, H., et al., 2015a. Development of a cost-effective and simple protocol for decellularization and preservation of human amniotic membrane as a soft tissue replacement and delivery system for bone marrow stromal cells. Adv. Healthc. Mater. 4, 918–926.

Gholipourmalekabadi, M., Mozafari, M., Salehi, M., Seifalian, A., Bandehpour, M., Ghanbarian, H., et al., 2015b. Development of a cost-effective and simple protocol for decellularization and preservation of human amniotic membrane as a soft tissue replacement and delivery system for bone marrow stromal cells. Adv. Healthc. Mater.

Gruessner, A., Gruessner, R., 2011. Pancreas transplant outcomes for united states and non united states cases as reported to the united network for organ sharing and the international pancreas transplant registry as of December 2011. Clin. Transpl. 23–40.

Guariguata, L., Whiting, D., Hambleton, I., Beagley, J., Linnenkamp, U., Shaw, J., 2014. Global estimates of diabetes prevalence for 2013 and projections for 2035. Diabetes Res. Clin. Pract. 103, 137–149.

Hakim, N.S., 2006. Whole organ pancreas transplantation. Liver and Pancreatic Diseases Management. Springer, Netherlands, pp. 95–105.

Han, J., Kim, E.-H., Choi, W., Jun, H.-S., 2012. Glucose-responsive artificial promoter-mediated insulin gene transfer improves glucose control in diabetic mice. World J. Gastroenterol. 18, 6420.

Harrison, B.S., Eberli, D., Lee, S.J., Atala, A., Yoo, J.J., 2007. Oxygen producing biomaterials for tissue regeneration. Biomaterials 28, 4628–4634.

Hasse, J.M., Di Cecco, S.R., Skipper, A. 1998. Solid organ transplantation. Dietician's Handbook of Enteral and Parenteral Nutrition, Gatetherburg, Maryland, 295–323.

Hench, L.L., Polak, J.M., 2002. Third-generation biomedical materials. Science 295, 1014–1017.

Herold, K.C., Pescovitz, M.D., Mcgee, P., Krause-Steinrauf, H., Spain, L.M., Bourcier, K., et al., 2011. Increased T cell proliferative responses to islet antigens identify clinical responders to anti-CD20 monoclonal antibody (rituximab) therapy in type 1 diabetes. J. Immunol. 187, 1998–2005.

Hopfner, U., Schenck, T.-L., Chávez, M.-N., Machens, H.-G., Bohne, A.-V., Nickelsen, J., et al., 2014. Development of photosynthetic biomaterials for *in vitro* tissue engineering. Acta Biomater. 10, 2712–2717.

Hopt, U.T., Drognitz, O., 2000. Pancreas organ transplantation. Langenbeck's Arch Surg. 385, 379–389.

Hoshino, A., Fujioka, K., Oku, T., Suga, M., Sasaki, Y.F., Ohta, T., et al., 2004. Physicochemical properties and cellular toxicity of nanocrystal quantum dots depend on their surface modification. Nano Lett. 4, 2163–2169.

Hu, F.B., 2011. Globalization of diabetes the role of diet, lifestyle, and genes. Diabetes Care 34, 1249–1257.

Huang, J., Lin, X., Shi, Y., Liu, W., 2015. Tissue engineering and regenerative medicine in basic research: a year in review of 2014. Tissue Eng Part B Rev 21, 177–186.

Inzucchi, S.E., Bergenstal, R.M., Buse, J.B., Diamant, M., Ferrannini, E., Nauck, M., et al., 2012. Management of hyperglycemia in type 2 diabetes: a patient-centered approach position statement of the American Diabetes Association (ADA) and the European Association for the Study of Diabetes (EASD). Diabetes Care 35, 1364–1379.

Jain, K.K., 2003. Nanodiagnostics: application of nanotechnology in molecular diagnostics. Expert Rev. Mol. Diagn. 3, 153–161.

Jajarmi, V., Bandehpour, M., Kazemi, B., 2013. Regulation of insulin biosynthesis in non-beta cells by a heat shock promoter. J. Biosci. Bioeng. 116, 147–151.

Juang, J.Y., Bogy, D.B., 2005. Nanotechnology advances and applications in information storage. Microsyst. Technol. 11, 950–957.

Jung, H.S., Chung, K.W., Won Kim, J., Kim, J., Komatsu, M., Tanaka, K., et al., 2008. Loss of autophagy diminishes pancreatic β cell mass and function with resultant hyperglycemia. Cell Metab. 8, 318–324.

Kaigler, D., Wang, Z., Horger, K., Mooney, D.J., Krebsbach, P.H., 2006. VEGF scaffolds enhance angiogenesis and bone regeneration in irradiated osseous defects. J. Bone Miner. Res. 21, 735–744.

Katz, D.L., 2014. Diet and diabetes: lines and dots. J. Nutr. 144, 567S–570S.

Kelly, C., Parke, H.G., Mccluskey, J.T., Flatt, P.R., Mcclenaghan, N.H., 2010. The role of glucagon- and somatostatin-secreting cells in the regulation of insulin release and beta-cell function in heterotypic pseudoislets. Diabetes Metab. Res. Rev. 26, 525–533.

Khademhosseini, A., Langer, R., Borenstein, J., Vacanti, J.P., 2006. Microscale technologies for tissue engineering and biology. Proc. Natl Acad. Sci. U.S.A. 103, 2480–2487.
Khattak, S.F., Chin, K.S., Bhatia, S.R., Roberts, S.C., 2007. Enhancing oxygen tension and cellular function in alginate cell encapsulation devices through the use of perfluorocarbons. Biotechnol. Bioeng. 96, 156–166.
Kotton, C.N., Kumar, D., Caliendo, A.M., Åsberg, A., Chou, S., Snydman, D.R., et al., 2010. International consensus guidelines on the management of cytomegalovirus in solid organ transplantation. Transplantation 89, 779–795.
Kozlowski, M., Olson, D.E., Rubin, J., Lyszkowicz, D., Campbell, A., Thulé, P.M., 2007. Adeno-associated viral delivery of a metabolically regulated insulin transgene to hepatocytes. Mol. Cell. Endocrinol. 273, 6–15.
Langer, R., Vacanti, J.P., 1993. Tissue engineering Science. 260, 920–926.
Lanza, R., Langer, R., Vacanti, J.P., 2007. Principles of Tissue Engineering. Academic Press, San Diego, CA.
Li, Z., Guo, X., Guan, J., 2012. An oxygen release system to augment cardiac progenitor cell survival and differentiation under hypoxic condition. Biomaterials 33, 5914–5923.
Liao, S., Chan, C.K., Ramakrishna, S., 2008. Stem cells and biomimetic materials strategies for tissue engineering. Mater. Sci. Eng. C 28, 1189–1202.
Lin, C.-C., Anseth, K.S., 2011. Cell–cell communication mimicry with poly (ethylene glycol) hydrogels for enhancing β-cell function. Proc. Natl Acad. Sci. 108, 6380–6385.
Liu, X., Ma, P.X., 2004. Polymeric scaffolds for bone tissue engineering: on musculoskeletal bioengineering. Ann. Biomed. Eng. 32, 477–486.
Liu, H., Webster, T.J., 2007. Nanomedicine for implants: a review of studies and necessary experimental tools. Biomaterials 28, 354–369.
Ludwig, B., Zimerman, B., Steffen, A., Yavriants, K., Azarov, D., Reichel, A., et al., 2010. A novel device for islet transplantation providing immune protection and oxygen supply. Horm. Metab. Res. 42, 918–922.
Ma, P.X., 2004. Scaffolds for tissue fabrication. Mater. Today 7, 30–40.
Ma, P.X., 2008. Biomimetic materials for tissue engineering. Adv. Drug Deliv. Rev. 60, 184–198.
Ma, P.X., Langer, R., 1995. Degradation, structure and properties of fibrous nonwoven poly (glycolic acid) scaffolds for tissue engineering. Mater. Res. Soc. Symp. Proc. Polym. Med. Pharm. 394, 99–104.
Ma, P.X., Zhang, R., Xiao, G., Franceschi, R., 2000. Engineering new bone tissue *in vitro* on highly porous poly (α-hydroxyl acids)/hydroxyapatite composite scaffolds. J. Biomed. Mater. Res. 54, 284–293.
Medintz, I.L., Uyeda, H.T., Goldman, E.R., Mattoussi, H., 2005. Quantum dot bioconjugates for imaging, labelling and sensing. Nat. Mater. 4, 435–446.
Mikos, A.G., Herring, S.W., Ochareon, P., Elisseeff, J., Lu, H.H., Kandel, R., et al., 2006. Engineering complex tissues. Tissue Eng. 12, 3307–3339.
Mobini, S., Solati-Hashjin, M., Peirovi, H., Osman, N.A.A., Gholipourmalekabadi, M., Barati, M., et al., 2013. Bioactivity and biocompatibility studies on silk-based scaffold for bone tissue engineering. J. Med. Biol. Eng. 33, 207–213.
Montanya, E., 2004. Islet- and stem-cell-based tissue engineering in diabetes. Curr. Opin. Biotechnol. 15, 435–440.
Mooney, D.J., Baldwin, D.F., Suh, N.P., Vacanti, J.P., Langer, R., 1996. Novel approach to fabricate porous sponges of poly (D, L-lactic-co-glycolic acid) without the use of organic solvents. Biomaterials 17, 1417–1422.

Morrissey, S., 2006. Nanotechnology in food and agriculture. Chem. Eng. News 84, 31–31.

Mozafari, M., Gholipourmalekabadi, M., Chauhan, N., Jalali, N., Asgari, S., Caicedoa, J., et al., 2015. Synthesis and characterization of nanocrystalline forsterite coated poly (L-lactide-co-β-malic acid) scaffolds for bone tissue engineering applications. Mater. Sci. Eng. C.

Nathan, D.M., Buse, J.B., Davidson, M.B., Ferrannini, E., Holman, R.R., Sherwin, R., et al., 2009. Medical management of hyperglycemia in type 2 diabetes: a consensus algorithm for the initiation and adjustment of therapy a consensus statement of the american diabetes association and the european association for the study of diabetes. Diabetes Care 32, 193–203.

Nezafati, N., Moztarzadeh, F., Hesaraki, S., Mozafari, M., Samadikuchaksaraei, A., Hajibaki, L., et al., 2012. Effect of silver concentration on bioactivity and antibacterial properties of SiO2-CaO-P2O5 sol-gel derived bioactive glass. Key Eng. Mater. 493, 74–79.

Nomi, M., Atala, A., Coppi, P.D., Soker, S., 2002. Principals of neovascularization for tissue engineering. Mol. Aspects Med. 23, 463–483.

Norris, S.A., Osmond, C., Gigante, D., Kuzawa, C.W., Ramakrishnan, L., Lee, N.R., et al., 2012. Size at birth, weight gain in infancy and childhood, and adult diabetes risk in five low-or middle-income country birth cohorts. Diabetes Care 35, 72–79.

Oh, S., Brammer, K.S., Li, Y.S.J., Teng, D., Engler, A.J., Chien, S., et al., 2009a. Stem cell fate dictated solely by altered nanotube dimension. Proc. Natl Acad. Sci. 106, 2130–2135.

Oh, S.H., Ward, C.L., Atala, A., Yoo, J.J., Harrison, B.S., 2009b. Oxygen generating scaffolds for enhancing engineered tissue survival. Biomaterials 30, 757–762.

Olson, D.E., Paveglio, S.A., Huey, P.U., Porter, M.H., Thulé, P.M., 2003. Glucose-responsive hepatic insulin gene therapy of spontaneously diabetic BB/Wor rats. Hum. Gene Ther. 14, 1401–1413.

Papa, G., Fedele, V., Rizzo, M.R., Fioravanti, M., Leotta, C., Solerte, S.B., et al., 2006. Safety of type 2 diabetes treatment with repaglinide compared with glibenclamide in elderly people a randomized, open-label, two-period, cross-over trial. Diabetes Care 29, 1918–1920.

Paya, C.V., 1993. Fungal infections in solid-organ transplantation. Clin. Infect. Dis. 16, 677–688.

Pedraza, E., Coronel, M.M., Fraker, C.A., Ricordi, C., Stabler, C.L., 2012. Preventing hypoxia-induced cell death in beta cells and islets via hydrolytically activated, oxygen-generating biomaterials. Proc. Natl Acad. Sci. 109, 4245–4250.

Peng, S., Cho, K., 2000. Chemical control of nanotube electronics. Nanotechnology 11, 57.

Peppas, N.A., 2004. Intelligent therapeutics: biomimetic systems and nanotechnology in drug delivery. Adv. Drug Deliv. Rev. 56, 1529.

Pera, M.F., Reubinoff, B., Trounson, A., 2000. Human embryonic stem cells. J. Cell Sci. 113, 5–10.

Pileggi, A., Molano, R.D., Ricordi, C., Zahr, E., Collins, J., Valdes, R., et al., 2006. Reversal of diabetes by pancreatic islet transplantation into a subcutaneous, neovascularized device. Transplantation 81, 1318–1324.

Pitale, S.U., Abraira, C., Emanuele, N.V., Mccarren, M., Henderson, W.G., Pacold, I., et al., 2000. Two years of intensive glycemic control and left ventricular function in the Veterans Affairs Cooperative Study in Type 2 Diabetes Mellitus (VA CSDM). Diabetes Care 23, 1316–1320.

Reynolds, T.Y., Rockwell, S., Glazer, P.M., 1996. Genetic instability induced by the tumor microenvironment. Cancer Res. 56, 5754–5757.

Rice, M.A., Dodson, B.T., Arthur, J.A., Anseth, K.S., 2005. Cell-based therapies and tissue engineering. Otolaryngol. Clin. North Am. 38, 199–214.

Robertson, R.P., Harmon, J., Tran, P.O., Tanaka, Y., Takahashi, H., 2003. Glucose toxicity in β-cells: type 2 diabetes, good radicals gone bad, and the glutathione connection. Diabetes 52, 581–587.

Robertson, R.P., Harmon, J., Tran, P.O.T., Poitout, V., 2004. β-Cell glucose toxicity, lipotoxicity, and chronic oxidative stress in type 2 diabetes. Diabetes 53, S119–S124.

Sahoo, S.K., Labhasetwar, V., 2003. Nanotech approaches to drug delivery and imaging. Drug Discov. Today 8, 1112–1120.

Samadikuchaksaraei, A., 2006. Stem cell therapy for acute myocardial infarction. Hellenic. J. Cardiol. 47, 100–111.

Sato, N., Meijer, L., Skaltsounis, L., Greengard, P., Brivanlou, A.H., 2003. Maintenance of pluripotency in human and mouse embryonic stem cells through activation of Wnt signaling by a pharmacological GSK-3-specific inhibitor. Nat. Med. 10, 55–63.

Seifu, D.G., Isimjan, T.T., Mequanint, K., 2011. Tissue engineering scaffolds containing embedded fluorinated-zeolite oxygen vectors. Acta Biomater. 7, 3670–3678.

Shapiro, A.J., Lakey, J.R., Ryan, E.A., Korbutt, G.S., Toth, E., Warnock, G.L., et al., 2000. Islet transplantation in seven patients with type 1 diabetes mellitus using a glucocorticoid-free immunosuppressive regimen. N. Engl. J. Med. 343, 230–238.

Shin, H., Jo, S., Mikos, A.G., 2003. Biomimetic materials for tissue engineering. Biomaterials 24, 4353–4364.

Siegel, R.W., Fougere, G.E., 1995. Mechanical properties of nanophase metals. Nanostruct. Mater. 6, 205–216.

Sinensky, M., Leiser, A., Babich, H., 1995. Oxidative stress aspects of the cytotoxicity of carbamide peroxide: *in vitro* studies. Toxicol. Lett. 75, 101–109.

Skarja, G., Woodhouse, K., 2001. *In vitro* degradation and erosion of degradable, segmented polyurethanes containing an amino acid-based chain extender. J. Biomater. Sci. Polym. Ed. 12, 851–873.

Snydman, D., 1999. Infection in solid organ transplantation. Transpl. Infect. Dis. 1, 21–28.

Soleymani, M., Moheb, A., Babakhani, D., 2011. Hydrogen peroxide decomposition over nanosized La1–xCaxMnO3 ($0 \leq X \leq 0.6$) perovskite oxides. Chem. Eng. Technol. 34, 49–55.

Strain, A.J., Neuberger, J.M., 2002. A bioartificial liver—state of the art. Science 295, 1005–1009.

Stupp, S.I., Ciegler, G.W., 2004. Organoapatites: materials for artificial bone. I. Synthesis and microstructure. J. Biomed. Mater. Res. 26, 169–183.

Stupp, S.I., Lebonheur, V., Walker, K., Li, L.S., Huggins, K.E., Keser, M., et al., 1997. Supramolecular materials: self-organized nanostructures. Science 276, 384–389.

Thomson, J.A., 2001. Embryonal carcinoma cells as embryonic stem cells. Stem Cell Biol. 40, 231.

Turner, R., Stratton, I., Horton, V., Manley, S., Zimmet, P., Mackay, I.R., et al., 1997. UKPDS 25: autoantibodies to islet-cell cytoplasm and glutamic acid decarboxylase for prediction of insulin requirement in type 2 diabetes. The Lancet 350, 1288–1293.

Uchegbu, I.F., 2006. Pharmaceutical nanotechnology: polymeric vesicles for drug and gene delivery. Expert. Opin. Drug Deliv. 350, 1288–1293.

Verge, C.F., Gianani, R., Kawasaki, E., Yu, L., Pietropaolo, M., Chase, H.P., et al., 1996. Prediction of type I diabetes in first-degree relatives using a combination of insulin, GAD, and ICA512bdc/IA-2 autoantibodies. Diabetes 45, 926–933.

Vijan, S., Hofer, T.P., Hayward, R.A., 1997. Estimated benefits of glycemic control in microvascular complications in type 2 diabetes. Ann. Intern. Med. 127, 788–795.

Waite, A.J., Bonner, J.S., Autenrieth, R., 1999. Kinetics and stoichiometry of oxygen release from solid peroxides. Environ. Eng. Sci. 16, 187–199.

Wang, G.L., Semenza, G.L., 1993. General involvement of hypoxia-inducible factor 1 in transcriptional response to hypoxia. Proc. Natl Acad. Sci. 90, 4304–4308.

Wang, X., Yang, L., Chen, Z.G., Shin, D.M., 2008. Application of nanotechnology in cancer therapy and imaging. CA Cancer J. Clin. 58, 97–110.

Wang, X., Liu, L.H., Ramström, O., Yan, M., 2009. Engineering nanomaterial surfaces for biomedical applications. Exp. Biol. Med. 234, 1128–1139.

Wang, J., Zhu, Y., Bawa, H.K., Ng, G., Wu, Y., et al., 2010. Oxygen-generating nanofiber cell scaffolds with antimicrobial properties. ACS Appl. Mater. Interfaces 3, 67–73.

Ward, C.L., Corona, B.T., Yoo, J.J., Harrison, B.S., Christ, G.J., 2013. Oxygen generating biomaterials preserve skeletal muscle homeostasis under hypoxic and ischemic conditions. PloS One 8, e72485.

Weber, L.M., Cheung, C.Y., Anseth, K.S., 2007a. Multifunctional pancreatic islet encapsulation barriers achieved via multilayer PEG hydrogels. Cell Transplant. 16, 1049–1057.

Weber, L.M., Hayda, K.N., Haskins, K., Anseth, K.S., 2007b. The effects of cell–matrix interactions on encapsulated β-cell function within hydrogels functionalized with matrix-derived adhesive peptides. Biomaterials 28, 3004–3011.

Weinzimer, S.A., Ahern, J.H., Doyle, E.A., Vincent, M.R., Dziura, J., Steffen, A.T., et al., 2004. Persistence of benefits of continuous subcutaneous insulin infusion in very young children with type 1 diabetes: a follow-up report. Pediatrics 114, 1601–1605.

Weissman, I.L., 2000. Stem cells: units of development, review units of regeneration, and units in evolution. Cell 100, 157–168.

White, D.M., Irvine, R.L., Woolard, C.R., 1998. The use of solid peroxides to stimulate growth of aerobic microbes in tundra. J. Hazard. Mater. 57, 71–78.

Willi, S.M., Planton, J., Egede, L., Schwarz, S., 2003. Benefits of continuous subcutaneous insulin infusion in children with type 1 diabetes. J. Pediatr. 143, 796–801.

Won, J.C., Rhee, B.D., Ko, K.S., 2009. Glucose-responsive gene expression system for gene therapy. Adv. Drug Deliv. Rev. 61, 633–640.

Wu, H., Avgoustiniatos, E.S., Swette, L., Bonner-Weir, S., Weir, G.C., Colton, C.K., 1999. *In situ* electrochemical oxygen generation with an immunoisolation device. Ann. N. Y. Acad. Sci. 875, 105–125.

Ye, Z., Mahato, R.I., 2008. Role of nanomedicines in cell-based therapeutics. Nanomedicine 3, 5.

Zhang, L., Webster, T.J., 2009. Nanotechnology and nanomaterials: promises for improved tissue regeneration. Nano Today 4, 66–80.

Zisch, A.H., Lutolf, M.P., Ehrbar, M., Raeber, G.P., Rizzi, S.C., Davies, N., et al., 2003. Cell-demanded release of VEGF from synthetic, biointeractive cell ingrowth matrices for vascularized tissue growth. FASEB J. 17, 2260–2262.

CHAPTER

Advances in the field of soft tissue engineering: from pure regenerative to integrative solutions

13

Denisa Ficai[1], Madalina Georgiana Albu[3], Maria Sonmez[2,3], Anton Ficai[4] and Ecaterina Andronescu[4]

[1]Department of Inorganic Chemistry, Faculty of Applied Chemistry and Materials Science, University Politehnica of Bucharest, Bucharest, Romania [2]University Politehnica of Bucharest, Bucharest, Romania [3]National Research & Development Institute for Textiles and Leather (INCDTP) – Leather and Footwear Research Institute, Bucharest, Romania [4]Department of Science and Engineering of Oxide Materials and Nanomaterials, Faculty of Applied Chemistry and Materials Science, University Politehnica of Bucharest, Bucharest, Romania

13.1 SOFT TISSUE ENGINEERING

Tissue engineering aims to replace or regenerate destroyed tissues as a result of various accidents or hereditary diseases. In order to help the regeneration of the injured tissue or to substitute damaged tissue and finally to repair the functionality of these tissues or organs, tissue engineering uses combinations of cells, bioactive factors, and supporting structures (Yang, 2011). For regeneration or tissue reconstruction, tissue engineering uses various materials (from monoliths to composite materials) with suitable biochemical and physiochemical properties in order to heal the damaged tissue. The most studied and used materials in soft tissue engineering are: chitosan and its derivatives, collagen, gelatin, polyvinyl alcohol (PVA), polycaprolactone (PCL), poly(lactic acid) and its derivatives, etc. as well as some of their combinations.

An ideal material used for fabricating tissue-engineered scaffolds is expected to provide structural and functional issues (Yang, 2011). Tissue/scaffolds can be applied both to soft and hard components of the body, the used materials being adapted function on the envisaged application. Soft tissues play a crucial functional role in the body. Based on this premise various studies on regeneration or reconstruction of various tissues such as liver (Feng et al., 2009), lung (Mondrinos et al., 2008), muscles (Beier et al., 2009), skin (Adekogbe and Ghanem, 2005), nerves (Amado et al., 2008), blood vessels (Zhang et al., 2006a), cornea (Rafat et al.,

Nanobiomaterials in Soft Tissue Engineering. DOI: http://dx.doi.org/10.1016/B978-0-323-42865-1.00013-1

Table 13.1 Applications of the Materials in Soft Tissue Engineering

Scaffold	Application—Effect	Reference
Chitosan–hyaluronan	Ligaments—cellular adhesion, cell proliferation, ECM and production	Funakoshi et al. (2005b)
Chitosan/gelatin	Skin—cell survival	Yang et al. (2010)
Chitosan/gelatin	Blood vessels—cell growth, cell migration	Zhang et al. (2006a)
Collagen, type I	Skin—wound healing	Kojima et al. (1998)
	Salivary gland—branching morphogenesis	Yang and Young (2008b)
	Ligament—cell proliferation	Funakoshi et al. (2005b)
	Vessel—cell phenotype	Funakoshi et al. (2005a)
	Tendon—cell ECM production	Zhu et al. (2009)
Collagen, type III	Skin—wound healing	Kojima et al. (1998)
	Glands—branching morphogenesis	Yang and Young (2008b)
	Ligaments—cell phenotypes	Shao et al. (2010)
Collagen, type IV	Skin—wound healing	Kojima et al. (1998)
Glycosaminoglycan	Vessel—cell phenotype	Zhu et al. (2009)

2008), heart valves (Schleicher et al., 2009), trachea (Yamashita et al., 2007), and adipose tissues (Wu et al., 2007) have been realized, worldwide. Various polymeric scaffolds (Arca and Şenel, 2008) have been investigated for soft tissue engineering, some of the most important are summarized in Table 13.1.

13.1.1 COLLAGEN

Collagen is a major extracellular matrix (ECM) protein, accounting for about 25% of total body protein—skin and bone (Tang et al., 2014; Vishwakarma et al., 2015; Feng et al., 2015). It has an active role in cell adhesion, differentiation, and migration owing to its specific recognition interaction with cells (Feng et al., 2015). Being biocompatible and having low immunogenicity, collagen scaffolds are considered to be ideal for tissue engineering.

In order to understand skin regeneration we have to understand 3D tissue organization and its biosynthesis from gene to tissue (Nath et al., 2004; Wood, 2014).

Collagen biosynthesis is a complex process which starts with gene transcription and ends with aggregation of fibrils in fibers—components of ECM (Koide and Nagata, 2005; Yamada et al., 1983; Sicari et al., 2015). The collagen biosynthesis starts in fibroblasts and takes place into two steps: intra- and extracellular, as shown in Figure 13.1 (Alberts et al., 1994).

Besides biosynthesis of globular protein, the procollagen is synthesized in lumen of the endoplasmic reticulum (Trandafir et al., 2007). Collagenic polypeptide chains (α-pro) are synthesized on ribosomes bonded on membrane, as

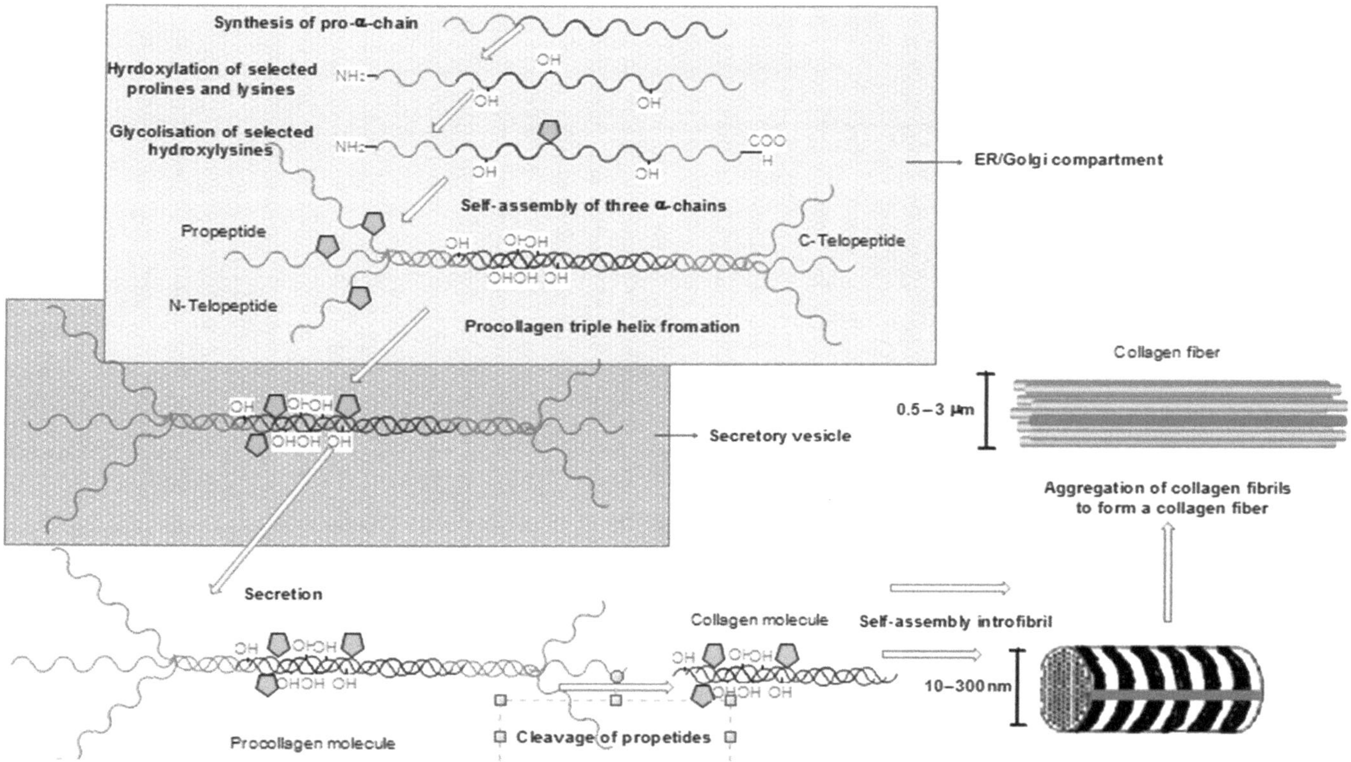

FIGURE 13.1

Intra- and extracellular steps involved in collagen biosynthesis (Alberts et al., 1994).

precursors. Thus, messenger ribonucleic acid (mRNA—a molecule with the role of copying genetic information of a DNA side chain) bonded on ribosome is translated at amino acids which have a signal sequence on the N-terminal of the peptide which interact with a signal recognition particle (SRP). The complex ribosome–mRNA–amino acid–SRP is sent into the RE lumen. These precursors contain not only short peptide signal amino-terminals requested for direct newly formed peptide to RE, but also additional amino acids with amino and carboxyl endings.

The remaining proline and lysine are hydroxylated in RE lumen forming hydroxyproline and hydroxylysine. Prolil–hydroxylase and lysil–hydroxylase are specific enzymes responsible for these changes. A part of hydroxylysine rests are glycosylated with galactosyltransferase, respectively glucosyltransferase. Each glycosylated α-pro chain will then combine with two others by hydrogen bonding and form a triple helical molecule known as a procollagen.

The formed procollagen molecule is then transported in the Golgi apparatus and secreted out of the cell for extracellular processing and fibril formation. Procollagenic aggregates are secreted in extracellular space, where N- and C-terminal propeptides of procollagen are cleaved by specific proteolytical enzymes, obtaining insoluble collagen molecules in physiological conditions. After propeptide cleaving, collagen molecules are self-assembled in fibrillar suprastructures (von der Mark, 1981) forming quarter-staggered arrangements by hydrophobic and electrostatic iterations, leading to microfibrils and then long fibrils (Batemann et al., 1996; Veis and Payne, 1988; Silver et al., 1992). This forms specific quaternary superstructures, depending on connective tissue: in tendons, for example, type I collagen fibrils are arranged parallel and form fibers, meanwhile in skin the orientation is similar, with a complex network of plain fibrils (Rossert and Crombrugghe, 2002). Moreover, molecular arrangement in fibrils is stabilized by formation of covalent intermolecular bonding, which finally contributes to the mechanical resistance of connective tissue (Simon et al., 2008).

Collagen fibrils are consolidated and stabilized by intra- and intermolecular crosslinking.

Collagen, as such or in association with other molecules of ECM, has an important role in physiology and behavior of cells in connective tissues (Iordăchescu and Stan, 2004). The keratocytes and fibroblasts are key cells involved in skin lesion healing. Thus, collagen is used as scaffolds for adherence, migration, growth, and differentiation of cells in normal conditions.

The interaction between collagen and blood platelets plays an important role in the mechanism of hemostat induction. The platelets adhere to the collagen surface and their adhesion and aggregation activates coagulation and hemostasis starts.

The interactions between collagen and cells are important phenomena in the process of lesion healing and remodeling of adult tissues, with collagen inducing differentiation and maintaining unchanged cell phenotype (Sassi et al., 2000; Kleimann et al., 1981). These collagen–cell interactions are important in tissue engineering of connective tissue as well as in the investigation of *in vivo* cell behavior (Miyata and Taira, 1992).

13.1.2 CHITOSAN

Chitosan [poly-(β-1/4)-2-amino-2-deoxy-D-glucopyranose] is the most abundant natural polymer, except cellulose, and is found in the shells of crustaceans and walls of fungi (Wang et al., 2005; Feng et al., 2009; Senel and McClure, 2004; Yang et al., 2009). Chitosan is a copolymer that can be obtained through alkaline deacetylation of chitin, where D-glucosamine and *N*-acetyl-D-glucosamine coexist, glucosamine being the predominant repeating unit of the structure.

13.1.2.1 Structure–proprieties relationship

The presence of the OH group on the chitosan structure differentiates it from chitin. The $3NH_2$ and 3OH groups give many special properties to chitosan, making it useful in many areas and easily available for chemical reactions. Chitosan is safe, non-toxic and can interact with polyanions to form complexes and gels (Agnihotri et al., 2004; Sunil et al., 2013; Se and Niranjan, 2005).

Chitosan with protonated amino groups can interact with a variety of natural or synthetic anionic species (Madihally and Matthew, 1999; Croisier and Jerome, 2013) such as lipids, proteins, DNA, and some negatively charge polymers like poly(acrylic acid), poly(lactic acid) (Madihally and Matthew, 1999; Aranaz et al., 2010; Pavinatto et al., 2010; Takahashi et al., 1990; Kim et al., 2007).

Through the $3NH_2$ and 3OH groups, chitosan can form stable covalent bondings with other species by etherification and esterification reactions (Rinaudo, 2006). The amino group of D-glucosamine residues may react with aldehyde functions under mild conditions through reductive amination (Rinaudo, 2006). By this technique, various functional groups can be linked onto the chitosan backbone in order to further extend the field of application of chitosan.

According to the literature the degree of deacetylation (DD) represents the proportion of D-glucosamine units reported to the total number of units indicating the free amine groups along the chitosan backbone. The difference between chitin and chitosan depends on the value of the DD. Chitin with a DD of up to 65–70% or above is generally known as chitosan. The molecular weight of chitosan may range between 10,000 and 2,000,000 Da (Senel and McClure, 2004; Seo et al., 2006). Also, the DD changes the physicochemical properties, such as chain conformation, solubility, mechanical, and electrostatic properties (Seo et al., 2006; Lin et al., 2007b; Kim et al., 2008).

Thein-Han et al. showed that 95% deacetylated chitosan showed better mechanical property than 88% deacetylated chitosan due to good nerve affinity of the polymer (Jiankang et al., 2009) to chitosan of similar molecular weight. They also showed that the cytocompatibility and morphology were similar for different deacetylated chitosans (Thein-Han and Kitiyanant, 2007).

For the construction of artificial skin tissue, chitosan with different deacetylation degrees (Adekogbe and Ghanem, 2005) was considered. Adekogbe and Ghanem observed that no significant differences in the proliferation rate of the fibroblasts in contrast with the mechanical properties which were changed significantly. It was also observed that with increasing degrees of acetylation and quantity acetylation agent (dimethyl 3-3,dithio-bispropionimidate [DTBP]), the tensile strength and elastic modulus were increased (Adekogbe and Ghanem, 2005). Although chitosan is a promising scaffold material, it has still some limitations. Zhao et al. have shown a lack of long-term stability (Zhao et al., 2009). Wang et al. reported that the degradation products of chitosan can significantly change the angiogenic behavior of endothelial cells at cellular and molecular levels (Wang et al., 2008). Chen et al. reported that chitosan has poor solubility (Chen et al., 2005), and the mechanical strength of chitosan scaffolds needs to be improved. In order to achieve the mechanical properties of chitosan scaffolds or tissue, chitosan blended with various bioceramics, such as hydroxyapatite (Nie and Wang, 2007; Malafaya and Reis, 2009; Thein-Han and Misra, 2009; Li et al., 2009), or calcium phosphate (Martins et al., 2009); or biomaterials like gelatin (Jiankang et al., 2009; Zhang et al., 2006b), collagen (Rafat et al., 2008; Chen et al., 2005), alginate (Zhao and Chang, 2004), or inorganic material such as wollastonite (Adekogbe and Ghanem, 2005; Cao et al., 2008) can be used. Also, chitosan is blended with other biomaterials to create scaffolds that are more appropriate for directing the desired cell behaviors.

13.1.2.2 Applications of chitosan in tissue engineering

At tissue level, chitosan has proved to be a promoter of regeneration of dermal tissues and an accelerator of healing, which formed the basis of studies that have used chitosan for simple bandages to matrix-type artificial leather (Esmaeili et al., 2010). Esmaeili et al. proved that the tissue regeneration properties of chitosan can be improved by incorporation of basic fibroblast growth factor (bFGF), resulting in chitosan-based films, chitosan–alginate, or sulfonamides (sulfadiazine), or copolymers of chitosan and glycosaminoglycans (hyaluronic acid, chondroitin sulfate, dermatan sulfate, heparin).

Chitosan can be easily processed and manufactured in a variety of forms including fibers, films, sponges, and hydrogels. This wide range of forms makes this polymer a principal candidate for tissue repair and regeneration (Vázquez et al., 2015).

Also, chitosan provides the ability to mimic the shape of the damaged tissue. Moreover, the chemical structure of chitosan and its derivatives offers the possibility of being chemically modified in order to adapt structurally and functionally to the host tissue, due to its previously described properties that allow for the ability to regenerate primary tissue cells and even stem cells (Kim et al., 2008; Kumar, 2000; Dang and Leong, 2006; Muzzarelli, 2009).

Mei et al. (2012) synthesized a series of chitosan/silica particle (SiO_2) membranes and showed that the membranes demonstrated no cytotoxicity against

L-929 cells after 24 h of culture. In addition, the macroporous membrane exhibited excellent cellular adhesion and proliferation after 24 and 48 h of culturing, which is why the developed scaffold might be adequate for skin tissue engineering (Mei et al., 2012).

Gobin et al. used chitosan in repair and regeneration of the abdominal wall in ventral hernias. They investigated the feasibility of using silk fibroin and chitosan blend scaffolds for ventral hernia repair in guinea pigs due to the properties that chitosan has shown in reduction and prevention of postoperative intraperitoneal adhesion (Gobin et al., 2006). They compared the blended scaffold with a biodegradable human acellular dermal matrix and a non-biodegradable polypropylene mesh. The study showed that the silk fibroin and chitosan blend scaffold present good tissue remodeling ability in all three dimensions, with seamless integration at the interface with adjacent native tissue, the mechanical strength of the silk fibroin and chitosan blend scaffold was similar to that of the native abdominal wall, the scaffold promoted the deposition of new ECM, uniform vascularization, and cellular infiltration in the repair sites, which contributed to the increase in mechanical strength of the regenerated tissue. Thus, this scaffold is potentially useful in reconstruction and regeneration of the abdominal wall (Gobin et al., 2006). Based on these studies, simple collagen or blended with various compounds can be used in ventral hernia and in inguinal hernia repair and other types of herniation, and in the repair of certain congenital defects such as omphalocele or gastroschisis, although to date there are still no studies to prove its effectiveness in the treatment of these types of defects in the human (Vázquez et al., 2015).

Zakhem et al. (2012) used chitosan as a biomaterial in intestinal tissue engineering applications. They showed that the use of aligned smooth muscle constructs is beneficial to the restoration of intestinal motility and elimination of the intestinal content. They investigated the biocompatibility of chitosan by growing rabbit colonic circular smooth muscle cells on chitosan-coated plates. They showed that the cells maintained their spindle-like morphology and preserved their smooth muscle phenotypic markers. The muscle constructs contracted in response to acetylcholine and potassium chloride and they relaxed in response to vasoactive intestinal peptide (VIP). The evidence of functionality of the smooth muscle constructs, after being placed around the composite chitosan scaffold, suggests the potential use of this biomaterial to produce a functional tissue (Zakhem et al., 2012).

Inas and Kawkab (2012) studied the effect of chitosan powder on the stimulation of healing of full-thickness skin wounds. For this reason, 12 apparently healthy male dogs of nearly the same age and weight were considered. Full-thickness, equal longitudinal skin incision wounds were created on each dog's dorsal side. A comparative study was done between wounds treated with chitosan powder and control wounds washed only in saline solution. The results have shown rapid regeneration and re-epithelialization of the wounds treated with chitosan powder compared with those treated with saline solution. From a clinical point of view, complete healing was achieved for the wounds treated with the chitosan after 3 weeks, compared with 7 weeks for the wounds treated with saline solution.

Also, complete regeneration of epidermal cells with the keratin layer occurred, which was similar to the normal skin associated with dermal connective tissue proliferation and the fibroblast cells laid down a network of collagen fibers, which appeared as wavy collagen bundles surrounding the neovasculature of the wounds, whereas, in the control group, hyalinosis of subcutaneous granulation tissue and haphazardly arranged collagen fibers were observed (Inas and Kawkab, 2012).

The good nerve affinity to the chitosan for different cell types like neutral stem cells (Wang et al., 2006a), PC-12 cells (Pfister et al., 2008), neuro-2a neuroblastoma cells (Qiang et al., 2005), or N1E-115 cells, derived from mouse neuroblastoma C-1300 (Amado et al., 2008), makes this polymer a potential candidate material for nerve tissue engineering (Haipeng et al., 2000).

Lyophilized chitosan-derived oligosaccharide has exhibit good cell attachment and proliferation, and promotes PC-12 cell differentiation to a neuron-like morphology and neurite outgrowth (Yang et al., 2009). Similarly, freeze-dried chitosan γ-glycidoxypropyltrimethoxysilane exhibit significant improvement of post-traumatic regrowth and functional recovery against N1E-115 cells (Amado et al., 2008).

13.1.2.3 Preparation of chitosan

Chitosan is a promising scaffold material that has been obtained in different ways (Wang et al., 2005; Gao et al., 2008; Alves da Silva et al., 2010). The most commonly used processing routes for chitosan-based scaffolds for soft tissue engineering are lyophilization, drying by heat, reverse micellar method, electrospinning, and ionic gelation methods (Arca and Şenel, 2008).

13.1.2.3.1 Ionic crosslinking methods

Chitosan nanoparticles can be prepared by ionic crosslinking methods. This method consists of ionic crosslinking through self-assembly of chitosan or chitosan derivatives and oppositely charged macromolecules or by addition of a low-molecular-weight anionic crosslinker, such as tripolyphosphate (TPP), sodium sulfate, or cyclodextrin (CD) (Amidi et al., 2010). Due to its excellent properties and its ability to form gels through ionic interactions in the presence of different agents, TPP has often been used to prepare chitosan nanoparticles. The ionic interaction can be controlled by the charge density of TPP and chitosan, which is dependent on the pH of the solution (Nasti et al., 2009). Nasti et al. (2009) studied the influence of pH, concentration, ratios of components, and method of mixing, on the preparation of chitosan/TPP nanoparticles, while Lin et al. (2007a) studied the relationship between free amino groups on the surface and the characteristics of chitosan nanoparticles prepared by the ionic gelation method.

The complexation between chitosan-based polymers and oppositely charged macromolecules can be used in order to prepare micro/nanoparticles suitable for drug delivery.

13.1.2.3.2 Electrospinning methods

Electrospinning methods are used to obtain chitosan nanofibers. Electrospinning is influenced by several parameters, such as the viscosity, the operating voltage, the temperature, the pressure, and the flow rate. Viscosity is a key parameter in electrospinning because it is related to the extent that the polymer molecule chain is entangled within the solution (Ramakrishna et al., 2005).

Ohkawa et al. successfully prepared an electrospun non-woven fabric of chitosan (Ohkawa et al., 2004). They studied the effects of the electrospinning solvent and the chitosan concentration on the morphology of the resulting non-woven fabrics. They demonstrated that trifluoroacetic acid (TFA) was the most successful solvent because the amino group moieties of chitosan form salts with TFA (Hasegawa et al., 1992), which can effectively destroy the rigid interactions between the chitosan molecules. As the chitosan concentration was increased, the morphology of the deposition on the collector changed from spherical beads to interconnected fibrous networks.

Torres-Giner et al. (2008) developed electrospun chitosan nanofibers using TFA and dichloromethane as solvent. In addition, they developed porous electrospun chitosan nanofibers using pure trichloromethane as solvent. Geng et al. (2005) reported the manufacture of chitosan nanofibers in concentrated aqueous acetic acid solutions by varying acetic acid concentration.

Nanofibers were also produced by electrospinning of chitin solutions using 1,1,1,3,3,3-hexafluoro-2-propanol (HFIP) as the spinning solvent (Min et al., 2004).

13.1.2.3.3 Reverse micellar method

Using a reverse micellar route, ultrafine polymeric nanoparticles can be prepared (Zhao et al., 2011). Brunel et al., 2009 used the reverse micellar method in order to prepare chitosan nanoparticles.

Mansouri et al. (2010) prepared bovine serum albumin (BSA)-loaded chitosan nanoparticles with size in the range of 143–428 nm, using the reverse micellar method. This method can be used for encapsulation of BSA into the chitosan nanoparticles. They showed that by increasing the chitosan solution concentration, the release of BSA decreases, regardless of BSA loading (10% and 20%).

13.1.2.3.4 Lyophilization

The most commonly used method is lyophilization based on freeze-evaporation of the solvent from previously frozen chitosan solution. In function of the process conditions (especially concentration), the production of materials with controlled porosity and specific pore size was reported. By adding additives to systems such as PCL, PVA, or using fillers such as calcium- and phosphate-based compounds the properties and applications can also be modified from soft to hard tissue engineering. Fillers based on calcium and phosphate are designed to stimulate the process of osteogenesis (Mucha et al., 2012), these materials being designed for bone tissue engineering.

13.1.3 OTHER POLYMERS

Chitin is the second most abundant natural polymer after chitosan. Chitin is commonly found in the exoskeletons of crustacean, insects, and the cell walls of fungi. Most chitin applications are based on its deacetylated form, chitosan.

Chitin-based materials have been widely used in the biomedical field due to the good biocompatibility and approval for human use (Yang, 2011). Chitin-based materials can be prepared into various forms of tissue, including hydrogels, microcapsules, membranous films, sponges, tubes, and a variety of three-dimensional porous structures (Jiang et al., 2008; Berger et al., 2004). Over other materials, chitin-based materials have been widely used for injured skin regeneration or reconstruction, due to the special properties such as the promotion of cell infiltration, ECM production, antimicrobial properties, and maintenance of homeostasis (Ueno et al., 1999; Cho et al., 1999; Jayakumar et al., 2011). In addition, chitin-based biomaterials have demonstrated superior capacity in tissue adhesion and gas permeability, which helps to improve wound healing.

13.1.4 GELATIN

Gelatin is a mixture of water-soluble protein fragments, comprised of the same amino acid sequences as collagen, from which it is derived. Collagen differs from gelatin in that it contains far more tertiary structures, leading to lower aqueous solubility (Coppoolse et al., 2014).

This is a natural protein present in the tendons, ligaments, and other tissues of mammalians. It is produced by boiling the connective tissues, bones, and skins of animals, usually cows and pigs. Gelatin's ability to form strong, transparent gels and flexible films that are easily digested and soluble in hot water make it a valuable material for food processing, pharmaceuticals, photography, and paper production.

Gelatin is used successfully in the pharmaceutical industry, as a soft or hard capsule for drugs, in surgical applications such as wound dressings, surgical sponges, sealants, and glues, as a coating on cell culture plates for the culture of endothelial cells, muscle cells, and embryonic stem cells, and as a scaffold for tissue engineering applications (as a component in bone composite materials, articular cartilage and as guiding conduits for nerve regeneration) (Maleknia and Majdi, 2014; Audoly, 2006; Boran, 2013).

13.1.5 HYALURONAN

Hyaluronan is a polysaccharide with a high density of negative charge (favorable for water retention) and the ability to act as a binding site for molecules, making it an attractive biomaterial for drug delivery and tissue engineering (Toole, 1990; Allison and Grande-Allen, 2006; Luo et al., 2000). Due to these proprieties, Shu et al. synthesized a gelatin–hyaluronan composite by incorporation of thiol functional groups into both gelatin and hyaluronan scaffolds to allow the crosslinking (Shu et al., 2003). Incorporation of gelatin into hyaluronan scaffolds increases the seeded cell proliferation in a dose-dependent fashion (Shu et al., 2003).

Peattie et al. have incorporated thiolated heparin into the gelatin–hyaluronan matrix (Peattie et al., 2008) in order to facilitate the controlled delivery of growth factors from these composite hydrogels. These scaffolds were successful in delivering a wide variety of growth factors over at least 2 weeks, and the incorporation of gelatin increased the drug delivery rate.

13.1.6 SILK

Silk is a protein-based polymer produced by insects and spiders, which has been studied in tissue engineering as a lightweight, tough biomaterial (Wang et al., 2006b). In tissue engineering, silk has been used to reinforce gelatin scaffolds, resulting in greater tensile and bending strength (Shubhra et al., 2011). Mandal et al. synthesized gelatin–silk composites that can be loaded with water-soluble drug and fabricated in stackable layers (Mandal et al., 2009) in order to release drugs for at least 25 days.

13.1.6.1 Drug delivery systems

Drug delivery systems were found to be very effective in many industrial and medical applications. Certainly, the medical applications are the most important.

13.1.6.2 DDS designed for faster skin regeneration

Living bodies have the capability to heal minor defects in reasonable time, regardless of the nature of the tissue (hard or soft tissue). If the defect is larger than a critical size, the intervention of a medical doctor is strongly recommended due to the many associated risks, the main risks being infections. Faster skin regeneration can be easily achieved by the addition of proper ternary components. Faster regeneration is usually achieved by using growth factors and other molecules as well as stem cells (Dreifke et al., 2015; Xie et al., 2013). The healing rate is dependent on many factors including composition and morphology of the support materials as well as the concentration and delivery rate of these factors.

Xie et al. developed a new dual growth factor releasing multifunctional nanofiber system for wound healing based on chitosan and poly(ethylene oxide) with different mixing ratio, as well as PLGA nanoparticle-loaded CS/PEO nanofibers further loaded with VEGF (vascular endothelial growth factor) and PDGF-BB (platelet-derived growth factor-BB) (Xie et al., 2013). Electrospinning was used in order to mimic as much as possible the ECM. The growth factors were used because during all (superposing) phases of healing (initial inflammation, tissue regeneration to fill the wound bed and tissue remodeling to regain skin functionalities), many cytokines and growth factors are produced and assist the healing. Based on this experiment, Xie et al. demonstrated that the dual growth factor releasing multifunctional nanofiber system led to faster wound healing from both an angiogenesis and a re-epithelialization point of view, while the granulation of new tissue is close to normal.

Kobsa et al. developed multifunctional systems capable of faster regeneration, especially due to the controlled delivery of bioactive substances, like nucleic acid (Kobsa et al., 2013). For this purpose, a dual-component polymer system (poly[L-lactide] [PLA] and polycaprolactone [PCL]) was obtained by electrospinning; the as-prepared system being chosen because is well known from the literature, is non-toxic, can be easily obtained, and offers good mechanical properties. As active components, these electrospun fibers were loaded with keratinocyte growth factor (KGF). The as-obtained engineered PLA/PCL scaffolds loaded with KGF proved to be highly efficient in DNA delivery and the *in vivo* tests reveal that, based on re-epithelialization, keratinocyte proliferation, and granulation response, these materials are promising for the treatment of skin wounds.

A relatively new trend in the field of electrospun fibers (core–shell nanofibers) is the synthesis of core–shell structures (Ficai et al., 2015). Two strategies of loading are used for these systems. The easiest way is for the active components to be dispersed/dissolved into the polymer solution (either inner or outer polymer layer) and then electrospun to assure the desired characteristics. The second way is to absorb the desired components from solutions. Both synthesis routes have advantages and disadvantages and are strongly dependent on the stability of the active component in the polymer solutions. Jin et al. developed core–shell nanofibers loaded with multiple epidermal induction factors for skin regeneration (Jin et al., 2013). As epidermal induction factors they used epidermal growth factor (EGF), insulin, hydrocortisone, and retinoic acid (RA), while as support they used gelatin and poly(L-lactic acid)-*co*-poly-(ε-caprolactone). The properties of the as-obtained systems are strongly dependent on morphology and consequently the influence of the morphology was studied by the authors (the morphologies of the two structures are presented in Figure 13.2). Based on

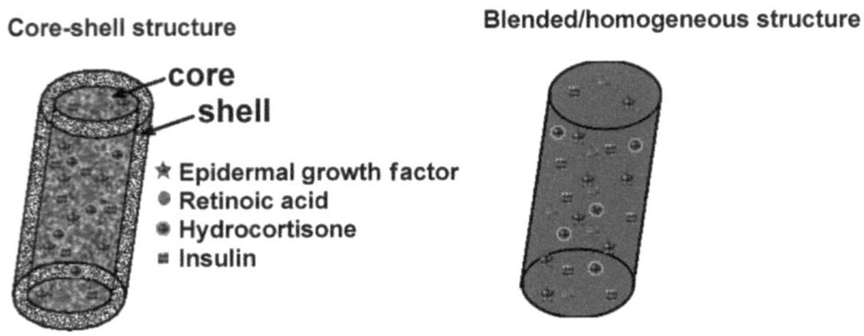

FIGURE 13.2

Characteristics of core–shell versus blended electrospun fibers.

this study, the delivery rate of these epidermal induction factors (as cumulative release, %) was strongly dependent on the morphology. In the case of core–shell structure, the delivery was sustained, even in the first few days (8.3% in the first 3 days and 50.9% after 14 days) while, in the case of the homogeneous structure, a burst release occurs during the first 3–6 days followed by sustained release for the next 8 days (44.9% in the first 3 days and 77.8% after 14 days). The long-term delivery could be further exploited and could reduce the frequency of changing the wound-dressing materials obtained via the core–shell route. A general conclusion of this study is related to the "new opportunities for transplantation of wound-healing mediators containing nanofibrous scaffolds as skin graft for skin tissue engineering."

13.1.6.3 DDS designed for the treatment of skin infections

The treatment protocols are strongly dependent on the health status of the patient. When no infections are identified, the wound dressing should not contain anti-infectious agents if the patient is exposed to limited or no risk of infections. If the risks of infections are high (for instance, unhygienic conditions, contact with outbreaks of infection, etc.) the treatment protocols must involve the use of anti-infective agents. The administration route should be either systemic or locoregional. The locoregional administration route is strongly recommended because systemic toxicity is avoided. In most skin injuries, locoregional administration of anti-infective agents is possible and brings advantages against the systemic route. If no open wound is present, the main limitation of the topical administration is skin permeability, which can strongly differ compared with the permeability of healthy skin.

Antibiotics play a very important role in the fight against microbes, in both preventive and eradication steps (Friberg and Bodin, 2013). It is well known that, over 2 billion years microbes were able to live and evolve on the earth without any obstacles. A crucial turn happened in the twentieth century, with the discovery of antibiotics. Since then, the use of antibiotics has been extremely useful in the treatment of many infections but, about 50 years ago, methicillin-resistant *Staphylococcus aureus* (MRSA) was first reported (Moellering, 2012). This event radically changed the general approaches related to antibiotics. To overcome the resistance of micro-organisms against antibiotics, the available solutions are to develop new antibiotics and especially to rationalize their use. The use of antibiotic delivery systems is of great importance because they can reduce the amount of antibiotics, thus limiting the systemic side effects and decreasing the amount of administered drug because of the better, locoregional administration route. Many antibiotic delivery systems were developed for various applications from skin delivery (Mori et al., 2014a, 2014b) to bone (Noel et al., 2010; Ordikhani and Simchi, 2014); gastric (Nogueira et al., 2013), pulmonary (Patil et al., 2015; Mehanna et al., 2014), or even to the brain (Ong et al., 2014).

At the soft tissue level, many drug delivery systems were developed because skin is an important barrier against microbial invasion. For this purpose, many antibiotic delivery wound dressings were developed and tested. For instance, Almeida et al. proved that collagen vascular graft implants loaded with gentamicin sulfate reduce surgical site infection in vascular surgery (Almeida et al., 2014) because the controlled delivery of the antibiotic is efficient and it acts locally at the most exposed site. Based on their results, the incidence of the infections associated with the surgical intervention decrease from about 20% to 0% when gentamicin-loaded collagen implants are used compared with pure collagen implants.

The same results were reported by Gomez et al., 1999 who highlighted that gentamicin-loaded collagen sponge reduces the infection risks in the treatment of "dirty" abdominal wounds. For this reason, 73 patients were randomized into two groups, the first group (32 patients) a control group with open wounds, was treated, with local cleansing, metronidazole (administered only on day 4, from 20 to 40 mg/kg) and gentamicin, while the second group (34 patients), was treated with primary closure with a collagen–gentamicin implant and metronidazole (administered only on day 4, from 20 to 40 mg/kg). In both groups, a similar number of patients with acute appendicitis, colon perforation, and gallbladder perforation were selected. Based on these results, polymicrobial infections were observed predominantly in the first group—14 patients comparing with only three from the second group, which means that a gentamicin-loaded collagen implant is effective and well tolerated in the treatment of "dirty" surgical abdominal wounds. Also important to mention is that 21 patients from the second group and only six from the first group were healed within 7 days.

Zhang et al. developed carboxyl-modified PVA-crosslinked chitosan hydrogel films for wound-dressing application. The synthesis of the crosslinked network occurs due to the intermolecular dehydration of the amino groups of CS and the carboxyl groups of COOH-PVA. The as-obtained films proved to be strong enough for the wound-dressing applications, with a higher swelling ratio compared with pure components (65–87%) being able to absorb a high content of liquid and thus the replacement frequency may be reduced while the water vapor and oxygen permeability are suitable for use on skin. In order to increase the native antimicrobial activity of the pure CS, these systems were loaded with gentamicin sulfate. The delivery efficiency was compared with pure CS or PVA/CS and the authors concluded that better delivery occurs for the COOH-PVA/CS systems. Based on the 48-h delivery study, less than 60% was released for the CS and PVA/CS samples while in the case of PVA-COOH/CS up to 87% was released. It is also important to mention that almost 25% of gentamicin was released in the first 2 h, which assure early protection after applying the wound dressing. The antimicrobial activity was studied against *Staphylococcus aureus* and *Escherichia coli* and proves that these films suppress the bacterial proliferation at 6, 12, and 24 h after incubation.

Besides the benefits of the antibiotic-loaded DDS the risk of resistance development led to special attention to the opportunity of using alternative ways instead of the antibiotic-loaded DDS. In this context, many alternative anti-infectious agents were tested for their efficiency in the prevention or eradication of infections. Many nanoparticles were proved to be effective in infection prevention or eradication, of these, by far the most studied were silver, zinc oxide, titanium dioxide, and copper nanoparticles (Sahin et al., 2014; Oprea et al., 2014; Nedelcu et al., 2014; Ficai et al., 2014; Spoiala et al., 2013; Guran et al., 2013; Das et al., 2014; Ren et al., 2009; Udayabhanu et al., 2015; Othman et al., 2014; Reddy et al., 2014; Cheng et al., 2014; Palza, 2015). Starting from these nanoparticles. different antimicrobial systems were developed for medical, environmental, or many industrial applications. The mechanism of action differs very much comparing with antibiotics and consequently these nanoparticles can be effective even on MRSA (Diez-Pascual and Diez-Vicente, 2014). Two major antimicrobial mechanisms can be identified based on metal reduction potential and metal donor atom selectivity (Palza, 2015). Table 13.2 presents the best-known metal-support pairs and its potential main applications in anti-infective applications.

In the field of soft tissue engineering, chitosan, collagen, alginate, and poly (lactic acid) are extensively used, as purely regenerative, as well as curative, drug delivery systems.

Silver nanoparticles can be used in many anti-infective applications because they are active against over 650 pathogens, including MRSA (when antibiotics are no more effective), have low systemic toxicity, and even good anti-inflammatory properties (Cortivo et al., 2010). Silver nanoparticles are extensively used in many applications from medical to industrial and environmental applications. This general trend is also happening in the field of tissue engineering. The use of silver nanoparticles induces antimicrobial activity and affords more protection to wounds against infection. Many silver-based materials were obtained and tested as wound-dressing materials, perhaps collagen, chitosan, and chitin-based materials are the most important (Madhumathi et al., 2010; Patrascu et al., 2015). The anti-infective activity of the silver nanoparticles is size- and shape-dependent, so the role of nanotechnology is essential in providing nanoparticles with good properties.

Poly(L-lactic acid) and its derivatives are extensively used in biomedical applications as grafting materials or drug delivery systems. Pantani et al., 2013 obtained PLA–ZnO nanocomposite films and tested their antimicrobial properties as well as water vapor barrier, two characteristic properties for food package materials but also for wound dressings. An extensive research paper was recently published also on a novel antibacterial electrospun mat based on poly(D,L-lactide) nanofibers and zinc oxide nanoparticles, these materials being potential candidates for many applications, including wound dressings (Rodriguez-Tobias et al., 2014). Four types of mats were obtained, as presented in Table 13.3. It can be seen that the presence of 3–5 wt.% of ZnO leads to improved mechanical properties but also improved antimicrobial activity. The addition of 5% ZnO compared with the sample with only 3% brings only marginal improvement.

Zinc oxide–silver nanoparticles stabilized by cellulose nanocrystals as filler in PVA/chitosan matrix were also obtained and tested for medical applications

Table 13.2 Various Blending Capabilities and Resulting Applications

Chitosan Combination	Scaffold Obtained	Applications
Chitosan alone	Tubes	Nerve (Tanaka et al., 2015; Vázquez et al., 2015)
Chitosan alone	Viscous solution and a monolayer rigid physical hydrogel	Skin (Boucard et al., 2007; Vázquez et al., 2015)
Chitosan alone	Membrane embryos	Salivary gland (Yang and Young, 2008a; Vázquez et al., 2015)
Collagen–chitosan + fibrin glue	Asymmetric porous	Skin (Han et al., 2010; Vázquez et al., 2015)
Chitosan + calcium phosphate	Cement chitosan microspheres	Bone (Meng et al., 2015; Vázquez et al., 2015)
Chitosan + layer of chitosan/gelatin	Sandwich tubular scaffold	Blood vessel (Zhang et al., 2006a; Vázquez et al., 2015)
Chitosan + aloe vera	Blended membrane, bovine	Skin (Silva et al., 2013; Vázquez et al., 2015)
Collagen alone	Cell attachment, proliferation Preadipocytes	Adipocyte (Wu et al., 2007; Arca and Şenel, 2008)
Hydroxypropyl CS/gelatin/chondroitin sulfate	Monolayer formation, similar cell adhesion and growth, significantly lower cytosolic enzyme release, rabbit corneal epithelial cells	Corneal tissue engineering (Gao et al., 2008; Arca and Şenel, 2008)
CS/gelatin	Good biocompatibility, allowed cell attachment formation of large colonies in hepatic chambers on hepatocyte cells	Liver tissue engineering (Jiankang et al., 2009; Arca and Şenel, 2008)
Titania/CS	No significant difference in liver-specific functions, long-term capability of metabolic activity Cell attachment: 81.2% HL-7702 cells	Liver tissue engineering (Zhao et al., 2009; Arca and Şenel, 2008)
Silk fibroin/chitosan	Significantly higher cell viability and attachment on hepatocyte cells	Liver tissue engineering (She et al., 2009; Arca and Şenel, 2008)

(Azizi et al., 2014). This complex system is interesting because both mechanical and antimicrobial activities are improved (Coppoolse et al., 2014). The improved antimicrobial activity is assured by the three antimicrobial components (chitosan, Ag, and ZnO) while the mechanical properties are obtained due to special

Table 13.3 Characteristics and Properties of Antimicrobial Electrospun Mats Based on Poly(D,L-lactide)/ZnO (Rodriguez-Tobias et al., 2014)

	Porosity (%)		Pore Size Based on Hg Porosity (μm)		Mechanical Properties		Antibacterial Activity	
ZnO Content (wt.%)	a	SEM	Average size	Range	Tensile Strength (N)	Young's Modulus (MPa)	*E. coli* (CFU/ml)	*S. aureus* (CFU/ml)
0	50	54	44	7–250	7.1 ± 0.5	13.9 ± 1.0	2.60×10^6	1.70×10^6
1	49	57	51	7–250	5.3 ± 0.3	11.5 ± 0.2	2.65×10^6	0.20×10^6
3	59	58	42	6–230	17.9 ± 1.4	37.9 ± 5.4	1.20×10^6	0.15×10^6
5	55	61	46	8–240	11.4 ± 1.1	31.6 ± 1.8	1.70×10^6	0.10×10^6

[a]*Based on mercury intrusion porosimetry measurements.*

reinforcing with cellulose nanocrystals. When the content of the reinforcing agent content increase from 0 to 5 wt.%, the tensile yield strength and Young's modulus increased from 0.055 to 0.205 GPa, representing a ~272% enhancement, and the tensile modulus increased from 0.395 to 1.2 GPa, indicating a ~203% increase. These changes suggest that the incorporation of the filler into the PVA–CS matrix restricts the relative motion of the fibers related to the matrix, promoting rigidity as a consequence of the strong interactions between the filler and the matrix. The antimicrobial activity gradually increased from 4.6 to 5.8, 7.1, and finally to 8.3 mm in the case of the *S. aureus* and from 3.7 to 4.1, 5.6, and finally to 6.0 mm in the case of *S. choleraesuis* after increasing the ZnO content from 1.0 to 3.0, 5.0, and finally 7.0%. Based also on other works, the CS/Ag/ZnO materials can be interesting also for their increased photocatalytic activity compared to pure ZnO (Simonescu et al., 2014).

Copper and copper oxide exhibit good antimicrobial activity and consequently can be used for antimicrobial applications (Haider et al., 2015; Gouda and Hebeish, 2010). Fibrillar materials are also attractive for wound dressings due to the relative high surface–volume ratio as well as due to the better biocompatibility induced by the fibrillar morphology. PLGA/CuO hybrid nanofiber scaffolds with a content of 0.5% CuO were obtained by an electrospinning method from THF-DMF 1:3 solvent, the PLGA content of the solution being 5–20 wt.%. The as-obtained scaffolds exhibit remarkable antibacterial activity against *E. coli* and *S. aureus* strains as well as good biocompatibility, as determined by the MT assay after 1 and 3 days. The Cu^{2+} release is very important because the antimicrobial activity of this ion is based on the ability of the Cu^{2+} to oxidize the thiol group of cysteine to disulfide group, with the formation of cystine. Based on the data obtained by Haider et al., 2015 the Cu^{2+} release is slow enough to ensure long-term antimicrobial activity (Table 13.4).

Table 13.4 Metal/Support Pair for Antimicrobial Fighting

No.	Metal	Support	Applications
1.	Ag	Zeolite	Antibacterial activity, silver can be directly reduced *in situ* and in this case the size and shape of the nanoparticles are highly controlled, the antimicrobial activity being directly correlated with these characteristics (Palza, 2015; Nedelcu et al., 2014; Madhumathi et al., 2010)
2.		Collagen	
3.		Chitin/chitosan	
4.		Poly(acrylamide-*co*-acrylic acid)	
5.		Poly(vinyl pyrrolidone)-based interpenetrating polymer network (IPN) hydrogel	
6.		Superabsorbant PVA/alginate hydrogels	
7.	Cu/CuO	Cotton fibers	Broad-spectrum antimicrobial and antimite activities (Palza, 2015; Haider et al., 2015)
8.		Latex	
9.		PE	
10.		Alginate–cotton cellulose	
11.	ZnO	Polyvinylpyrrolidone	ZnO was embedded/deposited into/on various support materials to ensure good antimicrobial activity against a wide variety of pathological micro-organisms (Oprea et al., 2014; Rahman et al., 2015; El-Nahhal et al., 2013; Pantani et al., 2013; Doumbia et al., 2015; Diez-Pascual and Diez-Vicente, 2014; Rodriguez-Tobias et al., 2014)
12.		Chitosan	
13.		Cotton	
14.		PLA	
15.		Poly(3-hydroxybutyrate-*co*-3-hydroxyvalerate)	
16.	ZnO–Ag	Chitosan	The use of two antimicrobial agents can be beneficial because these new materials exhibit broader antimicrobial activity and, due to the cumulative activity also induce stronger antimicrobial activity compared with the samples containing only one antimicrobial agent (Busila et al., 2015; Azizi et al., 2014)
17.		PVA–CS reinforced with cellulose nanocrystals	

13.1.6.4 DDS designed for the treatment of skin cancer

Polymer-based materials are extensively used in soft tissue engineering. Even if polymers exhibit excellent properties which make them suitable for a large range of applications, many drug delivery systems were developed in order to enlarge the applicability range. In this context, the influence of additional component(s) with regenerative purposes, as well as the addition of various drugs, was successfully tested. The added drugs can induce protective or curative roles, as presented in Table 13.3.

In cancer treatment, a wide variety of active components were tested, from metallic nanoparticles to complexes, synthetic or natural organic compounds, and so on. Curcumin is a natural compound which was proved to have high antitumoral activity against many cancer cells but lower cytotoxic effect comparing with the cytostatics. This makes it very attractive for anticancer formulations (Park et al., 2013). Chitosan-based carriers were also intensively studied by many researchers. Zhou et al., 2013 used galactosylated chitosan–PCL nanoparticles for hepatocyte-targeted delivery of curcumin. The support was prepared by grafting PCL onto the galactosylated chitosan (degree of galactosylation was $10.3 \pm 0.39\%$) at 45°C for 12 h, under stirring and nitrogen flow. The loading of the support with curcumin involves the dissolution of galactosylated chitosan–PCL nanoparticles into 0.5% acetic acid (final concentration 0.15 wt.%) followed by mixing of 30 ml of this solution with 0.5% ethanolic solution of curcumin. The formation of the curcumin-loaded galactosylated chitosan–PCL nanoparticles was obtained when 20 ml of sodium tripolyphosphate was slowly added to the as-obtained solution, under vigorous stirring (6000 rpm, 3 min). Two main parameters were modified in order to control the properties of the drug delivery systems: content of PCL (19.6 ± 2.1; 28.5 ± 2.3; 38.2 ± 1.9 and 37.6 ± 2.2) and TPP (0.06, 0.07, and 0.08%, w/v). By changing these parameters particles within 100 and 24 nm were obtained and zeta potential was between 19.3 and 30.7 mV. The encapsulation efficiency was found to be proportional with the content of PCL and concentration of sodium tripolyphosphate. Curcumin delivery is dependent on the synthesis parameters and especially on the delivery content of PCL and concentration of sodium tripolyphosphate. The curcumin uptake is better in the case of the curcumin-loaded galactosylated chitosan–PCL nanoparticles compared with the free curcumin. The antitumoral activity against HepG2 cells was found to be sixfold higher than the same amount of free curcumin, so the galactosylated chitosan–PCL nanoparticles are promising carriers for hepatocyte-targeted delivery of curcumin, especially due to the improved bioavailability.

Nanoparticles can be successfully used as carriers for various drugs, including most of the cancer forms. Both organic and inorganic nanoparticles were found to be suitable for targeted drug delivery. Liposomes, solid lipid nanoparticles (SLN), polymeric micelles and nanospheres, dendrimers, mesoporous silica, various quantum dots, nanotubes, superparamagnetic iron oxide nanoparticles (SPIONs), or metal nanoparticles were tested for cancer treatment, including for skin cancer treatment (Dianzani et al., 2014).

Glutathione-stabilized gold nanoparticles was non-covalently modified with doxorubicin (Au-GSH-Dox) and used for the treatment of feline injection-site sarcomas (malignant skin tumors of mesenchymal origin) (Wojcik et al., 2015). The use of Au-GSH-Dox instead of free doxorubicin was found to be more cytotoxic on all four studied feline fibrosarcoma cell lines (FFS1WAW, FFS1, FFS3, FFS5). Based on these data, Au-GSH-Dox may be considered a potential therapeutic agent being more efficient than the free drug and overcoming the resistance to doxorubicin. The IC50 of free doxicycline decreased in the case of the Au-GSH-Dox for three of the four studied lines from 69.66 to 30.62 μg/ml (FFS1WAW), from 35.39 to 2.82 μg/ml (FFS1), and from 18.09 to 2.57 μg/ml (FFS3), while slightly increasing from 8.67 to 10.22 μg/ml (FFS5).

Squamous cell carcinoma, a common skin cancer, was treated using 5-aminolevulinic acid polylactic-*co*-glycolic acid (PLGA) nanoparticle-mediated photodynamic therapy (Wang et al., 2015). Photodynamic therapy can be a valuable way of treating various localized diseases, especially close to the surface. In this study tumor-bearing male SKH-1 hairless mice (6–8 weeks old, Jackson Laboratories) and a total of 10 visible tumors, of size 61.6–96.28 mm^3 were considered. Aminolevulinic acid was loaded into PLGA nanoparticles using a modified double-emulsion solvent-evaporation method followed by freeze-drying and was further used for preparing the cream by mixing it with oil-in-water cream and applied onto the tumors. The irradiation protocol involved helium-neon laser (632.8 nm), at a power density of 8.6 mW/cm^2 and energy density of 15 J/cm^2 and was repeated once a week for 4 weeks. The mice were kept in dark. The four groups (control, without any treatment; aminolevulinic acid treated group; 0.8% aminolevulinic acid group exposed to photodynamic treatment; and 0.8% aminolevulinic-acid-loaded PLGA nanoparticles group exposed to photodynamic treatment) were comparatively analyzed after the treatment. Except the 0.8% aminolevulinic-acid-loaded PLGA nanoparticles group exposed to photodynamic treatment where the average tumor size decreased in all the other groups, the average tumor size increased, which means no or only limited efficiency. In fact, a slight decrease compared only with the control group also occurs in the group photodynamically treated with 0.8% aminolevulinic acid. Based on these results it can be concluded that topical application of the cream containing 0.8% aminolevulinic-acid-loaded PLGA nanoparticles involves an accumulation of the photosensitizer at the tumor level and the use of adequate laser radiation leads to the destruction of the tumor. To obtain better transdermal delivery of aminolevulinic-acid-loaded PLGA nanoparticles a microneedeling procedure may be used at the skin/tumor level (Table 13.5).

13.2 CONCLUSIONS AND PERSPECTIVES

Tissue engineering is a multidisciplinary field used to replace or augment damaged or defective tissues and organs. From literature data, chitosan and its derivatives, collagen, alginate, as well as some synthetic polymers like poly(lactic acid), PCL, PVA, etc. seems to be potential scaffold materials for soft tissues such as skin, adipose, cornea, liver, nerve, and blood vessel.

Due to their good biocompatibility, non-toxicity, antimicrobial activity, mechanical and chemical stability, chitosan and its derivatives are used in many biomedical applications. For soft tissue engineering, different types of chitosan with different molecular weights and deacetylation degrees can be used. Combinations with other polymers are also possible to enhance the properties of the systems.

Another polymer used in reconstruction or replacement of damaged tissue is collagen. The use of collagen in tissue engineering is recommended due to the excellent biocompatibility and biodegradability. However, due to its fast biodegradation and low mechanical strength, collagen is used in tissue engineering mixed with other polymers (chitosan, PCL, poly[lactic acid], etc.).

Table 13.5 The Influence of Third Components on the Properties of Different Polymeric Grafts

No.	Support Materials	Active Components	Roles
1.	Blends of polymers	–	Only pure regenerative role
2.	Chitosan	Growth factors (GF)	Only regenerative purposes but, due to the delivery of GF faster regeneration is expected (Dreifke et al., 2015)
3.	Multifunctional CS/PEO nanofibers loaded with PLGA nanoparticles	VEGF and PDGF-BB	The fibrillar morphology of the electrospun system as well as the dual growth factors system assure fast healing due to a faster angiogenesis and re-epithelialization without affecting the normal granulation of the new tissue (Xie et al., 2013)
4.	PLA–PCL	KGF	The system ensures early epithelialization of the skin wounds due to the support/KGF drug delivery system which is important because the fluid and electrolyte losses are avoided and due to the rapid epithelialization the barrier is formed and prevents infections
5.	PVA-COOH/CS	Gentamicin sulfate	The delivery rate of gentamicin can be controlled by the PVA:CS ratio, the increasing content of CS leading to a slower delivery (Zhang et al., 2015)
6.	Collagen	Antibiotics (gentamicin, doxycycline, etc.)	Antimicrobial wound dressing or antimicrobial skin grafts (Albu et al., 2010)
7.	Alginate	Tobramycin	Tobramycin is effective against *Pseudomonas aeruginosa* pulmonary infections (Deacon et al., 2015)
8.	Dextrin/poly (2-hydroxy-ethyl methylacrylate)	Ciprofloxacin	The synergism of the support and the broad-spectrum antibiotic is essential. This system is important because up to 3 months delivery of ciprofloxacin is assured (Das and Pal, 2015)
9.	Dextran- and chitosan-based hydrogels	Vancomycin	Promising drug delivery system of vancomycin was obtained by using natural polymers instead of the well-known and used polyethylene glycol (synthetic, non-biodegradable polymer) with delivery rate control induced by composition (Wang et al., 2014)
10.	Chitosan-based nanoemulsion	Acyclovir	Acyclovir-based nanoemulsion hydrogen is active against herpes simplex viral infection (Al-Subaie et al., 2015)

(Continued)

Table 13.5 The Influence of Third Components on the Properties of Different Polymeric Grafts *Continued*

No.	Support Materials	Active Components	Roles
11.	PCL–PEG	Curcumin	Curcumin is a natural product and a very promising anticancer agent and was tested for various cancers, in various formulations (Bui et al., 2014; Zamarioli et al., 2015; Zhou et al., 2013; Bora-Tatar and Erdem-Yurter, 2014)
12.	Solid lipid nanocapsules (SLNs)	Curcumin	
13.	Galactosylated chitosan–PCL nanoparticles	Curcumin	
14.	Glutathione-stabilized gold nanoparticles (Au-GSH)	Doxorubicin	Cytostatics use in the treatment of various cancers are essential but due to their high toxicity the DDS administration could be efficient in reducing the systemic toxicity (Wojcik et al., 2015)

The use of smart drug delivery systems is a key tool for tissue engineering. The use of biologically active components can improve some characteristics of the pure support (i.e., can induce faster healing, safer healing, etc.) or can even induce new functionalities (i.e., antimicrobial, analgesic, antitumoral activity). It is expected that novel drug delivery systems will be developed in the forthcoming years. These novel DDS will be able to release the active components in a more controlled way and even increase the bioavailability of these components at the targeted site.

ACKNOWLEDGMENTS

The authors recognize financial support from the UEFISCDI through PN-II-PT-PCCA-2013-4-0270 project: "Ligament reconstruction by using advanced structural materials based on natural and synthetic polymers – LigaSint."

REFERENCES

Adekogbe, I., Ghanem, A., 2005. Fabrication and characterization of DTBP-crosslinked chitosan scaffolds for skin tissue engineering. Biomaterials 26, 7241–7250.

Agnihotri, S.A., Mallikarjuna, N.N., Aminabhavi, T.M., 2004. Recent advances on chitosan-based micro- and nanoparticles in drug delivery. J. Control. Release 100, 5–28.

Al-Subaie, M.M., Hosny, K.M., El-Say, K.M., Ahmed, T.A., Aljaeid, B.M., 2015. Utilization of nanotechnology to enhance percutaneous absorption of acyclovir in the treatment of herpes simplex viral infections. Int. J. Nanomed. 10, 3973–3985.

Alberts, B., Bray, D., Lewis, J., Raff, M., Roberts, K., Watson, J.D., 1994. Molecular Biology of the Cell. Garland Publishing, New York, NY.

Albu, M.G., Ghica, M.V., Ficai, A., Titorencu, I., Popa, L. 2010. Influence of freeze-drying process on porosity and kinetics release of collagen–doxycycline matrices. In: Proceedings of the 3rd International Conference on Advanced Materials and Systems, pp. 181–186.

Allison, D.D., Grande-Allen, K.J., 2006. Review. Hyaluronan: a powerful tissue engineering tool. Tissue Eng. 12, 2131–2140.

Almeida, C.E.P.C., Reis, L., Carvalho, L., Almeida, C.M.C., 2014. Collagen implant with gentamicin sulphate reduces surgical site infection in vascular surgery: a prospective cohort study. Int. J. Surg. 12, 1100–1104.

Alves da Silva, M.L., Crawford, A., Mundy, J.M., Correlo, V.M., Sol, P., Bhattacharya, M., et al., 2010. Chitosan/polyesterbased scaffolds for cartilage tissue engineering: assessment of extracellular matrix formation. Acta Biomater. 6, 1149.

Amado, S., Simoes, M.J., Da Silva, P.A.S.A., Luis, A.L., Shirosaki, Y., Lopes, M.A., et al., 2008. Use of hybrid chitosan membranes and N1E-115 cells for promoting nerve regeneration in an axonotmesis rat model. Biomaterials 29, 4409–4419.

Amidi, M., Mastrobattista, E., Jiskoot, W., Hennink, W.E., 2010. Chitosan-based delivery systems for protein therapeutics and antigens. Adv. Drug Deliv. Rev. 62, 59–82.

Aranaz, I., Harris, R., Heras, A., 2010. Chitosan amphiphilic derivatives. Chem. Appl. Curr. Org. Chem. 14, 308–330.

Arca, H.Ç., Şenel, S., 2008. Chitosan based systems for tissue Engineering part II. Soft Tissues J. Pharm. Sci 33, 211–216s.

Audoly, S., 2006. Gelatin in Pharmaceutical Applications.

Azizi, S., Ahmad, B.I.N., Hussein, M., Ibrahim, M.Z., Namvar, N.A., 2014. Preparation and properties of poly(vinyl alcohol)/chitosan blend bionanocomposites reinforced with cellulose nanocrystals/ZnO–Ag multifunctional nanosized filler. Int. J. Nanomed. 9, 1909–1917.

Batemann, J.F., Lamande, S.R., Ramshaw, J.A.M., 1996. Collagen superfamily în Extracellular Matrix. Academic Press, Melbourne.

Beier, J.P., Klumpp, D., Rudisile, M., Dersch, R., Wendorff, J.H., Bleiziffer, O., et al., 2009. Collagen matrices from sponge to nano: new perspectives for tissue engineering of skeletal muscle. BMC Biotechnol. 9.

Berger, J., Reist, M., Mayer, J.M., Felt, O., Gurny, R., 2004. Structure and interactions in chitosan hydrogels formed by complexation or aggregation for biomedical applications. Eur. J. Pharm. Biopharm. 57, 35–52.

Bora-Tatar, G., Erdem-Yurter, H., 2014. Investigations of curcumin and resveratrol on neurite outgrowth: perspectives on spinal muscular atrophy. Biomed. Res. Int. 2014, (Article ID 709108, 8 pages). Available from: http://dx.doi.org/10.1155/2014/709108.

Boran, G., (Ed.), 2013. Gelatin: Production, Applications and Health Implications.

Boucard, N., Viton, C., Agay, D., Mari, E., Roger, T., Chancerelle, Y., et al., 2007. The use of physical hydrogels of chitosan for skin regeneration following third-degree burns. Biomaterials 28, 3478–3488.

Brunel, F., Veron, L., Ladaviere, C., David, L., Domard, A., Delair, T., 2009. Synthesis and structural characterization of chitosan nanogels. Langmuir 25, 8935–8943.

Bui, H.T., Chung, O.H., Dela Cruz, J., Park, J.S., 2014. Fabrication and characterization of electrospun curcumin-loaded polycaprolactone–polyethylene glycol nanofibers for enhanced wound healing. Macromol. Res. 22, 1288–1296.

Busila, M., Musat, V., Textor, T., Mahltig, B., 2015. Synthesis and characterization of antimicrobial textile finishing based on Ag:ZnO nanoparticles/chitosan biocomposites. Rsc Adv. 5, 21562–21571.

Cao, B., Zhou, D., Xue, M., Li, G., Weizhong, Y., Long, Q., et al., 2008. Study on surface modification of porous apatite-wollastonite bioactive glass ceramic scaffold. Appl. Surf. Sci. 255, 505–508.

Chen, J.S., Li, Q.H., Xu, J.T., Huang, Y.X., Ding, Y., Deng, H.W., et al., 2005. Study on biocompatibility of complexes of collagen–chitosan–sodium hyaluronate and cornea. Artif. Organs. 29, 104–113.

Cheng, H., Li, Y., Huo, K.F., Gao, B., Xiong, W., 2014. Long-lasting *in vivo* and *in vitro* antibacterial ability of nanostructured titania coating incorporated with silver nanoparticles. J. Biomed. Mater. Res. A 102, 3488–3499.

Cho, Y.W., Cho, Y.N., Chung, S.H., Yoo, G., Ko, S.W., 1999. Water-soluble chitin as a wound healing accelerator. Biomaterials 20, 2139–2145.

Coppoolse, J.M.S., Van Kooten, T.G., Heris, H.K., Mongeau, L., Li, N.Y.K., Thibeault, S.L., et al., 2014. An *in vivo* study of composite microgels based on hyaluronic acid and gelatin for the reconstruction of surgically injured rat vocal folds. J. Speech Lang. Hear. Res. 57, S658–S673.

Cortivo, R., Vindigni, V., Iacobellis, L., Abatangelo, G., Pinton, P., Zavan, B., 2010. Nanoscale particle therapies for wounds and ulcers. Nanomedicine 5, 641–656.

Croisier, F., Jerome, C., 2013. Chitosan-based biomaterials for tissue engineering. Eur. Polym. J. 49, 780–792.

Dang, J.M., Leong, K.W., 2006. Natural polymers for gene delivery and tissue engineering. Adv. Drug Deliv. Rev. 58, 487–499.

Das, D., Pal, S., 2015. Dextrin/poly (HEMA): pH responsive porous hydrogel for controlled release of ciprofloxacin. Int. J. Biol. Macromol. 72, 171–178.

Das, G., Kalita, R.D., Gogoi, P., Buragohain, A.K., Karak, N., 2014. Antibacterial activities of copper nanoparticle-decorated organically modified montmorillonite/epoxy nanocomposites. Appl. Clay Sci. 90, 18–26.

Deacon, J., Abdelghany, S.M., Quinn, D.J., Schmid, D., Megaw, J., Donnelly, R.F., et al., 2015. Antimicrobial efficacy of tobramycin polymeric nanoparticles for *Pseudomonas aeruginosa* infections in cystic fibrosis: formulation, characterisation and functionalisation with dornase alfa (DNase). J. Control. Release 198, 55–61.

Dianzani, C., Zara, G.P., Maina, G., Pettazzoni, P., Pizzimenti, S., Rossi, F., et al., 2014. Drug delivery nanoparticles in skin cancers. Biomed. Res. Int.

Diez-Pascual, A.M., Diez-Vicente, A.L., 2014. ZnO-reinforced poly(3-hydroxybutyrate-*co*-3-hydroxyvalerate) bionanocomposites with antimicrobial function for food packaging. ACS Appl. Mater. Interfaces 6, 9822–9834.

Doumbia, A.S., Vezin, H., Ferreira, M., Campagne, C., Devaux, E., 2015. Studies of polylactide/zinc oxide nanocomposites: influence of surface treatment on zinc oxide antibacterial activities in textile nanocomposites. J. Appl. Polym. Sci. 132.

Dreifke, M.B., Jayasuriya, A.A., Jayasuriya, A.C., 2015. Current wound healing procedures and potential care. Mater. Sci. Eng. C Mater. Biol. Appl. 48, 651–662.

El-Nahhal, I.M., Zourab, S.M., Kodeh, F.S., Elmanama, A.A., Selmane, M., Genois, I., et al., 2013. Nano-structured zinc oxide-cotton fibers: synthesis, characterization and applications. J. Mater. Sci. Mater. Electron. 24, 3970–3975.

Esmaeili, F., Heuking, S., Junginger, H.E., Borchard, G., 2010. Progress in chitosan-based vaccine delivery systems. J. Drug Deliv. Sci. Technol. 20, 53–61.

Feng, W., Mingbo, W., Zhending, S., Kunwu, F., Cheng, X., Bin, C., et al., 2015. Collagen/chitosan based two-compartment and bi-functional dermal scaffolds for skin regeneration. Mater. Sci. Eng. C 52, 155–162.

Feng, Z.Q., Chu, X.H., Huang, N.P., Wang, T., Wang, Y.C., Shi, X.L., et al., 2009. The effect of nanofibrous galactosylated chitosan scaffolds on the formation of rat primary hepatocyte aggregates and the maintenance of liver function. Biomaterials 30, 2753–2763.

Ficai, D., Oprea, O., Ficai, A., Holban, A.M., 2014. Metal oxide nanoparticles: potential uses in biomedical applications. Curr. Proteomics 11, 139–149.

Ficai, D., Ficai, A., Dinu, E., Oprea, O., Sonmez, M., Keler, M.K., et al., 2015. Magnetic core shell structures: from 0D to 1D assembling. Curr. Pharm. Des.

Friberg, O., Bodin, L., 2013. Collagen gentamicin for prevention of sternal wound infection: effective or not? Thorac. Cardiovasc. Surg. 61, 185–193.

Funakoshi, T., Majima, T., Iwasaki, N., Suenaga, N., Sawaguchi, N., Shimode, K., et al., 2005a. Application of tissue engineering techniques for rotator cuff regeneration using a chitosan-based hyaluronan hybrid fiber scaffold. Am. J. Sports Med. 33, 1193–1201.

Funakoshi, T., Majima, T., Iwasaki, N., Yamane, S., Masuko, T., Minami, A., et al., 2005b. Novel chitosan-based hyaluronan hybrid polymer fibers as a scaffold in ligament tissue engineering. J. Biomed. Mater. Res. A 74A, 338–346.

Gao, X., Liu, W., Han, B., Wei, X., Yang, C., 2008. Preparation and properties of a chitosan-based carrier of corneal endothelial cells. J. Mater. Sci. Mater. Med. 19, 3611–3619.

Geng, X.Y., Kwon, O.H., Jang, J.H., 2005. Electrospinning of chitosan dissolved in concentrated acetic acid solution. Biomaterials 26, 5427–5432.

Gobin, A.S., Butler, C.E., Mathur, A.B., 2006. Repair and regeneration of the abdominal wall musculofascial defect using silk fibroin-chitosan blend. Tissue Eng. 12, 3383–3394.

Gomez, G.G.V., Guerrero, T.S., Lluck, M.C., Delgado, F.J., 1999. Effectiveness of collagen-gentamicin implant for treatment of "dirty" abdominal wounds. World J. Surg. 23, 123–127.

Gouda, M., Hebeish, A., 2010. Preparation and evaluation of cuo/chitosan nanocomposite for antibacterial finishing cotton fabric. J. Ind. Textiles 39, 203–214.

Guran, C., Pica, A., Ficai, D., Ficai, A., Comanescu, C., 2013. Antimicrobial coatings—obtaining and characterization. Bull. Mater. Sci. 36, 183–188.

Haider, A., Kwak, S., Gupta, K.C., Kang, I.K., 2015. Antibacterial activity and cytocompatibility of PLGA/CuO hybrid nanofiber scaffolds prepared by electrospinning. J. Nanomater.

Haipeng, G., Yinghui, Z., Jianchun, L., Yandao, G., Nanming, Z., Xiufang, Z., 2000. Studies on nerve cell affinity of chitosan-derived materials. J. Biomed. Mater. Res. 52, 285–295.

Han, C.M., Zhang, L.P., Sun, J.Z., Shi, H.F., Zhou, J., Gao, C.Y., 2010. Application of collagen–chitosan/fibrin glue asymmetric scaffolds in skin tissue engineering. J. Zhejiang Univ. Sci. B 11, 524–530.

Hasegawa, M., Isogai, A., Onabe, F., Usuda, M., Atalla, R.H., 1992. Characterization of cellulose chitosan blend films. J. Appl. Polym. Sci. 45, 1873–1879.

Inas, N.E., Kawkab, A.A., 2012. Application of chitosan for wound repair in dogs. Life Sci. J. Acta Zhengzhou Univ. Overseas Ed. 9, 196–203.

Iordăchescu, D.A.C., Stan, C., 2004. Modelarea matricei extracelulare. Aplicaţii în ingineria tisulară, Pro-Transilvania, Bucureşti.

Jayakumar, R., Prabaharan, M., Kumar, P.T.S., Nair, S.V., Tamura, H., 2011. Biomaterials based on chitin and chitosan in wound dressing applications. Biotechnol. Adv. 29, 322–337.

Jiang, T., Kumbar, S.G., Nair, L.S., Laurencin, C.T., 2008. Biologically active chitosan systems for tissue engineering and regenerative medicine. Curr. Top. Med. Chem. 8, 354–364.

Jiankang, H., Dichen, L., Yaxiong, L., Bo, Y., Hanxiang, Z., Qin, L., et al., 2009. Preparation of chitosangelatin hybrid scaffolds with well-organized microstructures for hepatic tissue engineering. Acta Biomater. 5, 453–461.

Jin, G.R., Prabhakaran, M.P., Kai, D., Ramakrishna, S., 2013. Controlled release of multiple epidermal induction factors through core–shell nanofibers for skin regeneration. Eur. J. Pharma. Biopharm. 85, 689–698.

Kim, I.Y., Seo, S.J., Moon, H.S., Yoo, M.K., Park, I.Y., Kim, B.C., et al., 2008. Chitosan and its derivatives for tissue engineering applications. Biotechnol. Adv. 26, 1–21.

Kim, T.H., Jiang, H.L., Jere, D., Park, I.K., Cho, M.H., Nah, J.W., et al., 2007. Chemical modification of chitosan as a gene carrier *in vitro* and *in vivo*. Prog. Polym. Sci. 32, 726–753.

Kleimann, H.K., Klebe, R.J., Martin, G.R., 1981. Role of collagenous matrices in the adhesion and growth of cells. J. Cell Biol. 88, 473–485.

Kobsa, S., Kristofik, N.J., Sawyer, A.J., Bothwell, A.L.M., Kyriakides, T.R., Saltzman, W.M., 2013. An electrospun scaffold integrating nucleic acid delivery for treatment of full-thickness wounds. Biomaterials 34, 3891–3901.

Koide, T., Nagata, K., 2005. Collagen biosynthesis. Collagen 247, 85–114.

Kojima, K., Okamoto, Y., Miyatake, K., Kitamura, Y., Minami, S., 1998. Collagen typing of granulation tissue induced by chitin and chitosan. Carbohydr. Polym. 37, 109–113.

Kumar, M.N.V.R., 2000. A review of chitin and chitosan applications. Reactive Funct. Polym. 46, 1–27.

Li, J., Dou, Y., Yang, J., Yin, Y., Zhang, H., Yao, F., et al., 2009. Surface characterization and biocompatibility of micro- and nanohydroxyapatite/chitosan–gelatin network films. Mater. Sci. Eng. C 29, 1207.

Lin, A.H., Liu, Y.M., Ping, Q.N., 2007a. Free amino groups on the surface of chitosan nanoparticles and its characteristics. Yao Xue Xue Bao 42, 323–328.

Lin, H.R., Chen, K.S., Chen, S.C., Lee, C.H., Chiou, S.H., Chang, T.L., et al., 2007b. Attachment of stem cells on porous chitosan scaffold crosslinked by $Na_5P_3O_{10}$. Mater. Sci. Eng. C Biomim. Supramolecular Syst. 27, 280–284.

Luo, Y., Kirker, K.R., Prestwich, G.D., 2000. Cross-linked hyaluronic acid hydrogel films: new biomaterials for drug delivery. J. Control. Release 69, 169–184.

Madhumathi, K., Kumar, P.T.S., Abhilash, S., Sreeja, V., Tamura, H., Manzoor, K., et al., 2010. Development of novel chitin/nanosilver composite scaffolds for wound dressing applications. J. Mater. Sci. Mater. Med. 21, 807–813.

Madihally, S.V., Matthew, H.W.T., 1999. Porous chitosan scaffolds for tissue engineering. Biomaterials 20, 1133–1142.

Malafaya, P.B., Reis, R.L., 2009. Bilayered chitosan-based scaffolds for osteochondral tissue engineering: influence of hydroxyapatite on *in vitro* cytotoxicity and dynamic bioactivity studies in a specific double-chamber bioreactor. Acta Biomater. 5, 644–660.

Maleknia, L., Majdi, Z.R., 2014. Electrospinning of gelatin nanofiber for biomedical application. Oriental J. Chem. 30, 2043–2048.

Mandal, B.B., Mann, J.K., Kundu, S.C., 2009. Silk fibroin/gelatin multilayered films as amodel system for controlled drug release. Eur. J. Pharm. Sci. 37 (2), 160–171.

Mansouri, M., Khorram, M., Samimi, A., Osfouri, S. 2010. Preparation of bovine serum albumin loaded chitosan nanoparticles using reverse micelle method. http://www.chisa.cz/2010/admin/contrib_get_abst.

Martins, A.M., Pham, Q.P., Malafaya, P.B., Raphael, R.M., Kasper, F.K., Reis, R.L., et al., 2009. Natural stimulus responsive scaffolds/cells for bone tissue engineering: influence of lysozyme upon scaffold degradation and osteogenic differentiation of cultured marrow stromal cells induced by CaP coatings. Tissue Eng. A.

Mehanna, M.M., Mohyeldin, S.M., Elgindy, N.A., 2014. Respirable nanocarriers as a promising strategy for antitubercular drug delivery. J. Control. Release 187, 183–197.

Mei, L.Q., Hu, D.Y., Ma, J.F., Wang, X.P., Yang, Y.Z., Liu, J.S., 2012. Preparation, characterization and evaluation of chitosan macroporous for potential application in skin tissue engineering. Int. J. Biol. Macromol. 51, 992–997.

Meng, D., Dong, L.M., Wen, Y., Xie, Q.F., 2015. Effects of adding resorbable chitosan microspheres to calcium phosphate cements for bone regeneration. Mater. Sci. Eng. C Mater. Biol. Appl. 47, 266–272.

Min, B.M., Lee, S.W., Lim, J.N., You, Y., Lee, T.S., Kang, P.H., et al., 2004. Chitin and chitosan nanofibers: electrospinning of chitin and deacetylation of chitin nanofibers. Polymer 45, 7137–7142.

Miyata, T., Taira, T., 1992. Collagen engineering for biomaterial use. Clinical Materials, 9.

Moellering, R.C., 2012. MRSA: the first half century. J. Antimicrob. Chemother. 67, 4–11.

Mondrinos, M.J., Koutzaki, S.H., Poblete, H.M., Crisanti, M.C., Lelkes, P.I., Finck, C.M., 2008. *In vivo* pulmonary tissue engineering: contribution of donor-derived endothelial cells to construct vascularization. Tissue Eng. A 14, 361–368.

Mori, M., Almeida, P.V., Cola, M., Anselmi, G., Makila, E., Correia, A., et al., 2014a. *In vitro* assessment of biopolymer-modified porous silicon microparticles for wound healing applications. Eur. J. Pharm. Biopharm. 88, 635–642.

Mori, M., Rossi, S., Bonferoni, M.C., Ferrari, F., Sandri, G., Riva, F., et al., 2014b. Calcium alginate particles for the combined delivery of platelet lysate and vancomycin hydrochloride in chronic skin ulcers. Int. J. Pharm. 461, 505–513.

Mucha, M., Michalak, I., Balcerzak, J., Tylman, M., 2012. Chitosan scaffolds, films and microgranules for medical application—preparation and drug release studies. Polimery 57, 714–721.

Muzzarelli, R.A.A., 2009. Chitins and chitosans for the repair of wounded skin, nerve, cartilage and bone. Carbohydr. Polym. 76, 167–182.

Nasti, A., Zaki, N.M., De Leonardis, P., Ungphaiboon, S., Sansongsak, P., Rimoli, M.G., et al., 2009. Chitosan/Tpp and chitosan/Tpp-hyaluronic acid nanoparticles: systematic optimisation of the preparative process and preliminary biological evaluation. Pharm. Res. 26, 1918–1930.

Nath, N., Hyun, J., Ma, H., Chilkoti, A., 2004. Surface engineering strategies for control of protein and cell interactions. Surf. Sci. 570, 98–110.

Nedelcu, I.A., Ficai, A., Sonmez, M., Ficai, D., Oprea, O., Andronescu, E., 2014. Silver based materials for biomedical applications. Curr. Organ. Chem. 18, 173–184.

Nie, H.M., Wang, C.H., 2007. Fabrication and characterization of PLGA/HAp scaffolds for delivery of BMP-2 plasmid composite DNA. J. Control. Release 120, 111–121.

Noel, S.P., Courtney, H.S., Bumgardner, J.D., Haggard, W.O., 2010. Chitosan sponges to locally deliver amikacin and vancomycin a pilot *in vitro* evaluation. Clin. Orthop. Relat. Res. 468, 2074–2080.

Nogueira, F., Goncalves, I.C., Martins, M.C.L., 2013. Effect of gastric environment on *Helicobacter pylori* adhesion to a mucoadhesive polymer. Acta Biomater. 9, 5208–5215.

Ohkawa, K., Cha, D.I., Kim, H., Nishida, A., Yamamoto, H., 2004. Electrospinning of chitosan. Macromol. Rapid Commun. 25, 1600–1605.

Ong, W.Y., Shalini, S.M., Costantino, L., 2014. Nose-to-brain drug delivery by nanoparticles in the treatment of neurological disorders. Curr. Med. Chem. 21, 4247–4256.

Oprea, O., Andronescu, E., Ficai, D., Ficai, A., Oktar, F.N., Yetmez, M., 2014. ZnO applications and challenges. Curr. Organ. Chem. 18, 192–203.

Ordikhani, F., Simchi, A., 2014. Long-term antibiotic delivery by chitosan-based composite coatings with bone regenerative potential. Appl. Surf. Sci. 317, 56–66.

Othman, S.H., Salam, A.B.D., Zainal, N., Basha, R.K., Talib, R.A., 2014. Antimicrobial activity of TiO_2 nanoparticle-coated film for potential food packaging applications. Int. J. Photoenergy.

Palza, H., 2015. Antimicrobial polymers with metal nanoparticles. Int. J. Mol. Sci. 16, 2099–2116.

Pantani, R., Gorrasi, G., Vigliotta, G., Murariu, M., Dubois, P., 2013. PLA–ZnO nanocomposite films: water vapor barrier properties and specific end-use characteristics. Eur. Polym. J. 49, 3471–3482.

Park, W., Amin, A.R.M.R., Chen, Z.G., Shin, D.M., 2013. New perspectives of curcumin in cancer prevention. Cancer Prev. Res. 6, 387–400.

Patil, J.S., Devi, K., Devi, K., Suresh, S., 2015. Formulation and evaluation of novel spray-dried alginate microspheres as pulmonary delivery systems of rifampicin in rats. Indian J. Pharma. Educ. Res. 49, 320–328.

Patrascu, J.M., Nedelcu, I.A., Sonmez, M., Ficai, D., Ficai, A., Vasile, B.S., et al., 2015. Composite scaffolds based on silver nanoparticles for biomedical applications. J. Nanomater. Article ID 587989.

Pavinatto, F.J., Caseli, L., Oliveira, O.N., 2010. Chitosan in nanostructured thin films. Biomacromolecules 11, 1897–1908.

Peattie, R.A., Pike, D.B., Yu, B., Cai, S., Shu, X.Z., Prestwich, G.D., et al., 2008. Effect of gelatin on heparin regulation of cytokine release from hyaluronan-based hydrogels. Drug Deliv. 15, 389–397.

Pfister, L.A., Alther, E., Papaloizos, M.L., Merkle, H.P., Gander, B., 2008. Controlled nerve growth factor release from multiply alginate/chitosan-based nerve conduits. Eur. J. Pharma. Biopharm. 69, 563–572.

Qiang, A.O., Wang, A., Cao, W., Zhao, C., Gong, Y., Zhao, N., et al., 2005. Fabrication and characterization of chitosan nerve conduits with microtubular architectures. Tsinghua Sci. Technol. 10, 435–438.

Rafat, M., Li, F.F., Fagerholm, P., Lagali, N.S., Watsky, M.A., Munger, R., et al., 2008. PEG-stabilized carbodiimide crosslinked collagen–chitosan hydrogels for corneal tissue engineering. Biomaterials 29, 3960–3972.

Rahman, P.M., Muraleedaran, K., Mujeeb, V.M.A., 2015. Applications of chitosan powder with *in situ* synthesized nano ZnO particles as an antimicrobial agent. Int. J. Biol. Macromol. 77, 266–272.

Ramakrishna, S., Fujihara, K., Teo, W.E., Lim, T.C., Ma, Z.H. 2005. An Introduction to Electrospinning and Nanofibers.

Reddy, L.S., Nisha, M.M., Joice, M., Shilpa, P.N., 2014. Antimicrobial activity of zinc oxide (ZnO) nanoparticle against *Klebsiella pneumoniae*. Pharm. Biol. 52, 1388–1397.

Ren, G.G., Hu, D.W., Cheng, E.W.C., Vargas-Reus, M.A., Reip, P., Allaker, R.P., 2009. Characterisation of copper oxide nanoparticles for antimicrobial applications. Int. J. Antimicrob. Agents 33, 587–590.

Rinaudo, M., 2006. Chitin and chitosan: properties and applications. Prog. Polym. Sci. 31, 603–632.

Rodriguez-Tobias, H., Morales, G., Ledezma, A., Romero, J., Grande, D., 2014. Novel antibacterial electrospun mats based on poly(D,L-lactide) nanofibers and zinc oxide nanoparticles. J. Mater. Sci. 49, 8373–8385.

Rossert, J., Crombrugghe, B.D.E., 2002. Type I collagen: structure, synthesis and regulation. Principles in Bone Biology. Academic Press, Orlando.

Sahin, Y.M., Yetmez, M., Oktar, F.N., Gunduz, O., Agathopoulos, S., Andronescu, E., et al., 2014. Nanostructured biomaterials with antimicrobial properties. Curr. Med. Chem. 21, 3391–3404.

Sassi, M.L., Eriksen, H., Risteli, L., Niemi, S., Mansell, J., Gowen, M., et al., 2000. Immunochemical characterization of assay for carboxyterminal telopeptide of human type I collagen: loss of antigenicity by treatment with cathepsin K. Bone 26, 367–373.

Schleicher, M., Wendel, H.P., Fritze, O., Stock, U.A., 2009. *In vivo* tissue engineering of heart valves: evolution of a novel concept. Regen. Med. 4, 613–619.

Se, K.K., Niranjan, R., 2005. Enzymatic production and biological activities of chitosan oligosaccharides (COS): a review. Carbohydr. Polym. 62, 357–368.

Senel, S., McClure, S.J., 2004. Potential applications of chitosan in veterinary medicine. Adv. Drug Deliv. Rev. 56, 1467–1480.

Seo, S.J., Kim, I.Y., Choi, Y.J., Akaike, T., Cho, C.S., 2006. Enhanced liver functions of hepatocytes cocultured with NIH 3T3 in the alginate/galactosylated chitosan scaffold. Biomaterials 27, 1487–1495.

Shao, H.J., Chen, C.S., Lee, Y.T., Wang, J.H., Young, T.H., 2010. The phenotypic responses of human anterior cruciate ligament cells cultured on poly(epsilon-caprolactone) and chitosan. J. Biomed. Mater. Res. A 93A, 1297–1305.

She, Z.D., Liu, W.Q., Feng, Q.L., 2009. Self-assembly model, hepatocytes attachment and inflammatory response for silk fibroin/chitosan scaffolds. Biomed. Mater. 4.

Shu, X.Z., Liu, Y.C., Palumbo, F., Prestwich, G.D., 2003. Disulfide-crosslinked hyaluronangelatin hydrogel films: a covalent mimic of the extracellular matrix for *in vitro* cell growth. Biomater. Sci. 24 (21), 3825–3834.

Shubhra, Q.T.H., Alam, A.K.M.M., Beg, M.D.H., 2011. Mechanical and degradation characteristics of natural silk fiber reinforced gelatin composites. Mater. Lett. 65, 333–336.

Sicari, B.M., Londono, R., Badylak, S.F., 2015. Extracellular matrix as a bioscaffold for tissue engineering. Tissue Engineering. Elsevier, New York, Academic Press.

Silva, S.S., Caridade, S.G., Mano, J.F., Reis, R.L., 2013. Effect of crosslinking in chitosan/aloe vera-based membranes for biomedical applications. Carbohydr. Polym. 98, 581–588.

Silver, D., Miller, J., Harrison, R., Prockop, D.J., 1992. Helical model of nucleation and propagation to account for the growth of type I collagen fibrils from symmetrical pointed tips: a special exemple of self-assembly of rod-like monomers. Proc. Natl. Acad. Sci. U.S.A. 89, 9860–9864.

Simon, Y.T., Alok, D.S., Vashishth, D., 2008. Effects of collagen crosslinking on tissue fragility. Clin. Biomech 23, 122–123.

Simonescu, C.M., Szekely, A.C., Perniu, D., Capatina, C., 2014. Characterization and antimicrobial activity of chitosan/ZnO/Ag system. Revista De Chimie 65, 871–875.

Spoiala, A., Nedelcu, I.A., Ficai, D., Ficai, A., Andronescu, E., 2013. Zinc based antibacterial formulations for cosmetic applications. Dig. J. Nanomater. Biostruct. 8, 1235–1242.

Sunil, D., 2013. Recennt advances on Chitosan-Metal Oxide Nanoparticles and their biological application. Mater. Sci. Forum 754, 99–108.

Takahashi, T., Takayama, K., Machida, Y., Nagai, T., 1990. Characteristics of polyion complexes of chitosan with sodium alginate and sodium polyacrylate. Int. J. Pharm. 61, 35–41.

Tanaka, N., Matsumoto, I., Suzuki, M., Kaneko, M., Nitta, K., Seguchi, R., et al., 2015. Chitosan tubes can restore the function of resected phrenic nerves. Interact. Cardiovasc. Thorac. Surg. 21, 8–13.

Tang, X., Thankappan, S.K., Lee, P.W., Fard, S.E., Harmon, M.D., Tran, K., et al., 2014. Polymeric Biomaterials in Tissue Engineering and Regenerative Medicine in Natural and Synthetic Biomedical Polymers. Elsevier.

Thein-Han, W.W., Kitiyanant, Y., 2007. Chitosan scaffolds for *in vitro* buffalo embryonic stem-like cell culture: an approach to tissue engineering. J. Biomed. Mater. Res. B Appl. Biomater. 80B, 92–101.

Thein-Han, W.W., Misra, R.D.K., 2009. Biomimetic chitosan–nanohydroxyapatite composite scaffolds for bone tissue engineering. Acta Biomater. 5, 1182–1197.

Toole, B.P., 1990. Hyaluronan and its binding proteins, the hyaladherins. Curr. Opin. Cell Biol. 2, 839–844.

Torres-Giner, S., Gimenez, E., Lagarona, J.M., 2008. Characterization of the morphology and thermal properties of zein prolamine nanostructures obtained by electrospinning. Food Hydrocolloids 22, 601–614.

Trandafir, V., Popescu, G., Albu, M.G., Iovu, H., Georgescu, M. 2007. Bioproduse pe bază de colagen, Bucureşti, Editura Ars Docendi.

Udayabhanu, C.G., Nethravathi, P.C., Kumar, M.A.P., Suresh, D., Lingaraju, K., Rajanaika, H., et al., 2015. Tinospora cordifolia mediated facile green synthesis of cupric oxide nanoparticles and their photocatalytic, antioxidant and antibacterial properties. Mater. Sci. Semiconductor Process 33, 81–88.

Ueno, H., Yamada, H., Tanaka, I., Kaba, N., Matsuura, M., Okumura, M., et al., 1999. Accelerating effects of chitosan for healing at early phase of experimental open wound in dogs. Biomaterials 20, 1407–1414.

Vázquez, M.R., Ruiz, B.V., Zúñiga, R.R., Koppel, D.A.S., Olvera, L.F.Q., 2015. Chitosan and its potential use as a scaffold fortissue engineering in regenerative medicine. BioMed Res. Int.

Veis, A., Payne, K., 1988. Collagen fibrillogenesis în "Collagen Biochemistry". CRC Press, Boca Raton, FL.

Vishwakarma, A., Sharpe, P., Shi, S., Ramalingam, M., 2015. An introduction to stem cell biology and tissue engineering. In: Stem Cell Biology and Tissue Engineering in Dental Sciences.

von der Mark, K., 1981. Localization of collagen types in tissues. Int. Rev. Connect. Tissue Res. 9, 265–324.

Wang, A., Ao, Q., Cao, W., Zhao, C., Gong, Y.Z.N., Zhang, X., 2005. Fiber-based chitosan tubular scaffolds for soft tissue engineering: fabrication and *in vitro* evaluation. Tsinghua Sci. Technol. 10 (4), 449–453.

Wang, A., Ao, Q., He, Q., Gong, X., Gong, K., Gong, Y., et al., 2006a. Neural stem cell affinity of chitosan and feasibility of chitosan-based porous conduits as scaffolds for nerve tissue engineering. Tsinghua Sci. Technol. 11, 415–420.

Wang, J.Y., Chen, Y.W., Ding, Y.L., Shi, G.Q., Wan, C.X., 2008. Research of the degradation products of chitosan's angiogenic function. Appl. Surf. Sci. 255, 260–262.

Wang, M.H., Wang, X.Q., Yue, Q., Zhang, Y., Wang, C., Chen, J., et al., 2014. Templated fabrication of core–shell magnetic mesoporous carbon microspheres in 3-dimensional ordered macroporous silicas. Chem. Mater. 26, 3316–3321.

Wang, X.J., Shi, L., Tu, Q.F., Wang, H.W., Zhang, H.Y., Wang, P.R., et al., 2015. Treating cutaneous squamous cell carcinoma using ALA PLGA nanoparticle-mediated photodynamic therapy in a mouse model. Biophotonics Immune Responses X, 9324.

Wang, Y.Z., Kim, H.J., Vunjak-Novakovic, G., Kaplan, D.L., 2006b. Stem cell-based tissue engineering with silk biomaterials. Biomaterials 27, 6064–6082.

Wojcik, M., Lewandowski, W., Krol, M., Pawlowski, K., Mieczkowski, J., Lechowski, R., et al., 2015. Enhancing anti-tumor efficacy of doxorubicin by non-covalent conjugation to gold nanoparticles—*in vitro* studies on feline fibrosarcoma cell lines. PLoS One, 10.

Wood, F.M., 2014. Skin regeneration: the complexities of translation into clinical practise. Int. J. Biochem. Cell Biol. 56, 133–140.

Wu, X.M., Black, L., Santacana-Laffitte, G., Patrick, C.W., 2007. Preparation and assessment of glutaraldehyde-crosslinked collagen–chitosan hydrogels for adipose tissue engineering. J. Biomed. Mater. Res. A 81A, 59–65.

Xie, Z.W., Paras, C.B., Weng, H., Punnakitikashem, P., Su, L.C., Vu, K., et al., 2013. Dual growth factor releasing multi-functional nanofibers for wound healing. Acta Biomater. 9, 9351–9359.

Yamada, Y., Mudryj, M., de Crombrugghe, B., 1983. A uniquely conserved regulatory signal is found around the translation initiation site in three different collagen genes. J. Biol. Chem. 258, 14914–14919.

Yamashita, M., Kanemaru, S., Hirano, S., Magrufov, A., Tamaki, H., Tamura, Y., et al., 2007. Tracheal regeneration after partial resection: a tissue engineering approach. Laryngoscope 117, 497–502.

Yang, J., Woo, S.L., Yang, G.H., Wang, J.M., Cui, L., Liu, W., et al., 2010. Construction and clinical application of a human tissue-engineered epidermal membrane. Plast. Reconstr. Surg. 125, 901–909.

Yang, T.L., 2011. Chitin-based materials in tissue engineering: applications in soft tissue and epithelial organ. Int. J. Mol. Sci. 12, 1936–1963.

Yang, T.-L., Young, T.-H., 2008a. The enhancement of submandibular gland branch formation on chitosan membranes. Biomaterials 29, 2501–2508.

Yang, T.L., Young, T.H., 2008b. The enhancement of submandibular gland branch formation on chitosan membranes. Biomaterials 29, 2501–2508.

Yang, Y.M., Liu, M., Gu, Y., Lin, S.Y., Ding, F., Gu, X.S., 2009. Effect of chitooligosaccharide on neuronal differentiation of PC-12 cells. Cell Biol. Int. 33, 352–356.

Zakhem, E., Raghavan, S., Gilmont, R.R., Bitar, K.N., 2012. Chitosan-based scaffolds for the support of smooth muscle constructs in intestinal tissue engineering. Biomaterials 33, 4810–4817.

Zamarioli, C.M., Martinsh, R.M., Carvalho, E.C., Freitas, L.A.P., 2015. Nanoparticles containing curcuminoids (*Curcuma longa*): development of topical delivery formulation. Rev. Bras. Farmacognosia-Braz. J. Pharma. 25, 53–60.

Zhang, D., Zhou, W., Wei, B., Wang, X., Tang, R.P., Nie, J.M., et al., 2015. Carboxyl-modified poly(vinyl alcohol)-crosslinked chitosan hydrogel films for potential wound dressing. Carbohydr. Polym. 125, 189–199.

Zhang, L., Ao, Q., Wang, A.J., Lu, G.Y., Kong, L.J., Gong, Y.D., et al., 2006a. A sandwich tubular scaffold derived from chitosan for blood vessel tissue engineering. J. Biomed. Mater. Res. A 77A, 277–284.

Zhang, L., Gao, Y., Kong, L., Gong, Y., Zhao, N., Zhang, X., 2006b. Compatibility of chitosan–gelatin films with adipose tissue derived stromal cells. Tsinghua Sci. Technol. 7, 421–426.

Zhao, L., Chang, J., 2004. Preparation and characterization of macroporous chitosan/wollastonite composite scaffolds for tissue engineering. J. Mater. Sci. Mater. Med. 15, 625–629.

Zhao, L., Chang, J., Zhai, W.Y., 2009. Preparation and HL-7702 cell functionality of titania/chitosan composite scaffolds. J. Mater. Sci. Mater. Med. 20, 949–957.

Zhao, L.M., Shi, L.E., Zhang, Z.L., Chen, J.M., Shi, D.D., Yang, J., et al., 2011. Preparation and application of chitosan nanoparticles and nanofibers. Braz. J. Chem. Eng. 28, 353–362.

Zhou, N., Zan, X.L., Wang, Z., Wu, H., Yin, D.K., Liao, C.Y., et al., 2013. Galactosylated chitosan–polycaprolactone nanoparticles for hepatocyte-targeted delivery of curcumin. Carbohydr. Polym. 94, 420–429.

Zhu, C.H., Fan, D.D., Duan, Z.Z., Xue, W.J., Shang, L.A., Chen, F.L., et al., 2009. Initial investigation of novel human-like collagen/chitosan scaffold for vascular tissue engineering. J. Biomed. Mater. Res. A 89A, 829–840.

CHAPTER

14 Tissue engineering: use of electrospinning technique for recreating physiological functions

Vaishali Bambole[1] and Jatinder Vir Yakhmi[2]

[1]*Department of Physics, University of Mumbai, Santacruz (E), Mumbai, India*

[2]*HomiBhabha National Institute (DAE), Mumbai, India*

LIST OF ABBREVIATIONS

BCP	Biphasic calcium phosphate
BG	Bioactive glass
CP	Calcium phosphate
ECM	Extracellular matrix
HA	Hyaluronic acid
HAP	Hydroxyapatite
HMW	High molecular weight
LDI	Lysine diisocyanate
PAA	Poly(acrylic acid)
PAam	Polyacrylamide
PANi	Polyaniline
PAN-MA	Polyacrlonitrile-co-Methyacrylate
PBT	Polybutylene terephthalate
PCA	Polycyanoacrylate
PCL	Poly(ε-caprolactone)
PCLTMC	Poly(caprolactone-co-trimethylene carbonate)
PDLLA	Poly(DL-lactide)
PDLLA-CL	Poly(D,L-lactide-co-caprolactone)
PDMAEM	Poly(dimethylaminoethylmethacrylate hydrochloride)
PDMS	Polydimethylsiloxane
PDO	Polydioxanone
PEDOT	Polyethylene Dioxy Thiophene
PEE	Poly(ether ester)
PEG	Poly(ethylene glycol)
PEO	Poly(ethylene oxide)
PEU	Poly(ester urethane)

Nanobiomaterials in Soft Tissue Engineering. DOI: http://dx.doi.org/10.1016/B978-0-323-42865-1.00014-3

PEVA	Poly(ethylene-co-vinylacetate)
PGA	Polyglycolide
PGCL	Poly(glycolide-co-ε-caprolactone)
PGS	Polyglycerol Sebacate
PHA	Polyhydroxyalkanoates
PHBHV	Poly(3-hydroxybutyrate)3-hydroxyvalerate
PHEMA	Polyhydroxy Ethyl Methacrylate
PLA	Polylactide
PLAGA	Poly(lactic acid-glycolic acid)
PLCL	Poly(l-lactide-co-caprolactone)
PLDLA	Poly-L/D-lactide
PLGA	Poly(l-lactide-co-glycolide)
PLLA	Poly(L-lactic acid)
PLLA-CL	Poly(l-lactide-co-ε-caprolactone)
PMMA	Polymethylmethacrylate
PNIPAAm	Poly(N-isopropylacrylamide)
POE	Poly(ortho ester)
PP	Polypropylene
PPF	Poly(propylene fumarate)
PPy	Polypyrrole
PS	Polysulfone
PTFE	Polytetrafluoroethylene
PTMC	Poly(trimethylene carbonate)
PU	Polyurethane
PVA	Polyvinyl alcohol
TCP	Tricalcium phosphate
TCP	Tricalcium phosphate

14.1 INTRODUCTION

The science of bionanotechnology is all-pervasive and promises a sustainable alternative for restoring and recreating physiological functions with a "systems approach" comprising of structural and functional forms. Bionanotechnology spans several disciplines such as physical sciences, molecular engineering, biotechnology, nanotechnology, chemistry, and medicine. It takes advantage of the knowledge of features acquired by living organisms in the course of evolution for technological purposes. It derives inspiration from human physiology to evolve complex artificial systems, through the fusion of biological systems with nanotechnology.

The central concept of bionanotechnology is to design molecular machinery to atomic specifications. Micro-observational studies of the cells reveal atomically precise molecule-sized motors, girders, random access memory, sensors, and a host of other useful mechanisms, all ready to be harnessed by bionanotechnology. The technology for designing and constructing these machines/devices in bulk is fully developed for medical therapeutics applications worldwide (Goodsell,

2004). Bionanotechnology applies the concept and techniques of molecular biology to engineering objectives, fabricating devices at the nanoscale, thus giving us the ability to mimic biological structures with molecular-level precision.

The relevance of bionanotechnology lies in the emergence of "artificial organs" fabricated from the cells of patients' own bodies. Although synthetic materials have served as implants in the past, they have their own limitations in terms of supply, sustainability, feasibility, and compatibility. For example, the current average lifespan of an orthopedic implant is only 15–20 years. Similarly, the functional integrity of valvular grafts for the cardiovascular system degrades gradually over a decade. The compatibility of a kidney transplant may be compromised in situations where blood groups do not match. Artificial organs produced from nanobiomaterials are a promising alternative, not just because of the ability of nanobiomaterials to simulate dimensions of proteins that comprise tissues, but also because of their higher reactivity for interactions of proteins that control cell adhesion and, thus providing an ability to regenerate tissues—also called "tissue engineering" (TE).

TE at the nanoscale has evolved to develop viable substitutes, which can restore, maintain, or improve the function of human tissue. The science of tissue engineering thus holds the promise to replace conventional treatments like organ transplants or artificial implants. Although patients suffering from disease and injured organs may be treated with transplanted organs, there is a severe shortage of donor organs that is worsening year after years, given the increasing proportion of the geriatric age-group in the population. Scientists in the field of regenerative medicine and tissue engineering apply the principles of cell transplantation, material science, and bioengineering to construct biological substitutes that will restore and maintain normal function in diseased and injured tissues. TE can provide definitive solutions for the development of *in vitro* and *in vivo* tissue regeneration. Regeneration of a healthy tissue can be achieved by using nanobiomaterials to convey signals to surrounding tissues for recruiting cells that promote inherent regeneration or by using cells or nanobiomaterials with scaffolds to act as a framework for developing tissue.

Nanomaterials such as nanofibers plays a vital role in tissue engineering. Three different approaches toward the formation of nanofibrous materials have emerged; namely self-assembly, phase separation, and electrospinning. Each of these approaches can lead to the development of a scaffolding system, for example, self-assembly can generate small-diameter nanofibers in the lowest end of natural extracellular matrix (ECM) collagen while electrospinning is more useful in generating large-diameter nanofibers at the upper end of the range of natural ECM collagen. Phase separation on the other hand generates nanofibers in the same range as natural ECM collagen and allows for design of macropore structures (Reisner, 2009). Electrospinning is a laboratory-based technique yielding uninterrupted fibers of diameters ranging from submicrometers to nanometers. This technique is easily adaptable and facilitates easy customization in the setup design. The properties of these fibers depend upon the physical variables, notably, applied potential, the distance between the two electrodes and the viscosity of the solution. Scaffolds are pivotal structures wherein cells are often implanted or seeded into an artificial structure capable of supporting three-dimensional (3D) tissue formations both *in vitro* and *in vivo*. It can also simulate intracellular and extracellular milieu influencing the microenvironments of the cells.

TE finds immediate application in recreation of bone, liver, nerve grafts, cartilage, retina, heart, pancreas, and blood vessels. A great deal of research findings are already implemented in skin diseases, cancers, and drug delivery.

Another new horizon, which has also opened up, is that of providing creative insights for evolving various *in vitro* human models contributing to artificial life in recreation of human physiology. These would facilitate identification and comprehension of the factors that drive cellular processes. The complex system that constitutes the cellular microenvironment needs to be differentiated into its chemical, mechanical, and physical factors and studied in detail so as to recreate such *in vitro* human models (Sala et al., 2013). Additionally, diseases such as cardiac arrhythmia (Thompson et al., 2012), skin fibrosis (Moulin, 2013) and wound healing (Bellas et al., 2012; Krishnan et al., 2012; Van den Broek et al., 2012; Li et al., 2013), blood–brain barrier (Lippmann et al., 2013), and mammary gland development (Wang et al., 2010) need to be immediately addressed applying the principles of TE. TE is still in its nascent stage and faces inherent critical challenges. Some important challenges are maintaining a high surface-to-volume ratio, continued cell sustainability, easy accessibility, matching macro- and microenvironments, with host cells and preventing collapse of the scaffolds.

14.2 TISSUE ENGINEERING

14.2.1 CONCEPTS AND APPLICATIONS

According to Langer and Vacanti (1993), TE is defined as "the application of principles and methods of engineering and life sciences toward fundamental understanding of structure–function relationships in normal and pathological mammalian tissues and the development of biological substitutes to restore, maintain, or improve tissue function."

In other words, TE is the restoration of pathologically damaged tissues/body organs using artificially designed biological substitutes prepared by applying the principles of physiology, engineering, and life sciences. It is thus an emerging interdisciplinary field which can be referred to as applied physiology or regenerative medicine, with an aim to prepare viable substitutes for restoration, maintenance, and improvement of tissue functionality. This may also be applied to phenomena outside the body such as construction of tissue for *in vitro* experimentation.

TE typically involves the culturing of living human cells, usually in a biocompatible polymer constituting to a scaffold, *ex vivo* and subsequently allowing them to develop into a 3D tissue. TE is poised to revolutionize the methods we adopt to improve human health and the quality of life of millions of people worldwide, by restoring, maintaining, or enhancing tissue and organ function. It holds the phenomenal ability to accurately mimic the natural physiological conditions of a tissue, native to a particular organ as well as living cells in a variety of ways. This fundamental ability happens to be the answer to why tissue engineering finds a variety of applications in regenerative medicine for either therapeutic or diagnostic applications. The tissue-engineered medical therapies have proved to be life-saving and have improved the quality of life in countless numbers of patients. Besides having therapeutic applications, where the tissue is either grown inside or outside the patient's body and transplanted, TE can have diagnostic applications where the tissue is made *in vitro* and used for testing drug metabolism and uptake, toxicity, and pathogenicity. These diagnostic applications of tissue engineering thus evolve as a set of biomedical parameters which would prove critical not only for the study of human physiology and physiopathology but also contributing to toxicology, medical devices, tissue replacement, repair, and regeneration.

Nevertheless, the challenges associated with TE need to be addressed judiciously. For example, in organ transplants the prevalence of transplant rejection and lack of donors to cover the worldwide demand is very well documented. Moreover, mechanical devices show restricted abilities to restore entire functions of a tissue or an organ and thus fail to prevent progressive deterioration in patients. Similarly, surgical reconstruction can result in unforeseen long-term problems due to complexity in human life (Lalan et al., 2001). Therefore, TE evolves from the need to provide more sustainable definitive solutions to tissue repair in medical sciences.

TE research comprises of extensive investigations on the following:

1. *Biomaterials*: These include novel materials that are systematically pharmacologically inert, which can be utilized in combinations of substances for implantation or incorporation within a living system to supplement or replace the functions of living organs or tissue.

   During the process of formation of functional tissue these biomaterials play an important role in growth and differentiation of cells by providing both physical and chemical cues. The examples of biological cues are cell adhesive ligands which enhance attachments. The examples of physical cues are the topography that influences the cell morphology and alignment.
2. *Cells*: Includes the techniques for controlling proliferation and differentiation of cells to specific phenotypes, determination of the appropriate cell type, identification of appropriate sources of cell such as autologous cells, allogeneic cells, xenogenic cells, stem cells, genetically engineered cells, isolation, purification, and cultivation techniques, and immunological manipulation.

3. *Biomolecules*: Includes stimulation of growth and differentiation, different ways of application, regulation of activity, growth factors (GFs), differentiation factors, angiogenic factors, hormones, bones, morphogenic hormones, iRNA, etc.
4. *Engineering design aspects*: Includes a range of different specifically designed bioreactors to culture the cells into 2D expansions, 3D tissue growth, seeding and implantation, vascularization, and finally tissue preservation and shipping.
5. *Biomedical aspects of design*: Includes identification of properties of native tissues, design of adequate scaffolds, and selection of adequate materials and routes to process them, identification of minimum properties required of engineered tissues such as porosity, interconnectivity, hydrophilicity, surface characteristics, mechanical signals regulating engineered tissues, use of animal models to test for therapeutic effect, and safety of engineered tissue.
6. *Informatics to support TE*: Includes standardization of experimental data, integration into a centralized database, use of data-mining tools such as artificial neural networks and decision trees, which can predict the results of tissue engineering strategies, development of algorithms, validation of efficacy with animal experiments, gene and protein sequencing and analysis, cellular image analysis, cell modeling, digital tissue manufacturing, and clinical informatics. Finally, all the related ethical issues especially those pertaining to use of stem cell and animal studies.

14.2.2 PRINCIPLE OF TISSUE ENGINEERING

TE is a five-step process: (i) Removal (isolation) of cells, (ii) expansion of number of culture through cell cultivation and proliferation, (iii) seeding into appropriate scaffolds with GFs, (iv) placing into culture (*in vitro*), and (v) re-implantation of engineered tissue into the body (Figure 14.1).

14.2.3 TISSUE ENGINEERING TRIAD

The combination of cells, growth-stimulating signals, and scaffolds is often referred to as the "tissue engineering triad." When cells are amassed into a complex formation, such as a whole organ, they must create systems for the nutrients' transportation, growth regulation, and other processes. The growth-stimulating signals include GFs such as morphogenes and regulatory biomolecules to speed up the regulation of tissues. The proliferation and differentiation of cells is regulated by morphogenes and scaffolds serve as a carrier and delivery system for the morphogenes and simultaneously produce and influence the microenvironment (Lyons et al., 2010). Scaffolds that are made up of biocompatible polymeric materials provide the structural framework to support the cell adhesion and cell growth, finally leading to tissue development. Figure 14.2 describes the tissue engineering triad factors that needs to be considered while designing a suitable structure for tissue engineering applications.

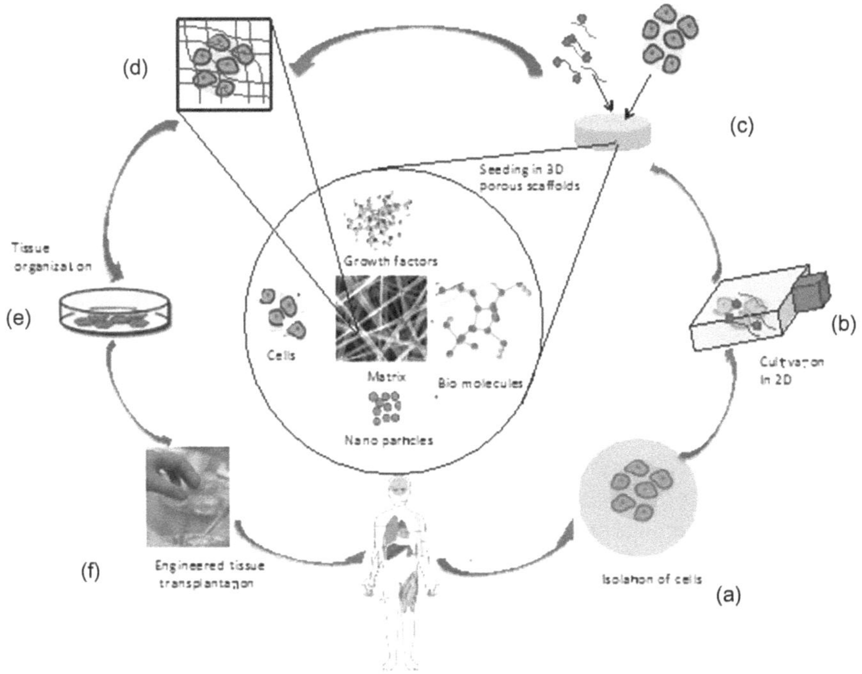

FIGURE 14.1

Principles of tissue engineering.

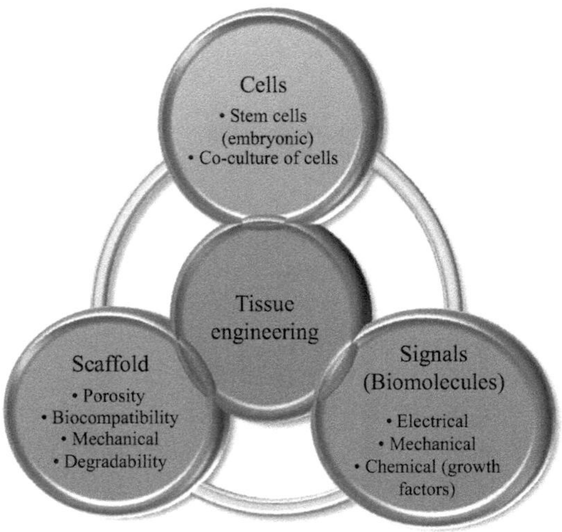

FIGURE 14.2

The tissue engineering triad.

14.2.3.1 Cells

Selection of the most appropriate source of cells is a strategic decision while designing tissue-engineered materials. The selected cells should fulfill a basic criterion, that is, they should integrate themselves in the specific tissue and secrete various GFs and cytokines, activating the endogenous tissue regeneration program.

In this process, a donor tissue source is disintegrated into singular cells, which can either be directly seeded into the host matrix or expanded in scaffold-supported culture and then reimplanted into the host. The source of donor tissue can either be heterologous, allogeneic, or autologous. Of these, the autologous cells are most preferred since this avoids rejection and the deleterious side effects of immunosuppressive medications. However, in terminally ill patients, there are not enough normal cells available for growth and proliferation. In such circumstances, pluripotent human embryonic stem cells (ESCs) or adult stem cells (ASCs) are a feasible option since they possess the ability to self-renew while maintaining the proliferative potential. However, the use of ESCs is highly restricted due to ethical controversies and their potential to produce teratomas. On the other hand, ASCs are multipotent, undifferentiated cells and can be identified mainly in brain, bone marrow (Clifford et al., 2012), blood vessels, skeletal muscles, skin, teeth, heart, gut, liver, ovarian epithalamus, testis, and umbilical cord (Weber et al., 2011). Induced pluripotent stem cells (iPSCs), which were first generated by Yamanaka and collaborators (Takahashi and Yamanaka, 2006) from mouse fibroblasts, are also being derived from adult human cells (Takahashi et al., 2006; Yu, 2007). iPSCs characteristically exhibit autologous character, differentiation capacity, robustness, and simplicity of reprogramming procedure.

14.2.3.1.1 Cell culture

Human tissues have a natural inherent healing capacity, when injured. A tissue when injured triggers complex biochemical mechanisms within the body systems, which initiates the process of tissue repair instantly. The entire repair is aided by active participation of all concerned tissues, cells, and immune bodies. Tissue damage (e.g., severe burns)/diseases (cardiomyopathy) or mechanical injuries can be fatal, while in some immune-compromised patients there may be permanent damage leading to organ failure. There is a significant shortage of organs available for transplantation. At times the damage to the tissue is nonsevere and there is a partial lack of organ functionality. The patient condition in such cases is not life-threatening and may not require an organ transplant, but these conditions have a high impact on the patient's quality of life and constitute a source of high cost over a period of time. Organ rejections due to incompatibility and ethical issues are additional considerations in this regard. Tissue regeneration or transplantation therapies then offer a solution to such challenging situations. This requires a donor tissue source from animals (heterologous), or the same species but different individuals (allogeneic), or from the same individual (autologous). Amongst the donor tissue sources, autologous cell sources are most suitable as they are immunocompatible. Therefore, regeneration of cells using bionanotechnology emerges as a cost-effective solution (Chester and Atala, 2004). Thus, growth of cells *in vitro* leads to creation of functional tissues promoting survival and growth of the organ or the body system. This mechanism, known as "cell culture" is influenced by factors such as pH, humidity, temperature, availability of oxygen, and maintenance of osmotic pressure. Cells are grown and maintained at an appropriate temperature and gas mixture (typically 37 °C, 5% CO_2 for mammalian cells) in a cell incubator. Culture conditions vary widely for each cell type, and variation of conditions for a particular cell type can result in different phenotypes. In TE, a 3D cell culture where cells assume a more natural morphology and physiology replaces the traditional cell culture technology. The sustainability of these cell cultures often requires booster components such as hormones, GFs, micronutrients, chemical and physical stimuli, which can be accomplished in a "bioreactor."

14.2.3.1.2 Bioreactors in tissue engineering

A system that attempts to simulate a physiological environment for creating and preconditioning of cells for tissues *in vitro*, is known as a bioreactor. Bioreactors are designed for facilitation of tissue culture in a controlled, environmentally monitored state, which ensures total simulation of organ growth as in the human body. This is achieved by various processes, chemical as well as biological, which are carried out in a vessel in an anaerobic or aerobic condition involving organisms or biochemical substances exuded from these organisms. The growth and productivity of the organisms is controlled by monitoring the environmental conditions inside the bioreactor, such as temperature, nutrient concentrations, pH, and dissolved gases (e.g., oxygen for aerobic fermentations). The scaffolds around the growing tissue must be able to maintain a constant flow of the nutrients and subsequent waste exchange.

There are numerous types of bioreactors in use which include: (i) perfusion bioreactors, (ii) rotary wall bioreactors, (iii) spinner flask bioreactors, (iv) controlled mechanics bioreactors, and (v) hollow-fiber bioreactors (Figure 14.3). Bioreactors rely on forced media flow through and/or around the scaffold to provide nutrient and waste exchange within the scaffold. Scaffolds are suspended in a medium due to opposing gravitational and drag forces and the medium is stirred using a magnetic stirrer to improve nutrient delivery to the scaffold.

14.2.3.2 Biomolecules

A biomolecule, for the purposes of TE, is any signaling molecule that is present in living organisms, including large macromolecules such as proteins, polysaccharides, lipids, and nucleic acids, as well as small molecules such as primary metabolites, secondary metabolites, and natural products. It can also be components present in the cellular milieu, in which the presence and gradient of

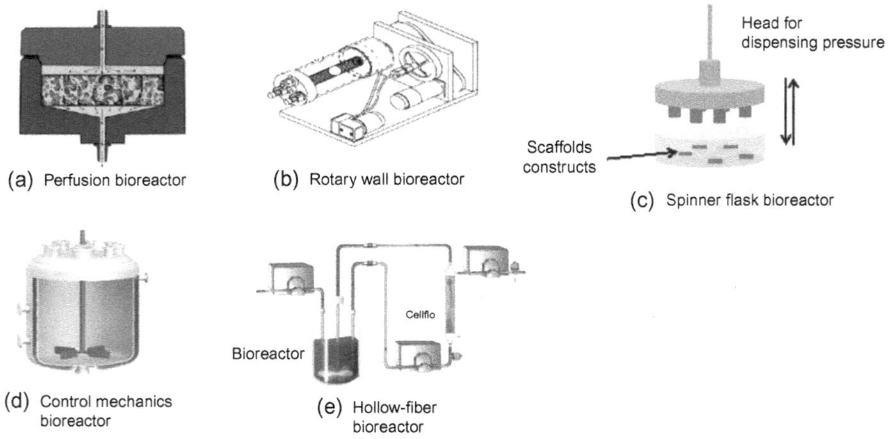

FIGURE 14.3

Types of bioreactors.

soluble factors such as GFs, chemokines, and cytokines play an important role in biological phenomena such as chemotaxis, morphogenesis, and wound healing. The regulatory biomolecules, such as GFs and cytokines, may be targeted at a particular cell to carry out a specific reaction (e.g., proliferation and differentiation). Many types of cells, such as endocrine, autocrine, juxtacrine, or intracrine, paracine, release regulatory biomolecules. In many cases, GF is used as a synonym for cytokines and describes factors associated with those cells that are involved in the immune system. A GF binding to target cells generates a "cellular signal" that reaches the nucleus, in turn producing a biological response. In particular these signals are tightly controlled and unique to each organ. In TE such signaling should stimulate the controlled proliferation and proper differentiation of the seeded cells in the scaffolds. Additionally it should also enhance the migration, differentiation, and proliferation of cells from the edges to the treated defects. Thus GFs have two important functions. First is to optimize tissue-engineered cell-scaffold *in vitro* and second to improve their integration and performance *in vivo*. In a nutshell, the function of a biomolecule is to regenerate damaged tissue and develop *in vitro* human models. This has regenerative implications in bone, cartilage, pancreas, and vascular TE.

14.2.3.3 Scaffolds

Scaffolds are analogous of naturally existing ECM present in human tissue. These are typically made of polymeric biomaterials which replicate the functions as well as the microenvironment of the ECM. They are biologically active and provide physical and structural support to the cells, serving as a matrix, so that the cells can attach themselves, proliferate, and differentiate. It thus supports neo-tissue genesis and ECM deposition (Ma et al., 2008; Holzwarth and Ma, 2011; Liu et al., 2012b). The main role of scaffold is regeneration and repair of the tissues. In TE, scaffolds can either be derived from the natural source, like human or animal tissue, or it can be synthetically made from biocompatible polymers. Scaffolds, which are polymeric, are made up of network of nanofibers which can be designed to match the optimum characteristics of the natural ECM, in terms of their strength, geometry, porosity, rate of degradation, the microenvironment, and the ease with which it can be reproduced in the laboratory. This network serves as an instructive background to signal and guide cell behavior (Liao et al., 2006; Jiang et al., 2010).

In TE strategies, porous 3D biodegradable scaffolds evolve into a template for tissue formation hosting the regenerative tissue. This template is then impregnated with isolated healthy cells along with the stimulant factors such as growth hormones, or biophysical, mechanical, and chemical triggers from the bioreactors. This brings about biological cohesion of the cells leading to maturation and subsequent regeneration of the tissue (Du and Yarema, 2010).

14.2.3.3.1 ECM and scaffolds—an analogy

Almost all cells in the human body, other than the blood cells, anchor themselves in a semisolid matrix called the ECM. The ECM characteristics and features are different in different tissues. Their main role is to provide a medium which supports the mechanical and biochemical functions of the growing tissue. By virtue of these functions, tissue obtains its mechanical characteristics in terms of rigidity, flexibility, elasticity, and tensile strength. Furthermore, it also provides a medium for facilitating intra- and intercellular electrolyte and nutrient exchange, monitoring the fluid dynamics of the tissue, which is essential for physiological function. It also acts as a source of biochemical stimulants, such as GFs and other hormones. It inherently has regenerative properties, wherein it mortifies so as to allow neogenesis, vascularization, and restructuring of cells. Therefore, the major challenge in TE is to design and fabricate a suitable scaffold to mimic functions analogous to those of the native ECM. Scaffolds are a fabricated "replica," which fosters cell attachment and migration, and diffusion of biochemical factors and nutrients. Thus, scaffolds for an engineered tissue are expected to acquire the microenvironment of the target tissue in its physiological state (Chan and Leong, 2008).

In order to obtain successful synergy between the cells and scaffolds a number of design parameters need to be considered such as the interconnectivity, mechanical strength, porosity, surface properties, density of cells, different filler materials, permeability, confinements, mechanical strength, and geometric properties which affect the transport of oxygen and nutrients throughout the tissue scaffolds. The scaffolds should simulate the appropriate biomechanical, biochemical, and biophysical cues which help the cell's maintenance, function, proliferation, and differentiation (Batorsky et al., 2005). The closely selected highly porous nanostructure offers suitable anchorage to the cell along with a 3D microenvironment which helps in regulating transport of ions and molecules. Biophysical and biochemical signals contribute fundamentally by facilitating the seeding of GFs, enzymes, ions, and molecules called the "binding effect." These signals control the diffusion, local concentration of molecules, ions, and nutrients, maintaining the balance of the electrolytes for normal metabolic activity. It also stimulates recognition by cellular adhesion receptors. As a result the ECM integrates itself with the intracellular signaling pathways. As a consequence the cell generates mechanical signals. A "mechano-transduction" phenomenon thus produces a chemical signal, which leads directly to cell differentiation (Broom and Poole, 1982; Borschel et al., 2005; Brodie et al., 2005).

Regardless of the tissue type, an ideally mimicked tissue-engineered scaffold should satisfy the following requirements:

1. *Biocompatibility*: The scaffold should be biocompatible and biodegradable. The cells must function normally, adhere and migrate onto the surface, and begin to proliferate before laying down the new matrix. The construct must not give any immune reaction leading to rejection by the body.
2. *Biodegradability*: Since the scaffolds are not intended to be permanent implants, they must therefore degrade themselves and their debris should be nontoxic and able to exit the body without interfering with other organs.
3. *Clinical compliance*: The scaffold must be clinically compliant, satisfying good manufacturing practices (GMP) to ensure successful translation of tissue-engineering strategies to the clinic.
4. *Mechanical properties*: The scaffold architecture should be consistent and compatible with the native anatomical site into which it is to be implanted. A critical balance between the mechanical integrity and high porosity to allow cell infiltration and vascularization has to be achieved for the successful scaffold architecture. A highly porous architecture with interconnected pore structure facilitates diffusion of nutrients to the cells seeded in the scaffolds. It provides channels for the diffusion of the waste products out of the scaffolds without interfering with other organs and surrounding tissue.

A scaffold for TE can be categorized as natural polymer-based and synthetic polymer-based depending upon its origin.

Natural polymer-based scaffolds: These make use of collagen, alginate, chitosan, and various proteoglycans for producing scaffolds. The specific advantage to using them in scaffold design is that they are biodegradable, biologically active, and promote excellent cell growth, adhesion, and migration. The limitations that they offer are poor mechanical strength (poor load-bearing capacity in orthopedic applications). When natural polymers are of specific animal origin, their composition, isolation, and purification offer a major challenge for assay reproduction (Adams and Roughley, 2006; Chan et al., 2007a, 2007b, 2007c).

Synthetic polymer-based scaffolds: Commonly used synthetic polymers for scaffold architecture are poly-L-lactic acid (PLLA), polyglycolic acid (PGA), polystyrene, and poly-DL-lactic-co-glycolic acid (PLGA). These can be custom-tailored to mimic specific ECM properties thereby providing controlled cellular environment. They have some limitations due to low bioactivity. They are susceptible to rejection and some of these (e.g., PLLA and PGA) degrade by hydrolysis by releasing CO_2 gas which lowers the local pH resulting in cell and tissue neurosis. The challenges in evolving both natural and synthetic scaffolds are formidable in nature. Scaffolds thus present inherent limitations unless we are able to recreate an analogous physiological matrix environment, until then scaffolds only serve to hold and guide cells in 3D space (Chang et al., 1992; Chan et al., 2005; Adams and Roughley, 2006).

14.2.4 SCAFFOLDING TECHNIQUES IN TISSUE ENGINEERING

There are four major techniques of scaffold synthesis in TE, namely: (i) implanting cell-seeded premade porous scaffolds; (ii) implanting cell-seeded decellularized allograft or xenograft ECM; (iii) implanting laminated cell sheets with secreted ECM; and (iv) injecting cell encapsulated self-assembled hydrogels (Chan and Leong, 2008; Figure 14.4).

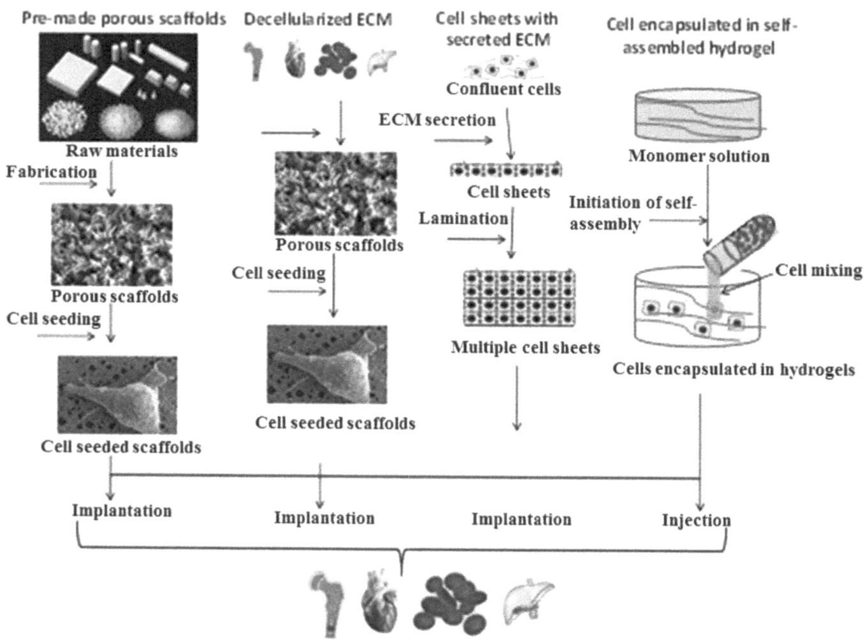

FIGURE 14.4

Different scaffolding approaches in tissue engineering.

14.2.4.1 Types of scaffolding techniques in tissue engineering

14.2.4.1.1 Pre-made porous scaffolds for cell seeding

Porous scaffolds are developed from natural or synthetic biomaterials. Naturally occurring biomaterials can be obtained from natural sources and include polysaccharides, polynucleotides, and lipids. They possess several advantages over synthetic biomaterials which include biocompatibility, biodegradability, and remodeling (Hubbell, 1995; Kim et al., 2000; Ratner and Bryant, 2004), but their load-bearing capacity is limited which can be improved by forming a composite with synthetic material and crosslinking (Chan et al., 2005, 2007a, 2007b, 2007c; Ifkovits and Burdick, 2007). Scaffold can also be allografts and/or xenograft-derived ECM, or can be in the form of small building blocks, which include inorganic ceramics such as calcium phosphates. Synthetic biomaterials, with better-controlled physical and mechanical properties, include inorganic substances like bioglasses, or organic substances, such as synthetic polymers. These can be used to tailor both soft and hard tissues; however, the difference in their structure and composition in comparison to the native tissue contributes to its antigenicity, thus limiting their capacity to remodel a tissue.

Porous scaffolds which balance cellular functions and allow better biopermeability are fabricated by various methods. These are: (i) use of porogenic materials in solid (e.g., sodium chloride), liquid (e.g., water), or gaseous (e.g., carbon dioxide) forms; (ii) solid free form using approaches based on computer-aided design (CAD) or rapid prototyping (RP) technologies; and (iii) techniques, mainly electrospinning, generating woven or nonwoven fibers (Chevalier et al., 2008). A porous scaffold can thus be formed by processing and eliminating porogens by sublimation, evaporation, and melting. Solvent casting and particulate leaching, gas foaming, freeze-drying, and phase separation are practical examples of such processes (Yang et al., 2002). Hierarchical porous structures can be formed by creating libraries of unit cells based on mathematical models aided by software (image-based design or CAD) (Hollister, 2005). Selective laser sintering, wax printing, stereo lithography, fused deposition modeling, bioplotter, and 3D printing are solid free-form fabrication technologies (Dhariwala et al., 2004; Hutmacher et al., 2004; Hollister, 2005). In another technique, woven and nonwoven fibers crosslink to form interpenetrating network structures using thermal energy or adhesives (Hutmacher et al., 2004). Electrospinning-generated nanofibers as well as microfibers are morphological mimics of fibrous elements of the ECM. Here a high voltage drives the polymer solution to emerge as a spinning fiber jet (Yang et al., 2002; Hollister, 2005; Chew et al., 2006, 2008a, 2008b; Pham et al., 2006; Chai and Leong, 2007; Dang and Leong, 2007; Bambole et al., 2010). Porous scaffolding techniques are, particularly, applicable to regenerate skeletal muscle structures intended for load-bearing functions in the human body. However, the mechanical strength compromises the penetrating ability of the cells. The drawbacks associated with this technique are time-consuming postfabrication cell seeding, low cell viability, and high cost. These drawbacks can be overruled by supplementing the fabrication technique with the process of agitation, perfusion, and enlarging the pore size.

14.2.4.1.2 Decellularized ECM from allogenic or xenogenic tissues for cell seeding

Decellularized ECM is synthesized from allogenic or xenogenic tissues by eliminating cellular antigens while preserving natural ECM components. For decellularization, allogenic, or xenogenic tissues are subjected to sequential physical and enzymatic treatments followed by treatment with appropriate detergents. Physical treatments such as freeze–thaw cycles or using ionic solutions such as hypo- or hypertonic solutions lyse the cells, whereas enzymatic treatment using trypsin/EDTA (Ethylene Diamine Tetraacytic Acid) separates the cellular components from the ECM. Solubilization and removal of cytoplasmic and nuclear cellular components is finally achieved by the use of appropriate detergents.

Optimization of process parameters during decellularization is very much essential whilst maintaining biochemical composition and mechanical properties. With the help of this scaffolding approach, heart valves (Knight et al., 2008), vessels (Borschel et al., 2005), nerves (Hall, 1997), tendons, and ligaments (Ingram et al., 2007) have been created. Researchers have documented the use of this approach to replace damaged analogous structural tissue, for example, use of decellularized blood vessels as allogenic vascular grafts (Batorsky et al., 2005; Borschel et al., 2005), which were well tolerated immunologically.

14.2.4.1.3 Cell sheets with self-secreted ECM

"Cell sheet engineering" comprises of cells that are cultured, until confluent, on thermoresponsive polymer, such as a poly(*N*-isopropylacrylamide)-coated culture dish. These cells, which secrete their own ECM upon confluence, are then detached by thermally regulating the hydrophobicity of the polymer coatings, without enzymatic treatment. Recently, thermosensitive chitosan has been investigated for its potential to prepare an aligned cell sheet (Dang and Leong, 2007). Such an approach can be repeated to obtain thicker matrix from multiple single-cell layers (Takezawa et al., 1990; Okano et al., 1993, 1995) and works excellently for epithelium, endothelium, and cell-dense tissues (Tsuda et al., 2007; Yang et al., 2007b), however, it renders difficulty in constructing thick tissues, as each layer is around 30 μm thick; although this proves less practical clinically due to the unlikely nature of multiple surgeries in patients and therefore, the need for preformed patches.

The cell sheet engineering approach has been utilized in the development and use of cornea (Nishida et al., 2004) in clinical trials and myocardium (Shimizu et al., 2003) in preclinical trials.

14.2.4.1.4 Cell encapsulation in self-assembled hydrogel matrix

In this method, living cells are entrapped either into a semipermeable membrane or within a homogeneous solid mass and thus are encapsulated. It can either be an injectable system where cells remain suspended in a liquid precursor solution and dispensed *in vivo* at the target site (Uludag et al., 2000; Orive et al., 2003, 2004) or a macromolecular precursor forming a gelatinous system. The most commonly used biomaterials for encapsulation are hydrogels. These hydrogels are elastic and rigid like tissue with crosslinking ability forming meshwork which can retain liquids. They dilate yet remain insoluble in water. These can be easily formed by covalent or ionic crosslinking of (a) water-soluble polymers such as polyvinylalcohol (PVA) (which are UV crosslinked) (Iwata et al., 1990), (b) biopolymers such as collagen, fibrin, polysaccharides derived from algae, such as sodium alginate (Batorsky et al., 2005), chitosan (Zielinski and Aebischer, 1994), and (c) synthetic materials such as poly(ethylene glycol) (PEG) (Nuttelman et al., 2005).

This technique has been advantageously used in xenogenic pancreatic cell transplantation for diabetes (Lanza et al., 1996; Gray, 2001). Applications for other disorders such as central nervous system insufficiency (Orive et al., 2003) and liver failure (hepatocytes and hematopoietic cells) (Chang et al., 1992) are also reported. In spite of their clinical relevance, the poor mechanical properties of the hydrogel materials limit its use for tissues with load-bearing functions (Chan and Leong, 2008).

The key scaffold characteristics can be tailored to suit an application by careful selection of polymers, additional scaffold components, and the fabrication technique. Typical scaffold designs have included meshes, fibers, sponges, and foams. This methodology promotes uniform cell distribution, diffusion of nutrients, and the growth of organized cell communities.

The fabrication technique for TE scaffolds (Dhandayuthapani et al., 2011) depends almost entirely on the bulk and surface properties of the material and the proposed function of the scaffold. Most techniques involve the application of heat and/or pressure to the polymer or dissolving it in an organic solvent to mold the material into its desired shape. While each method presents distinct advantages and disadvantages, the appropriate technique must be selected to meet the requirements for the specific type of tissue. Table 14.1 provides insights into the biomimicking process, highlighting different scaffold fabrication techniques.

14.2.5 A BRIEF OVERVIEW OF SCAFFOLD FABRICATION TECHNIQUES

The multidisciplinary field of tissue engineering is aimed at regenerating damaged tissue by the combination of cells from the body being seeded in highly porous, biomaterial "scaffolds." This functions as a template for regenerated tissue so as to guide the growth of newly developed tissue. Structurally, it should facilitate vascularization, development of new tissue, remodeling to support integration with host tissue after implantation. The natural or synthetic biomaterials used

Table 14.1 Insights into Bio-Mimicking Process: Different Scaffolds Fabrication Techniques

Types of Tissue	Methods of Fabrication	Polymers/Biomaterials	Synergistic Factors of Polymers/ Biomaterials	Application in Human Body	References
Epithelial tissue	Self-assembled process	Keratin	Biocompatibility, bioactive properties compatible with native cellular functions	Drug delivery, wound healing, soft tissue augmentation, synthetic skin, coatings for implants, and scaffolds for TE	Tachibana et al. (2002) Katoh et al. (2004)
	Nanofiber electrospinning process	PGA	Good mechanical properties	Drug delivery, wound healing, soft tissue synthetic skin, and scaffolds for TE	Doshi and Reneker (1995); Li (2003), Zeng et al. (2005)
		PLGA	Mesh-forming, biodegradable, high surface area		
		PCL	Long-term zero-order release		
		Collagen	Biocompatible with native ECM, injectable, fiber, and sheet forming		
		Elastin	Injectible, cell attachment and migration, mechanical strength		
	Microfiber wet-spinning process	PLGA	As mentioned above	Skin graft, reinforcement, vascular grafts, nonwetting textile surfaces, and scaffolds for tissue	Hirano et al. (2000), Pomfret et al. (2000), Okuzaki et al. (2009)
		Chitosan	Mechanical stability, biocompatibility, biodegradability, porous, durable, gel, and sponge forming		
		PLA	Biocompatible, biodegradable, mechanical, and thermoplastic properties		
		PCL	As mentioned earlier		

(*Continued*)

Table 14.1 Insights into Bio-Mimicking Process: Different Scaffolds Fabrication Techniques *Continued*

Types of Tissue	Methods of Fabrication	Polymers/Biomaterials	Synergistic Factors of Polymers/ Biomaterials	Application in Human Body	References
	GFs release process	Collagen	As mentioned earlier	Angiogenesis, bone regeneration, and wound healing	Wissink et al. (2001), Causa et al. (2007), Ho et al. (2009)
		Gelatin	As mentioned earlier		
		Chitosan	As mentioned earlier		
		PLGA	As mentioned earlier		
		PEG	Bioresorbable multibock		
		Fibrin	Mechanical properties, immunologic integrity		
		Alginate	Biocompatible, biodegradable, hydrogels, microspheres, microcapsules, sponges		
	Emulsification	Gelatin	As mentioned earlier	Sustainable and controllable drug delivery therapies, bioengineered skin equivalent	Peppas and Khare (1993), Alexakis et al. (1995), Reis et al. (2007)
		Collagen	As mentioned earlier		
		HA	Promote angiogenesis, sponge		
Connective tissue (ligament, bone, cartilage)	Solvent casting/ salt leaching method	PLLA	As mentioned earlier	Orthopedic fixation, bone, and cartilage tissue engineering, ligament replacement	Mikos et al. (1993), Mikos et al. (2004a), Ochi et al. (2003)
		PLGA	As mentioned earlier		
		Collagen	As mentioned earlier		
	Ice particle leaching method	PLLA	As mentioned earlier	Porous 3D scaffolds for bone TE	Holy et al. (2000), Karp et al. (2003), Kang et al. (2006)
		PLGA	As mentioned earlier		

	Solvent evaporation technique	PLGA	As mentioned earlier	Bone repair	Laurencin et al. (1996), Devin et al. (1996), Woo et al. (2001)
	Particle aggregated scaffold	Chitosan	As mentioned earlier	Bone, cartilage, or osteochondral TE	Borden et al. (2003), Malafaya et al. (2005), Malafaya et al. (2008)
	Ceramic-based injectable scaffolds	Ceramics TCP BCP BG CP	Porosity and biocompatibility	Cartilage TE	Blokhuis et al. (2000), Holland et al. (2004), Gauthier et al. (2005)
	Hydrogel-based injectable scaffolds	Combinations of PLA, PGA, PLGA, and PEG	Biocompatibility and cause minimal inflammatory responses, thrombosis, and tissue damage	Cartilage, bone TE, and drug delivery	Jeong et al. (1999), Ibusuki et al. (2003), Seong et al. (2005)
		PEO and PPO and polyoxamer			
		Alginates, collagen	As mentioned earlier		
		Chitosan, HA, fibroin	As mentioned earlier		
	Sponge replication method	PU sponge, PVA, TCP, BCP or	Interconnected porous ceramic scaffolds	Bone TE	Sepulveda and Binner (1999), Chen et al. (2006b), Jo et al. (2009)
		PVA, calcium sulfate	Mechanical strength and stiffness, adhesion		

(Continued)

Table 14.1 Insights into Bio-Mimicking Process: Different Scaffolds Fabrication Techniques *Continued*

Types of Tissue	Methods of Fabrication	Polymers/Biomaterials	Synergistic Factors of Polymers/ Biomaterials	Application in Human Body	References
	Simple calcium phosphate coating method	Coating on: metals, glasses, inorganic ceramics, and organic polymers (PLGA, PS, PP, silicone, and PTFE), collagens, fibers of silk, and hairs	Improve biocompatibility or enhance the bioreactivity	Orthopedic application	Li (2002), Chen et al. (2006a), Yang et al. (2008)
Muscle tissue	Electrospinning nano-fibrous scaffolding	HA	Fiber—mesh forming, tensile strength, flexibility, porosity, contractility	Muscle repair	Ramay and Zhang (2004), Bhattarai (2005), Uematsu et al. (2005)
	Freeze drying method	Chitosan	As mentioned earlier	Muscle repair	Webster (2005), Price et al. (2003)
	Magnetic force-based tissue engineering	PLGA	As mentioned earlier	Muscle repair	Fuzita (2010), Blan (2008)
	Target-specific biomaterials scaffolding system	Carbon, aluminum	Adhesion, proliferation, and migration	Muscle repair	In kap ko (2013)
	Angiogenic GF genesis	Magnelite incorporated myogenic cells	Biocompatible, flexible,	Skeletal muscle repairs	Kaully et al. (2010)
	Decellulerization microfabrication method (vesicular tissue)	Hematopoietic stem cell, MSC, Endothelical progenitor cells	Self-renewal and differentiation capacity	Muscle repair	Kaully et al. (2010)
		Hydrogells PLGA, bFGF with peptide amphiphile, solution	Angiogentic GF release property	Angiogenesis (cardiovascular systems)	Kaully et al. (2010)

Neural tissue	Self-assembly	Chitosan Chitan Algimate, collagen	Biocompatible, regenerative ECM	Axonal regeneration	
	Particulate leaching	PLGA, gelatin	Allogenic grafts	Nerve cell regeneration	
	Gas forming	PHB, polyhydroxy, ethylmetha acrylate (PHEMA)	Less inflammability, controlled biodegradability, nontoxic	Neuro-conductive property,	Anuradha Subramanian (2009)
	Freeze drying	Polyacrylonitrite-co-methacrylate (PAN-MA)	Controlled biodegradability, nontoxic	In diseases like stroke, spinal cord injury.	
	Phase separation	Polyethylene dioxythiophene	Nerve regeneration by controlled, ligament, high surface-to-volume ratio	Neuromas, neuro-degenerative diseases	
	Electrospinning	PHEMA, PAN-MA	Nerve regeneration by controlled alignment and high surface-to volume ratio		
	CAD	–			
	Injection moulding with solvent evaporation	–	Customized designs in congrons wth native ECM/tissue		
	Micropatterning	Polyethylene dioxy thiophene	Controlled regenerative designs	Nerve cell regenaration	Cullen (2011)
	Biohybridize neural electrical interface microsystem	Living 3D pre-engineered neural constructs (*in-vitro*)	Congruence with native ECM biocompatible		
	Axonal stretch growth technology				

(*Continued*)

Table 14.1 Insights into Bio-Mimicking Process: Different Scaffolds Fabrication Techniques *Continued*

Types of Tissue	Methods of Fabrication	Polymers/Biomaterials	Synergistic Factors of Polymers/ Biomaterials	Application in Human Body	References
Facilitators	Micromolding	Alginate, polymethylmethacrylate (PMMA), HA, PEG			Yeh et al. (2006), Fukuda et al. (2006), Khademhosseini et al. (2006)
	Photolithography	Chitosan, fibronectin, HA, PEG, PNIAAm Poly (N-isopropyl acrylamide) (PNIPAm), poly (acrylic acid), PMMA, polyacrylamide, and poly (dimethylaminoethylmethacrylate hydrochloride)	Biodegradable Micro-arrays Microbeads Valves and pumps forming Micro sensors Native ECM and biomedical property Biocompatible porous	Target specific hormones delivery (insulin growth hormones, estrogen, progesterone) Gene therapy Microreactors Cell separation Controlled drug delivery	Beebe et al. (2000), Liu and Bhatia (2002) Dendukuri et al. (2006)
	Microfluidics	Polyglycerol sebacate, PEG, calcium alginate, silicon, and PDMS			Nisisako et al. (2002), Burdick et al. (2004), Xu et al. (2005)
	Emulsifications	Gelatin, HA, and collagen			Peppas and Khare (1993), Alexakis et al. (1995), Reis et al. (2007)
	Decellularization	Biological tissues			Steinhoff et al. (2000), Zhao et al. (2003), Liang et al. (2004)
	Microfiber wet spring	PLGA, PLA, chitosan, and PCL	As mentioned earlier	Tissue engineering	Hirano et al. (2000), Pomfret et al. (2000), Okuzaki et al. (2009)

	Nonwoven fiber by melt blown process	Polymer, PGA, PDO (Poly dioxanone)	Porous, biocompatible	Vascular graft (wet spinning), filter action (renal tissues)	Lyons et al., 2004, Ellison et al. (2007), Kim et al. (2009)
	Inkjet printing process	Sodium algimate polymers	As mentioned earlier	Biochips	Lemmo et al. (1998), Calvert (2001), Yeong et al. (2006)
	Melt-based RP process	Biodegradable polymers	Honeycomb structure absorbing property	Biosensors (melt blown)	Mironov et al. (2003), Sun et al. (2004)
	CAD	–	Programmed algorithm	Organ specific scaffolds	Sun and Lal (2002), Sun et al. (2004)
	Organ printing	Tubular collagen gels	Microdeposition of cells	Printing 3D organs for simulation	Lalan et al. (2001), Boland et al. (2003)

must be compatible with the cells and the components of the engineered tissue, organs, and host tissue. It has to be highly porous so as to facilitate efficient nutrients and metabolite transport as well as biologically active to interact with the cellular components of the engineered tissue facilitating cell growth, adhesion, alignment and morphology, proliferation, differentiation, and migration. It may also serve as a vehicle for the delivery of GFs, chemokines, cytokines, enzymes, proteins, and DNA to promote tissue regeneration. Scaffold in many cases may be a decellularized ECM derived from allogenic or xenogenic tissue. These have been mainly suggested for heart valve TE, vessels, tendons, and ligaments (Hao et al., 2008). The major advantage here is that it is the closest mechanical and biological match with the native ECM so that the GFs preserved in such acellular matrix further enhances cell growth and helps in modeling. However, incomplete cell removal may damage the physical and biochemical properties leading to inhomogeneous distribution and inducing an immune reaction upon implantation.

Synthetic-based scaffolds facilitate development of "tailor-made" architecture under controlled conditions. The biocompatible polymers used here can be polymerized under controlled conditions so that the regular pore size, pore interconnectivity, and pore characters suitable for rapid nutrient diffusion and cell attachment can be obtained. To master mimicking of functional tissue and organs, which are embedded in a 3D body frame, a 3D approach toward tissue regeneration in the scaffolds is necessary.

The most commonly used scaffold fabrication techniques for potential tissue engineering applications are (i) solvent casting/particulate leaching; (ii) porogen leaching; (iii) gas foaming; (iv) melt-molding; (v) membrane lamination; (vi) emulsification/freeze-drying; (vii) fiber mesh/bonding; (viii) phase separation; (ix) rapid prototyping; (x) electrospinning; (xi) self-assembly; (xii) CAD/CAM technologies; and (xiii) laser-assisted bioprinting (LaBP). Each of these techniques has distinct advantages and limitations (Kundu et al., 2010) as described below.

1. *Solvent casting/particulate leaching*: Porosity, pore size, and crystallinity of the scaffolds can be controlled. However, mechanical strength may be compromised and residual solvent and porogen material may cause toxic effects, such as damage cells and nearby tissues. Such scaffolds find applications in bone and cartilage tissues (Xiang et al., 2006; Ma, 2008)
2. *Porogen leaching*: In the biomaterial scaffolds, since porosity and pore size play an important role both *in vitro* and *in vivo*, the porogen leaching method stands out compared to other methods of scaffold preparation, since here the porosity and the pore geometry can be precisely controlled. Here the porogens, either salt, sugar, or wax may either in the form of liquid particulates or powder materials be dispersed by the process of evaporation crosslinking. These porogens act as temporary placeholders for pores and

interconnection of these pores in the actual fabricated scaffolds. Such scaffolds find applications in bone regeneration and organ vascularization. The disadvantage is that only thin wafers (3 mm) can be produced and there is limited pore interconnectivity (Mano et al., 2007).

3. *Gas foaming*: Use of organic solvents or high temperature is not a desirable approach for scaffold fabrication as organic solvents may form harmful organic residues and polymer can degrade at high temperatures. The gas-foaming technique enables control over porosity and porous structure and is free from harmful organic residues. It promotes continuous processing of polymers and is not limited to batch processing. Here, highly pressurized CO_2 gas (800 psi) is used which, because of the formation of thermodynamic instability, forms clusters to minimize the free energy resulting in nucleation and growth of gas pores in the polymer matrix. This leads to the expansion of the polymer particles and hence decreases the polymeric density. Gas foaming thus results in the formation of a 3D porous structure. The porosity here is controlled by the use of porogens like wax, sugar, and salt particulates (Ikada, 2006). This technique is limited by poor mechanical property and pore interconnectivity.
4. *Melt molding*: The scaffolds here are prepared by melting polymers or ceramics in the presence of porogens (such as sodium chloride or sugar crystals). The desired porosity is obtained after cooling the mixture and dissolving the porogens in water.
   Thompson et al. (1995a) used the principle of compression modeling in polymers. Here teflon molds were filled with polymeric powder (PLGA) and gelatin microsphere. At high pressure and temperature (above glass transition temperature Tg of PLGA), the PLGA particles bond together (Thompson et al., 1995a). Once the mold is removed, the gelatin component can be leached out in water to obtain the desired scaffolds. The main advantages are control over pore geometry, size, and interconnectivity. The drawbacks are elevated temperatures in the case of nonamorphous polymers and some residues of porogens.
5. *Membrane lamination*: Membrane lamination offers a means of constructing 3D anatomical shapes necessary for regeneration of hard tissues, such as bone and cartilage, and also for the regeneration of tubular tissue, such as intestines (Mikos et al., 1993). The uniform porous structure of the original membrane needs to be preserved and, in addition, the boundaries between two layers must be fused and remain indistinguishable from the bulk of the device. Membrane lamination is prepared by solvent casting, particle leaching, and layer-by-layer protein and peptide deposition (Hutmacher, 2000, 2001). A 3D structure with continuous pores running vertically across the sheet can be obtained by stacking membranes layer by layer. The drawback is that stacking of thin sheets layer by layer is cumbersome, time-consuming and there is a chance of mismatching in pores of different

sheets leading to poor pore interconnectivity. Longer processing times are required.

6. *Emulsification/freeze-drying*: This technique uses the principle of sublimation. Porous scaffold geometries can be obtained by this method. Polymers are suspended in water or in organic solvents followed by emulsification with a water phase. The mixture is poured into molds and the solvents are removed by freeze-drying to obtain porous structures. Materials can also be freeze-dried under high vacuum. The frozen water in the materials is sublimed directly from the solid phase to the gas phase. A number of silk proteins, PLLA, PEG, and PLGA (polypropylene fumates) blends have been tried using these techniques (Boland et al., 2004; Mandal 2007; Mandal and Kundu, 2008a, 2008b).
7. *Fiber mesh and fiber bonding*: Here individual fibers are either woven or interweaved into a 3D pattern of variable pore size. This technique is one of the earliest method for scaffold construction. The nonwoven meshes of polymer fiber in three dimensions provide a large surface area, promoting cell growth and interactions. It is prepared by the deposition of the polymer solution (PLLA) over a nonwoven mesh of another polymer, such as PGA, followed by subsequent solvent evaporation. The composites thus formed are heated to temperatures above the melting point of both polymers (Mooney et al., 1996a, 1996b; Cen et al., 2002). One of the polymers (PLLA) melts first and fills all the voids left by the nonwoven fibers like PGA. This helps retain the spatial network of fibers. The foams formed here have high porosity of 80% and pore diameter of up to 500 nm (Mikos et al., 1993). Here, use of organic solvents imparts toxicity to the structure. Also, elevated temperature acts as a barrier for the bioactive materials, such as the GFs which are to be embedded in the scaffolds during fabrication.
8. *Phase separation*: This can control macro pore shape and size, inter-pore connectivity, and pore wall morphology, which ensures better dimensional stability of scaffolds (Smith et al., 2006). Another advantage is that it can easily combine with other fabrication techniques such as particulate leaching and RP technique. However, it is difficult to control scaffold morphology accurately.
9. *Rapid prototyping*: The scaffold is designed using a computer, equipped with CAD software so that 3D organs are automatically manufactured layer by layer according to the virtual design fed into the computer as per the patient's requirements. Patient needs are recorded to produce a database from the medical scans and the tissue-engineered organs are customized to match the data recorded. The different types of RP techniques used to obtain 3D organs, layer by layer are: fused deposition method, stereolithography, selective laser sintering, and 3D printing. RP is a solid free-form of technique. This technique is good for obtaining scaffolds with good mechanical integrity and controlled porosity. However, these scaffolds show low resolution of the struts that can deteriorate the initial cell attachment and

proliferation. When combined with an electrohydrodynamic system, it can generate highly roughened microsized threads for enhanced cellular behavior. However, it requires high temperature for nonamorphous polymer.

10. *Electrospinning*: This is a robust, highly versatile technique which ensures production of continuous fibers of submicrometer to nanometer diameters. Simplicity and ease of variation are an additional advantage which influences scaffold architecture. It is limited by inadequate mechanical strength and decreased thickness and pore size of fibers (Liang et al., 2007).
11. *Self-assembly*: This process mimics in scale and chemistry, natural *in vivo* ECM. It is suitable for designing complex engineered tissue. The nanofibers obtained here are much thinner than those obtained by electrospinning techniques. Moreover it is possible to obtain complex nanostructure with specific geometry and composition such as a coaxial nanotube. Another advantage of this technique is to avoid the use of organic solvent and reduce the cytotoxicity because it is carried out in aqueous salt solution or physiological media (Zhang, 2003; Zhang et al., 2006). The structural features of self-assembled scaffolds can be controlled by monitoring the molecular chemistry, kinetics, and assembly environment (e.g., salt addition, solvent, light, pH, and temperature). Some of the disadvantages in using this technique are its complicated process, difficulty controlling pore size, mechanical weakness (cannot sustain the to and fro transfer of mechanical loadings to the cells and surrounding tissues), expense, and it is time-consuming.
12. *CAD/CAM technologies*: This is a 3D plotting technique of scaffold generation, which can be utilized for obtaining a 3D structure using CAD software. This software provides structured algorithms for generating a scaffold as conceived by the designer. This involves use of polymer beads or polymer melt obtained through fused deposition modeling fed to an ink-jet printer.
13. *LaBP*: In this method, living cell suspensions are processed in a laser-assisted bioprinter which yields a 3D functional tissue. Here the micro details of the intricate ECM are retained because of the high-resolution quality of the device. It is useful for toxicology and drug discovery studies (Devillard et al., 2014).

14.2.5.1 Fibrous scaffold fabrication

To evolve an efficient functional tissue-engineered product with scaffold-based approaches, the artificial scaffold must mimic the structural and biological function of the native ECM in terms of the physical cues and chemical composition. Many extracellular proteins have a fibrous structure with a diameter at the nanometer or sub-micrometer scales. For example, collagen, the most abundant ECM protein in our body, has a fibrous structure with a fiber diameter that ranges from 50 to 500 nm. In this context, the fibrous scaffold fabrication technique emerges as the most advantageous feasible option.

Recently, much effort has been directed at understanding interactions between cells and the tissue microenvironment. Structurally, natural ECM consists of nanoscale-dimensional interwoven protein fibers with diameters ranging from tens to hundreds of nanometers (Wang et al., 2010). Nanotechnology offers preparation of nanoscale fibers with high surface-to-volume ratio that can potentially mimic the architecture of natural human tissue at the nanometer scale. Additionally, they offer a microporous structure, which facilitates cell adhesion, proliferation, migration, and differentiation, all of which are highly desired properties for tissue engineering applications (Bhattarai et al., 2004; Ma et al., 2005). Fabrication, characterization, and applications of nanofibrous systems as scaffolds for tissue engineering therefore lead the research in TE.

14.2.6 TECHNIQUES OF NANOFIBER SYNTHESIS

There are primarily three techniques for synthesis of nanofibers, phase separation, self-assembly, and electrospinning (Ma et al., 1999; Holmes et al., 2000; Holzwarth and Ma, 2011; Liu et al., 2011; Matson, 2011; Hartgerink et al., 2002; Wade and Burdick, 2012). Herein we elaborate the significance of the use of the electrospinning technique, in particular with reference to recreating human physiological functions through TE.

14.2.6.1 Self-assembly

Self-assembly is the spontaneous organization of molecules into a well-defined ordered structure required for a specific function (Zhang, 2003). It is a "bottom-up" approach for fabricating scaffolds. Here, the molecules assemble into structured, stable, noncovalently bonded aggregates. Self-assembly of natural or synthetic molecules produce nanofibers. The key elements in molecular self-assembly are structural compatibility and clinical compliance through noncovalent interactions. Several distinctive types of self-assembling peptide systems are reported, which are simple, versatile, and easy to produce. This is devoid of cytotoxicity since it is carried out in aqueous salt solutions or physiological media. The main disadvantage of this technique is that at times it can be complicated with elaborated processing.

The milestones in the technique of self-assembly are summarized in Table 14.2.

14.2.6.2 Phase separation

The technique of phase separation has been primarily devised to address the problem of drug delivery. In order to achieve this goal, the bioactive molecules must be incorporated into scaffold during manufacturing and the activity of the drug should not become lost due to exposure to strong chemicals and elevated thermal environments.

The scaffolds based on these techniques are designed by the formation of a gradient in temperature which separates the polymer into two phases: a

Table 14.2 Milestones of Self-Assembly of Scaffold Fabrication

S. No.	Technique	Reference
1.	Peptide amphiphile (PA)-based system was synthesized with dialkyl chain moiety that allows formation of thermally stable protein like molecular architectures (similar to human α (iv) collagen sequence)	Berndt et al. (1995)
2.	Dialkyl chain in PA was replaced with monoalkyl chain which increased thermal stability	Yu et al. (1996, 1999)
3.	Bioactivity of PA was determined by incorporating bioactive sequences, producing ordered structure of bioactive sequence, which provoked favorable cell response (cell adhesion, spreading proliferation)	Malkar et al. (2003)
4.	Discovery of PA structures with potential to be used as surface coating for biomaterials to improve biocompatibility	Fields et al. (1998)
5.	Di- and triblock PAs were designed that self-assembled into a rod-like architecture	Stupp et al. (1997)
6.	Peptide head group of the PA were engineered changing self-assembles of PA into nanofibers using PH control. The nanoscale orientation resembled PA crystals in mineralized ECM and collagen fiber of bone tissue	Hartgerink et al. (2001)
7.	Three different techniques were introduced: pH-controlled self-assembly, drying on surface SA, and divalent ion-induced SA. It produced good yield of nanofibers with low polydispersity	Hwang et al. (2002)

polymer-lean phase with low polymer concentration and a polymer-rich phase with high polymer concentration (Mikos et al., 2004b). In case of preparation of a phase-separated scaffold prepared by porous PLLA and poly(phosphoester) incorporated with hydrophilic and hydrophobic bioactive molecules, the following steps are involved:

1. Dissolving the polymer in a solvent of molten phenol or napthalene at the low temperature (53 °C for phenol and 85 °C for napthalene).
2. The bioactive molecules are dissolved to form a homogeneous solution. The resulting solution is cooled under controlled conditions until liquid–liquid phase separation is induced. Further quenching creates a two-phase solid. Solidified solvent is removed by sublimation to obtain a porous scaffold with bioactive molecules incorporated within the polymers (Hua et al., 2002; Sachlos and Czernuszka, 2003). A liquid–liquid phase-separated solution can be utilized for 3D nanofibrous structure of collagen type I (Ma and Zhang,

1999; Zhang and Ma, 2002). The main advantages of such techniques are that the activity of drug molecules for drug delivery systems (DDSs) can be retained. It is a simple, straightforward method with minimal requirements. This technique can be combined with other techniques (such as particulate leaching and RP) to form 3D network structure morphology suitable for DDSs (Smith et al., 2006). A few challenges remain unmet in the phase separation technique such as:

a. The incorporation and release of drug with large protein structure.
b. Little control over fiber diameter.
c. Orientation.
d. Time consuming.
e. Poor mechanical properties.

The three different approaches available for the fabrication of nanofibers are:

1. Molecular self-assembly;
2. Phase separation;
3. Electrospinning.

The electrospinning process has attracted much attention since it is a well-established and versatile process capable of producing fibers in the submicron to nano range. Such nanofibers can be further functionalized through incorporation with bioactive molecules, for example, DNA, enzymes, and GFs. Scaffolds fabricated from such fibers have better control of the proliferation and differentiation of cells.

14.2.6.3 Electrospinning of nanofibers

The most attractive feature of this technique is the ability to produce fiber based on polymeric biomaterials analogous to the fibrous structure of the native ECM. A wide range of fibers varying in thickness, geometry, and materials can be produced using an electrospinning technique that also offers an opportunity to control morphology, composition, and porosity, using simple, robust, and relatively unsophisticated equipment. This makes it very cost effective (Doshi and Renekar, 1995; Reneker and Chun, 1996; Dzenis, 2004; Jayaraman et al., 2004). Electrospinning can produce ultrafine fibers with special orientation, high aspect ratio, high surface area, and control over pore geometry. Cell seeding problems can be overcome by sacrificial biopolymers or cryospinning, allowing the creation of the desired size in electrospun matrices.

The notable quality of electrospun nanofibers is the high surface-to-volume ratio, high permeability, and 3D interlinkages. These features make them an appropriate choice of material for scaffold fabrication. The major advantage offered by electrospinning includes the ability to mimic the microprocesses happening at the cellular level as per human physiological tissues (Li et al., 2002a, 2002b; Smith and Ma, 2004; Khil et al., 2005; Ma et al., 2005).

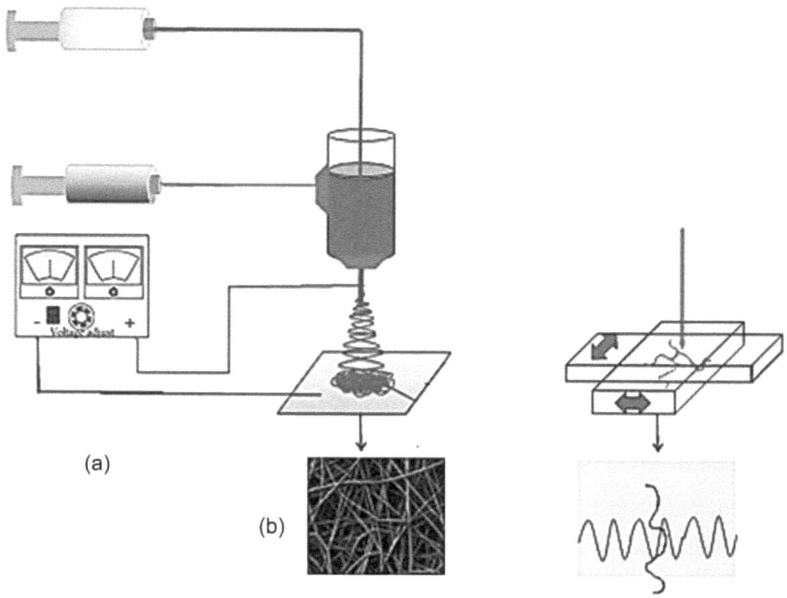

FIGURE 14.5

(a) Schematic of the electrospinning process. (b) Scanning electron micrograph of PLGA nanofibers synthesized using the electrospinning technique (scale bar = 10 μm).

Source: Katti et al. (2004).

A basic functional electrospinning setup consists of a high-voltage power supply (~20 kV), spinneret constituted by a glass capillary tube (syringe) or a needle of small diameter and a stationary or rotating metallic collector which is grounded (Figure 14.5).

The entire setup is housed in a chemical hood from where the organic vapors can be conveniently pumped out. This hood serves the purpose of shielding from air turbulence and humidity, and facilitates better control over the temperature. The polymeric solution, whose nanofibers are to be spun, is filled in a capillary. A high electrical field is applied across the capillary containing the polymer solution. The electric potential induces mutual charge repulsive force in the polymer solution, which in turn opposes the surface tension of the polymer fluid. When the applied electric potential overcomes this surface tension force, which is responsible for holding the polymeric liquid at the tip of the capillary, the polymeric fluid first elongates to form a "taylor cone" and is ejected out in the form of a jet, and eventually collects on the collector electrode in the form of a fiber mesh. The jet, which progresses from capillary toward the collector, experiences a forward pull due to forces from the external electric field, so it is accelerated and stretched. This results in jet thinning in air due to stretching and solvent evaporation. As the diameter of the jet becomes smaller and smaller the radial forces from the charge can become large enough to overcome the cohesive forces of the fibers and the fiber splits into two or more fragments. This fragmentation occurs several times in rapid succession producing a large number of charged fibers randomly moving toward the metallic collector (Zeleny, 1914; Reneker et al., 2000; Shin et al., 2001a, 2001b; Frenot and Chronakis, 2003).

The fibers repel each other due to the repulsive forces originating from the charged ions within the electrospinning jet. The technique originated from electrospraying where the conducting liquid produces a jet of fiber particles resembling a spray (Rayleigh, 1882; Zeleny, 1914). When polymer fluids are filled into the capillary the jet undergoes instability and thins to form nanofibers (due to the long chain-forming nature of polymers). Molten polymers as well as polymers (synthetic or natural) which can be dissolved in appropriate solvents are carefully chosen for electrospinning (Bambole et al., 2010). It is necessary to melt spun polymeric fibers under vacuum and at high temperature. The process governing parameters which govern the fabrication of electrospun fibers is:

1. Ambient parameters: Such as humidity, air velocity in surrounding, solution temperature.
2. Operational conditions: Shape of orifice of needle, hydrostatic pressure in the capillary (syringe), distance between the needle and the collector screen, motion of the collector determining pattern formation during fiber deposition.
3. Intrinsic solution properties: Surface tension, elasticity, conductivity, viscosity, molecular weight distribution of polymers.

The customized "tailor-made" nanofibers of desired shapes and sizes can be achieved by varying the different polymeric systems along with the governing parameters (Shin et al., 2001b; Zong et al., 2002).

Although it is expected that ideally fiber diameter must be uniform and consistent, the fiber surface defect free, the obtained fibers lack mechanical stability, thicknesses are nonuniform, and they lack orientation forming a nonwoven mesh or at times beads are formed.

Electrospinning a wide range of polymers (natural and synthetic) can yield water-soluble biopolymers or liquid crystalline polymers. Nanofibers produced from natural polymers such as hyaluronic acid (HA; Um et al., 2004), collagen (Huang et al., 2001; Matthews et al., 2002), chitosan (Bhattarai et al., 2005; Geng et al., 2005), silk fibroin (Jin et al., 2002, 2004; Gersbach et al., 2004; Shields et al., 2004), and gelatin (Zhang et al., 2005) have found applications in TE. Protein nanofibers (Li et al., 2005; Woerdeman et al., 2005) have also been found to be promising in TE. The synthetic polymers that are explored for the fabrication of nanofibers include polyurethane (PU; Verreck et al., 2003), poly(ethylene-co-vinyl acetate) (PEVA; Kenawy et al., 2002), poly(lactic acid) (PLA; Yang et al., 2004, 2005b), PLGA (Uematsu et al., 2005), poly(ε-caprolactone) (PCL; Reneker et al., 2002), and poly(l-lactide-co-ε-caprolactone) (Mo and Weber, 2004).

It is important to note that both synthetic and natural polymers have their own limitations. Synthetic polymers are inherently flexible, easy to make, with high mechanical strength, but because of their low hydrophilicity and absence of surface cell recognition sites, cell adhesion becomes difficult. Natural polymers, although biocompatible, display poor mechanical properties and processability. It therefore turns out that the best-suited strategy to mimic a natural nanofibrous scaffold would be to employ a composite of both, such that synthetic polymers provide the backbone and natural polymers facilitate cellular attachment, producing a bioactive surface with excellent mechanical properties.

14.2.6.3.1 Factors influencing electrospinning of nanofibers

Electrospun nanofibers can be "custom-made" by varying the different governing parameters in a number of ways, for example, the electric field of the polymer solution can be changed and hence the charge can be varied and trajectory of fiber can be controlled (Hohman et al., 2001a, 2001b). Oriented fibers can thus be obtained which helps in designing the scaffolds, which promote cell seeding and cell growth. Such axially oriented fibers would promote desired neuronal/axonal growth and thus be useful in regeneration of neural tissue (Yang et al., 2005b). Sundaray et al. (2004) used a rotating disk with sharpened edges for nanofiber alignment to facilitate deposition of the nanofibers on edge of the rotating disk resulting in aligned nanofibers (Theron et al., 2001; Lee et al., 2005; Yang et al., 2005b).

In another method, new variants such as near field and polymer melt have recently been invented. This gives better control over fiber alignment (Lyons et al., 2004; Chang et al., 2008; Teo et al., 2011). Here in the first case distance between the needle tip and collector is reduced and in the second, viscosity of polymer is raised, which stabilizes the spinning jet. These new variants, along with fast motion automated system, result in direct writing methods (Bisht et al., 2011; Brown et al., 2011; Lee et al., 2012). A new collector plate design generates a 3D fibrous structure for scaffold architecture (Li et al., 2003, 2004, 2005; Zhang et al., 2009).

Electrospun nanofibers can also be collected using patterned electrodes (Li et al., 2005). Introducing insulating gaps on the conductive collector giving uniaxially oriented nanofibers formed the patterning electrodes. Recently Dalton et al. (2013) reported additive manufacturing (AM) approaches with electrospinning. The AM produces complex 3D structures in a layer-by-layer process by CAD. Such hybrid electrospun scaffolds tailored with 3D micropatterns can be obtained using rapid prototype resin formed as template during the electrospinning process. Complex geometries such as sinosoidal wave and hexagons were also produced.

14.2.7 SCAFFOLD ARCHITECTURES USING ELECTROSPINNING

The structure, composition, and functions of tissues in different parts of the body are variable. It is important to understand the structural and biological properties of tissues in order to gain an insight into choosing the materials from which nanofibers could be made and the experimental conditions to obtain the architecture that best suits reconstruction of these tissues (Jang et al., 2009). Electrospinning exhibits great potential in the fabrication of fibrous scaffolds with controllable compositions and structures, enabling the fabrication of novel scaffolds incorporating various biomimetic characteristics at genetic, molecular, and nanometer scales (Ma et al., 2008).

Nanofibers can be electrospun in various patterns and geometries depending on the biomedical application. For example, core-shell fibers can facilitate drug delivery in which drugs will be encapsulated in a nonreactive coating and safely delivered to the target sites (Reddy et al., 2013). Biomimetic substitutes have been developed to replicate natural tissues for use in the repair of destroyed tissues such as skin, bone, dura mater, sciatic nerve, articular cartilage, and tendon in order to improve functional outcomes (Wang et al., 2010; Nguyen and Lee, 2012). In skin tissue regeneration, for example, nanofibers have shown great potential to mimic skin ECM in both morphology and composition, and thus may be promising tissue engineering scaffolds for skin substitutes (Huang et al., 2012). The high surface area of nanofibrous scaffolds allows oxygen permeability and prevents fluid accumulation at the wound site, making them ideal substrates for wound dressings (Reddy et al., 2013). Therefore, it is important to understand the structural and biological properties of tissues in order to gain an insight into choosing the materials that best suit reconstruction of these tissues (Jang et al., 2009). Bone tissue, as an example, has a hierarchical organization over length scales ranging from macro- to nano-structured (ECM) components. When designing biomimetic scaffolds for bone tissue engineering, the following aspects should be considered: They must (i) mimic the nanofibrous collagen ECM; (ii) be highly porous to allow for cell ingrowth and efficient mass transport of nutrients, oxygen, GFs, and waste products; and (iii) be able to withstand mechanical stresses during tissue neogenesis (Stevens, 2008; Deng et al., 2012).

14.2.7.1 Different geometries of nanofibrous scaffolds

14.2.7.1.1 Aligned nanofibrous scaffolds

A well-defined architecture is believed to be necessary in order to precisely imitate native ECM for guiding cell growth or tissue regeneration (Yang et al., 2005a; Kim et al., 2012). Different electrospun nanofibrous scaffold geometries such as axially aligned, random, tubular conduit, sheath yarn, and radially aligned nanofibers can be obtained by varying and controlling the systems as well as process parameters. The strategies for controlling electrospun nanofiber alignment include mechanical, electrostatic, and magnetic, depending on the type of forces involved (Matthews et al., 2002; Li et al., 2004; Yang et al., 2007b). The native ECMs are tissue-specific (e.g., sciatic nerve, heart, tendon, and blood vessel) and mostly display anisotropic architecture. Alignment of electrospun nanofibers in well-defined geometries would facilitate effective cell adhesion, migration, and differentiation, and thereby lead to superior quality and capacity of scaffold as compared to other types of scaffolds both *in vitro* and *in vivo* (Wan et al., 2009; Xie et al., 2010a).

Alignment of nanofibers can be uniaxial or uniquely biomimetic with 3D nanofibrous matrices having high spatial interconnectivity, high porosity, and controlled alignment, which ensures direct cell orientation and migration (Zhang et al., 2012). An aligned electrospun nanofibrous scaffold can effectively guide the migration and extension of cells which is immensely important in replicating the ECM for a specific tissue such as cardiac tissue, where the ventricular myocardium is composed of perpendicularly interwoven collagen strips (Engelmayr et al., 2008).

In this regard, Chew and coworkers introduced the concept of "Contact guidance," which highlights the advantage of orientation of aligned fibrous scaffolds. Contact guidance meticulously channels elongation and alignment of cells along the axes of the fibers (Chew et al., 2008a, 2008b), as was demonstrated by them for aligned electrospun PCL scaffolds which were able to provide contact guidance to cultured human Schwann cells (hSCs). The effect of contact guidance of aligned electrospun fibers on cell morphological changes was also evident in other cell types (e.g., neural stem cell (NSC)) (He et al., 2010). As shown in Figure 14.6, the effect of contact guidance provided by the aligned fibers appeared

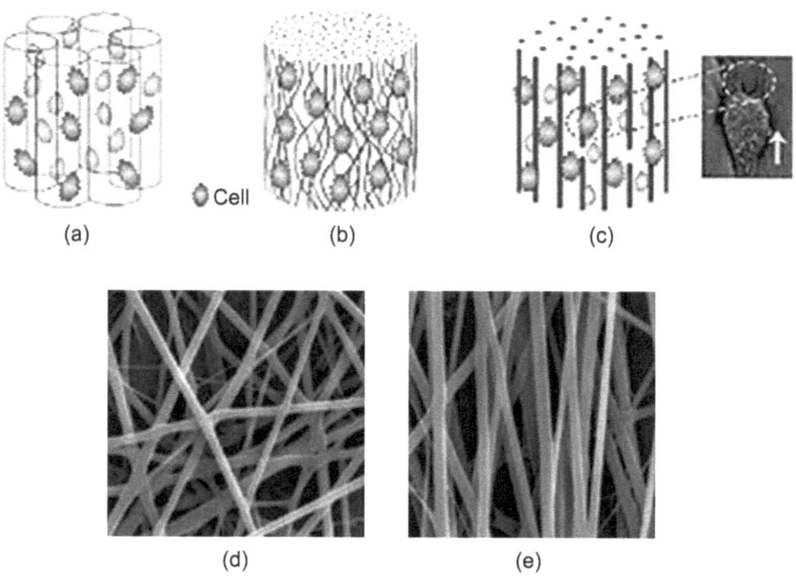

FIGURE 14.6

Schematic of nanofibers with (a) random orientation, (b) alignment in progress, (c) aligned nanofibers providing contact guidance facilitating cell migration and extension (SEM micrographs of PCL scaffolds for hSC culture), (d) randomly oriented, and (e) aligned PCL electrospun fibers.

Source: Chen et al. (2013).

to be more dramatic than the randomly oriented fibers. When cultured on aligned fibers, the cytoskeleton and nuclei align and elongate on the fiber axes.

Aligned nanofibrous structures such as tissue-engineered scaffolds find extensive applications for bone, cartilage, neural, dural, and other tissues.

14.2.7.1.2 Radial nanofibrous scaffolds

Xie et al. (2010a) developed a scaffold, which could serve as an artificial dural substitute or as biomedical patches or grafts for wound covering. The scaffold was made up of the PCL nanofibers, which are radially aligned. Such radial alignment of nanofiber is brought about by an electrospinning assembly wherein the collector is composed of a central point electrode and a peripheral ring electrode. The unique feature of such a scaffold is that it presents topographic cues at the nanoscale to the cultured cell by directing and enhancing their migration from the periphery to the center. The radial alignment also promotes faster cellular migration and population than nonwoven mats, which are unaligned. Figure 14.7 shows an electrospinning setup with pointed electrode for obtaining radially aligned nanofibers.

14.2.7.1.3 Mixed-aligned and random nanofibrous scaffolds

In another case, a combination of aligned and random (mixed) geometry on the same scaffold was demonstrated by Li et al. (2009), where the aligned portion could imitate the high level of alignment for collagen fibers in a normal tendon and the random portion could recapitulate the less ordered organization of

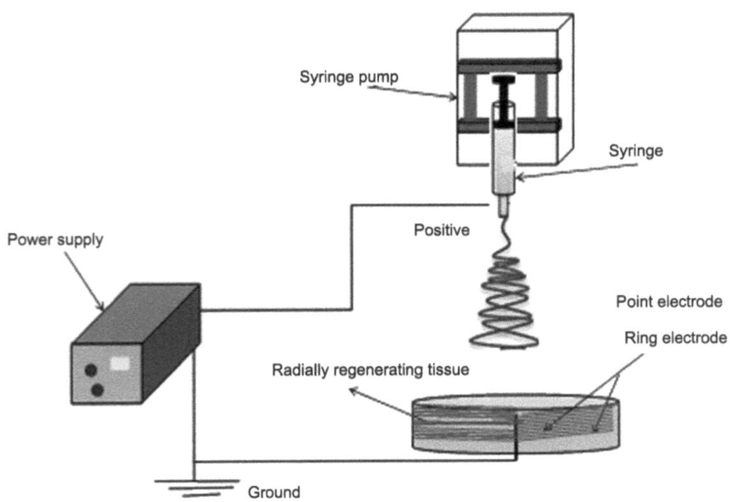

FIGURE 14.7

Electrospinning setup with pointed electrode for obtaining radially aligned nanofibers.

collagen fibers in a bone. Such a gradient in composition is a requisite to mimic a tendon-to-bone insertion site.

14.2.7.1.4 Spiral nanofibrous scaffolds

Some of the important features exhibited by the spiral nanofibrous scaffolds are open geometries, large surface areas, and porosity, which is helpful for improving nutrient transport and cell penetration into the scaffolds. The spiral walls are thinner than the walls of the tubular and cylindrical scaffolds and are subject to cellular invasion from both sides of the wall, and hence, have a greater ratio of interior to exterior cells than the other scaffolds. To mimic dynamic conditions spiral scaffolds represent better design when compared with other geometries. The spiral nanofibrous scaffold with its hierarchical architecture and mechanical characteristics similar to that of native tissue ECM is the most successful imitation of real bone tissue matrix and supports the vascularization of a large tissue construct (Deng et al., 2011; Lee et al., 2012). Deng and coworkers designed and constructed a 3D biomimetic scaffold by rolling electrospun nanofiber matrices in a concentric manner with an open central cavity to imitate native bone structurally and mechanically.

Cells could migrate through 250-μm-thick concentric fiber laminates from both the surfaces leading to a homogeneous ECM deposition and cellular activity throughout the biomimetic scaffold.

14.2.7.1.5 Tubular conduit nanofibrous scaffolds

A tubular conduit is one of the important geometries obtained by collecting electrospun nanofibers over a rotating rod of desired diameter (<5 mm) and length (15 cm). These can imitate and find resemblance to native ECM of an artery and microenvironment of vascular tissue, because of their hollow architecture. In addition, axial alignment of fibers can provide guidance for axonal growth (Yu et al., 2008). Thomas et al. (2009) demonstrated a trilayer tubular conduit of 20 cm length and 4 mm inner diameter which was fabricated by sequential electrospinning of blends of polydioxanone and proteins onto a small-diameter rod (4 mm), which imitates the complex matrix structure of native arteries. Seamless, nonwoven, bioresorbable vascular prosthetics composed of submicron fibers were fabricated using electrospinning (Sell and Bowlin, 2008) and electrospun collagen and elastin fibers showed promise in vascular tissue engineering. "Nerve repair" (Xie et al., 2010b) is another aspect where tubular conduit nanofibrous scaffolds show promising application. When direct suturing of two opposing nerve stumps during surgery is not feasible, scaffolds are often used to bridge the damaged nerve gap and to guide nerve regeneration (Bashur et al., 2006). It has been reported that electrospun fibers could support oriented neurite outgrowth and glial cell migration from dorsal root ganglia explants (Schnell et al., 2007). *In vivo* studies indicated that nerve conduits with an inner layer of aligned fibers led to improved peripheral nerve regeneration (Chew et al., 2007).

14.2.7.1.6 Sheath membrane–laminar nanofibrous scaffolds

Two-layer sheath membrane type geometry to replicate a hierarchical architecture and complex biologic functions of a native sheath can be obtained by a sequential electrospinning technique. The biomimic should consist of an outer antiadhesion layer and an inner lubricant layer. It can be used as a replica of a membrane-shaped tendon sheath used for repairing damaged tissues. It consists of an outer fibrotic layer and an inner synovial layer. The fibrotic layer prevents exogenous healing of the tendon as an effective biological barrier while the synovial layer secretes synovial fluid (e.g., HA) to enable tendon gliding (Sharma and Maffulli, 2005). HA-loaded PCL fibrous membrane as the inner layer and a PCL fibrous membrane as the outer layer, which imitates a native sheath, were first demonstrated by Liu et al. (2012a).

14.2.7.2 Biomimicry through electrospinning

The technique of electrospinning can be successfully applied for the fabrication of fascinating structures resembling natural objects (e.g., lotus leaf, silver ragwort leaf, rice leaf, honeycomb, polar bear fur, spider webs, soap-bubbles, ECM) (Lin et al., 2012). A multifold and continuous expansion of the electrospinning approach in biomimetic scaffold design in the coming decades is envisioned, wherein procuring artificial organs "off the shelf" would be a reality. This is a stimulant for further research and advances in the exciting field of tissue engineering.

14.2.7.3 Electrospinning techniques: limitations and scope

Electrospinning techniques for the preparation of tissue engineering scaffolds presents several limitations, such as control over the pore sizes, achievement of in-depth penetration of cells into scaffolds, significant improvement in biomechanical properties, and solvent toxicity (Agarwal et al., 2009). The electrospinning technique could, however, successfully establish itself as a promising method in tissue engineering for simulating the fibrillar structures of ECM, offering large surface areas, ease of functionalization, and controllable mechanical properties, all leading to improvements in the ability to provide a true biomimetic microenvironment to the developing tissue. Novel electrospinning/netting technique (Barakat et al., 2009; Wang et al., 2010; Ding et al., 2011) overcomes the bottleneck problem of electrospinning and offers a versatile method for generating spider-web-like nano-nets with ultrafine fiber diameter (less than 50 nm) while maintaining high porosity, which make nano-nets optimal candidates for the fabrication of tissue-engineering scaffolds. In the following section the application of nanofibers in tissue engineering for recreating the physiological functions is discussed citing different case studies.

14.2.8 TISSUE ENGINEERING FOR MODELING HUMAN PHYSIOLOGY

TE is a rapidly expanding field that necessitates the combined efforts of cell biologists, engineers, material scientists, mathematicians, geneticists, and clinicians toward the development of artificial organs for transplantation and basic research for drug development. The fundamental ethos of TE is to comprehend the complex cellular microenvironment and create a near-natural form of *in vitro* human body. This should have a capacity to biomimic all the *in vivo* molecular mechanisms governing human physiological and pathological processes in addition to predicting and responding to medical therapies.

It has emerged as a rapidly expanding approach to address the organ shortage problem, and recreate and regenerate tissue and organ substitution. The inspiration toward this has been drawn from the creative efforts of the scientists who have achieved breakthrough results in overcoming different disorders such as wound healing (Van den Broek et al., 2012; Li et al., 2013), skin fibrosis (Moulin, 2013), cardiac arrhythmia (Thompson et al., 2012), and the comprehension of biological function of healthy organs such as skin (Paquet et al., 2010; Bellas et al., 2012; Fernandez et al., 2012), blood–brain barrier, and mammary gland (Wang, 2010) development. Therefore, it is necessary to develop practical insights into the types, structures, and functions of human tissues (Figure 14.8 and Table 14.3).

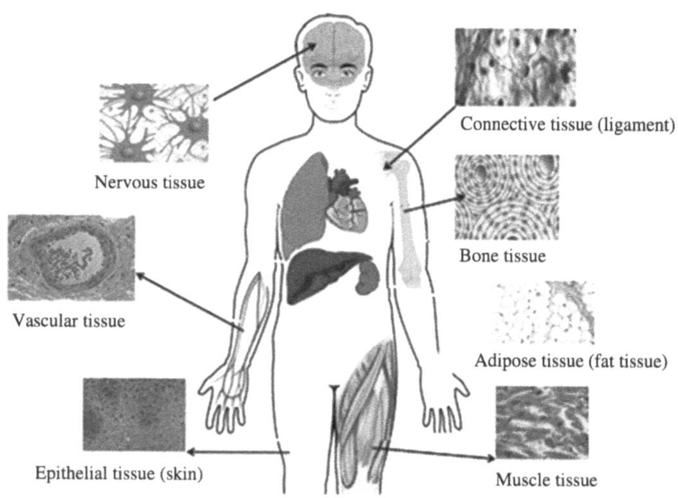

FIGURE 14.8

A photomicrograph of various body tissues. The figure depicts cross section of epithelial tissue, microfibrous connective tissue, areolar tissue, adipose tissue, and nervous tissue.

Table 14.3 Elementary Tissues of the Human Body

Sr. No.		Tissue	Functions
(I)		Epithelial	Protection Absorption Secretion Excretion
(II)	(i)	Connective areolar	Replacement by fibrosis during repairs
	(ii)	Adipose	Gives shape to limbs and body Protection to internal organs Regulation of body temperature stored energy of body
	(iii)	White fibrous (collagen)	Connect different tissues for mechanical strength
	(iv)	Yellow elastic	Ligaments of joints tensile strength Elastic recoil in blood vessels and lungs
	(v)	Reticular—endothelial	Protection of liver, lymph node, and spleen
	(vi)	Blood	Supply cells for defense against infection
	(vii)	Cartilage	Mechanical buffer, e.g., intervertebral disk
	(viii)	Jelly-like	Buffer gel in eyes and placental chord
	(ix)	Osseous (bone)	I. Attachment to muscles and tendons, healing of bone fracture II. Mechanical leverage to body III. Reservoir of calcium and phosphorus IV. Special function in each organ, e.g., bones of roof of mouth assist in speech; bone marrow forms blood
(III)		Muscle tissue	I. Movement of osseous joints, producing motion II. Body movement heat and fluid balance III. Contribute in provision of oxygen and elimination of CO_2 maintaining acid–base balance
(IV)		Nervous tissue	Reception, discharge of stimulus and transmission initiate neurochemical responses for higher functions.

14.2.8.1 Types of human physiological tissues

The structure, composition, and functions of tissues in different parts of the body are variable. These tissues essentially coordinate to execute different body functions, as directed through nervous stimuli. The characteristics of these tissues influence the concepts, process, and quality leading to the creation of tissue-engineered products. Table 14.3 lists the various body tissues and their functions.

14.2.9 CASE STUDIES IN RELATION TO ELEMENTARY TISSUES OF THE BODY

14.2.9.1 Neural tissues: nanofibers for neural tissue engineering

The nervous system of the human body predominantly consists of nervous tissue, as the brain, the cerebellum, the spinal cord, and the cranial nerves. The primary cell of the nervous tissue is the neuron, which has properties of reception, discharge, and transmission of stimulus giving directions to the various systems of the body. This vital function becomes a challenging task in preparation of a bio-mimicked nervous scaffold. Fine et al. (2000) highlighted that neural tissue injuries lead to neuronal cell losses, which are irreversible. This necessitates the use of genetically engineered cells and ECM equivalents along with potent synthetic tools such as biomaterials for scaffold design and/or DDSs. Yang et al. (2005b) have reported the use of randomly oriented nanofibers (150–350 nm) of PLLA to achieve effective NSC adhesion and differentiation. Their studies with aligned nanofibers have shown NSC elongation and neuritis outgrowth along the direction of the fiber orientation of the aligned nanofibers coupled with increased rates of differentiation along the alignment. To study 3D culture and cell entrapment, Semino et al. (2004) developed a self-assembling peptide scaffold and demonstrated its potential for regenerating neural tissue attributed to its ability to increase the migration of glial and neural cells. In addition, the use of entrapped cells collected from the migration zone to initiate new culture has led to the development of a technique for neural progenitor cell isolation and enrichment *in vitro*.

Kaplan et al. (2014) engineered rat tissue from cortical neurons that formed complex networks of functioning neurons, which behaved normally after an injury. The research team built a ring-shape scaffold out of fibroin, a protein found in silk. Six concentric scaffold circles—each seeded with a different neuronal cell type—represented the six layers of the mammalian cortex. To measure the lab-grown tissue's responses to injury, the researchers dropped a weight onto the scaffold. The subsequent chemical and electrical responses of the neurons were similar to what has been shown in animals.

3D constructs for neuro-regeneration are contemplated wherein tissue-engineered constructs are pre-engineered *in vitro* to directly replace lost axonal tracts to recapitulate the architecture of the lost neural tissue which directly replaces lost axonal tracts or to serve as living targeted scaffold axonal regeneration (Cullen et al., 2007).

14.2.9.2 Musculoskeletal tissue

14.2.9.2.1 Case study (i): Engineered muscle flap

Large soft tissue defects resulting from complex trauma cause significant tissue loss and essentially require surgical reconstruction. In such situations, autologous flaps are inadequate, and fabrication of a tissue-engineered muscle flap, being its own functional vascular pedicle for repair, is required to avoid harvesting autologous flaps and postoperative scarification. Keeping the pedicle intact ensures uninterrupted blood supply to the tissue through the conduits. Shandalov et al. (2014) engineered a muscle flap from a porous polymer scaffold which was seeded with endothelial cells, fibroblasts, and myoblasts of a mouse and cultured *in vitro*. This was then implanted around the femoral artery and veins along with its own vascular pedicle. The regenerated axial muscle flap was transplanted as a large soft tissue at the abdominal wall defect in the same mouse. The implanted engineered flap evolved as a tissue, rich in vascular density, within a span of 7 days. This integrated itself well with the host tissue ensuring perfusion and anastomosis with host vessels, apart from providing mechanical strength to support abdominal viscera. Many materials (natural and synthetic) have been explored as nanofibrous scaffolding materials for bone, cartilage, ligament, and skeletal muscle tissue engineering, including hydroxyapatite (HA; Ramay and Zhang, 2003), chitosan (Bhattarai et al., 2005), PLGA (Uematsu et al., 2005), carbon (Price et al., 2003), and aluminum nanofibers (Webster et al., 2005).

14.2.9.2.2 Case study (ii): Nanofibers for bone tissue engineering

The musculoskeletal system represents as an integrated unit in the human body, such as bone–ligament–bone, muscle–tendon–bone, and cartilage–bone. Thus, integrated tissue– tissue synchrony is important in musculoskeletal system applications. However, it requires a state-of-the-art complex scaffold design based on understanding of natural human physiological structures and functions. This approach is termed "strategic biomimicry" and will enable development of composite tissue systems. It holds promise of imparting integration and functional repair of soft tissue injuries in the native environment, and reconstruction of a joint or even the total limb.

Many materials (natural and synthetic) such as HA (Ramay and Zhang, 2003), chitosan (Bhattarai et al., 2005), PLGA (Uematsu et al., 2005), carbon (Price et al., 2003), and aluminum nanofibers (Webster et al., 2005) have been exploited as nanofibrous scaffolding materials for bone, cartilage, ligament, and skeletal muscle TE.

Grayson et al. (2009) selected the temporomandibular joint (TMJ) condyler bone as their tissue model. The TMJ is the connection between the jaw bone and the skull and has a complex shape. With the TE approach, an entire bone condyle with exact geometrical and anatomical shape was created *in vitro* using human mesenchymal stem cells (hMSCs) and a "biomimetic" scaffold—a bioreactor system with control of interstitial flow. Fully decellularized trabecular bone seeded with hMSCs, and cultured with interstitial flow of culture medium constituted the formation of anatomically shaped scaffolds. The chamber of the bioreactor was designed exactly in the shape of a human TMJ. Flow patterns associated with the complex geometry of the bone graft provided a unique opportunity to correlate the architecture of the bone under formation with interstitial flow characteristics, *in vitro* but under control conditions. After about 5 weeks of cultivation, clear signs of a viable bone graft of complex geometry such as TMJ were evident from the formation of confluent layers of lamellar-bone, there was also a remarkable increase in the volume of mineralized matrix and the formation of osteoids. Thus it is now viable to engineer complex geometries of anatomically shaped patient-specific bone grafts for craniofacial and orthopedic reconstruction.

14.2.9.3 Connective tissues

Connective tissues are of the following types: (i) areolar tissue, (ii) adipose tissue, (iii) collagen tissue, (iv) yellow elastic tissue, (v) recticular-endothelial tissue, (vi) blood or hematopoietic tissue, (vii) cartilage, and (viii) osseous tissue (bone). We present below case studies for tissue-engineering designs used in common connective tissue repairs and replacements.

14.2.9.3.1 Case study (i): Cartilage

The cartilage tissues are typically regenerated by using hydrogel-based culture medium, impregnated with specific micronutrients and growth ingredients. The living cells preferred in this process are adult human stem cells. However, these cells generate a relatively low-tensile cartilage, contrary to its anticipated load-bearing functions. Another alternative to ASCs is mesenchymal cells, which undergo a condensation process prior to induction into the culture medium. This technique successfully regenerated cartilage tissue with reasonable mechanical strength and flexibility to remodel into the required anatomical shapes as per the functional needs (Bhumiratna et al., 2014).

14.2.9.3.2 Case study (ii): Collagen tissue

The presence of collagen in all connective tissue makes collagen-based biomaterials most important for tissue engineering and regenerative medicine. Collagen, a fibrous protein, forms the major component of skin and bone. It can be extracted from various tissue sources and assembled in combination with the molecules of skin and bone. Collagen types I, II, III, V, and XI are fiber-forming collagens. Of these mostly type I collagen is used as a biomaterial in the field of tissue engineering. There are two prime methods in which collagen-based biomaterials can be formed. In the first, the collagen matrix is decellularized while preserving the original tissue shape and the ECM structure. In the second method the collagen can be extracted and purified or collagen and its diverse components can be polymerized to form a scaffold which is biologically fully functional.

Crosslinking methods of reinforcement and protocols can be subsequently applied to both the types. Gilbert, Sellaro, and Badylak proposed three methods for the production of acellular collagen matrix or ECM, namely: physical, chemical, and enzymatic (Gilbert et al., 2006). The extracted type of collagen-based biomaterial is obtained by processing a collagen solution with biomolecules like chitosan, elastin, and glycosaminoglycans (GAG) (Aprahamian et al., 1987). The collagen-based scaffolds serve as a basis for first-hand information for the researchers to study the cell behavior like cell proliferation, differentiation, migration, and phenotype expression.

Other collagen-based scaffolds offer themselves as the model to study the nervous system to visualize motor neuron myelination by Schwann cells (Gingras et al., 2008). 3D collagen scaffolds can be useful to study anticancer drugs since these can be analyzed to study the invasive character of cancer cells and interactions between cancer cells and other, healthy cells.

Collagen-based biomaterials are used for bone and cartilage (type II collagen) reconstruction, especially when osteochondral defects reach an important volume or when autografts need to be avoided. For bone regeneration the collagen is hardened either by mineralization with calcium phosphate or by crosslinking with a substance like HA or bushite. Osteochondral defects can be filled with sheet-like collagen scaffolds seeded with or without autologous cells.

14.2.9.3.3 Case study (iii): Vascular tissues

Two challenges need to be addressed when dealing with vascular malfunction diseases. The first is cardiovascular malfunction and the second is atherosclerosis. Collagen-based materials offer an impressive solution to cardiovascular tissue regeneration. Due to the problems with the autologous grafts, collagen- and elastin-based tissue-engineered vascular grafts can be an alternate source since they can be potentially remodeled, repaired, regrown and can adapt to local hemodynamic conditions and acquire the structural and mechanical characteristics of the vessel they replace.

They thus serve as a biocompatible component with tensile strength to provide mechanical support, compliance, and recoil. Acid-soluble type I collagen as a scaffold has proved that it neither enhances blood coagulation, interferes with viscoelastic properties of the blood, nor supports excessive platelet adhesion and aggregation (Boccafoschi et al., 2005). Electrospun silk fibroin fibers fabricated into tubular conduits promote vascular cell growth (Zhang et al., 2008). Cell sheets can be rolled up to form layered tubular structures offering sufficient mechanical strength and suturability (L'Huereux et al., 1998). A robust vascular network was formed when mesenchymal stem cells (MSCs) from human bone marrow were combined with human endothelial cells (Bischoff and Melero-Martin, 2008). The incorporation of different types of cells into a gel resulted in a self-organized tube-like structure resembling a network of small blood vessels. When such gels were implanted in mice, an intravascular connection was established between the host cells of mice and the blood vessels in the gels and blood coursed through the engineered human vessel for up to 4 weeks. The interesting result obtained here is that the stem cells acted here as "builders" to help organize "the building block" (in this case the endothelial cells) into a functional 3D network rather than functioning in typical stem cell capacity. That is, neither did they differentiate into the endothelial cells nor did they convert themselves into bone, cartilage, or fat that MSCs normally do. Collagen-based vascular tissue engineering grafts lacked mechanical integrity. This problem was overcome by using nanopatterned type I collagen films which were prepared by solvent casting on poly(dimethylsiloxane) (PDMS) templates. The films were rolled into tubular conduits and crosslinked.

The nanopatterns were estimated to guide the smooth muscle cells and the eventual secretion of ECM in a circumferential manner by these cells mimicking the natural ECM of the vessels (Zorlutuna et al., 2008).

14.2.9.3.4 Case study (iv): Yellow elastic tissues

Yellow elastic tissues present in the ligaments are bands of dense connective tissue that connect bones to other bones and are responsible for joint movements and stability. Although the ligaments are mechanical load-bearing elements in the body, they have a poor regeneration capacity. Rupture of ligaments causes irreversible damage to the surrounding tissue, leading to tissue-degenerative diseases which cannot be clinically addressed (Lin et al., 1999; Goutet et al., 2000). Induction of autografts and allografts is the clinical approach; however, each has its own limitations.

TE is a novel promising technique by which an ideal engineered ligament that allows immediate load-bearing and degrades at a comparable rate can be constructed. Additional clinical advantages offered by such tissue-engineered ligaments are simpler surgical techniques, rapid recovery to pre-injury functions, biodegradation at a rate that provides sufficient mechanical stability, minimal patient morbidity, host tissue ingrowth support system, cell adhesion, and matrix formation.

Different materials that have been used for the formation of tissue-engineered ligament are collagens, silk, HA, and ECM bioscaffolds such as urinary bladder membrane and intestine submucosa. Among synthetic polymers are PGA, PLLA, poly(ethylene oxide) (PEO), and poly(urethane urea).

In order to assemble a biomimic ligament-like tissue structure, different combinational geometries are mandatory. Such combinations may include knitting, braiding, stratifying, merging scaffolds with sponges, crosslinking of scaffolds along with the cells, functionalization of scaffold surfaces, addition of mechanical *ex vivo* stimulation, etc.

14.2.9.4 Epithelial tissues: skin and cornea

The tissue structures for skin and cornea are similar. Dermis and stroma are the connective tissue, epidermis and cornea being stratified epithelia. The epidermis of skin and the epithelium of the cornea are self-renewing tissue, since they house a permanent pool of stem cells, which ensures their homeostasis. Tissue engineering strategies can be successfully applied to construct a living biological substitute for the treatment of skin and corneal defects.

Thin sheets of living keratinocytes rich in fundamental epithelial cell population generate fully differentiated epidermis after grafting. These can be clinically used as wound dressings for burned patients. Tissue-engineered collagen is most common and is used as the first line of treatment in cases of burns and ulcers. Similarly for the treatment of limbal stem cell deficiency corneal stem cell cultures have been used. Different skin models applying the tissue engineering strategies were developed. These were demonstrated utilizing sensory innervation, dendritic cells (Bechetoille et al., 2007), capillary network (Tremblay et al., 2005), adipose tissue, and tissue reproducing psoriatic or sclerotic phenotypes. Natural and synthetic biomaterials have been used to regenerate dermis. Their physical form may vary from hydrogels to fibrous, sheet-like porous scaffolds. These can be engineered to mimic the native physical environment by controlling stiffness, porosity, architecture, and topography. These can further be functionalized to enable ECM proteins such as collagens, fibronectin, and ligands like arginine-glycine-aspartic acid peptides to mimic the microenvironment guiding the stem cell behavior *in vitro*. Autologous cultured skin substitute prevent the problems associated with rejection and can function as a permanent skin replacement. These can be developed by seeding fibroblasts in bovine collagen and GAG sponge, which are seeded with autologous keratinocytes to regenerate new skin. Edmonds (2009) reconstructed a living allogeneic skin which was commercialized as a temporary dressing for ulcer treatment. Advances in corneal scaffolds which are collagen-based, include the use of recombinant human collagen (Griffith et al., 2009), self-assembled fibroblast sheets which themselves secrete collagen, and modification of surface to reduce extensive endothelialization (Rafat et al., 2009). Human postnatal MSCs derived from adipose tissue can be used to reconstruct connective or adipose tissue *in vitro* (Vermette et al., 2007).

14.2.9.5 Nanofibers for controlled drug delivery

Nanofibers can be loaded with drug for drug delivery, targeted at a particular site. Such nanofiber-based DDSs are used to improve the performance and safety of the medicinal drug by delivering them to the site of action at a rate dictated by the need of the physiological environment. Also, bioactive molecule-laden polymer nanofibers that are electrospun have been tested as drug delivery vehicles as per the requirement of the specific application (Heller and Hoffman, 2004).

One of the early researches on this was reported by Kenawy et al. (2002). The drug to be delivered was chosen to be tetracycline hydrochloride for periodontal applications. The polymer mats were made from PLA, PEVA, or from a 50:50 blend of the two, using chloroform as the solvent. Studies were also reported on DDS which were fast-dissolving, implantable, transdermal, oral, and transmembrane.

The active pharmaceutical ingredients were used as model drugs, such as herbs, poorly water-soluble or highly water-soluble proteins, genes, vaccines, and DNA. Chew et al. (2005) reported delivery of human β-nerve growth factor (NGF) that was stabilized in the carrier protein, bovine serum albumin (BSA).

The polymer matrix in this case was a copolymer of ε-caprolactone and ethyl ethylene phosphate. The sustained release of NGF by diffusion was obtained for at least 3 months.

Luu et al. (2003) made use of a DNA/synthetic polymer (PLGA) and PLA-PEG block copolymer composition in gene delivery designed for tissue engineering. Maximum release of plasmid DNA occurred at approximately two hours, which could be sustained for a period of 20 days. The important finding of the study was that DNA was indeed intact, capable of cellular transfection, and successfully expressed the encoded protein β-galactosidase. Polymer nanofiber served as a drug delivery vehicle due to two governing reasons, first their high surface-to-volume ratio and second the profile of the drug released can be easily and finely controlled and tailored by modulating not only the composition of the nanofiber mats but also the morphology of nanofibers, the process, and the microstructure.

Core-sheath morphology is very versatile and utilized in many applications. Xu et al. (2006) reported core-sheath nanowires which were prepared by "emulsion electrospinning." The core here is of PEO and sheath of PEG-PLA. The diameter of the core can be controlled by varying emulsion composition and emulsion parameter.

Coaxial electrospinning is another approach where an initial burst effect is avoided. Here two or more polymer liquids are forced by an electrostatic potential. The resultant fiber is a coaxial fiber, which offers protection toward easily denatured biological agents and ability to wrap all substances in the core regardless of drug–polymer interaction. With this technique proteins, drugs, GFs, and even genes can be incorporated into nanofibers by dissolving them in the core solution. Nanofiber scaffolds serve as a drug delivery vehicle for both hydrophilic and hydrophobic drugs. Controlling the fiber morphology, porosity, and composition can monitor the drug release rate. The major achievement in this regard is that the peak concentration of the drug can be achieved in a shorter pulsating manner. This makes it target-oriented, with focused action on the organ or a system, for example, antibiotics. These can also function effectively in cases such as diabetes and chronic asthma where the optimal drug is to be delivered at a slow rate of absorption with distribution throughout the day.

14.2.9.6 Nanofibers for DNA, protein, and enzyme delivery

Electrospun scaffolds loaded with DNA, protein, or enzyme with all their versatilities could prove to be the next "magic-bullet" in the field of molecular drug delivery systems. Electrospun nanofibers possess special attributes, such as high aspect ratio and interconnected pores. This feature completely resembles the topology of ECM. These important attributes are essential for the transport of nutrients, oxygen, and excreting waste through the pores. Such assemblies of nanofibers loaded with bioactive molecules establish communication between the seeded cell and the ECM for cell growth, proliferation, and differentiation as well as to deliver a range of genes, drugs, DNA, and proteins. The initial study of Fang et al. (1997) demonstrated that DNA can be electrospun into nanofibers. However, the first demonstration of the use of electrospun nanofiber scaffold as a nonviral gene delivery vehicle by the use of plasmid DNA was reported by Hadjiargyrou et al. (2005). Biopolymers used for gene delivery are PVA, PEG, PLGA, and PLA-PEG copolymers. Electrospinning of nanofibers to form a scaffold can serve as a better platform for enzyme immobilization, because it offers a high aspect ratio, effective loading, reduced mass transfer resistance, and easier recycling. Physical parameters such as size and surface morphology, essential for enzyme immobilization, can be easily controlled during nanofiber fabrication.

Biocatalytic conjugates made up of electrospun polystyrene, poly(styrene co-maleic anhydride) nanofiber, when coated with trypsin, served as a stable nanobiocatalytic system (Lee et al., 2010). Fructose dehydrogenase was immobilized on gold nanofibers by Marx et al. (2011) to develop a biosensor which could detect both serum and popular beverages sweetened with high-fructose corn syrup. Nanofibers are also known to be protein-delivery vehicles. PVA nanofibers were uploaded with BSA or luciferase proteins. A chemical vapor deposition technique was used to coat them further by poly (p-xylene). The bioactivity of released protein was then studied for coated and uncoated PVA fibers (Zeng et al., 2005). The findings demonstrated that intact protein and enzyme were continuously released from both the nanofibers and their bioactivity was preserved after releasing from scaffolds.

14.3 APPLICATION OF TISSUE ENGINEERING IN ARTIFICIAL ORGANS

Recreation of artificial organs through tissue engineering is an invaluable achievement influencing the quality of human life. A functionally damaged vital organ causes high mortality unless it is replaced either by human transplant or by laboratory-based, artificially prepared organs. Lack of transplantable organs and the long waiting list adversely affect the patient's quality of life. In addition, the financial burden builds-up over a period of time on the individual and society. Organ transplants are associated with a high prevalence of immune-rejection. Also, organs could be subjected to ischemic damage during the time from removal from the donor to the time of transplantation into the recipient.

"Off-the-shelf" replacement organs offer many advantages, for example, surgical procedures are quicker, waiting lists can be cut, and health services can save money. However, our vital organs are complex and therefore very difficult to mimic using artificial materials; all artificial organs provide only a limited compromise in function. This section discusses artificial organ transplants in selective cases as representative examples. Figure 14.9 is a cartoon, illustrating the future in artificial organ recreation, leading to a remodeled human.

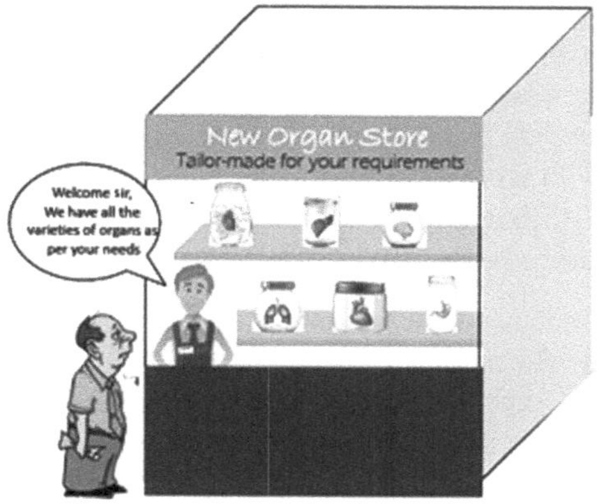

FIGURE 14.9

Future of human remodeling.

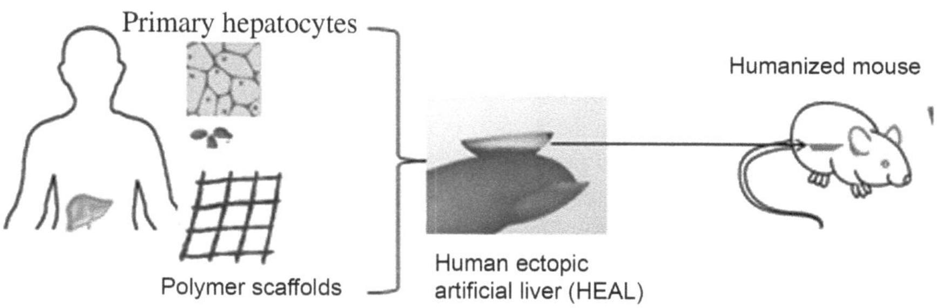

FIGURE 14.10

To the naked eye, a HEAL looks like a pink contact lens. Approximately 4/5 of an inch in diameter, the implant comprises half a million liver cells.

1. *Regenerating a new kidney*: The regeneration of a new kidney in the case of patients with end-stage renal failure is the last hope for survival of such patients. Researchers invented a new possibility by first stripping cells from a donor organ and using the remaining collagen scaffold to aid growth of new tissue. They regenerated kidney from patients' own cells by seeding kidney scaffolds with epithelial and endothelial cells. In the case of rats the regenerated kidney performed the physiological functions of clearance of metabolites, reabsorption of nutrients, and produced urine, both *in vitro* and *in vivo*. Thus the need for organ donation was circumvented, eliminating the constraints of donor organ shortages and the morbidity associated with immunosuppression in organ transplants.
2. *Implanting human liver in mice*: An engineered human liver tissue implanted in a mouse (Figure 14.10) has demonstrated the drug-metabolizing capacity

similar to humans while retaining the normal mice liver functions. This has paved the way for further studies on testing susceptibility to toxicity and demonstrating species-specific responses before clinical trials.

3. *Retinal cells printed by inkjet*: Organ printing TE is a modern and innovative approach of TE with a potential to provide a 3D environment to cells. Its success has been attributed to its property of not suffering from vascularization and cell organization limitation.

It involves the simultaneous deposition of assembly of cells and ECM elements so as to biomimic the functional organ to be reconstructed. Using CAD, biologically relevant materials such as molecules, cells, tissues, and biodegradable biomaterials can be deposited in a layer-by-layer fashion to fabricate a 3D vascularized functional living human organ (Mirononv et al., 2008). This time-efficient process finds applications in clinical implantation, pharmacological tests, histogenesis, and organogenesis (Mironov et al., 2011; Partridge et al., 2012). Organ printing finds its origin from the classical approach of designing hydrogel-based ECM with high cell density, essential for the fabrication of solid organ structures.

Two approaches have been devised to carryout organ printing: the first approach involves printing of proteins and cells (or small clusters of cells) over the ECM hydrogels using a commercial inkjet printer (Wilson and Boland, 2003). Here hydrogels work as "biopapers" and cell blocks or tissue spheroids work as a "bioink." Thus, during the biomanufacturing of viable tissue, biopapers mentioned above take the same shape and contours of the organ to be printed, whereas the cell spheroids serving as bioink vary in properties according to their composition, ensuring the functional aspect of the organ. Cells can sustain the temperature and the deposition conditional forces of the printer. In the second approach, mechanical extruders interfaced with computer that dictates the topology of the organ are used to print organs by fusing "bioink" particles into "biopapers." The advantage of this technique is that here cells are sorted and arranged to form a 3D tissue so that they reside in a more physiologically compatible environment. This establishes adhesive contacts with the neighboring host cells ensuring transmission of vital biomolecular signals. The inkjet printing and use of extruder for printing are biocompatible with RP. Greens (2013) demonstrated how to print healthy rat retinal cells. These printed retinal cells demonstrated an ability for retinal repairs. The printed retinal ganglion cells and glia were just as likely to survive as nonprinted cells. The findings generated an exciting possibility for a tissue-engineered functional eye with restoration of eyesight.

Biomanufacturing of organ printing needs to have control over two aspects of phase change of fluids dealing with viscoelastic properties of fluids that form hydrogels or biopaper. First, the fluid which carries cells and molecules should behave as a viscoelastic solid immediately after printing and, secondly, it must not solidify too much otherwise the cell spheroids cannot interact and hamper tissue growth. Thus, phase change has to be gradual without causing damage to the biochemical cells or biomolecular signals. Organ printing makes use of "state-of-art" devices like automated cell sorters, organ and cell bioreactors, robotic printers, extruders, etc. Organ printing holds promise to deliver high throughput of artificial organs and transforms tissue engineering into a commercially successful biomedical industry.

1. Human body compatible—artificial blood: Creating artificial blood of all types of blood group is the ultimate treatment modality in medical care. Akst (2014) have reported a revolutionary breakthrough in the creation of human artificial blood from fibroblasts. In this, the PSCs, integrated with dedifferentiated and reprogrammed fibroblasts, are impregnated into a cultured bone-marrow-like environment for about a month. Blood cells thus formed are then obtained from the cell culture. This technique has promising potential for mass production of blood, ensuring a continuous supply of artificial blood and could truly be a life-saving technology, especially during disasters and calamities when massive numbers of human lives are at stake.

It is important to note that the recipients of the blood group should have negative RH factor as this artificially generated blood will be classified as "O negative" blood group. The "O" blood group is also known as the "universal donor" blood group. As such, the availability of RH negative blood is inadequate in the general population, hence, the discovery would possibly raise the availability of blood for all hematological disorders such as thalassemia, sickle cell anemia, and blood cancers.

14.4 CHALLENGES IN TISSUE ENGINEERING

TE promises to deliver a complete, functional repair of human tissue which may be damaged either by disease or injury. With the advent of new inventions in stem cell biology it is now possible to direct the integration of transplanted cells into the damaged tissue, replacing such structures with the new tissue-engineered organs, developed *in vitro* using biomaterials such as cells, biomaterials imparting signals, and regenerating damaged structures by employing endogenous repair mechanisms *in vivo*.

TE has now emerged as an independent discipline in medical science since 1980. Although these methods have significantly improved the lifespan of patients, a number of challenges remain unaddressed. Certain therapeutic approaches and additional breakthroughs are still required until this is established as a fully fledged technology for organ regeneration with complete recreation of physiological functions. In a broader sense, the main disadvantages are shortage of matched organs for people who are waiting for the transplantation, constant immunosuppressant therapies which can damage the health of patients, challenging nerve transplantations, and the limited life of transplanted organs.

The challenges associated with the translation applications regarding soft tissue engineering strategies are listed below:

1. Mechanical challenges such as scaffold collapse and "on-the-shelf" availability.
2. Survival of cells after implantation.
3. Compositional considerations, such as microenvironment-related malignant behavior, cell exhaustion, or cell migration.

The major concern in translational applications is to maintain a high volume-to-surface ratio at all levels. This presents a constant threat to survival of cells due to the lack of a sufficient supply of oxygen and nutrient.

While addressing the volume restoration challenge the mechanical design of the scaffold would have to match the contours of the removed tissue and provide initial mechanical support to prevent collapse of the volume defect while being able to degrade completely and be replaced with soft tissue. Furthermore, the patterned microenvironment of the construct must provide a degradable porous conduit for tissue infiltration, provide a substrate for cell adherence and migration, mimic the optimal extracellular environment for the engineered tissue, and house the delivery vehicles for any desired bioactive compounds. For this, structural elements (i.e., porosity) and chemical makeup (i.e., ECM composition and cell adhesiveness characteristics) should be in congruence with each other.

Cell migration can be rectified by creating pull vectors and gradients, which can control the spatiotemporal distribution and micropatterning of the biological factors. Similarly, by the addition of tissue-type plasminogen activation or by the addition of enzymes, which help degrade matrix of the ECM, cell exhaustion can be prevented.

Another challenge to TE, which needs to be addressed when designing tissue *in vitro* vascularization, is the lack of a sufficient blood vessel system, causing insufficient supply of oxygen and nutrients to the engineered tissue. *In vivo*, in the host tissue there is an enormous supply of endothelial-cell-coated tubular networks. The new tissue engineering strategy is therefore based on developing endothelial cells as well as their ability to form new vessels known as neo-angiogenesis.

The California Institute for Regenerative Medicine (CIRM) organized a workshop on engineering strategies opportunities, challenges for tissue repair, and regeneration during January 2012. The workshop summarized various challenges to be met in the field of tissue engineering along with recommendations, including those listed below.

1. To support research using scaffolds, preseeded with cells for transplantation as well as cell-free scaffold approaches. Such methods should promote use of such scaffolds that would integrate itself with the transplant site in addition to providing a conducive microenvironment.
2. To support development of hydrogels that mimic the natural tissue properties. Devising appropriate hydrogels to give the best chance for an effective therapy.

3. To model stem cell niches *in vivo* to enhance the direct stem cell expansion *in vitro*.
4. To develop better quantitative tools for testing tissue-engineered products. These would help in the assessment of cell quality, scaling up of good manufacturing processes in clinical trials by using appropriate assays for validating the biological activity.
5. To develop materials that mitigate the immune response and enhance engraftment. Patients' immune systems must be the prime consideration in designing and application of tissue-engineered tools. In this regard, Frey-Vasconcells et al. (2012) reported that a small-animal model system may not yield sufficient insight to guide best practices in human, specifically in the context of predicting safety and efficacy of tissue-engineered organs. This is because although the small-animal models (Chu et al., 2010), like rat, rabbit, and mice, offer easy access to experimental material and genetically modified strains for *in vivo* studies, their immunity is higher, that is, they are inherently more resistant to infections than humans.
6. To help educate researchers about the translational considerations of cell–scaffold combination products.
7. To promote interactions between stem cells and biomaterial communities implies involving surgeons in the product development process as well as communicating with stakeholders, FDA interactions, communicating with patients, funders and advocates, nonscientists, and regulatory personnel.
8. Facilitating dialog with the FDA regarding regulations of tissue-engineered products.

It is important to bridge the "Valley of Death" (Finkbeiner, 2010). Biomedical breakthroughs or discoveries seldom reach the clinic or the market place either because of flaws in the technologies or due to other competing technologies. Most scientists are short of funds, and lack regulatory know-how and incentives to send their inventions to market. Tissue-engineering products from academia must reach industry through suitable business models.

In industry, quality control is the most important issue for the promotion of tissue engineering products. The establishment of quality control protocols and standard procedures manuals is necessary in this context. The standard protocols of GMP and FDA regulations should be complied with stringently. An international quality accreditation standards assessment organization should be established globally. All research in tissue engineering is subjected to approval by authorized ethics committees.

14.5 THE FUTURE

TE has tremendous scope. The impact of TE on society will be exemplary. It holds the promise of sustainable improvement in the quality of human life, with a reduction in the societal and economic cost associated with healthcare and life expectancy. It has potential to offer early detection of pathological conditions, reduce the severity of therapy and result in an improved clinical outcome for the patient. It may discover newer approaches for promotion of health and longevity. The ultimate goal is obviously comprehensive monitoring, repair, and improvement of all human biologic systems. Essentially, an enhanced and sustainable quality of life with "health" as the prime goal as defined by the "World Health Organization" (WHO defines health as a state of complete physical, mental, social, and spiritual well-being, and not merely the absence of disease).

In future, collaborative efforts amongst all countries are anticipated in evolving policies with reference to the development of tissue-engineered products. This will lead to development of "standard guidelines" on safety and efficacy which are acceptable worldwide. The formation of global and national committees to monitor the quality aspects of tissue-engineered products with international regulations is envisioned in this context. Networking and "big-data" communications between industry, medical professionals, and disease morbidity trends need to be established.

Newer terminologies such as "microphysiological systems research program" and "body on a chip" program have been coined with reference to the promotion of advanced research in TE. This initiative implies endorsement of a multidisciplinary approach, merging tissue engineering and systems biology—an integrative physiology—as an incredibly powerful combination for the future of the recreation of human physiological systems, in totality.

TE has great significance in regenerative medicine, which is an essential component of all surgical and allied specialties. Thus, it will have applications in dermatology, dentistry, general surgery, plastic surgery, pediatric surgery, oncology, gynecology, ophthalmology, gastrointestinal medicine and surgery, urology, neurosurgery, cardiovascular and thoracic surgery, ear-nose-throat surgery, and organ transplants. Amongst the nonsurgical specialties, it will have its applications in gastrointestinal medicine, general medicine, endocrinology, anesthesia, chest medicine, neurology, and geriatric medicine. This wide spectrum of medical therapeutic applications is a reality because of advances in the tissue-engineered targeted, controlled-release DDS. New horizons in the field of nanomedicine have now emerged as a promising futuristic technology. This will revolutionize medicine and its applied aspects in the fields of drug delivery, drug resistance, gene therapy, diagnostics, medical therapies, treatment protocols, immunomodulants or -simulants therapy, surgical interventions, and related research areas in the interests of quality patient care and medical research. The field of nanomedicine has also led to the evolution of the concept of the "submicroscopic laboratory," which facilitates handling of cell components, viruses, or pieces of DNA, using a range of tiny tools, robots, and tubes. It is needless to say that this revolution will also redefine the application of "epidemiological" principles to determine disease causation—the basis of medical research.

It implies that the potential for tissue-engineered bionanotechnology to mimic native ECM and related cells and tissues is a path-breaking revolutionary tool for alternative medical therapies.

The merger of bioengineering and medicine emphasizes the emergence of a multidisciplinary approach as the most advanced professional skill of the practitioners of medicine and surgery. The fusion induces formation of new functional tissues rather than just implanting spare parts. With the expanding avenues of tissue engineering, medical terms such as "impairment," "disability," and "handicap" will become obsolete, as the lost functions due to tissue damage will be restored in the body.

Human diseases which cause tissue damage are usually managed with clinical approaches which comprise of "early diagnosis and treatment" (secondary prevention) and "disability limitation" and "rehabilitation" (tertiary prevention). Tissue engineering is poised to dominate the spectrum of secondary and tertiary medical care in the future, including both medical and surgical interventions. The role of tissue engineering has already emerged in developing nutraceuticals (science of nutrients) for health promotion. This will then make tissue engineering as effective a tool even for primary health care (health promotion and specific protection). In fact, the future of medicine may witness development of a specialty branch called the "tissue engineer medicine specialist." Futuristic vision reflects bionanotechnology and tissue engineering applications as the crowning components of the medical therapy pyramid in medicine.

REFERENCES

Adams, M.A., Roughley, P.J., 2006. What is intervertebral disc degeneration, and what causes it? Spine 31 (18), 2151–2161.

Agarwal, S., et al., 2009. Progress in the field of electrospinning for tissue engineering applications. Adv. Mater. 21, 3343.

Akst, J., 2014. Artificial Blood Is Patient-Ready. University of Edinburgh, Edinburgh, http://www.the-cientist.com/?articles.view/articleNo/39718/title/Artificial-Blood-Is-Patient-Ready/.

Alexakis, T., Boadid, K., Guong, D., et al., 1995. Microencapsulation of DNA within alginate microspheres and cross linked chitosan membranes for *in vivo* application. Appl. Biochem. Biotechnol. 50 (1), 93–106.

Aprahamian, M., Lambert, A., Balboni, G., Lefebvre, F., Schmitthaeusler, R., Damge, C., et al., 1987. New reconstituted connective tissue matrix: preparation, biochemical, structural and mechanical studies. J. Biomed. Mater. Res. 21, 965–977.

Bambole, V.A., Mahanwar, P.A., Kulkarni, A., 2010. Electrospinning of polymers, their modeling and applications. Polym.-Plast. Technol. Eng. 49 (5), 427–441.

Barakat, N.A.M., et al., 2009. Polymer 50, 4389.

Bashur, C.A., et al., 2006. Biomaterials 27, 5681.

Batorsky, A., Liao, J., Lund, A.W., Plopper, G.E., Stegemann, J.P., 2005. Encapsulation of adult human mesenchymal stem cells within collagen-agarose microenvironments. Biotechnol. Bioeng. 92 (4), 492–500.

Bechetoille, N., Dezutter-Dambuyant, C., Damour, O., Andre, V., Orly, I., Perrier, E., 2007. Effects of solar ultraviolet radiation on engineered human skin equivalent containing both langerhans cells and dermal dendritic cells. Tissue Eng. 13, 2667–2679.

Beebe, D.J., Moore, J.S., Bauer, J.M., et al., 2000. Functional hydrogel structures for autonomous flow control inside microfluidic channels. Nature 404 (6778), 588–590.

Bellas, E., Seiberg, M., Garlick, J., Kaplan, D.L., 2012. *In vitro* 3D full-thickness skin-equivalent tissue model using silk and collagen biomaterials. Macromol. Biosci. 12, 1627–1636.

Berndt, P., Fields, G.B., Tirrell, M., 1995. Synthetic lipidation of peptides and amino acids: monolayer structure and prop. J. Am. Chem. Soc. 117, 9515–9522.

Bhattarai, S.R., Bhattarai, N., Yi, H.K., et al., 2004. Novel biodegradable electrospun membrane: scaffold for tissue engineering. Biomaterials 25, 259–5602.

Bhattarai, N., Edmondson, D., Veiseh, O., et al., 2005. Electrospun chitosan-based nanofibers and their cellular compatibility. Biomaterials. 26 (31), 6176–6184.

Bhumiratana, S., Ateshian, G.A., Vunjak-Novakovic G., 2014. Large, stratified, and mechanically functional human cartilage grown *in vitro* by mesenchymal condensation PNAS. 111 (19), 6940–6945.

Bischoff, J., Melero-Martin, J.M., 2008. An *in vivo* experimental model for postnatal vasculogenesis. Methods Enzymol. 445, 303–329.

Bisht, G.S., Canton, G., Mirsepassi, A., Kulinsky, L., Oh, S., Dunn-Rankin, D., et al., 2011. Controlled continuous patterning of polymeric nanofibers on three-dimensional substrates using low-voltage near-field electrospinning. Nano Lett. 11, 1831–1837.

Blan, N., Birla, K., 2008. Design and fabrication of heart muscle using scaffold-based tissue engineering. J. Biomed. Mater. Res. A 86A (1), 195–208.

Blokhuis, T.J., Termaat, M.F., Den Boer, F.C., Patka, P., Bakker, F.C., Haarman, H.J.T.M., 2000. Properties of calcium phosphate ceramics in relation to their *in vivo* behavior. J. Trauma Inj. Infect.Criti. Care 48 (1), 179–186.

Boccafoschi, F., Habermehl, J., Vesentini, S., et al., 2005. Biological performances of collagen-based scaffolds for vascular tissue engineering. Biomaterials 26 (35), 7410–7417.

Boland, T., Mironov, V., Gutowska, A., Roth, E.A., Markwald, R.R., 2003. Cell and organ printing 2: fusion of cell aggregates in three-dimensional gels. Anat. Rec. A 272 (2), 497–502.

Boland, E.D., Espy, P.G., Bowlin, G.L. 2004. Tissue engineering scaffolds. In Encyclopaedia of biomaterials and biomedical engineering. Wenk, G.E., Bowlin, G.L. (Eds). Richmong, Virginia, USA, pp. 1633-1635.

Borden, M., Attawia, M., Khan, Y., Laurencin, C.T., 2002. Tissue engineered microsphere-based matrices for bone repair: design and evaluation. Biomaterials 23 (2), 551–559.

Borden, M., El-Amin, S.F., Attawia, M., Laurencin, C.T., 2003. Structural and human cellular assessment of a novel microsphere-based tissue engineered scaffold for bone repair. Biomaterials 24 (4), 597–609.

Borschel, G.H., Huang, Y.C., Calve, S., Arruda, E.M., Lynch, J.B., Dow, D.E., et al., 2005. Tissue engineering of recellularized small-diameter vascular grafts. Tissue Eng. 11 (5–6), 778–786.

Brodie, J.C., Goldie, E., Connel, G., Merry, J., Grant, M.H., 2005. Osteoblast interactions with calcium phosphate ceramics modified by coating with type I collagen. J. Biomed. Mater. Res. A 73 (4), 409–421.

Broom, N.D., Poole, C.A., 1982. A functional-morphological study of the tidemark region of articular cartilage maintained in a non-viable physiological condition. J. Anat. 135 (1), 65–82.

Brown, T.D., Dalton, P.D., Hutmacher, D.W., 2011. Direct writing by way of melt electrospinnng. Adv. Mater. 23, 5651–5657.

Burdick, J.A., Khademhosseini, A., Langer, R., 2004. Fabrication of gradient hydrogels using a microfluidics/photopolymerization process. Langmuir 20 (13), 5153–5156.

Calvert, P., 2001. Inkjet printing for materials and devices. Chem. Mater. 13 (10), 3299–3305.

Causa, F., Netti, P.A., Ambrosio, L., 2007. A multi-functional scaffold for tissue regeneration: the need to engineer a tissue analogue. Biomaterials 28 (34), 5093–5099.

Chai, C., Leong, K.W., 2007. Biomaterials approach to expand and direct differentiation of stem cells. Mol. Ther. 15 (3), 467–480.

Chan, B.P., Leong, K.W., 2008. Scaffolding in tissue engineering: general approaches and tissue-specific considerations. Eur. Spine J. 17 (4), 467–479.

Chan, B.P., Chan, G.C.F., Wong, H.L., Cheung, P.T., Chan, D., Cheah, K., 2007a. Cell–matrix microsphere, associated products, methods for preparation and applications. Regular Patent Application 60/801,975 filed on 19 May 2007.

Chan, B.P., Hui, T.Y., Chan, O.C., So, K.F., Lu, W., Cheung, K.M., et al., 2007b. Photochemical cross-linking for collagen-based scaffolds: a study on optical properties, mechanical properties, stability, and hematocompatibility. Tissue Eng. 13 (1), 73–85.

Chan, B.P., Hui, T.Y., Yeung, C.W., Li, J., Mo, I., Chan, G.C.F., 2007c. Self-assembled collagen–human mesenchymal stem cell microspheres for regenerative medicine. Biomaterials 28, 4652–4666.

Chen, J., Chu, B., Hsiao, B.S., 2006a. Mineralization of hydroxyapatite in electrospun nanofibrous poly(L-lactic acid) scaffolds. J. Biomed. Mater. Res. A 79 (2), 307–317.

Chen, Q.Z., Thompson, I.D., Boccaccini, A.R., 2006b. 45S5 Bioglass®-derived glass-ceramic scaffolds for bone tissue engineering. Biomaterials 27 (11), 2414–2425.

Chester, J.K., Atala, A., 2004. Therapeutic cloning and tissue engineering. In: Schatten, G.P. (Ed.), Stem Cells in Development and Disease. Elsevier Academic Press, London, pp. 1–12.

Chevalier, E., Chulia, D., Pouget, C., Viana, M., 2008. Fabrication of porous substrates: a review of processes using pore forming agents in the biomaterial field. J. Pharm. Sci. 97 (3), 1135–1154.

Chew, S.Y., Wen, J., Yim, E.K.F., Leong, K.W., et al., 2005. Sustained release of proteins from electrospun biodegradable fibers. Biomacromolecules 6, 2017–2024.

Chew, S.Y., Wen, Y., Dzenis, Y., Leong, K.W., 2006. The role of electrospinning in the emerging field of nanomedicine. Curr. Pharm. Des. 12 (36), 4751–4770.

Chew, S.Y., et al., 2007. Adv. Funct. Mater 17, 1288.

Chew, S.Y., et al., 2008a. Biomaterials 29, 653.

Chew, S.Y., Mi, R., Hoke, A., Leong, K.W., 2008b. The effect of the alignment of electrospun fibrous scaffolds on schwann cell maturation. Biomaterials 29 (6), 653–661.

Chu, C.R., Szczodry, M., Bruno, S., 2010. Animal models for cartilage regeneration and repair. Tissue Eng. Part B 16 (1), 105–115.

Clifford, D.M., et al., 2012. Long-term effects of autologous bone marrow stem cell treatment in acute myocardial infarction: factors that may influence outcomes. PLoS One 7, e37373.

Cullen, D.K., et al., 2007. *In vitro* neural injury model for optimization of tissue engineered constructs. J. Neurosci. Res. 85 (16), 3642–3651.

Cullen, D.K., Pfister, B.J., 2011. State of the art and future challenges in neural engineering: neural interfaces. Crit. Rev. Biomed. Eng. 39 (1), 1–3.

Dalton, P.D., Vaquette, C., Farrugia, B.L., Gargaville, T., Brown, T.D., Hutmacher, D.W., 2013. Electrospinning and additive manufacturing: converging technologies. Biomater. Sci. 1, 171–185.

Dang, J.M., Leong, K.W., 2007. Myogenic induction of aligned mesenchymal stem cell sheets by culture on thermally responsive electrospun nanofibers. Adv. Mater. 19 (19), 2775–2779.

Dendukuri, D., Pregibon, D.C., Collins, J., Hatton, T.A., Doyle, P.S., 2006. Continuous-flow lithography for high-throughput microparticle synthesis. Nat. Mater. 5 (5), 365–369.

Deng, M., et al., 2011. Adv. Funct. Mater. 21, 2641.

Deng, M., et al., 2012. IEEE Trans. Nanobiosci. 11, 3.

Devillard, R., et al., 2014. Cell patterning by laser-assisted bioprinting. Methods Cell Biol. 119, 159–174.

Devin, J.E., Attawia, M.A., Laurencin, C.T., 1996. Three-dimensional degradable porous polymer-ceramic matrices for use in bone repair. J. Biomater. Sci. 7 (8), 661–669.

Dhandayuthapani, B., Yoshida, Y., Maekawa, T., Kumar, D.S., 2011. Polymeric scaffolds in tissue engineering application: a review. Int. J. Polym. Sci. 2011, Article ID 290602. Available from: http://dx.doi.org/10.1155/2011/290602.

Dhariwala, B., Hunt, E., Boland, T., 2004. Rapid prototyping of tissue-engineering constructs, using photopolymerizable hydrogels and stereolithography. Tissue Eng. 10 (9–10), 1316–1322.

Ding, B., et al., 2011. J. Mater. Chem. 21, 12784.

Doshi, J., Reneker, D.H., 1995. Electospinning process and application of electrospun fibers. J. Electrostat. 35, 51–60.

Du, J.A., Yarema, K.J., 2010. Adv. Drug. Deliv. Rev. 62, 671.

Dzenis, Y., 2004. Spinning continuous fibers for nanotechnology. Science 304, 1917–1919.

Edmonds, M., 2009. Apligraf in the treatment of neuropathic diabetic foot ulcers. Int. J. Low Extrem. Wounds 8, 11–18.

Ellison, C.J., Phatak, A., Giles, D.W., Macosko, C.W., Bates, F.S., 2007. Melt blown nanofibers: fiber diameter distributions and onset of fiber breakup. Polymer 48 (11), 3306–3316.

Engelmayr, G.C., et al., 2008. Nat. Mater. 7, 1003.

Fang, X., Reneker, D.H., et al., 1997. DNA fibers by electrospinning. J. Macromol. Sci. Phys. B 36 (2), 169–173.

Fernandez, T.L., Dawson, R.A., Van Lonkhuyzen, D.R., Kimlin, M.G., Upton, Z., 2012. A tan in a test tube—*in vitro* models for investigating ultraviolet radiation-induced damage in skin. Exp. Dermatol. 21, 404–410.

Fields, G.B., Lauer, J.L., Dori, Y., et al., 1998. Protein-like molecular architecture: biomaterial applications for inducing cellular receptor binding and signal transduction. Biopolymers 47, 143–151.

Fine, E.G., Valentini, R.F., Aebischer, P., 2000. Nerve regeneration. In: Lanza, R.P., Langer, R., Vacanti, J. (Eds.), Principles of Tissue Engineering, vol. 2. Academic Press, San Diego, pp. 785–796.

Finkbeiner, S., 2010. Bridging the Valley of Death of therapeutics for neurodegeneration. Nat. Med. 16, 1227–1232.

Frenot, A., Chronakis, I., 2003. Polymer nanofibers assembled by electrospinning. Curr. Opin. Coll. Inter. Sci. 8, 64–75.

Frey-Vasconcells, J., Whittlesey, K.J., Baum, E., Feigal, E.G., 2012. Translation of stem cell research: points to consider in designing preclinical animal studies. Stem Cells Translat. Med. 1, 16.

Fukuda, J., Khademhosseini, A., Yeo, Y., et al., 2006. Micromolding of photocrosslinkable chitosan hydrogel for spheroid microarray and co-cultures. Biomaterials 27 (30), 5259–5267.

Gauthier, O., Müller, R., Von Stechow, D., et al., 2005. *In vivo* bone regeneration with injectable calcium phosphate biomaterial: a three-dimensional micro-computed tomographic, biomechanical and SEM study. Biomaterials 26 (27), 5444–5453.

Geng, X., Kwon, O.H., Jang, J., 2005. Electrospinning of chitosan dissolved in concentrated acetic acid solution. Biomaterials 26, 5427–5432.

Gersbach, C.A., Byers, B.A., Pavlath, G.K., et al., 2004. Runx2/Cbfa1-genetically engineered skeletal myoblasts mineralize collagen scaffolds *in vitro*. Biotechnol. Bioeng. 88, 369–378.

Gilbert, T.W., Sellaro, T.L., Badylak, S.F., 2006. Decellularization of tissues and organs. Biomaterials 27, 3675–3683.

Gingras, M., Beaulieu, M.M., Gagnon, V., Durham, H.D., Berthod, F., 2008. *In vitro* study of axonal migration and myelination of motor neurons in a three-dimensional tissue-engineered model. Glia 56, 354–364.

Goodsell, D.S., 2004. Bionanotechnology—Lessons from Nature. Wiley-Liss, Inc., Hoboken, NJ.

Gray, D.W., 2001. An overview of the immune system with specific reference to membrane encapsulation and islet transplantation. Ann. N. Y. Acad. Sci. 944, 226–239.

Grayson, et al., 2009. Engineering anatomically shaped human bone grafts. Proc. Natl Acad. Sci. U.S.A. 107, 3299–3304.

Greens, K., 2013. Retinal Cells Printed by Inkjet. University of Cambridge, Cambridge.

Griffith, M., Jackson, W.B., Lagali, N., Merrett, K., Li, F., Fagerholm, P., 2009. Artificial corneas: a regenerative medicine approach. Eye (Lond.) 23, 1985–1989.

Hadjiargyrou, M., Chiu, J.B., et al., 2008. Enhanced composite electrospunnanofiber scaffolds for use in drug delivery. Expert. Opin. Drug Deliv. 5 (10), 1093–1106.

Hall, S., 1997. Axonal regeneration through acellular muscle grafts. J. Anat. 190 (1), 57–71.

Hao, H., Nian, G., Jia, S., Chao, G., Ping, H., 2008. Fabrication of biomatrix/polymer hybrid scaffold for heart valve tissue engineering *in vitro*. ASAIO J. 54 (6), 627–632.

Hartgerink, J.D., et al., 2002. Proc. Natl Acad. Sci. U.S.A. 99, 5133.

He, L., et al., 2010. Acta Biomater. 6, 2960.

Heller J., Hoffman, A.S., 2004. Drug delivery system. In: Ratner, B.D., Hoffman, A.S., Schoen, F.J., Lemons, J.E. (Eds.). Biomaterials Science: An Introduction to Materials in Medicine, 2nd ed. Elsevier Academic Press, San Francisco, CA, pp. 628–648.

Hirano, S., Zhang, M., Nakagawa, M., Miyata, T., 2000. Wet spun chitosan-collagen fibers, their chemical N-modifications, and blood compatibility. Biomaterials 21 (10), 997–1003. Available from: http://dx.doi.org/10.1016/S0142-9612(99)00258-6.

Ho, Y.C., Mi, F.L., Sung, H.W., Kuo, P.L., 2009. Heparin-functionalized chitosan-alginate scaffolds for controlled release of growth factor. Int. J. Pharm. 376 (1–2), 69–75.

Hohman, M.M., Shin, M., Rutledge, G., et al., 2001a. Electrospinning and electrically forced jets I. Stab. Theor. Phys Fluids 13, 2201–2220.

Hohman, M.M., Shin, M., Rutledge, G., et al., 2001b. Electrospinning and electrically forced jets II. Applications. Phys. Fluids 13, 1–16.

Holland, T.A., Tessmar, J.K.V., Tabata, Y., Mikos, A.G., 2004. Transforming growth factor-β1 release from oligo(poly(ethylene glycol) fumarate) hydrogels in conditions that model the cartilage wound healing environment. J. Control. Release 94 (1), 101–114. Available from: http://dx.doi.org/10.1016/j.jconrel.2003.09.007.

Hollister, S.J., 2005. Porous scaffold design for tissue engineering. Nat. Mater. 4 (7), 518–524.

Holmes, T.M., et al., 2000. Proc. Natl Acad. Sci. U.S.A. 97, 6728.

Holy, C.E., Shoichet, M.S., Davies, J.E., 2000. Engineering three dimensional bone tissue *in vitro* using biodegradable scaffolds: investigating initial cell-seeding density and culture period. J. Biomed. Mater. Res. 51 (3), 376–382. Available from: http://dx.doi.org/10.1002/1097-4636(20000905)51:3%3C376::AID JBM11%3E3.0.CO;2-G.

Holzwarth, J.M., Ma, P.X., 2011. Biomaterials 32, 9622.

Hua, F.J., Kim, G.E., Lee, J.D., Son, Y.K., Lee, D.S., 2002. Macroporous poly l-lactide scaffold 1. Preparation of a macroporous scaffold by liquid–liquid phase separation of a PLLA-dioxane-water system. J. Biomed. Mater. Res. 63, 61–167.

Huang, L., Nagapundi, K., Apkarian, R.P., et al., 2001. Engineered collagen-PEO nanofibers and fabrics. J. BioMater. Sci. Polym. (Ed.) 12, 979–993.

Huang, C.Y., et al., 2012. Biomaterials 33, 1791.

Hubbell, J.A., 1995. Biomaterials in tissue engineering. Bio-Technol. N. Y. 13 (6), 565–576.

Hutmacher, D.W., 2001. Scaffold design and fabrication technologies for engineering tissues-state of the art and future perspectives. J. Biomat. Sci. Polym. (Ed.) 12, 107–124.

Hutmacher, D.W., Sittinger, M., Risbud, M.V., 2004. Scaffold-based tissue engineering: rationale for computer-aided design and solid free-form fabrication systems. Trends Biotechnol. 22 (7), 354–362.

Hwang, J.J., Harrington, D.A., Klok, H.A., et al., 2002. Cell-synthetic surface interaction: self-assembling biomaterials. In: Atala, A., Lanza, R.P. (Eds.), Methods of Tissue Engineering. Academic Press, San Diego, CA, pp. 741–750.

Ibusuki, S., Fujii, Y., Iwamoto, Y., Matsuda, T., 2003. Tissue-engineered cartilage using an injectable and *in situ* gelable thermoresponsive gelatin: fabrication and *in vitro* performance. Tissue Eng. 9 (2), 371–384.

Ifkovits, J.L., Burdick, J.A., 2007. Review: photopolymerizable and degradable biomaterials for tissue engineering applications. Tissue Eng. 13 (10), 2369–2385.

Ikada, Y., 2006. Scope of tissue engineering. In: Ikada, Y. (Ed.), Tissue Engineering: Fundamental and Applications. Academic Press, San Diego, p. 29.

Ingram, J.H., Korossis, S., Howling, G., Fisher, J., Ingham, E., 2007. The use of ultrasonication to aid recellularization of acellular natural tissue scaffolds for use in anterior cruciate ligament reconstruction. Tissue Eng. 13 (7), 1561–1572.

Iwata, H., Amemiya, H., Hayashi, R., Fujii, S., Akutsu, T., 1990. The use of photocrosslinkable polyvinyl alcohol in the immunoisolation of pancreatic islets. Transplant. Proc. 22 (2), 797–799.

Jang, J.H., et al., 2009. Adv. Drug Deliv. Rev. 61, 1065.

Jayaraman, K., Kotaki, M., Zhang, Y., et al., 2004. Recent advances in polymer nanofibers. J. Nanosci. Nanotechnol. 4, 52–65.

Jeong, B., Bae, Y.H., Kim, S.M., 1999. Thermoreversible gelation of PEG-PLGA-PEG triblock copolymer aqueous solutions. Macromolecules 32 (21), 7064–7069.

Jiang, B.B., et al., 2010. Biomacromolecules 11, 3630.

Jin, H.J., Fridrikh, S.V., Rutledge, G.C., et al., 2002. Electrospinning bombyx mori silk with poly(ethylene oxide). Biomacromolecules 3, 1233–1239.

Jin, H.J., Chen, J., Karageorgiou, V., Altman, G.H., Kaplan, D.L., 2004. Human bone marrow stromal cell responses to electrospun silk fibroin mats. Biomaterials 25, 1039–1047.

Jo, I.H., Shin, K.H., Soon, Y.M., Koh, Y.H., Lee, J.H., Kim, H.E., 2009. Highly porous hydroxyapatite scaffolds with elongated pores using stretched polymeric sponges as novel template. Mater. Lett. 63 (20), 1702–1704.

Kang, H.G., Kim, S.Y., Lee, Y.M., 2006. Novel porous gelatin scaffolds by overrun/particle leaching process for tissue engineering applications. J. Biomed. Mater. Res. B 79 (2), 388–397.

Kaplan, T., Kafa, I.M., Cansev, M., Bekar, A., Karli, N., Taskapilioglu, M.O., et al., 2014. Investigation of the dose-dependency of citicoline effects on nerve regeneration and functional recovery in a rat model of sciatic nerve injury. Turk Neurosurg. 24, 54–62.

Karp, J.M., Shoichet, M.S., Davies, J.E., 2003. Bone formation on two-dimensional poly (DL-lactide-co-glycolide) (PLGA) films and three-dimensional PLGA tissue engineering scaffolds *in vitro*. J. Biomed. Mater. Res. A 64 (2), 388–396.

Katoh, K., Tanabe, T., Yamauchi, K., 2004. Novel approach to fabricate keratin sponge scaffolds with controlled pore size and porosity. Biomaterials 25 (18), 4255–4262.

Katti, D.S., Robinson, K.W., Ko, F.K., et al., 2004. Bioresorbable nanofiber based systems for wound healing and drug delivery: optimization of fabrication parameters. J. Biomed. Mater. Res. 70B, 286–296.

Kaully, T., Kaufman-Francis, K., Lesman, A., Levenberg, S., 2010. Vascularization: the conduit to viable engineered tissues. Adv. Tissue Eng. Angiogenesis, 17–27.

Kenawy, E.R., Bowlin, G.L., Mansfield, K., et al., 2002. Release of tetracycline hydrochloride from electrospun poly(ethylene-co-vinylacetate), poly(lactic acid), and a blend. J. Control Release 81, 57–64.

Khademhosseini, A., Eng, G., Yeh, J., et al., 2006. Micromolding of photocrosslinkable hyaluronic acid for cell encapsulation and entrapment. J. Biomed. Mater. Res. A 79 (3), 522–532.

Khil, M.S., Bhattarai, S.R., Kim, H.Y., et al., 2005. Novel fabricated matrix via electrospinning for tissue engineering. J. Biomed. Mater. Res. B Appl. Biomater. 72B, 117–124.

Kim, B.S., Baez, C.E., Atala, A., 2000. Biomaterials for tissue engineering. World J. Urol. 18 (1), 2–9.

Kim, K., Lee, C., Kim, I.W., Kim, J., 2009. Performance modification of a melt-blown filter medium via an additional nano-web layer prepared by electrospinning. Fibers Polym. 10 (1), 60–64.

Kim, T.G., et al., 2012. Adv. Funct. Mater. 22, 2446.

Knight, R.L., Wilcox, H.E., Korossis, S.A., Fisher, J., Ingham, E., 2008. The use of acellular matrices for the tissue engineering of cardiac valves. Proc. Inst. Mech. Eng. [H] 222 (1), 129–143.

Ko, I.K., Lee, S.J., Atala, A., Yoo, J.J., 2013. In situ tissue regeneration through host stem cell recruitment. Exp. Mol. Med. 45, e57.

Krishnan, R., Rajeswari, R., Venugopal, J., Sundarrajan, S., Sridhar, R., 2012. Polysaccharide nanofibrous scaffolds as a model for *in vitro* skin tissue regeneration. J. Mater. Sci. Mater. Med. 23, 1511–1519.

Kundu, S.C., Subia, B., Kundu, J., 2010. Biomaterial scaffold fabrication techniques for potential tissue engineering application. In: Daniel, E. (Ed.), Tissue Engineering. pp. 141–157, ISBN: 978-953-307-079-7, InTech. Available from: http://dx.doi.org/10.5772/8581.

L'Heureux, N., Pâquet, S., Labbé, R., Germain, L., Auger, F.A., 1998. A completely biological tissue-engineered human blood vessel. FASEB J. 12 (1), 47–56.

Lalan, S., Pomerantseva, I., Vacanti, J.P., 2001. Tissue engineering and its potential impact on surgery. World. J. Surg. 25 (11), 1458–1466.

Langer, R., Vacanti, J.P., 1993. Tissue Eng. Sci. 260, 920–926.

Lanza, R.P., Hayes, J.L., Chick, W.L., 1996. Encapsulated cell technology. Nat. Biotechnol. 14 (9), 1107–1111.

Laurencin, C.T., Attawia, M.A., Elgendy, H.E., Herbert, K.M., 1996. Tissue engineered bone-regeneration using degradable polymers: the formation of mineralized matrices. Bone 19 (1). Available from: http://dx.doi.org/10.1016/S8756-3282(96)00132-9.

Lee, C.H., Shin, H.J., Cho, I.H., et al., 2005. Nanofiber alignment and direction of mechanical strain affect the ECM production of human ACL fibro blast. Biomaterials 26, 1261–1270.

Lee, S.M., Nair, S., Ahn, H., Kim, B.S., Jun, S.H., An, H.J., et al., 2010. Property control of enzyme coatings on polymer nanofibres by varying the conjugation site concentration. Enzyme Microbial. Technol. 47 (5), 216–221.

Lee, J., Lee, S.Y., Jang, J., Jeong, Y.H., Cho, D.W., 2012. Fabrication of patterned nanofibrous mats using direct-write electrospinning. Langmuir 28, 7267–7275.

Lemmo, A.V., Rose, D.J., Tisone, T.C., 1998. Inkjet dispensing technology: applications in drug discovery. Curr. Opin. Biotechnol. 9 (6), 615–617.

Li, F., Feng, Q.L., Cui, F.Z., Li, H.D., Schubert, H., 2002a. A simple biomimetic method for calcium phosphate coating. Surf. Coat. Technol. 154 (1), 88–93.

Li, W.J., Laurencin, C.T., Caterson, E.J., et al., 2002b. Electrospun nanofibrous structure: a novel scaffold for tissue engineering. J. Biomed. Mater. Res. 60, 613–621.

Li, W.J., Danielson, K.G., Alexander, P.G., Tuan, R.S., 2003. Biological response of chondrocytes cultured in three-dimensional nanofibrous poly(ε-caprolactone) scaffolds. J. Biomed. Mater. Res. A 67 (4), 1105–1114.

Li, D., et al., 2004. Adv. Mater. 16, 361.

Li, D., Ouyang, G., McCann, J.T., et al., 2005. Collecting electrospun nanofibers with patterned electrodes. Nano. Lett. 5, 913–916.

Li, W.J., Tuan, R.S., 2009. Fabrication and application of nanofibrous scaffolds in tissue engineering. Curr. Protoc. Cell Biol. 25, Unit 25.2.

Li, Y.C., Chen, C.R., Young, T.H., 2013. Pearl extract enhances the migratory ability of fibroblasts in a wound healing model. Pharm. Biol. 51, 289–297.

Liang, H.C., Chang, Y., Hsu, C.K., Lee, M.H., Sung, H.W., 2004. Effects of crosslinking degree of an acellular biological tissue on its tissue regeneration pattern. Biomaterials 25 (17), 3541–3552.

Liang, D., Hsiao, B.S., Chu, B., 2007. Functional electrospun nanofibrous scaffolds for biomedical applications. Adv. Drug Deliv. Rev. 59, 1392–1412.

Liao, S., et al., 2006. Biomed. Mater. 1, R45.

Lin, V.S., Lee, M.C., O'Neal, S., et al., 1999. Ligament tissue engineering using synthetic biodegradable fiber scaffolds. Tissue. Eng. 5, 443–451.

Lin, J.Y., et al., 2012. Crit. Rev. Solid State Mater. Sci. 37, 94.

Lippmann, E.S., Al-Ahmad, A., Palecek, S.P., Shusta, E.V., 2013. Modeling the blood–brain barrier using stem cell sources. Fluids Barriers CNS 10, 2.
Liu, V.A., Bhatia, S.N., 2002. Three-dimensional photopatterning of hydrogels containing living cells. Biomed. Microdevices 4 (4), 257–266.
Liu, X.H., et al., 2011. Nat. Mater. 10, 398.
Liu, S., et al., 2012a. Biomacromolecules 13, 3611.
Liu, W., et al., 2012b. Adv. Health. Mater. 1, 10.
Luu, Y.K., Kim, K., Hsiao, B.S., Chu, B., Hadjiargyrou, M., et al., 2003. Development of a nanostructured DNA delivery scaffold via electrospinning of PLGA and PLAPEG block copolymers. J. Control Release 89, 341–353.
Lyons, J., Li, C., Ko, F., 2004. Melt-electrospinning—part I: processing parameters and geometric properties. Polymer 45 (22), 7597–7603.
Lyons, F., et al., 2010. Biomaterials 31 (35), 9232–9243.
Ma, P.X., 2008. Biomimetic materials for tissue engineering. Adv. Drug Deliv. Rev. 60, 184–198.
Ma, P.X., Zhang, R., 1999. Synthetic nano-scale fibrous extracellular matrix. J. Biomed. Mater. Res. 46, 60–72.
Ma, Z., Kotaki, M., Inai, R., et al., 2005. Potential of nanofiber matrix as tissue-engineering scaffolds. Tissue Eng. 11, 101–109.
Malafaya, P.B., Pedro, A.J., Peterbauer, A., Gabriel, C., Redl, H., Reis, R.L., 2005. Chitosan particles agglomerated scaffolds for cartilage and osteochondral tissue engineering approaches with adipose tissue derived stem cells. J. Mater. Sci. Mater. Med. 16 (12), 1077–1085.
Malafaya, P.B., Santos, T.C., Griensven, M.V., Reis, R.L., 2008. Morphology, mechanical characterization and *in vivo* neo-vascularization of chitosan particle aggregated scaffolds architectures. Biomaterials 29 (29), 3914–3926.
Malkar, N.B., Lauer-Fields, J.L., Juska, D., et al., 2003. Characterization of peptide-amphiphiles possessing cellular activation sequences. Biomacromolecules 4, 518–528.
Mandal, B.B., Kundu, S.C., 2008a. Non-bioengineered silk gland fibroin protein: characterization and evaluation of matrices for potential tissue engineering applications. Biotechnol. Bioeng. 100 (6), 1237–1250.
Mandal, B.B., Kundu, S.C., 2008b. Non-bioengineered high strength three-dimensional gland fibroin scaffolds from tropical non-mulberry silkworm for potential tissue engineering applications. Macromol. Biosci. 8, 807–818.
Mano, J.F., Silva, G.A., Azevedo, H.S., Malafaya, P.B., Sousa, R.A., Silva, S.S., et al., 2007. Natural origin biodegradable systems in tissue engineering and regenerative medicine: present status and some moving trends. J. R. Soc. Interface 4, 999–1030.
Marx, S., Jose, M.V., Anderson, J.D., Russel, A.J., et al., 2011. Electrospun gold nanofiber electrodes for biosensors. Biosens. Bioelectron. 26 (6), 2981–2986.
Matson, J.B., 2011. Curr. Opin. Solid State Mater. Sci. 15 (22), 225.
Matthews, J.A., Wnek, G.E., Simpson, D.G., et al., 2002. Electrospinning of collagen nanofibers. Biomacromolecules 3, 232–238.
Mikos, A.G., Sarakinos, G., Leite, S.M., Vacanti, J.P., Langer, R., 1993. Laminated three-dimensional biodegradable foams for use in tissue engineering. Biomaterials 14 (5), 323–330.
Mikos, A.J., Thorsen, A.J., Czerwonka, L.A., et al., 2004. Preparation and characterization of poly (l-lactic acid) foams. Polymer 35 (5), 1068–1077.

Mikos, A.G., Lu, L., Temenoff, J.S., Temmser, J.K., 2004. Synthetic bioresorbablepolymer scaffolds. In: Ratner, B.D., Hoffman, A.S., Schoen, F.J., Lemons, J.E. (Eds.), An Introduction to Material in Medicine. Elsevier Academic Press, San Diego, CA, p. 743.

Mironov, V., Boland, T., Trusk, T., Forgacs, G., Markwald, R.R., 2003. Organ printing: computer-aided jet-based 3D tissue engineering. Trends. Biotechnol. 21 (4), 157–161.

Mirononv, V., Kasyanov, V., Drake, C., Markwald, R.R., 2008. Organ printing: promises and challenges. Regen. Med. 3 (1), 93–103.

Mironov, V., Kasyanov, V., Markwald, R.R., 2011. Organ printing: from bioprinter to organ biofabrication line. Curr. Opin. Biotechnol. 22, 667–673.

Mo, X., Weber, H.J., 2004. Electrospinning P(LLA-CL) nanofiber: a tubular scaffold fabrication with circumferential alignment. Macromol. Symp. 217, 413–416.

Mooney, D.J., Baldwin, D.F., Suh, N.P., Vacanti, J.P., Langer, R., 1996a. Novel approach to fabricate porous sponges of poly(D,L-lactic-co-glycolic acid) without the use of organic solvents. Biomaterials 17 (14), 1417–1422.

Mooney, D.J., McNamara, K., Hern, D., Vacanti, J.P., Langer, R., 1996b. Stabilized polyglycolic acid fibre-based tubes for tissue engineering. Biomaterials 17, 115–124.

Moulin, V.J., 2013. Reconstitution of skin fibrosis development using a tissue engineering approach. Methods Mol. Biol. 961, 287–303.

Nguyen, T.B.L., Lee, B.T., 2012. J. Biomater. Appl. 27, 255.

Nishida, K., Yamato, M., Hayashida, Y., Watanabe, K., Yamamoto, K., Adachi, E., et al., 2004. Corneal reconstruction with tissue engineered cell sheets composed of autologous oral mucosal epithelium. N. Engl. J. Med. 351 (12), 1187–1196.

Nisisako, T., Torii, T., Higuchi, T., 2002. Droplet formation in amicrochannel network. Lab. Chip. Miniaturisat. Chem. Biol. 2 (1), 24–26.

Nuttelman, C.R., Tripodi, M.C., Anseth, K.S., 2005. Synthetic hydrogel niches that promote hMSC viability. Matrix Biol. 24 (3), 208–218.

Ochi, K., Chen, G., Ushida, T., et al., 2003. Use of isolated mature osteoblasts in abundance acts as desired-shaped bone regeneration in combination with a modified poly-DL-lactic-co-glycolic acid (PLGA)-collagen sponge. J. Cell. Physiol. 194 (1), 45–53.

Okano, T., Yamada, N., Sakai, H., Sakurai, Y., 1993. A novel recovery system for cultured cells using plasma-treated polystyrene dishes grafted with poly N-isopropylacrylamide. J. Biomed. Mater. Res. 27 (10), 1243–1251.

Okano, T., Yamada, N., Okuhara, M., Sakai, H., Sakurai, Y., 1995. Mechanism of cell detachment from temperature-modulated, hydrophilic–hydrophobic polymer surfaces. Biomaterials 16 (4), 297–303.

Okuzaki, H., Harashina, Y., Yan, H., 2009. Highly conductive PEDOT/PSS microfibers fabricated by wet-spinning and dip-treatment in ethylene glycol. Eur. Polym. J. 45 (1), 256–261.

Orive, G., Hernandez, R.M., Gascon, A.R., Calafiore, R., Chang, T.M., De Vos, P., et al., 2003. Cell encapsulation: promise and progress. Nat. Med. 9 (1), 104–107.

Orive, G., Hernandez, R.M., Rodnguez, G.A., Calafiore, R., Chang, T.M., De Vos, P., et al., 2004. History, challenges and perspectives of cell micro-encapsulation. Trends Biotechnol. 22 (2), 87–92.

Partridge, R., Conlisk, N., Davies, J.A., 2012. In-lab three-dimensional printing: an inexpensive tool for experimentation and visualization for the field of organogenesis. Organogenesis 8 (1), 22–27.

Paquet, C., Larouche, D., Bisson, F., Proulx, S., Simard, B.C., 2010. Tissue engineering of skin and cornea, development of new models for *in vitro* studies. Ann. N. Y. Acad. Sci. 1197, 166–177.

Peppas, N.A., Khare, A.R., 1993. Preparation, structure and diffusional behavior of hydrogels in controlled release. Adv. Drug Deliv. Rev. 11 (1-2), 1–35.

Pham, Q.P., Sharma, U., Mikos, A.G., 2006. Electrospinning of polymeric nanofibers for tissue engineering applications: a review. Tissue Eng. 12 (5), 1197–1211.

Pomfret, S.J., Adams, P.N., Comfort, N.P., Monkman, A.P., 2000. Electrical and mechanical properties of polyaniline fibres produced by a one-step wet spinning process. Polymer 41 (6), 2265–2269. Available from: http://dx.doi.org/10.1016/S0032-3861(99)00365-1.

Price, R.L., Waid, M.C., Haberstroh, K.M., et al., 2003. Selective bone cell adhesion on formulations containing carbon nanofibers. Biomaterials 24, 1877–1887.

Rafat, M., Matsuura, T., Li, F., Griffith, M., 2009. Surface modification of collagen-based artificial cornea for reduced endothelialization. J. Biomed. Mater. Res. 88, 755–768.

Ramay, H.R.R., Zhang, M., 2003. Preparation of porous hydroxyapatite scaffolds by combination of the gel casting and polymer sponge methods. Biomaterials 24, 3292–3302.

Ramay, H., Zhang, M., 2004. Biphasic calcium phosphate nanocomposite porous scaffolds for load-bearing bone tissue engineering. Biomaterials 25 (21), 5171–5180.

Ratner, B.D., Bryant, S.J., 2004. Biomaterials: where we have been and where we are going. Annu. Rev. Biomed. Eng. 6, 41–75.

Rayleigh, J.W.G., 1882. On the equilibrium of liquid conducting masses charged with electricity. Lond. Edinb. Dulin. Phil. Mag. 44, 184–186.

Reddy, V.J., et al., 2013. Wound Repair Regen. 21, 1.

Reis, C.P., Ribeiro, A.J., Neufeld, R.J., Veiga, F., 2007. Alginate microparticles as novel carrier for oral insulin delivery. Biotechnol. Bioeng. 96 (5), 977–989.

Reisner, D.E., 2009. Bionanotechnology: global Prospects. CRC Press, Taylor & Francis Group, London, New York.

Reneker, D.H., Chun, I., 1996. Nanometer diameter fibers of polymer produced by electrospinning. Nanotechnology 7, 216–223.

Reneker, D.H., Yarin, A.L., Fong, H., et al., 2000. Bending instability of electrically charged liquid jets of polymer solutions in electrospinning. J. Appl. Phys. 87, 4531–4547.

Reneker, D.H., Kataphinan, W., Theron, A., et al., 2002. Nanofiber garlands of polycaprolactone by electrospinning. Polymer 43, 6785–6794.

Sachlos, E., Czernuszka, J.T., 2003. 'Making tissue engineering scaffolds work'. Review on the application of solid free from fabrication technology to the production of tissue engineering scaffolds. Eur. Cells Mater. 5, 29–40.

Sala, C.C., Ribes, A.M., Fernandez, M.T., Sancho, R.L., Lopez, C.P., et al., 2013. Current applications of tissue engineering in biomedicine. J. Biochip. Tissue Chip S2, 004.

Schnell, E., et al., 2007. Biomaterials 28, 3012.

Sell, S.A., Bowlin, G.L., 2008. J. Mater. Chem. 18, 260.

Semino, C.E., Kasahara, J., Hayashi, Y., et al., 2004. Entrapment of migrating hippocampal neural cells in three-dimensional peptide nanofiber scaffold. Tissue Eng. 10, 643–655.

Seong, J.Y., Jun, Y.J., Jeong, B., Sohn, Y.S., 2005. New thermogelling poly(organophosphazenes) with methoxypoly(ethylene glycol) and oligopeptide as side groups. Polymer 46 (14), 5075–5081.

Sepulveda, P., Binner, J.G.P., 1999. Processing of cellular ceramics by foaming and in situ polymerisation of organic monomers. J. Eur. Ceram. Soc. 19 (12), 2059–2066.

Shandalov, Y., Egozi, D., Koffler, J., Dado-Rosenfeld, D., Ben-Shimol, D., Freiman, A., et al., 2014. An engineered muscle flap for reconstruction of large soft tissue defects. Proc. Natl. Acad. Sci. U.S.A. 111, 6010–6015. Available from: http://dx.doi.org/10.1073/pnas.1402679111.

Sharma, P., Maffulli, N.J., 2005. Bone Joint Surg. Am. 87A, 187.

Shields, K.J., Beckman, M.J., Bowlin, G.L., et al., 2004. Mechanical properties and cellular proliferation of electrospun collagen type II. Tissue Eng. 10, 1510–1517.

Shimizu, T., Yamato, M., Kikuchi, A., Okano, T., 2003. Cell sheet engineering for myocardial tissue reconstruction. Biomaterials 24 (13), 2309–2316.

Shin, Y.M., Hohman, M.M., Brenner, M.P., et al., 2001a. Electrospinning: a whipping fluid jet generates submicron polymer fibers. Appl. Phys. Lett. 78, 1–3.

Shin, Y.M., Hohman, M.M., Brenner, M.P., et al., 2001b. Experimental characterization of electrospinning: the electrically forced jet and instabilities. Polymer 42, 9955–9967.

Smith, L.A., Ma, P.X., 2004. Nanofibrous scaffolds for tissue engineering. Colloids Surf. B. Biointerfaces 39, 125–131.

Smith, L.A., Beck, J.A., Ma, P.X., 2006. Nano fibrous scaffolds and their biological effects. In: Kumar, C. (Ed.), Tissue Cell and Organ Engineering. Wiley-VCH, p. 195.

Steinhoff, G., Stock, U., Karim, N., et al., 2000. Tissue engineering of pulmonary heart valves on allogenic acellular matrix conduits: *in vivo* restoration of valve tissue. Circulation 102 (19), III50–III55.

Stevens, M.M., 2008. Mater. Today 11, 18.

Stupp, S.I., LeBonheur, V., Walker, K., et al., 1997. Supramolecular materials: self-organized nanostructures. Science 275, 384–389.

Subramanian, A., Maheswari Krishnan, U., Sethuraman, S., 2009. Development of biomaterial scaffold for nerve tissue engineering: biomaterial mediated neural regeneration. J. Biomed. Sci. 16, 108.

Sun, W., Lal, P., 2002. Recent development on computer aided tissue engineering—a review. Comput. Methods. Programs Biomed. 67 (2), 85–103.

Sundaray, B., Subramaniam, V., Natrajan, T.S., et al., 2004. Electrospinning of continuous aligned polymer fibers. Appl. Phys. Lett. 84, 1222–1224.

Tachibana, A., Furuta, Y., Takeshima, H., Tanabe, T., Yamauchi, K., 2002. Fabrication of wool keratin sponge scaffolds for long-term cell cultivation. J. Biotechnol. 93 (2), 165–170.

Takahashi, K., Yamanaka, S., 2006. Induction of pluripotent stem cells from mouse embryonic and adult fibroblast cultures by defined factors. Cell 126, 663–676.

Takezawa, T., Mori, Y., Yoshizato, K., 1990. Cell culture on a thermo-responsive polymer surface. Biotechnol. N. Y. 8 (9), 854–856.

Teo, W.-E., Inai, R., Ramakrishna, S., 2011. Technological advances in electrospinning of nanofibers. Sci. Technol. Adv. Mater. 12, 013002.

Theron, A., Zussman, V., Yarin, A.L., 2001. Electrospinning field-assisted alignment of electrospun nanofibers. Nanotechnology 12, 384–390.

Thomas, V., et al., 2009. Biotechnol. Bioeng. 104, 1025.

Thompson, R.C., Wake, M.C., Yaszemski, Mikos, A.G., 1995a. Biodegradable polymer scaffolds to regenerate organs. Adv. Polym. Sci. 122, 245–274, aton, FL. 173–195.

Thompson, R.C., Yaszembksi, M.J., Powers, J.M., Harrigan, T.P., Mikos, A.G., 1995b. Poly a-hydroxy ester/short fiber hydroxyapatite composite foams for orthopaedic applications. In: Mikos, A.G., Leong, K.W., Yaszemski, M.J. (Eds.), Polymers in Medicine and Pharmacy, vol. 394. Materials Research Society, Pittsburgh, PA, pp. 25–30, Materials Research Society Symposium Proceedings.

Thompson, S.A., Burridge, P.W., Lipke, E.A., Shamblott, M., Zambidis, E.T., et al., 2012. Engraftment of human embryonic stem cell derived cardiomyocytes improves conduction in an arrhythmogenic *in vitro* model. J. Mol. Cell. Cardiol. 53, 15–23.

Tremblay, P.L., Hudon, V., Berthod, F., Germain, L., Auger, F.A., 2005. Inosculation of tissueengineered capillaries with the host's vasculature in a reconstructed skin transplanted on mice. Am. J. Transplant. 5, 1002–1010.

Tsuda, Y., Shimizu, T., Yamato, M., Kikuchi, A., Sasagawa, T., Sekiya, S., et al., 2007. Cellular control of tissue architectures using a three-dimensional tissue fabrication technique. Biomaterials 28 (33), 4939–4946.

Uematsu, K., Hattori, K., Ishimoto, Y., et al., 2005. Cartilage regeneration using mesenchymal stem cells and a three-dimensional poly lactic-co-glycolic acid PLGA scaffold. Biomaterials 26, 4273–4279.

Uludag, H., De Vos, P., Tresco, P.A., 2000. Technology of mammalian cell encapsulation. Adv. Drug Delivery Rev. 42 (1–2), 29–64.

Um, I.C., Fang, D., Hsiao, B.S., et al., 2004. Electrospinning and electro-blowing of hyaluronic acid. Biomacromolecules 5, 1428–1436.

Van den Broek, L.J., Niessen, F.B., Scheper, R.J., Gibbs, S., 2012. Development, validation and testing of a human tissue engineered hypertrophic scar model. ALTEX 29, 389–402.

Vermette, M., Trottier, V., Menard, V., et al., 2007. Production of a new tissue-engineered adipose substitute from human adipose-derived stromal cells. Biomaterials 28, 2850–2860.

Verreck, G., Chun, I., Rosenblatt, J., et al., 2003b. Incorporation of drugs in an amorphous state into electrospun nanofibers composed of a water-insoluble, nonbiodegradable polymer. J. Control. Release 92, 349–360.

Wade, R.J., Burdick, J.A., 2012. Mater. Today 15, 454.

Wang, J.P., 2010. J. Biomed. Mater. Res Part A 93A, 753.

Wang, X., Reagan, M.R., Kaplan, D.L., 2010. Synthetic adipose tissue models for studying mammary gland development and breast tissue engineering. J. Mammary Gland Biol. Neoplasia 15, 365–376.

Weber, B., Zeisberger, S.M., Hoerstrup, S.P., 2011. Prenatally harvested cells for cardiovascular tissue engineering: fabrication of autologous implants prior to birth. Placenta 32 (Suppl.), 316–319.

Webster, T.J., Hellenmeyer, E.L., Price, R.L., 2005. Increased osteoblast function on theta + delta nanofiber alumina. Biomaterials 26, 953–960.

Wilson, C., Boland, T., 2003. Cell and organ printing 1: protein and cell printers. Anat. Rec. 272A, 491–496.

Wissink, M.J.B., Beernink, R., Pieper, J.S., et al., 2001. Binding and release of basic fibroblast growth factor from heparinized collagen matrices. Biomaterials 22 (16), 2291–2299.

Woerdeman, D.L., Ye, P., Shenoy, S., et al., 2005. Electrospun fibers from wheat protein: investigation of the interplay between molecular structure and the fluid dynamics of the electrospinning process. Biomacromolecules 6, 707–712.

Woo, B.H., Kostanski, J.W., Gebrekidan, S., Dani, B.A., Thanoo, B.C., DeLuca, P.P., 2001. Preparation, characterization and *in vivo* evaluation of 120-day poly(D,L-lactide) leuprolide microspheres. J. Control. Release 75 (3), 307–315.

Xiang, Z., Liao, R., Kelly, M.S., Spector, M., 2006. Collagen–GAG scaffolds grafted onto myocardial infarcts in a rat model: a delivery vehicle for mesenchymal stem cells. J. Tissue Eng. 12, 2467–2478.

Xie, J., et al., 2010a. ACS Nano. 4, 5027.

Xie, J.W., et al., 2010b. Nanoscale 2, 35.

Xu, S., Nie, Z., Seo, M., et al., 2005. Generation of monodisperse particles by using microfluidics: control over size, shape, and composition. Ange. Chem. Int. Ed. 44 (5), 724–728.

Xu, X., Zhuang, X., Chen, X., Wang, X., Yang, L., Jing, X., et al., 2006. Preparation of core-sheath composite nanofibers by emulsion electrospinning. Macromol. Rapid Commun. 27, 1637–1642.

Yang, S., Leong, K.F., Du, Z., Chua, C.K., 2002. The design of scaffolds for use in tissue engineering: part II. Rapid prototyping techniques. Tissue Eng. 8 (1), 1–11.

Yang, F., Xu, C.Y., Kotaki, M., et al., 2004. Characterization of neural stem cells on electrospun poly(L-lactic acid) nanofibrous scaffold. J. Biomat. Sci. Polym. (Ed.) 15, 1483–1497.

Yang, F., et al., 2005a. Biomaterials 26, 2603.

Yang, F., Murugan, R., Wang, S., et al., 2005b. Electrospinning of nano/micro scale poly L-lactic acid aligned fibers and their potential in neural tissue engineering. Biomaterials 26, 2603–2610.

Yang, D., et al., 2007a. Adv. Mater. 19, 3702.

Yang, J., Yamato, M., Shimizu, T., Sekine, H., Ohashi, K., Kanzaki, M., et al., 2007b. Reconstruction of functional tissues with cell sheet engineering. Biomaterials 28 (34), 5033–5043.

Yang, F., Wolke, J.G.C., Jansen, J.A., 2008. Biomimetic calcium phosphate mcoating on electrospun poly (ε-caprolactone) scaffolds for bone tissue engineering. Chem. Eng. J. 137 (1), 154–161.

Yeh, J., Ling, Y., Karp, J.M., et al., 2006. Micromolding of shape-controlled, harvestable cell-laden hydrogels. Biomaterials 27 (31), 5391–5398.

Yeong, W.Y., Chua, C.K., Leong, K.F., Chandrasekaran, M., Lee, M.W., 2006. Indirect fabrication of collagen scaffold based on inkjet printing technique. Rapid Prot. J. 12 (4), 229–237.

Yu, J., 2007. Induced pluripotent stem cell lines derived from human somatic cells. Science 318, 1917–1920.

Yu, Y.C., Berndt, P., Tirrell, M., et al., 1996. Self-assembling amphiphiles for construction of protein molecular architecture. J. Am. Chem. Soc. 118, 12515–12520.

Yu, Y.C., Roontga, V., Daragan, V.A., et al., 1999. Structure and dynamics of peptide-amphiphiles incorporating triple-helical protein-like molecular architecture. Biochemistry 38, 1659–1668.

Yu, L.M.Y., et al., 2008. Mater. Today 11, 36.

Zeleny, J., 2004. The electrical discharge from liquid points and a hydrostatic method of measuring the electric intensity at their surface. Phys. Rev. 3, 69–91.

Zeng, J., Aigner, A., Czubayko, F., Kissel, T., Wendorff, J.H., Greiner, A., 2005. Poly (vinyl alcohol) nanofibers by electrospinning as a protein delivery system and the retardation of enzyme release by additional polymer coatings. Biomacromolecules 6 (3), 1484–1488. Available from: http://dx.doi.org/10.1021/bm0492576.

Zhang, D., Chang, J., 2008. Electrospinning of three-dimensional nanofibrous tubes with controllable architectures. Nano Lett. 8, 3283–3287.

Zhang, K., Wang, X., Jing, D., Yang, Y., Zhu, M., 2009. Bionic electrospun ultrafine fibrous poly(L-lactic acid) scaffolds with a multi-scale structure. Biomed. Mater. 4, 1–6.

Zhang, S., 2003. Fabrication of novel biomaterial through molecular self-assembly. J. Nat. Biotechnol. 21, 1171–1178.

Zhang, S., Ellis-Behnke, R., Zhao, X., Spirio, L., 2005. Self-assembling peptide nanofiber scaffolds. In: Elisseeff, P.X., Ma, J. (Eds.), Scaffolding in Tissue Engineering. CRC, Boca Raton (FL), pp. 217–238.

Zhang, R., Ma, P.X., 2002. Processing of polymer scaffolds: phase separation. In: Atala, A., Lanza, R.P. (Eds.), Methods of Tissue Engineering. Academic Press, San Diego, CA, pp. 715–724.

Zhang, Y., Ouyang, H., Lim, C.T., et al., 2005. Electrospinning of gelatin fibers and gelatin/PCL composite fibrous scaffolds. J. Biomed. Mater. Res. Part B Appl. Biomater. 72B, 156–165.

Zhang, Z.P., et al., 2012. Adv. Drug Deliv. Rev. 64, 1129.

Zhao, D.E., Li, R.B., Liu, W.Y., et al., 2003. Tissue-engineered heart valve on acellular aortic valve scaffold: *in-vivo* study. Asian Cardiovasc. Thorac. Ann. 11 (2), 153–156.

Zielinski, B.A., Aebischer, P., 1994. Chitosan as a matrix for mammalian cell encapsulation. Biomaterials 15 (13), 1049–1056.

Zong, X., Kim, K., Fang, D., et al., 2002. Structure and process relationship of electrospun biodegradable nanofiber membrane. Polymer 43, 4403–4412.

Zorlutuna, P., Hasirci, N., Hasirci, V., 2008. Nanopatterned collagen tubes for vascular tissue engineering. J. Tissue Eng. Regen. Med. 2 (6), 373–377.

CHAPTER

In vivo microscopic and mechanical characteristics of bioengineered and biodegradable tissue scaffolds and nanomaterials

15

Kubíková Tereza[1], Kochová Petra[2], Holeček Miroslav[3], Plencner Martin[4], Prosecká Eva[4], Filová Eva[4], Rampichová Michaela[4] and Tonar Zbyněk[5]

[1]*Department of Histology and Embryology, Faculty of Medicine in Pilsen, Charles University, Prague, Czech Republic* [2]*European Centre of Excellence NTIS, Faculty of Applied Sciences, University of West Bohemia, Pilsen, Czech Re/public* [3]*New Technologies Research Centre, University of West Bohemia, Pilsen, Czech Republic* [4]*Department of Tissue Engineering, Institute of Experimental Medicine of the ASCR, v. v. i., Prague, Czech Republic* [5]*Biomedical Centre, Faculty of Medicine in Pilsen, Charles University, Prague, Czech Republic*

15.1 INTRODUCTION

The term "biomaterial" is used for a support tool designed for protection, strengthening, or replacement of tissues, organs, or bodily functions used in close contact with living tissue (Williams, 1987). Materials of animal or plant origin or inspired by nature are also sometimes referred as to biomaterials. The function of most biomaterials is to provide mechanical support of cells. They may be modified by using adhesion molecules to stimulate a cellular response. They may be designed to release growth factors during various phases of wound healing (Palsson and Bhatia, 2004). We expect biomaterials to be compatible with the recipient's tissues to induce an acceptable organ response. Histological examination is a suitable way to verify the effect of tissue scaffolds after *in vivo* application. The type of wound, as well as the healing phases, has to be considered when selecting a suitable biomaterial for a particular use.

Nanobiomaterials in Soft Tissue Engineering. DOI: http://dx.doi.org/10.1016/B978-0-323-42865-1.00015-5

15.2 WOUND HEALING

15.2.1 PHASES OF WOUND HEALING

Recovery of damaged homeostasis begins immediately after an injury. It is a continuous process; however, it can be categorized into three phases according to the prevailing type and activity of cells involved in the healing process. These phases are the inflammatory, the proliferative, and the remodeling phases.

The hallmark of the *inflammatory phase* is early invasion of granulocytes reaching its maximum 2–5 days after injury (Reinke and Sorg, 2012). Granulocytes are attracted to the wound by chemotactic stimuli (e.g., denatured proteins, lymphokines, thromboxanes) (Helpap, 1987). Fibronectin promotes adhesion and movement of fibroblasts, keratinocytes, and endothelial cells (EC) and is present in the wound 15 min after the injury (Kondo, 2007). Three days after injury (Reinke and Sorg, 2012) macrophages appear in the healing wound. Macrophages are significantly involved in the cellular histiocytic reaction by phagocytizing necrotic tissue (Leibovich and Wiseman, 1988). Fusion of macrophages that phagocytize the nondegradable remnants form multinucleated foreign bodies giant cells, called Langhans cells (Dettmeyer, 2011). In addition to phagocytosis of bacteria and necrotic tissue (debridement), white blood cells produce growth factors, thus preparing the wound for the proliferative phase.

In the *proliferative phase*, which takes place 3–10 days after injury (Reinke and Sorg, 2012), fibroblasts are prominent. Fibroblasts produce a provisional extracellular matrix (ECM), where newly formed blood vessels are abundant, forming a granulation tissue. the spatial structure of fibrin fibers, together with adhesive proteins, provides an environment suitable for cell adhesion and migration. The provisional matrix is a rich source of mitogens, chemoattractants, cytokines, and growth factors modulating cell division (Anderson, 2001). The ECM formed in the proliferation phase contains fibrin, fibronectin, first collagen fibers, and hyaluronic acid (HA). Type III collagen is formed within 2–3 days after injury. Type I collagen, which is significantly applied, e.g., during the healing in dermis, occurs in the matrix for 5 days (Kondo, 2007). Collagen type II is formed in healing hyaline and elastic cartilage; however, the regenerative potential of these tissues is strongly limited in adults. Type IV collagen and laminin are important parts of the basal lamina of epithelia; regeneration of the basal lamina is needed for re-epithelialization. The production of extremely hydrophilic glycosaminoglycans, such as HA, provides sufficient hydration. This facilitates cell migration and improves the local microcirculation of tissue fluid and substances. Moreover, HA itself induces the release of cytokines and chemokines and thus promotes cell proliferation and differentiation. Adhesive proteins also participate in organizing the ECM. Although representation of adhesive proteins in the matrix is minor, they regulate cellular interactions, and affect cell migration and shape (Masopust and Průša, 2003). Artificial modifications of biomaterials, such as using the CD44 adhesive protein, can mimic these effects on cell proliferation and migration. the standard type of CD44 binds HA, optional variants of CD44 bind fibronectin, laminin, and collagen.

The *remodeling phase* starts approximately 21 days after injury (Reinke and Sorg, 2012) and is characterized by intensive production of collagen fibers by myofibroblasts. Thus the primary scar is formed. Heavily vascularized tissue bulges initially, but later it is subjected to retraction due to the contractile myofibroblasts. The collagen undergoes remodeling into a more organized matrix of final scar.

15.2.2 REMODELING OF SCAR

During wound healing there are cellular responses in terms of hypertrophy, hyperplasia, atrophy, or metaplasia (Mačák and Mačáková, 2004), which are accompanied by changes in the ECM. After completion of the tissue repair processes, proliferation of myofibroblasts ceases and the excess cells undergo apoptosis. Without reducing the number and activity of myofibroblasts, fibrosis (excessive formation of connective tissue) of the wound occurs. It may suppress the healing of the functional parenchyma, the organ, or may be the cause of adhesions (Darby and Hewitson, 2007).

Problematic scars are classified as atrophic, hypertrophic, and keloid types. Atrophic scars are sunken below the line of the original injury. They arise, for example, after acne or after spontaneously healing decubitus. Hypertrophic scars can be palpated, but fundamentally do not exceed the line of the original injury. Keloid scars are only known in human. They exceed the original range of the wound (Litvik and Vantuchová, 2011). In the skin they lack the typical skin surface patterns, dermatoglyphs, and skin appendages. Women, adolescents, and darker skin phototypes with hyperpigmentation are more prone to the formation of keloid scars. Keloid scars do not occur in albinos (Litvik and Vantuchová, 2011). Keloid scars often emerge on the face, ears, neck, shoulders, neck, upper chest, and back (Seo and Sung, 2012).

The later phases of wound healing are strongly dependent on adequate nutritional support provided by the newly formed blood vessels. The formation of new blood vessels is based either on proliferation, migration, and remodeling of resident EC (angiogenesis), or on differentiation of progenitor cells into a new vascular network (vasculogenesis).

15.3 ANGIOGENESIS

15.3.1 PHASES OF ANGIOGENESIS

There are two distinct forms of neovascularization: vasculogenesis, where vessels arise de novo, and angiogenesis, in which the EC sprout from preexisting vessels. Vasculogenesis occurs mostly during embryogenesis; however, it may take part during wound healing as well (Velazquez, 2007). Angiogenesis is encountered under physiological conditions, such as growth, or under pathological conditions, such as wound healing or remodeling of tumors (Tichý et al., 2010). The blood vessels supply the provisional granulation tissue by providing trophic factors and oxygen and taking away various metabolites. Angiogenesis depends on signals from both the blood plasma and from the surrounding matrix (Risau, 1997). These signals are present already in the inflammatory phase of healing. Angiogenesis occurs only during the proliferation phase (Li et al., 2003).

Angiogenesis may be arbitrarily divided into several steps:

1. Expression of angiogenic factor receptors (fibroblast growth factor-receptor (FGF-R), vascular endothelial growth factor-receptor) on EC (Pepper, 2001).
2. Partial degradation of the basement membrane by EC followed by penetration of EC into the surrounding tissue matrix. This requires cooperation of plasminogen activator and matrix metalloproteinases (Mignatti and Rifkin, 1996).
3. Proliferation (budding, sprouting) and differentiation of EC. The vascular buds elongate and a new blood vessel lumen forms.

Establishing new capillary routes and reinforcement of the microvessels occurs with the basal membrane, pericytes, and smooth muscle cells (Yoo and Kwon, 2013) (Figure 15.1).

15.3.2 FACTORS AFFECTING WOUND HEALING AND ANGIOGENESIS

Angiogenesis as a part of wound healing is regulated by a number of growth and differentiation factors. These include the vascular endothelial growth factor (Keck et al., 1989), the fibroblast growth factor (Folkman and Klagsbrun, 1987), the angiopoietins (Suri et al., 1996), the platelet-derived growth factor, the epidermal growth factor, and the transforming growth factor beta (Yang and Moses, 1990). A selection of factors with most evidence and relevance to wound healing is given in Table 15.1.

15.3.3 PROMOTING ANGIOGENESIS IN BIOMATERIALS

Replacement and restoration of various parts of the body has been previously limited to either avascular tissues (such as cartilage) or thin-layered organs (epidermis, urinary bladder) (Atala et al., 2006; Jain, 2003; Oberpenning et al., 1999). Cell viability within these organs depends on oxygen and nutrient diffusion, the efficiency of which is limited to a few hundred microns. Cells more distant from the nearest capillaries suffer from hypoxia, which may result in their apoptosis.

Insufficient supply of oxygen and nutrients is a complication for wound healing. Diabetic ulcer is an example of chronic wounds. A reason for the formation of diabetic ulcers is inadequate blood supply with complicated healing leading to recurrent inflammation and infection (Steed, 2006). On the other side, uncontrolled

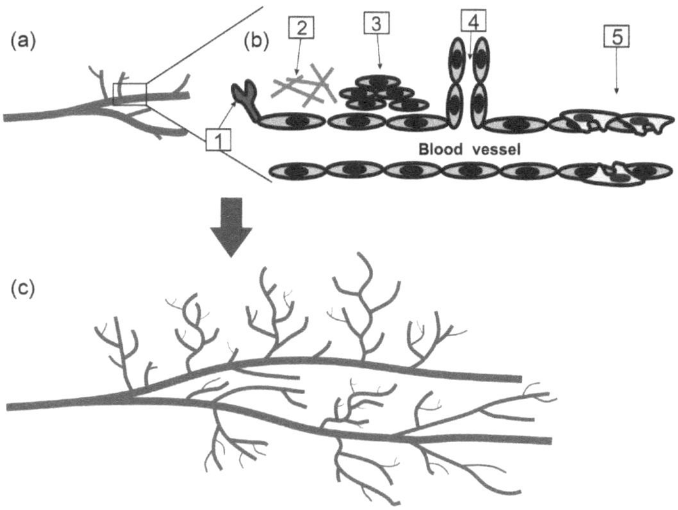

FIGURE 15.1

Angiogenesis. (a) Vascular network before wound healing; (b) phases of angiogenesis: (1) growth factors binding on endothelial cell receptors; (2) matrix metalloproteinases degrade the basal lamina; (3) EC proliferate and migrate; (4) vascular channels (tubes) are formed and undergo remodeling; (5) blood vessels are stabilized with pericytes; (c) vascular network after wound healing.

Redrawn and modified from Yoo and Kwon (2013).

angiogenesis also leads to severe pathological conditions, such as macular degeneration of the retina and tumor growth (Patel and Mikos, 2004). Controlled application of angiogenic or antiangiogenic factors delivered in scaffolds may support proper vascularization of healing wounds (Moon and West, 2008).

15.3.3.1 Modification of material to promote neovascularization

Scaffolds that underwent *ex vivo* prevascularization can be transplanted *in vivo* to integrate with the host microvasculature. This utilizes various biochemical signals embedded within scaffolds to simulation of the natural tissue microenvironment and to revitalize the angiogenic potential of seeded cells. These scaffolds are frequently modified with ECM proteins organized in micropatterns to provide a guiding network for angiogenesis. Into tissue may be delivered angiogenic factors, vascular cells, and other supporting cell types (Moon and West, 2008).

Modifications using ECM proteins or ECM-derived peptides—ECM proteins, such as collagen and fibronectin, often cover surfaces of biomaterials to augment their interaction with cells. An ECM coat on biomaterials can facilitate neovascularization *in vivo* (Moon and West, 2008).

Cellular interactions with ECM proteins are quite complex because these proteins present cells with multiple cell binding and growth factor binding domains.

Table 15.1 Growth and Differentiation Factors Involved in Wound Healing

Name of Factor	Origin	Function
PDGF (platelet-derived growth factor)	α Granules of platelets	The family of PDGF are mitogens and chemoattractants for fibroblasts (Ross et al., 1986; Seppä et al., 1982), smooth muscle cells (Grotendorst et al., 1982; Sjölund et al., 1988), and other cells of mesenchymal origin (Mutsaers et al., 1997)
		Chemotaxis of neutrophils and monocytes stimulates the activation of macrophages (Deuel et al., 1982; Tzeng et al., 1985)
		Regulates gene expression of fibronectin (Blatti et al., 1988), synthesis of protocollagen (Butt et al., 1995), and increases the activity of collagenase (Bauer et al., 1985)
TGF-β (transforming growth factor beta)	Fibroblasts, platelets, monocytes, chondrocytes, osteoblasts	TGF-β leads to the formation of fibronectin, type I and III collagen (Ferguson and O'Kane, 2004). Simultaneously it inhibits the formation of metalloproteainases in fibroblasts and thus prevents collagen degradation (a large quantity of TGF-β leads to creation of a hypertrophic scar) (Pakyari et al., 2013)
FGF (fibroblast growth factor)	Damage endothelial cells (EC) and macrophages	The family of FGF is mitogenic for EC, regulates migration and proliferation of EC (Folkman, 1987; Montesano, 1986)
		It is also mitogenic for keratinocytes (Ristow and Messmer, 1988)
EGF (epidermal growth factor)	Platelets and macrophages	The EGF family supports the mitoses of fibroblasts, keratinocytes, smooth muscle cells, and epithelial cells (Laato et al., 1987; Rheinwald and Green, 1977; Schreiber et al., 1986)

To overcome these issues, peptides, often only several amino acids long, have been derived from ECM proteins as the most basic subunits required for normal cell adhesion and proliferation (Moon and West, 2008).

Cellular interactions with ECM proteins are quite complex. For effective cell adhesion and proliferation to be sufficient often only several amino acids are derived from ECM proteins, such as Arg-Gly-Asp-Ser (RGDS) peptide derived from vitronectin and fibronectin and Tyr-Iso-Gly-Ser-Arg, YIGSR is a peptide sequence derived from laminin (Moon and West, 2008).

Micropatterning techniques to regulate angiogenesis—Micropatterning techniques such as photolithographic patterning, micromolding, microcontact printing, and laser photolithography can allow control over the presentation of angiogenic biomolecules at cellular-length scales (Moon and West, 2008). Photolithography provides a convenient method to micropattern molecules onto the surfaces of biomaterials. Microcontact printing commonly uses the strong interaction between thiol-containing moieties and a gold substrate to pattern different biomolecules. Micromolding processes have been applied to create complex tissue architectures in scaffold materials. Laser photolithography exploits selective photopolymerization of biomolecules with lasers to create internally complex 3D materials (Moon and West, 2008).

15.3.3.2 Controlled drug delivery from natural ECM polymers

Delivering angiogenic factors using a bolus injection is associated with negative side effects (hyperpermeable vessels, hypotension, uncontrolled angiogenesis, and stimulation of tumor growth) in surrounding nontarget tissues (Epstein et al., 2001). Therefore, the aim of tissue engineering is to provide a targeted and consistent delivery of angiogenic factors.

Simple loading—Interception of growth factors in scaffolds is an easy way to delivery drug (Moon and West, 2008). FGF-2 was added by Obara et al. (2003) during polymerization of chitosan hydrogels. Most of the added FGF-2 was released in a sustained fashion during *in vivo* degradation. Obara et al. (2003) observed increased capillary formation in healing-impaired diabetic mice model in a group with chitosan scaffold and addition of FGF-2 (Obara et al., 2003).

Ionic complexation—Using ionic complexation of growth factors with scaffolds is another way to deliver growth factors (Moon and West, 2008). Ionic interactions between positively charged growth factor and negatively charged polymers promote slow initial release of growth factors (Tabata and Ikada, 1999).

Heparin-mediated release—Modification of natural ECM proteins, such as heparin, conducts an increased angiogenic potential. Heparin binds to a number of growth factors and releases later on in response to cellular activities. Heparin also helps to protect growth factors from proteolytic degradation, thus increasing the presentation and availability of these factors (Sakiyama-Elbert and Hubbell, 2000).

15.4 BIOMATERIALS USED IN WOUND HEALING

15.4.1 ORIGIN OF BIOMATERIALS

Biomaterials are natural or synthetically produced. However, in both cases they are subjected to additional modifications of their composition, shape, texture, or surface using tissue engineering techniques. Natural biomaterials are usually glycoproteins, proteins, or polysaccharides. ECM is itself a very complex natural biomaterial, which provides mechanical support and affects the function and fate of cells.

The origin of natural materials is (Palsson and Bhatia, 2004):

- autologous—coming from other parts of the body of the same individual;
- isogenic—derived from a genetically identical individual;
- allogenic—originating from another individual of the same species;
- xenogenic—originating from other animal species.

Xenogenic and allogenic antigens induce an unwanted inflammatory response in the recipient's tissues. To prevent this, the antigens are removed from the grafts using decellularization. This may be done using physical factors (freeze), chemical substances (Triton X-100, hypotonic or hypertonic sodium EDTA) (Hrebikova et al., 2013), enzymes (trypsin, exonuclease), protease inhibitors (aprotinin), and antibiotics (penicillin, streptomycin) (Gilbert et al., 2006).

15.4.2 PROPERTIES OF BIOMATERIALS

The biological response to the presence of the biomaterial in the tissue is influenced by a combination of physical and chemical properties (surface area, size, chemical composition) and biological properties (immunoreactivity, adhesion to cells and intercellular matrix, etc.). The interaction between cells and the material is a combination of nonspecific and specific interactions reflecting the surface topography. The nonspecific interactions are due to van der Waals forces, electrostatic repulsion, hydration, and solvation forces. The biological interactions are due to adhesion molecules on the cell surfaces. For example, fibronectin as protein of ECM (Lewandowska et al., 1992) is a very effective cell-adhesive substance. Similarly, laminin, being a key component of the basement membrane, is a powerful cell-binding agent (Christopherson et al., 2009). In contrast, albumin is an effective nonadhesive biological coating on hydrophobic surfaces due to its irreversible strong adsorption and conformational change (Dekker et al., 1991).

The topology of the surface, stiffness of scaffold, size of the pores, and thickness of the biomaterial influence not only the cell adhesion, but also cell proliferation, migration, and function (Palsson and Bhatia, 2004). Uygun (2010) observed the growth of rat mesenchymal stem cells (MSCs) on chitosan membranes of various thicknesses. He detected significantly improved cell adhesion, spreading, and proliferation that was accompanied by increased membrane thickness. Similarly to the MSCs, rat hepatocytes also exhibited increased growth on the substrate with a thickened basal membrane (Uygun et al., 2010).

Zeltinger et al. (2001) followed the influence of pore size on the attachment, growth, and ECM deposition in several cell types. Canine dermal fibroblasts showed no preference for the pore sizes tested (for pores ranging from 38 to 150 μm). However, the growth of vascular smooth muscle cells and microvascular EC favored the scaffolds with larger pore size (Zeltinger et al., 2001).

Fibroblasts, epithelial cells, and EC showed increased proliferation on stiffer substrates. In contrast, neurons showed greater proliferation on softer substrates, which correlated with their natural environment in the brain (Engler et al., 2004).

Modifying the physical properties (e.g., the surface charge) on the biomaterial can significantly affect and control the growth of various types of cells (Hejcl et al., 2009).

15.4.2.1 Mechanical properties of biomaterials

This section summarizes the mechanical properties of various biomaterials used in medicine.

15.4.2.1.1 Polymers

Polymers are flexible, resistant to biochemical attack, have good compatibility, light weight, and are available in a wide variety of compositions with adequate physical and mechanical properties (Hench and Jones, 2005; Ifkovits and Burdick, 2007; Patel and Gohil, 2012; Pruitt and Chakravartula, 2011; Ratner, 2012; Seal, 2001; Wong and Bronzino, 2007). They can be easily shaped. Whereas the first medically used polymers were industrial polymers, new polymers have been specially synthesized for medical use. They are broadly used in tissue engineering, implantation of medical devices and artificial organs, prostheses, dentistry, bone repair, drug delivery and targeting into sites of inflammation or tumors, plastic tubing for intravenous infusion, bags for the transport of blood plasma, and catheters (Langer and Vacanti, 1993; Patel and Gohil, 2012).

Polymers can be amorphous, having no crystallinity, and exhibit glass-like properties (below glass transition temperature) as well as elastomeric properties (above glass transition temperature). Other forms are semicrystalline polymers that contain amorphous as well as crystalline regions. The mechanical parameters are highly influenced by the degree of crystallinity. The Young's modulus and yield stress generally increase with the degree of crystallinity, the ultimate elongation is reduced. Ultimate strength and fracture toughness may increase or decrease with crystallinity.

The currently used biomedical polymers cover a broad spectrum of polymers with various mechanical properties (Seal, 2001). Bioinert polymers cover poly(tetrafluoroethylene) (PTFE), poly(methylmethacrylate) (PMMA), polyethylene (PE), silicones, polyamides, poly(ethyleneterephthalate), and polyurethanes. Bioresorbable polymers, which are designed to degrade within the body after performing its function, cover polylactide, polyglycolide, poly(-3-hydroxybutyrate), polyhyaluronic acid esters, polydioxanone, and copolymers. Natural polymers, or polymers derived from living creatures, such as collagen, chitosan, HA, fibrin, and alginate, are also of great interest in the biomaterials field.

PTFE, a fluorocarbon-based polymer known as Teflon, is chemically extremely stable. It can be produced in various forms, such as woven into porous meshes, tubes, sheets (Goretex^{TM}), or as coatings (Dacron^{TM}). This makes it ideal for sutures, catheters, artificial vascular grafts, and mechanical heart valves. The limitations in use are due to relatively poor mechanical properties: low modulus of elasticity (0.5 MPa), low tensile strength (14–30 MPa), and low yield strength. The ultimate elongation is 120–350%.

PMMA is a hard, rigid, glassy but brittle polymer. PMMA has a modulus of elasticity of 2.2 GPa, tensile strength 30 MPa, and ultimate deformation 1.4%. Alone it is used in intraocular lenses and hard contact lenses, or it can be used as bone cementum in joint replacement surgery. The macromolecule composed of multiple PMMA molecules creates resins. Its physical properties are suitable for dental applications. The strength of an individual denture base resin is dependent on the composition of the resin, processing technique, conditions presented by the oral environment, and degree of polymerization. As the degree of polymerization increases, the strength of the resin increases.

PE is a polymer with low yield strength. It can be increased by crystallinity and by increasing molecular weight (Mw). It is stable and suitable for long-term implantation of joint (knee, ankle) replacements or as catheters. The ultra-high-molecular-weight PE has a modulus of elasticity of 4–12 GPa, tensile strength higher than 35 MPa, and ultimate deformation higher than 300%.

Collagen is a natural protein providing high strength to tissues. Collagen may also be processed into various forms, such as porous sponges, gels, and sheets. Chemical crosslinking of collagen increases its strength and stability. Collagen can have an effect causing alteration of cell behavior (e.g., changes in growth), it may have inopportune mechanical properties, or suffer shrinkage. Fortunately, it is possible to improve the mechanical properties of collagen by its combination with other biological or synthetic materials. Collagen combined with elastin and gelatin can be used to create scaffold for use in soft tissue engineering (Grover et al., 2012).

Chitosan is a natural polysaccharide that is derived from chitin present in hard exoskeletons of shellfish. It has controllable mechanical/biodegradation properties (such as porosity). Chitosan has broad possibilities for application, such as drug delivery, engineering of cartilage, nerve and liver tissue. Chitosan has low strength and inconsistent behavior with seeded cells, so alone chitosan cannot be used as a polymer scaffold in tissue engineering. However, chitosan may be easily combined with other materials to increase its strength and cell attachment potential (Nwe et al., 2009).

Alginate is a brown seaweed-derived polysaccharide. It has been tested for use in nerve, heart, liver, and cartilage tissue engineering. Alginate alone is mechanically weak and has poor cell adhesion. The strength of alginates has been increased by combining it with different polymer substances, such as agarose and chitosan (Kong et al., 2004; Sun and Tan, 2013).

15.4.2.1.2 Composites

Composite materials are a mixture of two or more phases (Burdick and Mauck, 2011; Hench and Jones, 2005; Ratner, 2012; Wang, 2003; Wong and Bronzino, 2007). The stress transfer occurs across the phase boundary. Composite biomaterials offer a variety of advantages in comparison with homogeneous materials. The individual homogeneous materials could have good properties such as lightness, easy production, but they could be limited by some mechanical properties. The combination of two or more materials together leads to an improvement of mechanical properties to emulate the mechanical properties of biological tissues. In particular, the properties of a composite material depend upon the shape of the heterogeneities, upon the volume fraction occupied by them, and upon the interface among the constituents. This has promising potential for stiff, strong, light-weight materials as well as for highly resilient and compliant materials. The material, mostly a polymer, is stiffened or hardened by the integration of the second-phase particulate inclusions. The elastic modulus of composite is significantly affected by the ratio of the second-phase modulus to the matrix modulus and volume fraction of the second-phase particles. It was found that the shape of the inclusion affects the stiffness of the composite. Stiff spherical particles are recommended to reach a stiff composite. The mechanical properties of composites could be isotropic, i.e., the same in all directions, or anisotropic, i.e., different properties in different directions. Note that billions of years of evolution led to development of almost always anisotropic biological materials.

Most natural structural biological materials are composites (Hench and Jones, 2005). The soft tissues are composed mostly from collagen fibers, elastic fibers, and amorphous ground substance among the matrix fibers. Elastin has tension strength about 1 MPa and ultimate elongation 100%. Collagen has a higher tensile strength between 50 and 100 MPa and lower ultimate elongation about 10%. Their composite in tendons with a low elastin content has ultimate strength 53 MPa, ultimate elongation about 10%, while in skin with a high elastin content the ultimate strength is about 8 MPa and ultimate elongation about 80%.

15.5 ANIMAL MODELS

Although some of the interactions between the biomaterials and organisms may be inferred from *in vitro* testing, further testing of the most promising materials requires the next stage of tests, i.e., *in vivo* tests. Animal models are used for *in vivo* evaluation of the interactions between tissues and tissue scaffolds. Biomaterial is implanted into an organ artificially damaged during the experiment under controlled conditions. Samples for analysis are taken away after different time intervals. The healing of the defect is then evaluated by noninvasive imaging methods such as X-ray examination, computed tomography, ultrasound sonography, magnetic resonance imaging (MRI), or histology, revealing microscopic changes in the defect. Table 15.2 reviews the model animals used for *in vivo* assays of biomaterials intended for healing of skin, cartilage, abdominal closure, and implanted arterial banding.

Table 15.2 Animal Models for *In Vivo* Evaluation of Biomaterials Designated for Healing of Skin, Cartilage, and Abdominal Closure and for Implantation of Arterial Banding; Typical Localization of Defects and Time Interval of Sampling of Individual Organs and Species

Area of Interest	Animal Model	Localization of Defect	Samples were Taken After
Healing of skin wounds	Rat	Back (Krasnov et al., 2012; Meruane et al., 2012)	1, 2, and 3 weeks (Meruane et al., 2012) 14 and 25 days (Krasnov et al., 2012)
	Rabbit	Back (Ananta et al., 2012; Ulubayram et al., 2001)	1, 3, and 5 weeks (Ananta et al., 2012.) 1, 2, and 3 weeks (Ulubayram et al., 2001)
Healing of hyaline cartilage	Dog	Knee (Breinan et al., 2001; Igarashi et al., 2012).	1.5, 3, 6, 12, and 18 months (Breinan et al., 2001.) 16 weeks (Igarashi et al., 2012)
	Pig	Knee (Cui et al., 2011; Filová et al., 2013)	12 months (Filová et al., 2013) 6 months (Cui et al., 2011)
	Rabbit	Knee (Fan et al., 2010; Filová et al., 2008)	8 weeks (Fan et al., 2010) 6 weeks (Filová et al., 2008)
Healing of abdominal closure	Rabbit	Fascia	6 weeks (Plencner et al., 2014)
	Chinchilla, rabbit	Abdominal wall	7, 21 days (Lambertz et al., 2014)
	Pig	Fascia	2, 4 weeks (Monteiro et al., 2013)
	Rat	Abdominal wall	5, 9 weeks (Song et al., 2013)
Implanted arterial banding	Pig	The pulmonary trunk about 1 cm above the valve; constrict to 70–80% of the original diameter	5 weeks (Nedorost et al., 2013)
	Mice	Aorta	14 days (Rockman et al., 1994)

15.6 *IN VIVO* MICROSCOPIC AND MECHANICAL CHARACTERIZATION OF BIOMATERIALS

To evaluate the suitability of the biomaterial we can combine mechanical tests with biochemical and histological analyses.

15.6.1 MECHANICAL CHARACTERIZATION OF BIOMATERIALS

The bioengineering and biodegradable tissue scaffolds and nanomaterials cover a broad spectrum of biomaterials (metals, ceramics, polymers, and composites) which replace a part or a function of various organs and tissues of the body (Hench and Jones, 2005; Jaffe et al., 2013; Pruitt and Chakravartula, 2011; Wong and Bronzino, 2007). These biomaterials and related devices have mechanical and performance requirements that originate from the usage in the body and the physical properties of the materials (Ratner, 2012; Ratner et al., 2012). A hip prosthesis has to be strong and rigid; a tendon material should be strong but flexible; an articular cartilage substitute should be soft and elastomeric; a heart valve leaflet should be flexible and tough; a dialysis membrane has to be strong and flexible.

Biomaterials have to have not only the special mechanical properties according to their usage but they also have to maintain them in *in vivo* conditions over a specific time (mechanical durability) (Parida, 2012; Ratner, 2012). A syringe needle is in contact with the body for only 1–2 s, and a tongue depressor 10 s, while contact lenses are in contact with the eye from 12 h up to 30 days; a bone plate or screw may fulfill its function for 6 months or longer, and a total hip replacement up to 20 years. The leaflets of heart valves must bend 60 times per minute without forming tears during the expected patient's lifetime (10 years at least). A hip joint must keep under heavy loads for more than 10 years. The intraocular lenses, which may fulfill their function for 30 and more years, are an extreme case. We have to take into account that the mechanical properties of the implanted biomaterials could differ before implantation, in *in vivo* conditions after implantation and could change in time through use. The biomaterials are therefore exposed to many mechanical and optical tests to assess their mechanical behavior (Jaffe et al., 2013; Pruitt and Chakravartula, 2011).

15.6.2 MECHANICAL TESTS

The biomaterials are in *in vivo* conditions exposed to mechanical loading (tension, pressure, shear, torsion; Figure 15.2) (Ratner, 2012). When a force is applied to a material, an opposite force causing a stress in the material exists within the material (Hench and Jones, 2005). The stress defined as the force per unit area (units Pa) causes the material to deform. The ratio between the actual deformation and original dimensions of material sample is called strain (dimensionless).

To find the mechanical behavior and the mechanical parameters (modulus of elasticity, yield strength, ultimate tensile strength, and deformation), the biomaterials are exposed to various loading tests (pulling, pushing, bending, or rotation; Figure 15.2) (Pruitt and Chakravartula, 2011; Ratner, 2012).

15.6.2.1 Tensile testing

The most frequent mechanical test is the uniaxial tensile test (Figure 15.2a). The material is loaded by a given force or elongation in one chosen direction. The loading leads to elongation or stress production in the direction of loading.

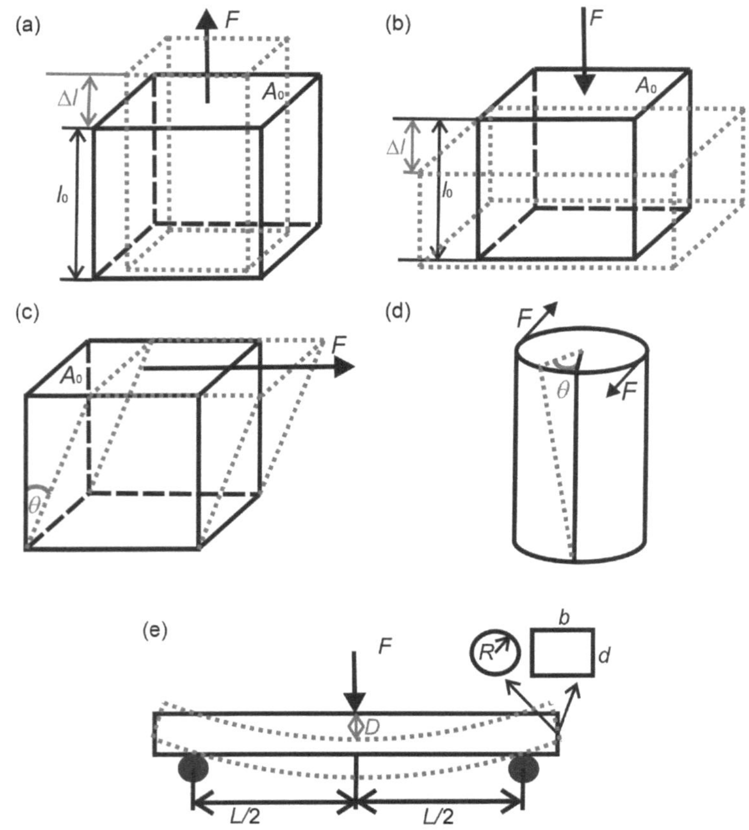

FIGURE 15.2

Types of loading: (a) tensile loading; (b) pressure loading; (c) shear loading; (d) torsion loading; (e) bending loading. F is the loading force, A_0 is the initial cross section area, l_0 is the initial dimension (length), Δl is the actual deformation, θ is the deformation angle, R is the cylinder radius, b, d are the width and thickness of the beam, respectively, L is the support span, and D is the deflection of the center of the beam.

The loading is applied perpendicularly to the cross section of the sample. The result of such a measurement is the *stress–strain curve* (Figure 15.3) plotted with strain on the x-axis and stress on the y-axis to show the relationship between the applied stress and strain. The stress–strain curve characterizes the mechanical performance of a material, such as yield strength, tensile strength, elastic modulus, elongation, and toughness.

The shape of the stress–strain curve differs between materials. Most materials initially have a linear proportion between stress and strain, whereas the slope (gradient) of this initial stress–strain curve is the *elastic modulus* or *Young's*

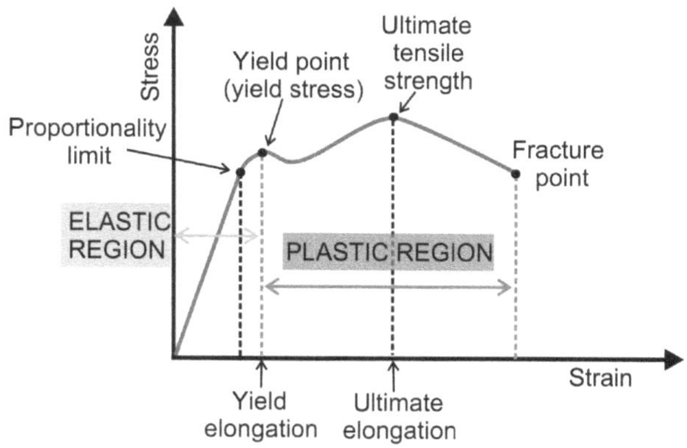

FIGURE 15.3

An example of a general stress–strain curve with typical features denoted.

modulus (*E*). A high elastic modulus corresponds with a greater rigidity of the material, that is, more stress is required to produce a given amount of strain. The linear relation is governed by Hooke's law = *E*. If the stress is removed during this stage of deformation, the material will return to its original dimensions. This process is repeatable, reversible, and is called *elastic deformation*. The *proportionality limit* on the stress–strain curve is the value of stress after which the material deformation no longer varies linearly with the applied stress.

Brittle materials, such as ceramics and glasses, break immediately after they undergo a critical (generally very small) amount of elastic deformation (Figure 15.4I). The plastic polymers and metals undergo, with increasing loading, the second stage of deformation called *plastic deformation* (Figure 15.3, Figure 15.4II—metals, Figure 15.4III—plastic polymers). The gradient of the stress–strain curve is changed in the plastic stage: a significant increase in strain is connected with little or no increase in stress. The point of change is called *yield point* (*yield strength*—σy, *yield point strain*—εyp). After the loading exceeds the yield point, when the material is unloaded, it does not return to its original dimensions, and a permanent plastic deformation remains. In metals, further increasing the strain loading after the yield point is characterized by the stress increasing very slowly and is followed by metal fracture. The stress–strain curve of plastic polymers differs from metals after the yield point. At high strain level, the stress is nearly independent of strain and shows a slight increase. For elastic polymers the stress increases very slowly with increasing strain even for small strains (Figure 15.4IV) and the fracture occurs at very high strain values.

The maximum tensile stress that can be applied to the material before rupture is called the *ultimate (maximum) tensile strength* (σUTS). The metals deform near this ultimate value usually so much that they have already failed to perform their function. The limitation factor for selecting metals for a given application is thus the yield strength and not the ultimate tensile strength.

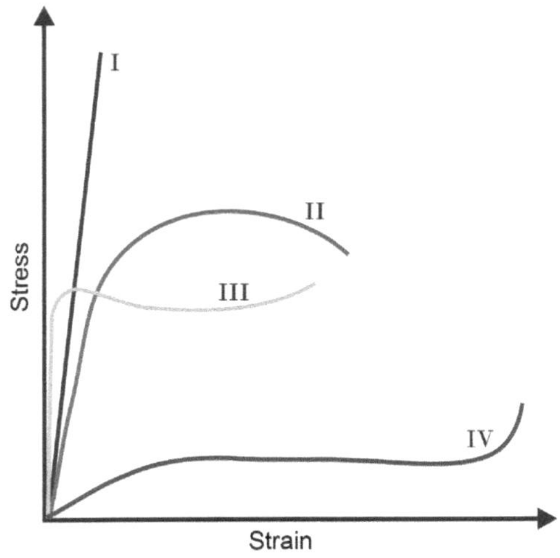

FIGURE 15.4

Stress–strain curve of ceramics (I), metals (II), plastic polymers (III), and elastic polymers (IV).

The other mechanical parameter obtained from the stress–strain curve is the *ultimate elongation* or the *ductility* of the material. In other words, the amount of strain that the material can undergo before rupture. The plastic strain could be quoted or the percentage changes in length of the fractured material to its original length. Note that the ultimate elongation cannot be used to predict the behavior of materials subjected to sudden or repeated loading.

Another mechanical parameter is the *toughness*. This is a measure of the resistance of a material to failure. The toughness is the area under the stress–strain curve. It corresponds to the energy required to fracture the material. Tough materials have a high value of toughness and are difficult to break. In contrast, brittle materials such as ceramics and glasses have a low value of toughness and the material is quite easily broken, often with little or no warning. Tough materials such as metals are also more resistant to impact loading or sudden changes of loading.

In order to match the mechanical properties of the surrounding tissue, it is important to note that the stress–strain curves of biological tissues are highly *nonlinear*. Such nonlinearity is much harder to quantify.

15.6.2.2 Compression testing

During compression test, the material is loaded by pressure in one chosen direction (Figure 15.2b). It is performed on biomaterials exposed to pressure in the body (bone, ligaments, or cartilage implants) and on biomaterials subjected to compressive forces during operation (orthopedic implants). The material is deformed according to a pressure loading and the relation between stress and deformation results in the stress–strain curve. The force is taken to be negative and the strain also reaches negative values. According to the tensile test the modulus of elasticity in pressure and the *compressive strength* are determined from the stress–strain curve. The *modulus of elasticity in pressure* is the slope of the linear part of the stress–strain curve. This is usually called the initial modulus of elasticity and is determined for strain between 2% and 10%. The compressive strength determines the capacity of material to withstand pressure loading until the rupture.

15.6.2.3 Shear and torsion testing

The shear (Figure 15.2c) and torsion (Figure 15.2d) test is applied to materials which undergo this kind of loading in the body (bone implants) and to brittle materials. In some cases, torsion forces may be applied to a sample instead of a pure shear.

During the shear test, the forces are parallel to the top and the bottom surfaces of the material sample. Shear stress (τ) is defined as the force divided by the original cross-sectional area of the sample. Shear strain (degree of rotation, γ, or angular displacement) is defined as the tangent of the deformation angle (θ). The relationship between shear stress and shear strain is plotted in the stress–strain curve. The slope of the linear part of the stress–strain under the proportionality limit is the *shear modulus* (G). The linear part is governed, analogically to the tensile test, by Hooke's law in the form $\tau = G\gamma$, where G is the shear modulus. The other mechanical parameters, elastic limit, yield strength, and ultimate strength can be obtained from the stress–strain curve analogically to the tensile test.

15.6.2.4 Bending testing

The three-point bending flexural test (Figure 15.2e) is mostly used to determine the modulus of elasticity in bending (flexural modulus, Ef), ultimate strength in bending, and toughness of the material. The tested specimen is a cylinder with radius (R), or a beam with rectangular cross section ($b \times d$, width $\times$ thickness). The parameters can again be obtained from the stress–strain curve. We denote by F the load at a given point on the load deflection curve, by L the support span, by D the deflection of the center of the beam, and by m the gradient (i.e., slope) of the initial straight-line portion of the load deflection curve. The flexural stress is defined as $\sigma f = 3FL/2bd^2$ (rectangular cross section) or $\sigma f = FL/\pi R^3$ (circular cross section), the flexural strain is defined as $\varepsilon f = 6Dd/L^2$. *Flexural modulus* is calculated as $Ef = L3m/4bd^3$. The *flexural strength* is the stress required to fracture the sample and is calculated as $\sigma mr = 3FL/2bd^2$, with F being here the smallest load that causes the fracture.

15.6.2.5 Fatigue testing

The biomaterials after implantation into the body very often undergo some type of cyclic loading (Pruitt and Chakravartula, 2011; Teoh, 2000). The progressive deterioration of the strength of a material or structural component during service means that a failure can occur at much lower stress levels than the ultimate stress of the material. This effect is called *fatigue*. Most alloys will fail at decreasing cycle stress amplitude as the number of stress cycles increases. The *fatigue limit* can be defined as the number of cycles that a material survives with a given stress amplitude. Alternatively, the *fatigue stress* can be defined as the stress that a material survives for some large number of cycles (10^7 or 10^8 cycles are typical). The fatigue stress is determined, i.e., for aluminum, magnesium, and most nonferrous metals. The aluminum has a fatigue stress typically one-third of the tensile strength of the alloy. Many steels and titanium alloys instead show a fatigue limit.

15.6.3 MICROSCOPIC CHARACTERIZATION OF BIOMATERIALS

15.6.3.1 Histological assessment

Histology provides information on the microscopic morphology, location, history, and current stage of healing, the formation of ECM, vascularization, tissue architectonics, inflammatory response to the presence of the biomaterial, and others. The most common processing of samples of soft tissue is by chemical fixation and paraffin embedding. The temperature during embedding samples to paraffin block (56 °C) leads to damage of thermo-labile materials. Alternatively, therefore, bypass the paraffin freezing process (ca. −25 °C) and take sections using a cryomicrotome.

One of the most challenging points in histological studies evaluating the impact of biomaterials *in vivo* is to choose appropriate technology and methods relevant to the original biological question of the experiment. It is possible to use scoring systems, in which the investigated parameters are classified using semiquantitative scoring scales. The scales might reflect the cellular morphology, positivity of the ECM ground substance to neutral or acidic glycosaminoglycans, surface regularity, structural integrity, thickness, degree of integration with the adjacent tissue, cellularity, clustering of chondrocytes, the presence of degenerative changes, or other morphological features (Filová et al., 2007; van Susante et al., 1999). A different strategy is to quantify the tissue composition using stereology and continuous variables that describe, e.g., cell number per unit volume, the length of the blood vessels or fibrous matrix structure, surface area, surface and volume fractions of the components of tissue, clustering and colocalization of microscopic objects. Many applications of quantitative microscopy are dominated by technique stereology. This way we can obtain information about the three-dimensional structure measurements made on the two-dimensional planar sections (Mouton, 2002).

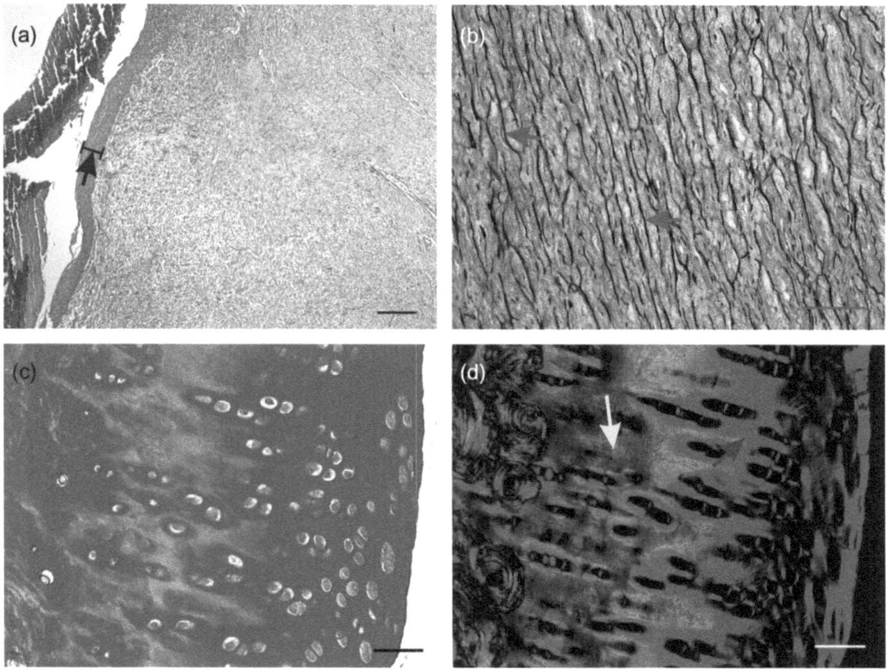

FIGURE 15.5

Microphotographs of stained tissue sections. (a) Epidermis (black arrow) newly formed during skin healing in rabbit, HE stain, scale bar 200 μm; (b) black elastic fibers and green collagen fibers within an elastic artery, Verhoeff's hematoxylin and green trichrome stain, scale bar 50 μm; (c) hyaline cartilage stained by picrosirius red and observed in a bright-field microscope, scale bar 50 μm; (d) hyaline cartilage stained by picrosirius red observed using polarized light, type I collagen appearing as red and yellow fibers (blue arrow), type III collagen appearing as green fibers (yellow arrow), scale bar 50 μm.

15.6.3.2 Biological importance of parameters from quantitative analysis

A high proportion of mature type I collagen fibers in a defect contributes to the mechanical resistance of the tissue (Fung, 1993; Screen, 2008). Increasing the ratio of collagen I/III means mechanically strong maturation of precursors of type III collagen into the type I collagen (Junge et al., 2004). A suitable method for differentiating the type I and type III collagen is the picrosirius red histological staining combined with circularly polarized light microscopy (Figure 15.5c and d) (Meruane et al., 2012). Type II collagen is present in ECM of hyaline and elastic cartilage. For detection of collagen II, immunohistochemistry applying an anticollagen II antibody may be used (Figure 15.6a; Rampichová et al., 2010).

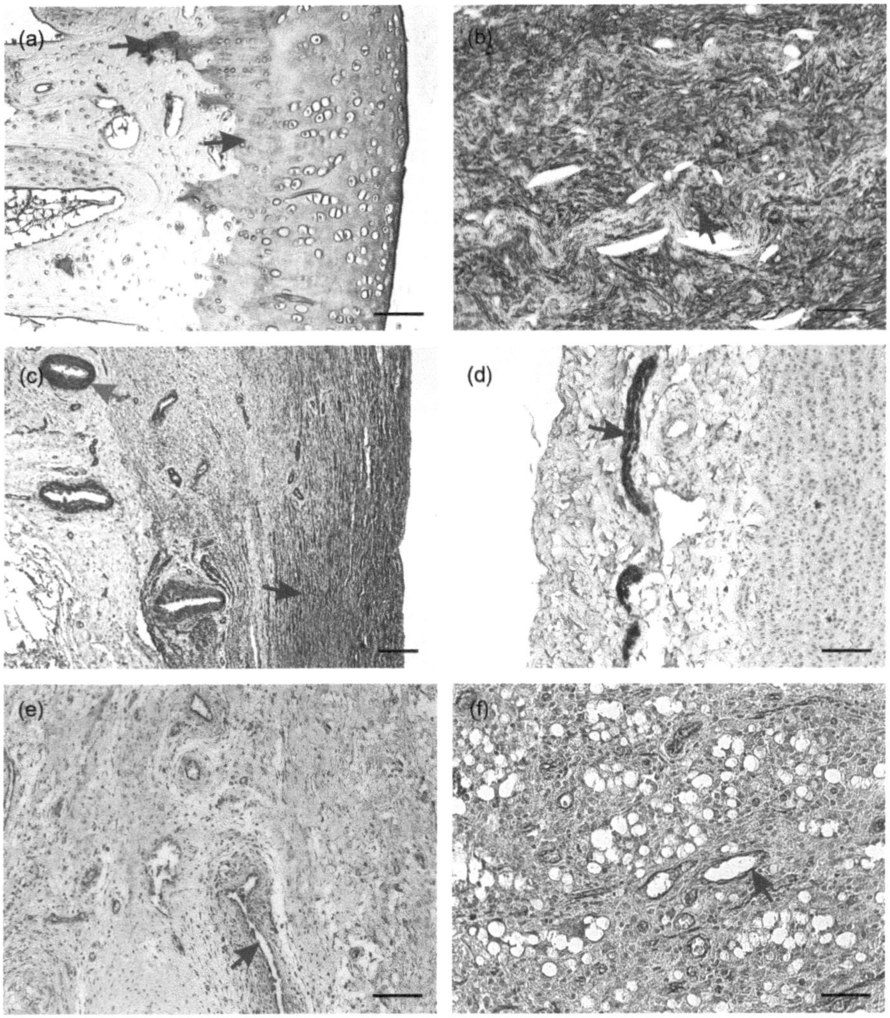

FIGURE 15.6

Microphotographs of tissue sections stained using immunohistochemistry. (a) Detection of type II collagen type (brown area, red arrow) within the extracellular matrix of hyaline cartilage using anticollagen II antibody, scale bar 100 μm. (b) Immunohistochemical detection of α-smooth muscle actin showing positive myofibroblasts (brown cytoplasm, red arrow) in healing abdominal incision, scale bar 100 μm. (c) Immunohistochemical detection of α-smooth muscle actin showing positive smooth muscle cells in tunica media of pulmonary artery (brown area, red arrow) and positive smooth muscle cells in the vasa vasorum (blue arrow), scale bar 200 μm. (d) Immunohistochemical detection of the neurofilament protein showing peripheral nerves (the nervi vasorum) within the tunica

(*Continued*)

A high proportion of elastin fibers in a defect contributes to the elasticity of the tissue (Fung, 1993). Modified green trichrome with Verhoeff's hematoxylin can be used to detect elastin fibers (Figure 15.5b; Kocová, 1970).

A high proportion of contractile myofibroblasts in the healing lesion contributes to wound contraction (Nowak et al., 2009; Van Beurden et al., 2005). Antibody antismooth muscle actin detects myofibroblasts (Figure 15.6b) and smooth muscle cells in media of vessels in tissues (Figure 15.6c; Plencner et al., 2014).

A high density of microvessels in a wound contributes to the regeneration and growth of tissue. Numerical and length density of microvessels in three dimensions, or the density of microvessel profiles in two dimensions, may be quantified. EC may be visualized using anti-von Willebrand factor antibody (Figure 15.6e; Meruane et al., 2012) or anti-CD31 antibody (Figure 15.6f; Plencner et al., 2014).

High numbers of inflammatory cells (leukocytes, macrophages) in a wound are linked to the immune response to injury (Adamson, 2009). Neutrophilic granulocytes react with antimyeloperoxidase antibody (Andrade et al., 2011). Macrophages react with anticapprotectin antibodies (Brandtzaeg et al., 1992; Marin et al., 1995), with anti-CD14 and anti-CD163 (Evans et al., 2013), and with anti-CD36 antibodies (Ortiz-Masià et al., 2012). Unfortunately, there is currently no single commercially available antibody that would be entirely specific for macrophages in all model animal species.

The thickness of newly formed epidermis is important for the evaluation of skin healing. The thickness of the epithelium layer is well visible even in routine stains, such as hematoxylin and eosin (HE) (Figure 15.5a) (Truong et al., 2005).

Arterial banding using textile bands can damage the nervi vasorum within the tunica adventitia of an artery. For detection of nerve fibers it is possible to use antibody antineurofilament protein (Figure 15.6d) (Nedorost et al., 2013).

15.7 TESTING AND ASSESSMENT OF DEGRADATION

Scaffolds from biodegradable polymers usually change their physical and chemical properties substantially after *in vivo* implantation. During evaluation of these changes we must pay attention to healing time and phases of degradation. In the first phase, we find changes of polymer surface, such as an increase in surface

◀ adventitia of pulmonary artery of a pig (brown area, red arrow), scale bar 100 μm. (e) Immunohistochemical detection of endothelial cells (EC) (red arrow) in newly formed vessels, anti-von Willebrand factor antibody, scale bar 100 μm. (f) Detection of EC (red arrow) in newly formed vessels, anti-CD31, scale bar 50 μm. Visualization was done using horseradish peroxidase/diaminobenzidine in all slides, counterstaining was done with Gill's hematoxylin in all slides.

roughness. Decomposition of molecular chains comes up during the next phase. This leads to a decrease in the polymer Mw and diffusion of large-molecular-weight fragments into the surrounding tissue. This results in a decrease in the tensile strength. In the last stage, the polymer matrix collapses and decreases its mean Mw. Mechanical properties decline due to disappearing crystallinity (Azevedo and Reis, 2005). The mechanism of degradation for different polymers depends on their Mw, morphology of each type of polymer, and environmental factors such as osmotic pressure, pH, temperature, etc. Degradation occurs mainly by hydrolysis, oxidation, or enzymatic reactions (Marin et al., 2013). The efficiency of polymeric material is affected by its stability (Uhrich et al., 1999). Therefore, understanding the mechanisms of degradation of a specific polymer is crucial to determine its suitable applications, but also limitations of its use.

Characteristics evaluating the polymer degradation are as follows: weight loss, crystallinity, molecular weight, morphology and dimensional changes, surface chemistry, isolation, and identification of degradation products and mechanical properties.

15.7.1 WEIGHT LOSS

Comparing the mass before implantation and after the degradation period we get information about changes of polymer weight. The initial weight of the sample is measured after drying of material to a constant mass. The degree of degradation is calculated as a percentage of weight loss (Azevedo and Reis, 2005), using the formula:

$$\%\ \text{Mass loss} = \frac{M_i - M_f}{M_i} \times 100$$

where M_f is the final mass and M_i is the initial mass (Lam et al., 2009).

15.7.2 MOLECULAR WEIGHT

The quantification of the polymer molecular weight (Mw) during the degradation is important for analyzing the degradation mechanisms of biomaterials. Mw influences many other properties, for example crystallinity, weight loss, mechanical properties, and morphology (Azevedo and Reis, 2005).

15.7.3 CRYSTALLINITY

The crystallinity of polymer affects its mechanical strength, opacity, and thermal properties. The changes in the crystallinity of polymer after degradation can be measured by using differential scanning calorimetry (Azevedo and Reis, 2005).

15.7.4 MORPHOLOGY AND DIMENSIONAL CHANGES OF BIOMATERIAL

Changes on the polymer surface are usually observed using light microscopy, scanning electron microscopy, and atomic force microscopy (Matheson et al., 2002). Scaffold porosity is measured as a ratio of the true volume to the apparent volume. The true volume or actual volume of material that makes up the scaffold was determined using a gas pycnometer. The apparent volume denotes the overall geometrical volume occupied by the whole sample. The porosity of the scaffolds (expressed as a percentage value) may be calculated according to the formula:

$$\%\ \text{Porosity} = \frac{V_a - V_t}{V_a} \times 100$$

where V_a is the apparent volume and V_t the true volume (Lam et al., 2009).

15.7.5 ISOLATION AND IDENTIFICATION OF PRODUCTS OF DEGRADATION

The safety of a biomaterial and its degradation products is essential for its use in medicine. Products of degradation of polymers can leach into surrounding tissues and may enter the circulation. Some of the products may be easily metabolized and can cause toxic effects (Griffiths et al., 1996). Therefore it is important to identify the products released at different stages of degradation, their lifespan and the kinetics of their formation. For qualitative and quantitative analysis of the degradation products within the tissue fluid, synovial fluid, or other body fluids, the following methods may be used: high-performance liquid chromatography, nuclear magnetic resonance, and mass spectroscopy (Azevedo and Reis, 2005).

15.7.6 MECHANICAL TESTING OF DEGRADATION OF BIOMATERIALS

As mentioned in Section 15.4.2.1, the mechanical properties of individual biomaterials can differ between a pure form and a composite, and the mechanical properties can change after implantation in the body. The inert biomaterials are less influenced. In contrast, the biological materials such as collagen could be influenced by the surrounding environment. Moreover, it is very important to observe the *in vivo* behavior of the biomaterial implants, healing of the tissue, and degradation of biomaterials implanted into body.

The classical mechanical tests cannot be directly used in the *in vivo* environment to determine the healing of the tissue, changes in mechanical properties after implantation, or to assess and observe the degradation process. One possibility is the frequently used animal model, where the tissue is removed from the body after a given time necessary for healing after implantation operation or after another specific time. In this case the cells, tissue matrix, and biomaterials are destroyed because this is a one-way journey of monitoring mechanical properties.

The second possibility is the *in vitro* test done on biomaterials themselves or biomaterials planted with stem cells, currently very popular in tissue engineering scaffolds. The classical tests (Section 16.5.2) can then be applied to determine the mechanical parameters. In both cases the *in vitro* environment corresponds as much as possible to the body environment. It includes the physiological liquid buffer, pH, light, temperature, oxygen, and nutrition support, etc.

Noninvasive *in vivo* measurements can be done by the *elasticity imaging methods*. They combine the tissue excitation techniques with methods for detection of tissue response. They can be static or dynamic. In static methods, the tissue is compressed slowly and the distribution of its displacement is measured with magnetic resonance, ultrasound, or optically. The dynamic methods rely on the wave equation, which in its differential form is local in character. Therefore, the distribution of dynamic displacement, a three-dimensional vector, and its second-order partial derivatives in time and space within a small region of the tissue is enough to completely characterize the shear moduli of the tissue in that region. The excitation could be done by direct application of a compression force (stress) on the skin to deform the tissue at the bottom. This is often done by simply pressing and holding a plate on the skin (in static approach) or vibrating the skin using a vibratory device (in dynamic approach). The tissue could also be excited internally and directly in the region of interest within tissue, that is, using the radiation force of an ultrasound beam. By this method we can reach a concentrated stress (or a point-like force) to probe the tissue point-by-point, directly and remotely within the region of interest.

15.7.6.1 Ultrasound elastography (elasticity imaging)

The ultrasound elasticity imaging is popular in noninvasive monitoring of cell growth, scaffold degradation, and tissue development technique (Carlsen et al., 2013; Gennisson et al., 2013; Ophir et al., 2002; Svensson and Amiras, 2006). It enables continuous monitoring of the *in vivo* regeneration of tissue, progressive biomaterial degradation, and progression of various diseases. The method is based on phase-sensitive speckle displacement.

When a tissue is mechanically excited by a weak quasistatic compression, the internal stresses are defined by the boundary conditions as well as by the structure and properties of the tissue. The local elastic properties of material under compression should be measured in three orthogonal spatial orientations relative to the ultrasonic beam.

When using ultrasound elasticity imaging it is important to use a small compression strain (less than 2%, typically 1%) to minimize the distortion of the signal due to compression. The tissue is insonified before loading and after loading. The strain is estimated from displacement from the time shift measurement by assuming a constant speed of sound. The local longitudinal strain in combination with the local longitudinal stress in the tissue generates quantitative images (elastograms) of local estimation of the elastic modulus. Original elastograms are gray-scaled, where black represents hard tissue, white represents soft tissue, and grays represent intermediate elasticity.

The ultrasound elasticity imaging requires a mechanical compression, which limits its application to areas where clear physical access can be achieved. The measured strain has to be normalized to overall strain applied to the body and this is the source of error.

An alternative to ultrasound elasticity is transient elastography (TE). In this method, a single transient shear wave is induced into tissue via a special transducer and the propagation of this wave is imaged using ultrasound. The propagation speed of the shear wave is related to the underlying tissue shear modulus. The results are used to calculate the absolute elastic modulus of the tissue. The TE can be combined with an optical method. For example, the photoaccoustic imaging combines optical excitation and ultrasound detection (Park et al., 2014) to also obtain the visualization of scaffold degradation.

15.7.6.2 Magnetic resonance elastography

Magnetic resonance elastography is a dynamic elasticity imaging-based noninvasive technique that is currently used to monitor *in vivo* regeneration of tissue, subsequent biomaterial degradation, and the progression of various diseases (Mariappan et al., 2010; Smith et al., 1997). It combines benefits of the acoustic shear waves and MRI. MRI has a high image resolution and is used to measure the displacement caused by shear waves. The measurable scale of displacement is 100 nm and greater.

The harmonic shear waves (vibrations) of acoustic-range frequencies (50–500 Hz) are induced using an external driver. The propagation of these vibrations in the tissue is captured using the MRI technique. The shear modulus of material (μ) is calculated using assumptions on tissue properties: to be linearly elastic, isotropic, and Hookean. Also, the quantitative images displaying the stiffness of material (tissue) can be generated.

15.7.6.3 Optical elastography

Optical coherence elastography (OCE) is a novel elastography technology used to determine tissue biomechanical properties *in vivo* using optical coherence tomography (Kennedy et al., 2014; Liang et al., 2010; Rogowska et al., 2004; Sun et al., 2011). The OCE is used for measuring and imaging biomechanical properties at the micron-scale tissue level, the cellular level, and even the molecular level. The tissue excitation can be static or dynamic (waves, pulse) and applied to the tissue either internally or externally: external compressive load, surface acoustic waves, shear waves, acoustic radiation force, magnetomotive, and swept-frequency loading. The tissue displacement and the resulting data are processed by a special algorithm to obtain the elastogram image reconstruction.

Tissue Doppler optical coherence elastography is another optical method to image tissue movements, strain rates, and strains of soft tissue *in vivo* in real time (Wang, 2006). The reaction on tissue excitation is measured with using Doppler

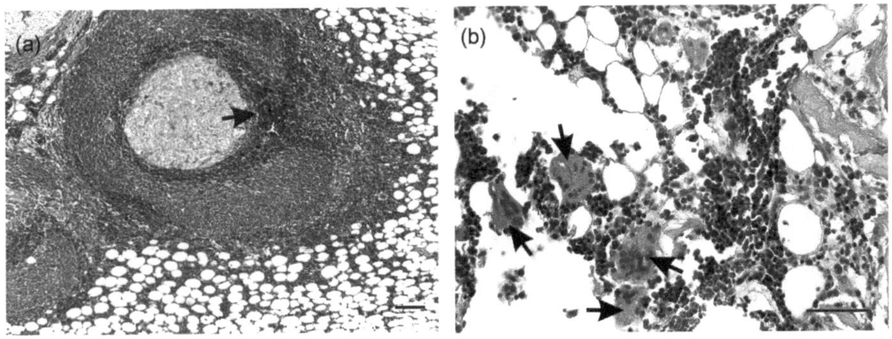

FIGURE 15.7

Microphotographs of tissue reaction to the presence of foreign materials (foreign bodies). (a) Recruitment of granulocytes within bone marrow as a reaction on implantation of calcium phosphate osteoinductive granules; hematoxylin–eosin (HE) stain, scale bar 100 μm. (b) Multinucleated giant cells from foreign bodies formed by fusion of a number of macrophages within the bone marrow close to a healing bone defect supported with a degradable tissue scaffold, HE stain, scale bar 50 μm.

effect in optical coherence interferograms induced by a tissue motion. The phase changes are measured between individual scans to resolve the instantaneous tissue displacement.

15.7.7 REACTION TO FOREIGN BODIES

Tissue reactions to the presence of foreign bodies comprise invasion of granulocytes (Figure 15.7a), recruitment of macrophages, and formation of multinucleated giant cells from foreign bodies (Figure 15.7b), which originated fusion of macrophages. A connective capsule may be formed around biomaterials as a result of synthesis of tissue matrix by fibroblasts. These findings may be evaluated after *in vivo* implantation of biomaterials using histological processing.

15.8 CONCLUSIONS

Histological methods are an irreplaceable part of the *in vivo* evaluation of the effect of biomaterials implanted into damage tissue. Application of quantitative histology provides us with information on distribution and spatial relationships among the scaffold, cells, ECM, and the process of angiogenesis and inflammation. Measuring of the biomechanical properties of biomaterials provides important results supplementary to those from morphological analysis. We use animal models for *in vivo* evaluation of biomaterials. Continuous morphometric variables are preferably used for microscopic quantification of tissue healing, so that biological hypotheses of the experiments in animal models may be tested using standard statistical tests.

ACKNOWLEDGMENTS

This work was supported by project ED.1.05/2.1.00/03.0076 from the European Regional Development Fund and by SVV 260 047 and PRVOUK P36 Projects of the Charles University in Prague. The biomechanical part of the study was supported by the ERDF project "NTIS—New Technologies for Information Society," European Centre of Excellence, CZ.1.05/1.1.00/02.0090. The contribution of PK was supported by the project LO1506 of the Czech Ministry of Education, Youth and Sports. One of the authors (MH) also received support from the project CENTEM No. CZ.1.05/2.1.00/03.0088, which was cofounded by the ERDF within the OP RDI program of the Ministry of Education, Youth and Sports of the Czech Republic.

REFERENCES

Adamson, R., 2009. Role of macrophages in normal wound healing: an overview. J. Wound Care 18, 349–351.

Ananta, M., Brown, R.A., Mudera, V., 2012. A rapid fabricated living dermal equivalent for skin tissue engineering: an in vivo evaluation in an acute wound model. Tissue Eng. A 18, 353–361.

Anderson, J.M., 2001. Biological responses to materials. Annu. Rev. Mater. Res. 31, 81–110.

Andrade, T.A.M., Iyer, A., Das, P.K., Foss, N.T., Garcia, S.B., Coutinho-Netto, J., et al., 2011. The inflammatory stimulus of a natural latex biomembrane improves healing in mice. Braz. J. Med. Biol. Res. Rev. Bras. Pesqui. Médicas E Biológicas Soc. Bras. Biofísica Al 44, 1036–1047.

Atala, A., Bauer, S.B., Soker, S., Yoo, J.J., Retik, A.B., 2006. Tissue-engineered autologous bladders for patients needing cystoplasty. Lancet 367, 1241–1246.

Azevedo, H., Reis, R., 2005. Understanding the enzymatic degradation of biodegradable polymers and strategies to control their degradation rate. In: Reis, R.L., Román, J.S. (Eds.), Biodegradable Systems in Tissue Engineering and Regenerative Medicine. CRC Press, Boca Raton, FL, pp. 177–202.

Bauer, E.A., Cooper, T.W., Huang, J.S., Altman, J., Deuel, T.F., 1985. Stimulation of in vitro human skin collagenase expression by platelet-derived growth factor. Proc. Natl. Acad. Sci. U.S.A. 82, 4132–4136.

Blatti, S.P., Foster, D.N., Ranganathan, G., Moses, H.L., Getz, M.J., 1988. Induction of fibronectin gene transcription and mRNA is a primary response to growth-factor stimulation of AKR-2B cells. Proc. Natl. Acad. Sci. U.S.A. 85, 1119–1123.

Brandtzaeg, P., Dale, I., Gabrielsen, T.O., 1992. The leucocyte protein L1 (calprotectin): usefulness as an immunohistochemical marker antigen and putative biological function. Histopathology 21, 191–196.

Breinan, H.A., Minas, T., Hsu, H.P., Nehrer, S., Shortkroff, S., Spector, M., 2001. Autologous chondrocyte implantation in a canine model: change in composition of reparative tissue with time. J. Orthop. Res. Off. Publ. Orthop. Res. Soc 19, 482–492. Available from: http://dx.doi.org/10.1016/S0736-0266(00)90015-9.

Burdick, J.A., Mauck, R.L., 2011. Biomaterials for Tissue Engineering Applications: A Review of the Past and Future Trends. Springer, Wien.

Butt, R.P., Laurent, G.J., Bishop, J.E., 1995. Collagen production and replication by cardiac fibroblasts is enhanced in response to diverse classes of growth factors. Eur. J. Cell Biol. 68, 330–335.

Carlsen, J., Ewertsen, C., Lönn, L., Nielsen, M., 2013. Strain elastography ultrasound: an overview with emphasis on breast cancer diagnosis. Diagnostics 3, 117–125.

Christopherson, G.T., Song, H., Mao, H.-Q., 2009. The influence of fiber diameter of electrospun substrates on neural stem cell differentiation and proliferation. Biomaterials 30, 556–564. Available from: http://dx.doi.org/10.1016/j.biomaterials.2008.10.004.

Cui, W., Wang, Q., Chen, G., Zhou, S., Chang, Q., Zuo, Q., et al., 2011. Repair of articular cartilage defects with tissue-engineered osteochondral composites in pigs. J. Biosci. Bioeng. 111, 493–500. Available from: http://dx.doi.org/10.1016/j.jbiosc.2010.11.023.

Darby, I.A., Hewitson, T.D., 2007. Fibroblast differentiation in wound healing and fibrosis. In: Jeon, K.W. (Ed.), International Review of Cytology. Academic Press, University of Tennesse, Knoxville, TN, USA, pp. 143–179.

Dekker, A., Beugeling, T., Wind, H., Poot, A., Bantjes, A., Feijen, J., et al., 1991. Deposition of cellular fibronectin and desorption of human serum albumin during adhesion and spreading of human endothelial cells on polymers. J. Mater. Sci. Mater. Med. 2, 227–233.

Dettmeyer, R.B., 2011. Forensic Histopathology: Fundamentals and Pespectives. Springer-Verlag, Berlin.

Deuel, T.F., Senior, R.M., Huang, J.S., Griffin, G.L., 1982. Chemotaxis of monocytes and neutrophils to platelet-derived growth factor. J. Clin. Invest. 69, 1046–1049.

Engler, A.J., Griffin, M.A., Sen, S., Bönnemann, C.G., Sweeney, H.L., Discher, D.E., 2004. Myotubes differentiate optimally on substrates with tissue-like stiffness: pathological implications for soft or stiff microenvironments. J. Cell Biol. 166, 877–887.

Epstein, S.E., Kornowski, R., Fuchs, S., Dvorak, H.F., 2001. Angiogenesis therapy: amidst the hype, the neglected potential for serious side effects. Circulation 104, 115–119.

Evans, B.J., Haskard, D.O., Sempowksi, G., Landis, R.C., 2013. Evolution of the macrophage CD163 phenotype and cytokine profiles in a human model of resolving inflammation. Int. J. Inflamm. 2013, 780502.

Fan, H., Tao, H., Wu, Y., Hu, Y., Yan, Y., Luo, Z., 2010. TGF-β3 immobilized PLGA-gelatin/chondroitin sulfate/hyaluronic acid hybrid scaffold for cartilage regeneration. J. Biomed. Mater. Res. A 95, 982–992. Available from: http://dx.doi.org/10.1002/jbm.a.32899.

Ferguson, M.W.J., O'Kane, S., 2004. Scar-free healing: from embryonic mechanisms to adult therapeutic intervention. Philos. Trans. R. Soc. Lond. B. Biol. Sci. 359, 839–850. Available from: http://dx.doi.org/10.1098/rstb.2004.1475.

Filová, E., Jelínek, F., Handl, M., Lytvynets, A., Rampichová, M., Varga, F., et al., 2008. Novel composite hyaluronan/type I collagen/fibrin scaffold enhances repair of osteochondral defect in rabbit knee. J. Biomed. Mater. Res. B. Appl. Biomater. 87, 415–424. Available from: http://dx.doi.org/10.1002/jbm.b.31119.

Filová, E., Rampichová, M., Handl, M., Lytvynets, A., Halouzka, R., Usvald, D., et al., 2007. Composite hyaluronate-type I collagen-fibrin scaffold in the therapy of osteochondral defects in miniature pigs. Physiol. Res. Acad. Sci. Bohemoslov. 56 (Suppl. 1), S5–S16.

Filová, E., Rampichová, M., Litvinec, A., Držík, M., Míčková, A., Buzgo, M., et al., 2013. A cell-free nanofiber composite scaffold regenerated osteochondral defects in miniature pigs. Int. J. Pharm. 447, 139–149. Available from: http://dx.doi.org/10.1016/j.ijpharm.2013.02.056.

Folkman, J., Klagsbrun, M., 1987. Angiogenic factors. Science 235, 442–447.

Fung, Y.C., 1993. Biomechanics: Mechanical Properties of Living Tissues, second ed. Springer-Verlag, New York, NY.

Gennisson, J.-L., Deffieux, T., Fink, M., Tanter, M., 2013. Ultrasound elastography: principles and techniques. Diagn. Interv. Imaging 94, 487–495.

Gilbert, T.W., Sellaro, T.L., Badylak, S.F., 2006. Decellularization of tissues and organs. Biomaterials 27, 3675–3683.

Griffiths, M.M., Langone, J.J., Lightfoote, M.M., 1996. Biomaterials and granulomas. Methods San Diego Calif. 9, 295–304.

Grotendorst, G.R., Chang, T., Seppä, H.E., Kleinman, H.K., Martin, G.R., 1982. Platelet-derived growth factor is a chemoattractant for vascular smooth muscle cells. J. Cell Physiol. 113, 261–266. Available from: http://dx.doi.org/10.1002/jcp.1041130213.

Grover, C.N., Cameron, R.E., Best, S.M., 2012. Investigating the morphological, mechanical and degradation properties of scaffolds comprising collagen, gelatin and elastin for use in soft tissue engineering. J. Mech. Behav. Biomed. Mater. 10, 62–74.

Hejcl, A., Lesný, P., Prádný, M., Sedý, J., Zámecník, J., Jendelová, P., et al., 2009. Macroporous hydrogels based on 2-hydroxyethyl methacrylate. Part 6: 3D hydrogels with positive and negative surface charges and polyelectrolyte complexes in spinal cord injury repair. J. Mater. Sci. Mater. Med. 20, 1571–1577.

Helpap, B., 1987. Leitfaden der Allgemeinen Entzündungslehre. Springer, Berlin.

Hench, L.L., Jones, J.R., 2005. Biomaterials, Artificial Organs and Tissue Engineering. Woodhead Publishing in Materials. CRC Press, Boca Raton, FL.

Hrebikova, H., Diaz, D., Mokry, J., 2013. Chemical decellularization: a promising approach for preparation of extracellular matrix. Biomed. Pap. 157, 12–17.

Ifkovits, J.L., Burdick, J.A., 2007. Review: photopolymerizable and degradable biomaterials for tissue engineering applications. Tissue Eng. 13, 2369–2385.

Igarashi, T., Iwasaki, N., Kawamura, D., Kasahara, Y., Tsukuda, Y., Ohzawa, N., et al., 2012. Repair of articular cartilage defects with a novel injectable in situ forming material in a canine model. J. Biomed. Mater. Res. A 100, 180–187. Available from: http://dx.doi.org/10.1002/jbm.a.33248.

Jaffe, M., Hammond, W., Tolias, P., Arinzeh, T., 2013. Characterization of Biomaterials. Woodhead Publishing, Oxford.

Jain, R.K., 2003. Molecular regulation of vessel maturation. Nat. Med. 9, 685–693.

Junge, K., Klinge, U., Rosch, R., Mertens, P.R., Kirch, J., Klosterhalfen, B., et al., 2004. Decreased collagen type I/III ratio in patients with recurring hernia after implantation of alloplastic prostheses. Langenbecks Arch. Surg. Dtsch. Ges. Für Chir. 389, 17–22.

Keck, P.J., Hauser, S.D., Krivi, G., Sanzo, K., Warren, T., Feder, J., et al., 1989. Vascular permeability factor, an endothelial cell mitogen related to PDGF. Science 246, 1309–1312.

Kennedy, B.F., McLaughlin, R.A., Kennedy, K.M., Chin, L., Curatolo, A., Tien, A., et al., 2014. Optical coherence micro-elastography: mechanical-contrast imaging of tissue microstructure. Biomed. Opt. Express 5, 2113–2124.

Kocová, J., 1970. Overall staining of connective tissue and the muscular layer of vessels. Folia Morphol. 18, 293–295.

Kondo, T., 2007. Timing of skin wounds. Leg. Med. Tokyo Jpn. 9, 109–114.

Kong, H.J., Kaigler, D., Kim, K., Mooney, D.J., 2004. Controlling rigidity and degradation of alginate hydrogels via molecular weight distribution. Biomacromolecules 5, 1720–1727.

Krasnov, M.S., Rybakova, E.Y., Tikhonov, V.E., Stretskii, G.M., Avdeenko, O.E., Shaikhaliev, A.I., et al., 2012. Burn-healing effects of a composition containing chitosan gel and a blood serum bioregulator. Bull. Exp. Biol. Med. 153, 550–553.

Laato, M., Kahari, V.M., Niinikoski, J., Vuorio, E., 1987. Epidermal growth factor increases collagen production in granulation tissue by stimulation of fibroblast proliferation and not by activation of procollagen genes. Biochem. J. 247, 385–388.

Lam, C.X.F., Hutmacher, D.W., Schantz, J.-T., Woodruff, M.A., Teoh, S.H., 2009. Evaluation of polycaprolactone scaffold degradation for 6 months *in vitro* and *in vivo*. J. Biomed. Mater. Res. A 90, 906–919.

Lambertz, A., Vogels, R.R.M., Busch, D., Schuster, P., Jockenhövel, S., Neumann, U.P., et al., 2015. Laparotomy closure using an elastic suture: a promising approach: laparotomy closure using an elastic suture. J. Biomed. Mater. Res. B. Appl. Biomater. 103, 417–423. Available from: http://dx.doi.org/10.1002/jbm.b.33222.

Langer, R., Vacanti, J.P., 1993. Tissue engineering. Science 260, 920–926.

Leibovich, S.J., Wiseman, D.M., 1988. Macrophages, wound repair and angiogenesis. Prog. Clin. Biol. Res. 266, 131–145.

Lewandowska, K., Pergament, E., Sukenik, C.N., Culp, L.A., 1992. Cell-type-specific adhesion mechanisms mediated by fibronectin adsorbed to chemically derivatized substrata. J. Biomed. Mater. Res. 26, 1343–1363. Available from: http://dx.doi.org/10.1002/jbm.820261007.

Li, J., Zhang, Y.-P., Kirsner, R.S., 2003. Angiogenesis in wound repair: angiogenic growth factors and the extracellular matrix. Microsc. Res. Tech. 60, 107–114.

Liang, X., Crecea, V., Boppart, S.A., 2010. Dynamic optical coherence elastography: a review. J. Innov. Opt. Health Sci. 3, 221–233.

Litvik, R., Vantuchová, Y., 2011. Hypertrofické a keloidní jizvy pohledem dermatologa. New EU Mag. Med. 2011, 15–17.

Mačák, J., Mačáková, J., 2004. Patologie. Grada, Praha.

Mariappan, Y.K., Glaser, K.J., Ehman, R.L., 2010. Magnetic resonance elastography: a review. Clin. Anat. 23, 497–511.

Marin, M.L., Veith, F.J., Cynamon, J., Sanchez, L.A., Bakal, C.W., Suggs, W.D., et al., 1995. Human transluminally placed endovascular stented grafts: preliminary histopathologic analysis of healing grafts in aortoiliac and femoral artery occlusive disease. J. Vasc. Surg. 21, 595–603, discussion 603–604.

Marin, E., Briceño, M.I., Caballero-George, C., 2013. Critical evaluation of biodegradable polymers used in nanodrugs. Int. J. Nanomed. 8, 3071–3090.

Masopust, J., Průša, R., 2003. Patobiochemie Buňky. ČSKB, 2.LF UK, Praha.

Matheson, L.A., Labow, R.S., Santerre, J.P., 2002. Biodegradation of polycarbonate-based polyurethanes by the human monocytes-derived macrophage and U937 cell systems. J. Biomed. Mater. Res. 61, 505–513.

Meruane, M.A., Rojas, M., Marcelain, K., 2012. The use of adipose tissue-derived stem cells within a dermal substitute improves skin regeneration by increasing neoangiogenesis and collagen synthesis. Plast. Reconstr. Surg. 130, 53–63.

Mignatti, P., Rifkin, D.B., 1996. Plasminogen activators and matrix metalloproteinases in angiogenesis. Enzyme Protein 49, 117–137.

Monteiro, G.A., Delossantos, A.I., Rodriguez, N.L., Patel, P., Franz, M.G., Wagner, C.T., 2013. Porcine incisional hernia model: evaluation of biologically derived intact extracellular matrix repairs. J. Tissue Eng, 4. Available from: http://dx.doi.org/10.1177/2041731413508771.

Montesano, R., Vassalli, J.D., Baird, A., Guillemin, R., Orci, L., 1986. Basic fibroblast growth factor induces angiogenesis in vitro. Proc. Natl. Acad. Sci. U.S.A. 83, 7297–7301.

Moon, J.J., West, J.L., 2008. Vascularization of engineered tissues: approaches to promote angio-genesis in biomaterials. Curr. Top. Med. Chem. 8, 300–310.

Mouton, P.R., 2002. Principles and Practices of Unbiased Stereology: An Introduction for Bioscientists. Johns Hopkins University Press, Baltimore, MD.

Mutsaers, S.E., McAnulty, R.J., Laurent, G.J., Versnel, M.A., Whitaker, D., Papadimitriou, J.M., 1997. Cytokine regulation of mesothelial cell proliferation in vitro and in vivo. Eur. J. Cell Biol. 72, 24–29.

Nedorost, L., Uemura, H., Furck, A., Saeed, I., Slavik, Z., Kobr, J., et al., 2013. Vascular histopathologic reaction to pulmonary artery banding in an *in vivo* growing porcine model. Pediatr. Cardiol. 34, 1652–1660.

Nowak, D., Popow-Woźniak, A., Raźnikiewicz, L., Malicka-Błaszkiewicz, M., 2009. Actin in the wound healing process. Postepy Biochem. 55, 138–144.

Nwe, N., Furuike, T., Tamura, H., 2009. The mechanical and biological properties of chitosan scaffolds for tissue regeneration templates are significantly enhanced by chitosan from gongronella butleri. Materials 2, 374–398.

Obara, K., Ishihara, M., Ishizuka, T., Fujita, M., Ozeki, Y., Maehara, T., et al., 2003. Photocrosslinkable chitosan hydrogel containing fibroblast growth factor-2 stimulates wound healing in healing-impaired db/db mice. Biomaterials 24, 3437–3444.

Oberpenning, F., Meng, J., Yoo, J.J., Atala, A., 1999. De novo reconstitution of a functional mammalian urinary bladder by tissue engineering. Nat. Biotechnol. 17, 149–155.

Ophir, J., Alam, S.K., Garra, B.S., Kallel, F., Konofagou, E.E., Krouskop, T., et al., 2002. Elastography: imaging the elastic properties of soft tissues with ultrasound. J. Med. Ultrason. 29, 155–171.

Ortiz-Masià, D., Díez, I., Calatayud, S., Hernández, C., Cosín-Roger, J., Hinojosa, J., et al., 2012. Induction of CD36 and thrombospondin-1 in macrophages by hypoxia-inducible factor 1 and its relevance in the inflammatory process. PLoS One 7, e48535.

Pakyari, M., Farrokhi, A., Maharlooei, M.K., Ghahary, A., 2013. Critical role of transforming growth factor beta in different phases of wound healing. Adv. Wound Care 2, 215–224. Available from: http://dx.doi.org/10.1089/wound.2012.0406.

Palsson, B., Bhatia, S., 2004. Tissue Engineering. Pearson Prentice Hall, Upper Saddle River, NJ.

Parida, P., 2012. Classification of biomaterials used in medicine. Int. J. Adv. Appl. Sci. IJAAS 3, 125–129.

Park, S., Lee, C., Kim, J., Kim, C., 2014. Acoustic resolution photoacoustic microscopy. Biomed. Eng. Lett. 4, 213–222.

Patel, N.R., Gohil, P.P., 2012. A review on biomaterials: scope, applications & human anatomy significance. Int. J. Emerg. Technol. Adv. Eng. 2 (4), 91–101.

Patel, Z.S., Mikos, A.G., 2004. Angiogenesis with biomaterial-based drug- and cell-delivery systems. J. Biomater. Sci. Polym. Ed. 15, 701–726.

Pepper, M.S., 2001. Role of the matrix metalloproteinase and plasminogen activator-plasmin systems in angiogenesis. Arterioscler. Thromb. Vasc. Biol. 21, 1104–1117.

Plencner, M., East, B., Tonar, Z., Otáhal, M., Prosecká, E., Rampichová, M., et al., 2014. Abdominal closure reinforcement by using polypropylene mesh functionalized with poly-ε-caprolactone nanofibers and growth factors for prevention of incisional hernia formation. Int. J. Nanomed. 9, 3263–3277.

Pruitt, L.A., Chakravartula, A.M., 2011. Mechanics of Biomaterials Fundamental Principles for Implant Design. Cambridge University Press, Cambridge, MA.

Rampichová, M., Filová, E., Varga, F., Lytvynets, A., Prosecká, E., Koláčná, L., et al., 2010. Fibrin/hyaluronic acid composite hydrogels as appropriate scaffolds for *in vivo* artificial cartilage implantation. ASAIO J. 56, 563–568.

Ratner, B.D., 2012. Biomaterials Science: An Introduction to Materials in Medicine, second ed. Academic Press, New York, NY.

Reinke, J.M., Sorg, H., 2012. Wound repair and regeneration. Eur. Surg. Res. 49, 35–43.

Rheinwald, J.G., Green, H., 1977. Epidermal growth factor and the multiplication of cultured human epidermal keratinocytes. Nature 265, 421–424.

Risau, W., 1997. Mechanisms of angiogenesis. Nature 386, 671–674.

Ristow, H.J., Messmer, T.O., 1988. Basic fibroblast growth factor and insulin-like growth factor I are strong mitogens for cultured mouse keratinocytes. J. Cell Physiol. 137, 277–284. Available from: http://dx.doi.org/10.1002/jcp.1041370210.

Rockman, H.A., Ono, S., Ross, R.S., Jones, L.R., Karimi, M., Bhargava, V., et al., 1994. Molecular and physiological alterations in murine ventricular dysfunction. Proc. Natl. Acad. Sci. U. S. A. 91, 2694–2698.

Rogowska, J., Patel, N.A., Fujimoto, J.G., Brezinski, M.E., 2004. Optical coherence tomographic elastography technique for measuring deformation and strain of atherosclerotic tissues. Heart Br. Card. Soc. 90, 556–562.

Ross, R., Raines, E.W., Bowen-Pope, D.F., 1986. The biology of platelet-derived growth factor. Cell 46, 155–169.

Sakiyama-Elbert, S.E., Hubbell, J.A., 2000. Development of fibrin derivatives for controlled release of heparin-binding growth factors. J. Control. Release Off. J. Control. Release Soc. 65, 389–402.

Schreiber, A.B., Winkler, M.E., Derynck, R., 1986. Transforming growth factor-alpha: a more potent angiogenic mediator than epidermal growth factor. Science 232, 1250–1253.

Screen, H.R.C., 2008. Investigating load relaxation mechanics in tendon. J. Mech. Behav. Biomed. Mater. 1, 51–58.

Seal, B., 2001. Polymeric biomaterials for tissue and organ regeneration. Mater. Sci. Eng. R Rep. 34, 147–230.

Seo, S.-H., Sung, H.-W., 2012. Treatment of keloids and hypertrophic scars using topical and intralesional mitomycin C. J. Eur. Acad. Dermatol. Venereol. JEADV 26, 634–638.

Seppä, H., Grotendorst, G., Seppä, S., Schiffmann, E., Martin, G.R., 1982. Platelet-derived growth factor in chemotactic for fibroblasts. J. Cell Biol. 92, 584–588.

Sjölund, M., Hedin, U., Sejersen, T., Heldin, C.H., Thyberg, J., 1988. Arterial smooth muscle cells express platelet-derived growth factor (PDGF) A chain mRNA, secrete a

PDGF-like mitogen, and bind exogenous PDGF in a phenotype- and growth state-dependent manner. J. Cell Biol. 106, 403–413.

Smith, J.A., Muthupillai, R., Rossman, P.J., Hulshizer, T.C., Greenleaf, J.F., Ehman, R.L., 1997. Characterization of biomaterials using magnetic resonance elastography. In: Thompson, D.O., Chimenti, D.E. (Eds.), Review of Progress in Quantitative Nondestructive Evaluation, Review of Progress in Quantitative Nondestructive Evaluation. Springer, Springer Science, New York, US, pp. 1323–1330.

Song, Z., Peng, Z., Liu, Z., Yang, J., Tang, R., Gu, Y., 2013. Reconstruction of abdominal wall musculofascial defects with small intestinal submucosa scaffolds seeded with tenocytes in rats. Tissue Eng. A 19, 1543–1553. Available from: http://dx.doi.org/10.1089/ten.tea.2011.0748.

Steed, D.L., 2006. Clinical evaluation of recombinant human platelet-derived growth factor for the treatment of lower extremity ulcers. Plast. Reconstr. Surg. 117, 143S–151S.

Sun, J., Tan, H., 2013. Alginate-based biomaterials for regenerative medicine applications. Materials 6, 1285–1309.

Sun, C., Standish, B., Yang, V.X.D., 2011. Optical coherence elastography: current status and future applications. J. Biomed. Opt. 16, 043001–043001–12.

Suri, C., Jones, P.F., Patan, S., Bartunkova, S., Maisonpierre, P.C., Davis, S., et al., 1996. Requisite role of angiopoietin-1, a ligand for the TIE2 receptor, during embryonic angiogenesis. Cell 87, 1171–1180.

Svensson, W.E., Amiras, D., 2006. Ultrasound elasticity imaging. Breast Cancer Online 9, 1–7.

Tabata, Y., Ikada, Y., 1999. Vascularization effect of basic fibroblast growth factor released from gelatin hydrogels with different biodegradabilities. Biomaterials 20, 2169–2175.

Teoh, S.H., 2000. Fatigue of biomaterials: a review. Int. J. Fatigue 22, 825–837.

Tichý, M., Tichá, V., Ščudla, V., Šváchová, M., Zapletalová, J., 2010. Analýza angiogeneze v kostní dřeni u plazmocytárního myelomu. Čes.-Slov. Patol. 2010, 15–19.

Truong, A.-T.N., Kowal-Vern, A., Latenser, B.A., Wiley, D.E., Walter, R.J., 2005. Comparison of dermal substitutes in wound healing utilizing a nude mouse model. J. Burns Wounds 4, e4.

Tzeng, D.Y., Deuel, T.F., Huang, J.S., Baehner, R.L., 1985. Platelet-derived growth factor promotes human peripheral monocyte activation. Blood 66, 179–183.

Uhrich, K.E., Cannizzaro, S.M., Langer, R.S., Shakesheff, K.M., 1999. Polymeric systems for controlled drug release. Chem. Rev. 99, 3181–3198.

Ulubayram, K., Nur Cakar, A., Korkusuz, P., Ertan, C., Hasirci, N., 2001. EGF containing gelatin-based wound dressings. Biomaterials 22, 1345–1356.

Uygun, B.E., Soto-Gutierrez, A., Yagi, H., Izamis, M.-L., Guzzardi, M.A., Shulman, C., et al., 2010. Organ reengineering through development of a transplantable recellularized liver graft using decellularized liver matrix. Nat. Med. 16, 814–820. Available from: http://dx.doi.org/10.1038/nm.2170.

Van Beurden, H.E., Von den Hoff, J.W., Torensma, R., Maltha, J.C., Kuijpers-Jagtman, A.M., 2005. Myofibroblasts in palatal wound healing: prospects for the reduction of wound contraction after cleft palate repair. J. Dent. Res. 84, 871–880.

Van Susante, J.L., Buma, P., Schuman, L., Homminga, G.N., van den Berg, W.B., Veth, R.P., 1999. Resurfacing potential of heterologous chondrocytes suspended in fibrin glue in large full-thickness defects of femoral articular cartilage: an experimental study in the goat. Biomaterials 20, 1167–1175.

Velazquez, O.C., 2007. Angiogenesis & vasculogenesis: inducing the growth of new blood vessels and wound healing by stimulation of bone marrow derived progenitor cell mobilization and homing. J. Vasc. Surg. 45, A39–A47.

Wang, M., 2003. Developing bioactive composite materials for tissue replacement. Biomaterials 24, 2133–2151.

Wang, R.K., 2006. Tissue doppler optical coherence elastography for real time strain rate and strain mapping of soft tissue. Appl. Phys. Lett. 13, 144103–144103-3.

Williams, D.F., 1987. Definitions in Biomaterials. Elsevier Science Ltd., Amsterdam.

Wong, J.Y., Bronzino, J.D., 2007. Biomaterials. CRC Press, Boca Raton, FL.

Yang, E.Y., Moses, H.L., 1990. Transforming growth factor beta 1-induced changes in cell migration, proliferation, and angiogenesis in the chicken chorioallantoic membrane. J. Cell Biol. 111, 731–741.

Yoo, S.Y., Kwon, S.M., 2013. Angiogenesis and its therapeutic opportunities. Mediators Inflamm. 2013, 127170.

Zeltinger, J., Sherwood, J.K., Graham, D.A., Müeller, R., Griffith, L.G., 2001. Effect of pore size and void fraction on cellular adhesion, proliferation, and matrix deposition. Tissue Eng. 7, 557–572.

Index

Note: Page numbers followed by "*f*" and "*t*" refer to figures and tables, respectively.

A

B

C

F

G

K

L

M

FSC
www.fsc.org
MIX
Papier | Fördert
gute Waldnutzung
FSC® C083411

Kolibri 360 GmbH
Ferdinand-Jühlke-Straße 7
99095 Erfurt, Deutschland
produktsicherheit@kolibri360.de